# Med-Surg Success

## A Course Review Applying Critical Thinking to Test Taking

# Med-Surg Success
## A Course Review Applying Critical Thinking to Test Taking

**Kathryn Cadenhead Colgrove** RN, MS, CNS, OCN
Trinity Valley Community College
Kaufman, Texas

**Judy Callicoatt** RN, MS, CNS
Trinity Valley Community College
Kaufman, Texas

**Consultant:**
**Ray A. Hargrove-Huttel** RN, PhD
Trinity Valley Community College
Kaufman, Texas

 **F. A. DAVIS COMPANY** • Philadelphia

F. A. Davis Company
1915 Arch Street
Philadelphia, PA 19103
www.fadavis.com

Printed in the United States of America

Last digit indicates print number: 10 9 8 7 6 5 4 3

*Publisher, Nursing:* Robert G. Martone
*Content Development Manager:* Darlene D. Pedersen
*Project Editor:* Thomas A. Ciavarella
*Art and Design Manager:* Carolyn O'Brien

As new scientific information becomes available through basic and clinical research, recommended treatments and drug therapies undergo changes. The author(s) and publisher have done everything possible to make this book accurate, up to date, and in accord with accepted standards at the time of publication. The author(s), editors, and publisher are not responsible for errors or omissions or for consequences from application of the book, and make no warranty, expressed or implied, in regard to the contents of the book. Any practice described in this book should be applied by the reader in accordance with professional standards of care used in regard to the unique circumstances that may apply in each situation. The reader is advised always to check product information (package inserts) for changes and new information regarding dose and contraindications before administering any drug. Caution is especially urged when using new or infrequently ordered drugs.

ISBN 13: 978-0-8036-1576-2
ISBN 10: 0-8036-1576-0

# Dedication

The authors would like to dedicate this book to the Trinity Valley Community College Associate Degree nursing students who graduated in 2005 and 2006. Thank you for giving of your time to pilot the questions and provide us constructive feedback. We would like to thank Bob Martone for giving us the opportunity to embark on this endeavor. Our appreciation goes to Barbara Tchabovsky for her assistance in editing the book and answering our numerous questions via e-mail, which is a wonderful invention. Our thanks go to Tom Ciavarella for supporting us through the maze of publishing this book. This book would not be possible without the unbelievable computer skills of Glada Norris.

**—The Authors**

I would like to dedicate this book to the memory of my mother, Mary Cadenhead, and grandmother, Elsie Rogers. They always told me that I could accomplish anything I wanted to accomplish. I would like to dedicate this book to my husband, Larry, daughter Laurie and son-in-law Todd, and son Larry Jr. and daughter-in-law Mai, and grandchildren Chris, Ashley, Justin C., Justin A., and Connor. Without their support and patience, the book would not have been possible.

**—Kathryn Colgrove**

This book is dedicated to my husband, George; my family, and my friends, who love and support me. Many thanks are given to the students who teach me and inspire me by persevering through the difficulties of nursing school. I want to extend my gratitude to members of the profession of nursing, both faculty and staff who share their art with nursing students.

**—Judy Callicoatt**

This book is dedicated to the memory of my husband, Bill, and my parents, T/Sgt. Leo and Nancy Hargrove, who are the rocks on which my life is built. I would like to thank my sisters, Gail and Debbie; my nephew Benjamin; and Paula for their support and encouragement through the good times and the bad. My children, Teresa and Aaron, are the most important people in my life and I want to thank them for always believing in me.

**—Ray Hargrove-Huttel**

# Reviewers

Freda Black, MSN, RN, ANP-BC
Assistant Professor
Ivy Tech State College
Gary, Indiana

Anne Dunphy, RN, MA, CS
Nursing Instructor
Delaware Technical & Community College
Newark, Delaware

Judy R. Hembd, RN, BSN, MSN
Assistant Professor
Montana State University-Northern
Department of Nursing
Havre, Montana

Linda Ann Kucher, BSN, MSN
Assistant Professor of Nursing
Gordon College
Barnesville, Georgia

Regina M. O'Drobinak, MSN, RN, ANP-BC
Assistant Professor, Associate of Science in Nursing
Ivy Tech State College
Gary, Indiana

Elizabeth Palmer, PhD, RN
Assistant Professor of Nursing
Indiana University of Pennsylvania
Indiana, Pennsylvania

# Editors and Contributors

**Joan L. Consullo, RN, MS, CNRN**
Advanced Clinical Nurse, Neuroscience
St. Luke's Episcopal Hospital
Houston, Texas

**Michelle L. Edwards, RN, MSN, ACNP, FNP**
Advanced Practice Nurse, Cardiology
Acute Care Nurse Practitioner/Family Nurse Practitioner
St. Luke's Episcopal Hospital
Houston, Texas

**Gail F. Graham, APRN, MS, NP-C**
Advanced Practice Nurse, Internal Medicine
Adult Nurse Practitioner
St. Luke's Episcopal Hospital
Houston, Texas

**Elester E. Stewart, RRT, RN, MSN, FNP**
Advanced Practice Nurse, Pulmonary
Family Nurse Practitioner
St. Luke's Episcopal Hospital
Houston, Texas

**Leslie Prater, RN, MS, CNS, CDE**
Clinical Diabetes Educator
Associate Degree Nursing Instructor
Trinity Valley Community College
Kaufman, Texas

**Helen Reid, RN, PhD**
Dean, Health Occupations
Trinity Valley Community College
Kaufman, Texas

# Contents

# Fundamentals of Critical Thinking Related to Test Taking: The RACE Model

This book is the second in a series of books, published by the F. A. Davis Company, designed to assist the student nurse in being successful in nursing school and in taking examinations, particularly the NCLEX-RN examination for licensure as a registered nurse.

*Med-Surg Success: A Course Review Applying Critical Thinking to Test Taking* focuses, as its name implies, on critical thinking as it pertains to test-taking skills for examinations in the nursing field. It contains the usual practice test questions found in review books, but it also provides important test-taking hints to help in analyzing questions and determining the correct answers. It follows book one of this series— *Fundamentals Success: A Course Review Applying Critical Thinking to Test Taking* by Patricia Nugent, RN, MA, MS, EdD, and Barbara Vitale, RN, MA—which defines critical thinking and the RACE model for applying critical thinking to test taking, but it does not repeat the same specific topics. Rather, it focuses on how to use the thinking processes and test-taking skills in answering questions on topics specifically addressed in the NCLEX-RN exam and in other nursing exams.

Test-taking skills and hints are valuable, but the student and future test taker must remember that the most important aspect of taking any examination is to become knowledgeable about the subject matter the test will cover. **There is no substitute for studying the material.**

## GUIDELINES FOR USING THIS BOOK

This book contains 19 chapters and a final comprehensive examination. This introductory chapter on test taking focuses on guidelines for studying and preparing for an examination, specifics about the nature of the NCLEX-RN test and the types of questions contained in it, and approaches to analyzing the questions and determining the correct answer using the RACE model.

Thirteen chapters (Chapters 2–14) focus on disorders affecting the different major body systems. Each of these chapters is divided into four major sections: Practice Questions, Practice Questions Answers and Rationales, a Comprehensive Examination, and Comprehensive Examination Answers and Rationales. Key words and abbreviations are also included in each chapter.

Different types of multiple-choice questions about disorders that affect a specific body system help the test taker to more easily identify specific content. The answers to these questions, the explanations for the correct answers, and the reasons why other possible answer options are wrong or not the best choice reinforce the test taker's knowledge and ability to discern subtle points in the question. Finally, the test-taking hints provide some clues and tips for answering the specific question. The Comprehensive Examination includes questions about the disorders covered in the practice section and questions about other diseases/disorders that may affect the particular body system. Answers and rationales for these examination questions are given, but test-taking hints are not.

Chapters 15–18 follow the same pattern but focus on emergency nursing, perioperative nursing, cultural nursing and alternative health care, and end-of-life issues.

Chapter 19, the pharmacology chapter, deals specifically with what the student nurse should know about the administration of medications, provides test-taking tips specific to pharmacology questions, and provides questions and answers.

A final 100-question comprehensive examination completes the main part of the book.

# PREPARING FOR LECTURE

To prepare for attending a class on a specific topic, students should read the assignment in the textbook and prepare notes to take to class. Highlight any information the test taker does not understand so that the information may be clarified during class or, if the instructor does not cover it in class, after the lecture.

Writing a prep sheet while reading (studying) is very useful. A single sheet of paper divided into categories of information, as shown in the following, should be sufficient for learning about most disease processes. If students cannot limit the information to one page, they are probably not being discriminatory when reading. The idea is not to rewrite the textbook; the idea is to glean from the textbook the important, need-to-know information.

Sample Prep Sheet

---

**Medical Diagnosis:**                    **Definition:**

Diagnostic Tests:            Signs and Symptoms            Nursing Interventions:
(List normal values)                                      (Include Teaching)

Procedures and Nursing
Implications:

                             Medical Interventions:

---

Complete the prep sheet in one color ink. Take the prep sheet to class along with a pen with different color ink or a pencil and a highlighter. Highlight on the prep sheet whatever the instructor emphasizes during the lecture. Write in different color ink or with a pencil any information the instructor emphasizes in lecture that the student did not include on the prep sheet. After the lecture, reread the information in the textbook that was included in the lecture but not on the student's prep sheet.

By using this method when studying for the exam, the test taker will be able to identify the information obtained from the textbook and the information obtained in class. The information on the prep sheet that is highlighted represents information that the test taker thought was important from reading the textbook and that the instructor emphasized during lecture. This is need-to know-information for the examination. Please note, however, that the instructor may not emphasize laboratory tests and values but still expect the student to realize the importance of this information.

Carry the completed prep sheets in a folder so that it can be reviewed any time there is a minute that is spent idly, such as during children's sports practices or when waiting for an appointment. This is learning to make the most of limited time. The prep sheets also should be carried to clinical assignments to use when caring for clients in the hospital.

If students are prepared prior to attending class, they will find the lecture easier to understand and, as a result, will be more successful during examinations. Being prepared allows students to listen to the instructor and not sit in class trying to write every word from the overhead presentation.

Test takers should recognize the importance of the instructor's hints during the lecture. The instructor may emphasize information by highlighting areas on overhead slides, by repeating information, or by emphasizing a particular fact. This usually means the instructor thinks the information is very important. *Important information usually finds its way onto tests at some point.*

## PREPARING FOR AN EXAMINATION

There are several steps that the test taker should take in preparing for an examination—some during the course of the class and some immediately before the day of the test.

### Study, Identify Weaknesses, and Practice

The test taker should plan to study three (3) hours for every one (1) hour of class. For example, a course that is three (3) hours of credit requires nine (9) hours of study a week. Cramming immediately prior to the test usually places the test taker at risk for being unsuccessful. The information acquired during cramming is not really learned and is quickly forgotten. And remember: Nursing examinations include material required by the registered nurse when caring for clients at the bedside.

The first time many students realize they do not understand some information is during the examination or, in other words, when it is too late. Nursing examinations contain high-level application questions requiring the test taker to have memorized information and to be able to interpret the data and make a judgment as to the correct course of action. The test taker must recognize areas of weakness prior to seeing the examination for the first time. This book is designed to provide assistance in identifying areas of weakness prior to the examination.

Two to 3 days prior to the examination the test taker should compose a practice test or take any practice questions or comprehensive exams in this book that have not already been answered. If a specific topic of study—say, the circulatory system and its disorders—proves to be an area of strength, as evidenced by selecting the correct answers to the questions on that system, then the test taker should proceed to study other areas identified as areas of weakness because of incorrect answers in those areas. Prospective test takers who do not understand the rationale for the correct answer should read the appropriate part of the textbook and try to understand the rationale for the correct answer. However, test takers should be cautious when reading the rationale for the incorrect answer options because during the actual examination, the student may remember reading the information and become confused about whether the information applied to the correct answer or to the incorrect option.

### The Night Before the Exam

The night before the examination the test taker should stop studying by 6:00 P.M. or 7:00 P.M. and then do something fun or relaxing until bedtime. Don't make bedtime too late: A good night's rest is essential prior to taking the examination. Studying until bedtime or an all-night cram session will leave the test taker tired and sleepy during the examination, just when the mind should be at its top performance.

### The Day of the Exam

Eat a meal before an examination. A source of carbohydrate for energy, along with a protein source, make a good meal prior to an examination. Skipping a meal before the examination leaves the brain without nourishment. A glass of milk and a bagel with peanut butter is an excellent meal; it provides a source of protein and a sustained release of carbohydrates. Do not eat donuts or other junk food or drink soft drinks. They provide energy that is quickly available but will not last throughout the time required for an examination. Excessive fluid intake may cause the need to urinate during the examination and make it hard for students to concentrate.

## Test-Taking Anxiety

Test takers who have test-taking anxiety should arrive at the testing site 45 minutes prior to the examination. Find a seat for the examination and place books there to reserve the desk. Walk for 15 minutes at a fast pace away from the testing site and then turn and walk back. This exercise literally walks anxiety away.

If other test takers' getting up and leaving the room is bothersome, try to get a desk away from the group, in front of the room or facing a wall. Most schools allow students to wear hunter's earplugs during a test if noise bothers them. Most RN-NCLEX test sites will provide earplugs if the test taker requests them.

## TAKING THE EXAM

The NCLEX-RN examination is a computerized exam. Tests given in nursing schools in specific subject areas may be computerized or pen and pencil. Both formats include multiple-choice questions and may include several types of alternate questions: a fill-in-the-blank question that tests math abilities; a select-all-that-apply question that requires the test taker to select more than one option as the correct answer; a prioritizing question that requires the test taker to prioritize the answers 1, 2, 3, 4, and 5 in the order of when the nurse would implement the intervention; and, in the computerized version, a click-and-drag question that requires the test taker to identify a specific area of the body as the correct answer. Examples of all types of questions are included in this book. In an attempt to illustrate the click-and-drag question, this book has pictures with lines to delineate choices A, B, C, or D.

Refer to the National Council of State Boards of Nursing for additional information on the NCLEX-RN examination (http://www.ncsbn.org).

### Pen-and-Pencil Exam

A test taker taking a pen-and-pencil examination in nursing school who finds a question that contains totally unknown information should circle the question and skip it. Another question may help to answer the skipped question. Not moving on and worrying over a question will place success on the next few questions in jeopardy. The mind will not let go of the worry, and this may lead to missing important information in subsequent questions.

### Computerized Test

The computerized NCLEX-RN test is composed of from 75 (the minimum number of questions) to 265 questions. The computer determines with a 95% certainty whether the test taker's ability is above the passing standard before the examination concludes.

During the NCLEX-RN computerized test, take some deep breaths and then select an answer. The computer does not allow the test taker to return to a question. Test takers who become anxious during an examination should stop, put their hands in their lap, close their eyes, and take a minimum of five deep breaths before resuming the examination. Test takers must become aware of personal body signals that indicate increasing stress levels. Some people get gastrointestinal symptoms and others feel a tightening of muscles.

Test takers should not be overly concerned if they possess only rudimentary computer skills. Simply use the mouse to select the correct answer. Every question asks for a confirmation before being submitted as the correct answer.

In addition to typing in pertinent personal information, test takers must be able to type numbers and use the drop-down computer calculator. However, test takers can request an erasable slate to calculate math problems by hand.

Practice taking tests on the computer before taking the NCLEX-RN examination. Many textbooks contain computer disks with test questions, and there are many on-line review opportunities.

# UNDERSTANDING THE TYPES OF NURSING QUESTIONS

## Components of a Multiple-Choice Question

A multiple-choice question is called an **item.** Each item has two parts. The **stem** is the part that contains the information that identifies the topic and its parameters and then asks a question. The second part consists of one or more possible responses, which are called **options.** One of the options is the **correct answer;** the others are the wrong answers and are called **distracters.**

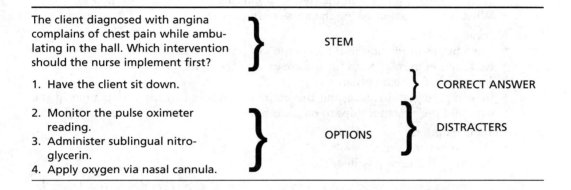

## Cognitive Levels of Nursing Questions

Questions on nursing examinations reflect a variety of thinking processes that nurses use when caring for clients. These thinking processes are part of the cognitive domain, and they progress from the simple to the complex, from the concrete to the abstract, and from the tangible to the intangible. There are four types of thinking processes represented by nursing questions.

1. Knowledge Questions—These questions emphasize recalling information that has been learned/studied.
2. Comprehension Questions—These questions emphasize understanding the meaning and intent of remembered information.
3. Application Questions—These questions emphasize the use of remembered and understood information in new situations.
4. Analysis Questions—These questions emphasize comparing and contrasting a variety of elements of information.

# THE RACE MODEL: THE APPLICATION OF CRITICAL THINKING TO MULTIPLE-CHOICE QUESTIONS

Answering a test question is like participating in a race. Of course, each test taker wants to come in first and be the winner. However, the thing to remember about a race is that success is not just based on speed but also on strategy and tactics. The same is true about nursing examinations. Although speed may be a variable that must be considered when taking a timed test so that the amount of time spent on each question is factored into the test strategy, the emphasis on RACE is the use of critical-thinking techniques to answer multiple-choice questions.

The **RACE Model** presented here is a critical-thinking strategy to use when answering multiple-choice questions concerning nursing. If the test taker follows the **RACE Model** every time when looking at and analyzing a test question, its use will become second nature.

This methodical approach will improve the ability to critically analyze a test question and improve the chances of selecting the correct answer.

The **RACE Model** has four steps to answering a test question. The best way to remember the four steps is to refer to the acronym **RACE**.

**R** — **R**ecognize
- What information is in the stem.
- The key words in the stem.
- Who the client is in the stem.
- What the topic is about.

**A** — **A**sk
- What is the question asking?
- What are the key words in the stem that indicate the need for a response?
- What is the question asking the nurse to implement?

**C** — **C**ritically analyze
- The options in relation to the question asked in the stem.
- Each option in relation to the information in the stem.
- A rationale for each option.
- By comparing and contrasting the options in relation to the information in the stem and their relationships to one another.

**E** — **E**liminate options
- One option at a time.
- As many options as possible.

The text *Fundamentals Success: Course Review Applying Critical Thinking to Test Taking* by Patricia Nugent and Barbara Vitale includes a discussion exploring the **RACE Model** in depth and its relation to the thinking processes used in multiple-choice questions in the field of nursing.

# 2

*The first step toward knowledge is to know that we are not ignorant.*—Richard Cecil

# Neurological Disorders

Test-taking hints are useful to discriminate information, but they cannot substitute for knowledge. The student should refer to Chapter 1 for assistance in preparing for class, studying, and taking an examination.

This chapter focuses on disorders that affect the neurological system. It provides a list of keywords and abbreviations, practice questions focused on disease processes, and a comprehensive examination that includes other content areas involving the neurological system and the disease processes addressed in the practice questions. Answers and reasons why the answer options provided are either correct or incorrect are also provided as are some test-taking hints. The following chapters (Chapters 3–12) focus on disorders that affect other body systems and function.

## KEYWORDS

agnosia
akinesia
aphasia
apraxia
areflexia
ataxia
autonomic dysreflexia
bradykinesia
decarboxylase
diplopia
dysarthria
dysphagia
echolalia
epilepsy
papilledema
paralysis
paresthesia
paroxysms
penumbra
postictal

## ABBREVIATIONS

Activities of Daily Living (ADLs)
Amyotrophic Lateral Sclerosis (ALS)
As Soon As Possible (ASAP)
Blood Pressure (BP)
Cerebrovascular Accident (CVA)
Computed Tomography (CT)
Electroencephalogram (EEG)
Electromyelogram (EMG)
Emergency Department (ED)
Enzyme-Linked Immunoassay (ELISA)
Health-Care Provider (HCP)
Intracranial Pressure (ICP)
Intensive Care Department (ICD)
Intravenous (IV)
Magnetic Resonance Imaging (MRI)
Nonsteroidal Anti-Inflammatory Drug (NSAID)
Nothing By Mouth (NPO)
Parkinson's Disease (PD)
Pulse (P)
Range of Motion (ROM)
Respiration (R)
Rule Out (R/O)
Spinal Cord Injury (SCI)
STAT—immediately (STAT)
Temperature (T)
Transient Ischemic Attack (TIA)
Traumatic Brain Injury (TBI)
Unlicensed Assistive Personnel (UAP)

**Please note:** The term health-care provider, as used in this text, refers to a nurse practitioner (NP), physician (MD), osteopath (DO), or physician assistant (PA) who has prescriptive authority. These providers are responsible for directing the care and providing orders for the clients.

## Cerebrovascular Accident (Stroke)

1. A 78-year-old client is admitted to the emergency department with numbness and weakness of the left arm and slurred speech. Which nursing intervention is priority?
   1. Prepare to administer recombinant tissue plasminogen activator (rt-PA).
   2. Discuss the precipitating factors that caused the symptoms.
   3. Schedule for a STAT computed tomography (CT) scan of head.
   4. Notify the speech pathologist for an emergency consult.

2. The nurse is assessing a client experiencing motor loss as a result of a left-sided cerebrovascular accident (CVA). Which clinical manifestations would the nurse document?
   1. Hemiparesis of the client's left arm and apraxia.
   2. Paralysis of the right side of the body and ataxia.
   3. Homonymous hemianopsia and diplopia.
   4. Impulsive behavior and hostility toward family.

3. Which client would the nurse identify as being most at risk for experiencing a CVA?
   1. A 55-year-old African American male.
   2. An 84-year-old Japanese female.
   3. A 67-year-old Caucasian male.
   4. A 39-year-old pregnant female.

4. The client diagnosed with a right-sided cerebrovascular accident is admitted to the rehabilitation unit. Which interventions should be included in the nursing care plan? Select all that apply.
   1. Position the client to prevent shoulder adduction.
   2. Turn and reposition the client every shift.
   3. Encourage the client to move the affected side.
   4. Perform quadriceps exercises three (3) times a day.
   5. Instruct the client to hold the fingers in a fist.

5. The nurse is planning care for a client experiencing agnosia secondary to a cerebrovascular accident. Which collaborative intervention will be included in the plan of care?
   1. Observing the client swallowing for possible aspiration.
   2. Positioning the client in a semi-Fowler's position when sleeping.
   3. Placing a suction set-up at the client's bedside during meals.
   4. Referring the client to an occupational therapist for evaluation.

6. The nurse and an unlicensed assistive personnel (UAP) are caring for a client with right-sided paralysis. Which action by the UAP requires the nurse to intervene?
   1. The assistant places a gait belt around the client's waist prior to ambulating.
   2. The assistant places the client on the back with the client's head to the side.
   3. The assistant places her hand under the client's right axilla to help him/her move up in bed.
   4. The assistant praises the client for attempting to perform ADLs independently.

7. The client diagnosed with atrial fibrillation has experienced a transient ischemic attack (TIA). Which medication would the nurse anticipate being ordered for the client on discharge?
   1. An oral anticoagulant medication.
   2. A beta-blocker medication.
   3. An anti-hyperuricemic medication.
   4. A thrombolytic medication.

8. The client has been diagnosed with a cerebrovascular accident (stroke). The client's wife is concerned about her husband's generalized weakness. Which home modification should the nurse suggest to the wife prior to discharge?
   1. Obtain a rubber mat to place under the dinner plate.
   2. Purchase a long-handled bath sponge for showering.
   3. Purchase clothes with Velcro closure devices.
   4. Obtain a raised toilet seat for the client's bathroom.

9. The client is diagnosed with expressive aphasia. Which psychosocial client problem would the nurse include in the plan of care?
   1. Potential for injury.
   2. Powerlessness.
   3. Disturbed thought processes.
   4. Sexual dysfunction.

10. Which assessment data would indicate to the nurse that the client would be at risk for a hemorrhagic stroke?
    1. A blood glucose level of 480 mg/dL.
    2. A right-sided carotid bruit.
    3. A blood pressure of 220/120 mm Hg.
    4. The presence of bronchogenic carcinoma.

11. The 85-year-old client diagnosed with a stroke is complaining of a severe headache. Which intervention should the nurse implement first?
    1. Administer a nonnarcotic analgesic.
    2. Prepare for STAT magnetic resonance imaging (MRI).
    3. Start an intravenous line with $D_5W$ at 100 mL/hr.
    4. Complete a neurological assessment.

12. A client diagnosed with a subarachnoid hemorrhage has undergone a craniotomy for repair of a ruptured aneurysm. Which intervention will the intensive care nurse implement?
    1. Administer a stool softener BID.
    2. Encourage the client to cough hourly.
    3. Monitor neurological status every shift.
    4. Maintain the dopamine drip to keep BP at 160/90.

## Head Injury

13. The client diagnosed with a mild concussion is being discharged from the emergency department. Which discharge instruction should the nurse teach the client's significant other?
    1. Awaken the client every two (2) hours.
    2. Monitor for increased intracranial pressure.
    3. Observe frequently for hypervigilance.
    4. Offer the client food every three (3) to four (4) hours.

14. The resident in a long-term care facility fell during the previous shift and has a laceration in the occipital area that has been closed with Steri-Strips™. Which signs/symptoms would warrant transferring the resident to the emergency department?
    1. A 4-cm area of bright red drainage on the dressing.
    2. A weak pulse, shallow respirations, and cool pale skin.
    3. Pupils that are equal, react to light, and accommodate.
    4. Complaints of a headache that resolves with medication.

15. The nurse is caring for the following clients. Which client would the nurse assess first after receiving the shift report?
    1. The 22-year-old male client diagnosed with a concussion who is complaining someone is waking him up every two (2) hours.
    2. The 36-year-old female client admitted with complaints of left-sided weakness who is scheduled for a magnetic resonance imaging (MRI) scan.
    3. The 45-year-old client admitted with blunt trauma to the head after a motorcycle accident who has a Glasgow Coma Scale score of 6.
    4. The 62-year-old client diagnosed with a cerebrovascular accident (CVA) who has expressive aphasia.

16. The client has sustained a severe closed head injury and the neurosurgeon is determining if the client is "brain dead." Which data support that the client is brain dead?
    1. When the client's head is turned to the right, the eyes turn to the right.
    2. The electroencephalogram (EEG) has identifiable waveforms.
    3. There is no eye activity when the cold caloric test is performed.
    4. The client assumes decorticate posturing when painful stimuli are applied.

17. The client is admitted to the medical floor with a diagnosis of closed head injury. Which nursing intervention has priority?
    1. Assess neurological status.
    2. Monitor pulse, respiration, and blood pressure.
    3. Initiate an intravenous access.
    4. Maintain an adequate airway.

18. The client diagnosed with a closed head injury is admitted to the rehabilitation department. Which medication order would the nurse question?
    1. A subcutaneous anticoagulant.
    2. An intravenous osmotic diuretic.
    3. An oral anticonvulsant.
    4. An oral proton pump inhibitor.

19. The client diagnosed with a gunshot wound to the head assumes decorticate posturing when the nurse applies painful stimuli. Which assessment data obtained three (3) hours later would indicate the client is improving?
    1. Purposeless movement in response to painful stimuli.
    2. Flaccid paralysis in all four extremities.
    3. Decerebrate posturing when painful stimuli are applied.
    4. Pupils that are 6 mm in size and nonreactive on painful stimuli.

20. The nurse is caring for a client diagnosed with an epidural hematoma. Which nursing interventions should the nurse implement? Select all that apply.
    1. Maintain the head of the bed at 60 degrees of elevation.
    2. Administer stool softeners daily.
    3. Ensure that pulse oximeter reading is higher than 93%.
    4. Perform deep nasal suction every two (2) hours.
    5. Administer mild sedatives.

21. The client with a closed head injury has clear fluid draining from the nose. Which action should the nurse implement first?
    1. Notify the health-care provider immediately.
    2. Prepare to administer an antihistamine.
    3. Test the drainage for presence of glucose.
    4. Place 2 × 2 gauze under the nose to collect drainage.

22. The nurse is enjoying a day out at the lake and witnesses a water skier hit the boat ramp. The water skier is in the water not responding to verbal stimuli. The nurse is the first health-care provider to respond to the accident. Which intervention should be implemented first?
    1. Assess the client's level of consciousness.
    2. Organize onlookers to remove the client from the lake.
    3. Perform a head-to-toe assessment to determine injuries.
    4. Stabilize the client's cervical spine.

23. The client is diagnosed with a closed head injury and is in a coma. The nurse writes the client problem as "high risk for immobility complications." Which intervention would be included in the plan of care?
    1. Position the client with the head of the bed elevated at intervals.
    2. Perform active range of motion exercises every four (4) hours.
    3. Turn the client every shift and massage bony prominences.
    4. Explain all procedures to the client before performing them.

24. The 29-year-old client that was employed as a forklift operator sustains a traumatic brain injury secondary to a motor vehicle accident. The client is being discharged from the rehabilitation unit after three (3) months and has cognitive deficits. Which goal would be most realistic for this client?
    1. The client will return to work within six (6) months.
    2. The client is able to focus and stay on task for ten (10) minutes.
    3. The client will be able to dress self without assistance.
    4. The client will regain bowel and bladder control.

## Spinal Cord Injury (SCI)

25. The nurse driving down the highway witnesses a one-car motor vehicle accident and stops to render aid. The driver of the car is unconscious. Which action should the nurse take first?
    1. Carefully remove the driver from the car.
    2. Assess the client's pupils for reaction.
    3. Stabilize the client's cervical spine.
    4. Attempt to wake the client up by shaking him.

26. In assessing a client with a T-12 SCI, which clinical manifestations would the nurse expect to find to support the diagnosis of spinal shock?
    1. No reflex activity below the waist.
    2. Inability to move upper extremities.
    3. Complaints of a pounding headache.
    4. Hypertension and bradycardia.

27. The rehabilitation nurse caring for the client with an L-1 SCI is developing the nursing care plan. Which intervention should the nurse implement?
    1. Keep oxygen on via nasal cannula on at all times.
    2. Administer low-dose subcutaneous anticoagulants.
    3. Perform active lower-extremity ROM exercises.
    4. Refer to a speech therapist for ventilator-assisted speech.

28. The nurse in the neurointensive care unit is caring for a client with a new C-6 SCI who is breathing independently. Which nursing interventions should be implemented? Select all that apply.
    1. Monitor the pulse oximetry reading.
    2. Provide pureed foods six (6) times a day.
    3. Encourage coughing and deep breathing.
    4. Assess for autonomic dysreflexia.
    5. Administer intravenously corticosteroids.

29. The home health nurse is caring for a 28-year-old client with a T-10 SCI who says, "I can't do anything. Why am I so worthless?" Which statement by the nurse would be the most therapeutic?
    1. "This must be very hard for you. You're feeling worthless?"
    2. "You shouldn't feel worthless—you are still alive."
    3. "Why do you feel worthless? You still have the use of your arms."
    4. "If you attended a work rehab program you wouldn't feel worthless."

30. The client is diagnosed with an SCI and is scheduled for a magnetic resonance imaging (MRI) scan. Which question would be most appropriate for the nurse to ask prior to taking the client to the diagnostic test?
    1. "Do you have trouble hearing?"
    2. "Are you allergic to any type of dairy products?"
    3. "Have you had anything to eat in the last eight (8) hours?"
    4. "Are you uncomfortable in closed spaces?"

31. The client with a C-6 SCI is admitted to the emergency department complaining of a severe pounding headache and has a BP of 180/110. Which intervention should the emergency department nurse implement?
    1. Keep the client flat in bed.
    2. Dim the lights in the room.
    3. Assess for bladder distention.
    4. Administer a narcotic analgesic.

32. The client with a cervical fracture is being discharged in a halo device. Which teaching instruction should the nurse discuss with the client?
    1. Discuss how to remove insertion pins correctly.
    2. Instruct the client to report reddened or irritated skin areas.
    3. Inform the client that the vest liner cannot be changed.
    4. Encourage the client to remain in the recliner as much as possible.

33. The intensive care nurse is caring for a client with a T-1 SCI. When the nurse elevates the head of the bed 30 degrees, the client complains of lightheadedness and dizziness. The client's vital signs are T 99.2°F, P 98, R 24, and BP 84/40. Which action should the nurse implement?
    1. Notify the health-care provider ASAP.
    2. Calm the client down by talking therapeutically.
    3. Increase the IV rate by 50 mL/hour.
    4. Lower the head of the bed immediately.

34. The nurse on the rehabilitation unit is caring for the following clients. Which client should the nurse assess first after receiving the change of shift report?
    1. The client with a C-6 SCI who is complaining of dyspnea and has crackles in the lungs.
    2. The client with an L-4 SCI who is crying and very upset about being discharged home.
    3. The client with an L-2 SCI who is complaining of a headache and feeling very hot.
    4. The client with a T-4 SCI who is unable to move the lower extremities.

35. Which nursing task would be most appropriate for the nurse to delegate to the unlicensed nursing assistant?
    1. To teach the Crede maneuver to the client needing to void.
    2. To administer the tube feeding to the client who is quadriplegic.
    3. To assist with bowel training by placing the client on the bedside commode.
    4. To observe the client demonstrating self-catheterization technique.

36. The 34-year-old male client with an SCI is sharing with the nurse that he is worried about finding employment after being discharged from the rehabilitation unit. Which intervention should the nurse implement?
    1. Refer the client to the American Spinal Cord Injury Association (ASIA).
    2. Refer the client to the state rehabilitation commission.
    3. Ask the social worker about applying for disability.
    4. Suggest that the client talk with his significant other about this concern.

## Seizures

37. The male client is sitting in the chair and his entire body is rigid with his arms and legs contracting and relaxing. The client is not aware of what is going on and is making guttural sounds. Which action should the nurse implement first?
    1. Push aside any furniture.
    2. Place the client on his side
    3. Assess the client's vital signs.
    4. Ease the client to the floor.

38. The occupational health nurse is concerned about preventing occupation-related acquired seizures. Which intervention should the nurse implement?
    1. Ensure that helmets are worn in appropriate areas.
    2. Implement daily exercise programs for the staff.
    3. Provide healthy foods in the cafeteria.
    4. Encourage employees to wear safety glasses.

39. The client is scheduled for an electroencephalogram (EEG) to help diagnose a seizure disorder. Which preprocedure teaching should the nurse implement?
    1. Tell the client to take any routine anti-seizure medication prior to the EEG.
    2. Tell the client not to eat anything for eight (8) hours prior to the procedure.
    3. Instruct the client to stay awake 24 hours prior to the EEG.
    4. Explain to the client that there will be some discomfort during the procedure.

40. The nurse enters the room as the client is beginning to have a tonic-clonic seizure. What action should the nurse implement first?
    1. Note the first thing the client does in the seizure.
    2. Assess the size of the client's pupils.
    3. Determine if the client is incontinent of urine or stool.
    4. Provide the client with privacy during the seizure.

41. The client that just had a three (3)-minute seizure has no apparent injuries and is oriented to name, place, and time but is very lethargic and just wants to sleep. Which intervention should the nurse implement?
    1. Perform a complete neurological assessment.
    2. Awaken the client every 30 minutes.
    3. Turn the client to the side and allow him to sleep.
    4. Interview the client to find out what caused the seizure.

42. The unlicensed nursing assistant is attempting to put an oral airway in the mouth of a client having a tonic-clonic seizure. Which action should the primary nurse take?
    1. Help the assistant to insert the oral airway in the mouth.
    2. Tell the assistant to stop trying to insert anything in the mouth.
    3. Take no action because the assistant is handling the situation.
    4. Notify the charge nurse of the situation immediately.

43. The client is prescribed phenytoin (Dilantin), an anticonvulsant, for a seizure disorder. Which statement indicates the client understands the discharge teaching concerning this medication?
    1. "I will brush my teeth after every meal."
    2. "I will check my Dilantin level daily."
    3. "My urine will turn orange while on Dilantin."
    4. "I won't have any seizures while on this medication."

44. The client is admitted to the intensive care department (ICD) experiencing status epilepticus. Which collaborative intervention should the nurse anticipate?
    1. Assess the client's neurological status every hour.
    2. Monitor the client's heart rhythm via telemetry.
    3. Administer an anticonvulsant medication intravenous push.
    4. Prepare to administer a glucocorticosteroid orally.

45. The client has been newly diagnosed with epilepsy. Which discharge instructions should be taught to the client? Select all that apply.
    1. Keep a record of seizure activity.
    2. Take tub baths only; do not take showers.
    3. Avoid over-the-counter medications.
    4. Have anticonvulsant medication serum levels checked regularly.
    5. Do not drive alone; have someone in the car.

46. Which statement by the female client indicates that the client understands factors that may precipitate seizure activity?
    1. "It is all right for me to drink coffee for breakfast."
    2. "My menstrual cycle will not affect my seizure disorder."
    3. "I am going to take a class in stress management."
    4. "I should wear dark glasses when I am out in the sun."

47. The nurse asks the male client with epilepsy if he has auras with his seizures. The client says, "I don't know what you mean. What are auras?" Which statement by the nurse would be the best response?
    1. "Some people have a warning that the seizure is about to start."
    2. "Auras occur when you are physically and psychologically exhausted."
    3. "You're concerned that you do not have auras before your seizures?"
    4. "Auras usually cause you to be sleepy after you have a seizure."

48. The nurse educator is presenting an in-service on seizures. Which disease process is the leading cause of seizures in the elderly?
    1. Alzheimer's disease.
    2. Parkinson's disease.
    3. Cerebral vascular accident (stroke).
    4. Brain atrophy due to aging.

## Brain Tumors

49. The client is being admitted to rule out a brain tumor. Which classic triad of symptoms supports a diagnosis of brain tumor?
    1. Nervousness, metastasis to the lungs, and seizures.
    2. Headache, vomiting, and papilledema.
    3. Hypotension, tachycardia, and tachypnea.
    4. Abrupt loss of motor function, diarrhea, and changes in taste.

50. The client has been diagnosed with a brain tumor. Which presenting signs and symptoms help to localize the tumor position?
    1. Widening pulse pressure and bounding pulse.
    2. Diplopia and decreased visual acuity.
    3. Bradykinesia and scanning speech.
    4. Hemiparesis and personality changes.

51. The male client diagnosed with a brain tumor is scheduled for a magnetic resonance imaging (MRI) scan in the morning. The client tells the nurse that he is scared. Which response by the nurse indicates an appropriate therapeutic response?
    1. "MRIs are loud but there will not be any invasive procedure done."
    2. "You're scared. Tell me about what is scaring you."
    3. "This is the least thing to be scared about—there will be worse."
    4. "I can call the MRI tech to come and talk to you about the scan."

52. The client diagnosed with breast cancer has developed metastasis to the brain. Which prophylactic measure should the nurse implement?
    1. Institute aspiration precautions.
    2. Refer the client to Reach to Recovery.
    3. Initiate seizure precautions.
    4. Teach the client about mastectomy care.

53. The significant other of a client diagnosed with a brain tumor asks the nurse for help identifying resources. Which would be the most appropriate referral for the nurse to make?
    1. Social worker.
    2. Chaplain.
    3. Health-care provider.
    4. Occupational therapist.

54. The nurse has written a care plan for a client diagnosed with a brain tumor. Which is an important goal regarding self-care deficit?
    1. The client will maintain body weight within two (2) pounds.
    2. The client will execute an advance directive.
    3. The client will be able to perform three ADLs with assistance.
    4. The client will verbalize feeling of loss by the end of the shift.

55. The client diagnosed with a brain tumor was admitted to the intensive care unit with decorticate posturing. Which indicates that the client's condition is becoming worse?
    1. The client has purposeful movement with painful stimuli.
    2. The client has assumed adduction of the upper extremities.
    3. The client is aimlessly thrashing in the bed.
    4. The client has become flaccid and does not respond to stimuli.

56. The client is diagnosed with a pituitary tumor and is scheduled for a transsphenoidal hypophysectomy. Which pre-op instruction is important for the nurse to teach?
    1. There will be a large turban dressing around the skull after surgery.
    2. The client will not be able to eat for four (4) or five (5) days post-op.
    3. The client should not blow the nose for two (2) weeks after surgery.
    4. The client will have to lie flat for 24 hours following the surgery.

57. The client has undergone a craniotomy for a brain tumor. Which data indicate a complication of this surgery?
    1. The client complains of a headache at a 3–4 on a 1–10 scale.
    2. The client has an intake of 1000 mL and an output of 3500 mL.
    3. The client complains of a raspy sore throat.
    4. The client experiences dizziness when trying to get up too quickly.

58. The client diagnosed with a brain tumor has a diminished gag response. Which intervention should the nurse implement?
    1. Make the client NPO until seen by the health-care provider
    2. Position the client in low Fowler's position for all meals.
    3. Place the client on a mechanically ground diet.
    4. Teach the client to direct food and fluid toward the unaffected side.

59. The client is diagnosed with a metastatic brain tumor, and radiation therapy is scheduled. The client asks the nurse, "Why not try chemotherapy first? It has helped my other tumors." The nurse's response is based on which scientific rationale?
    1. Chemotherapy is only used as a last resort in caring for clients with brain tumors.
    2. The blood–brain barrier prevents medications from reaching the brain.
    3. Radiation therapy will have fewer side effects than chemotherapy.
    4. Metastatic tumors become resistant to chemotherapy and it becomes useless.

60. The client is being discharged following a transsphenoidal hypophysectomy. Which discharge instructions should the nurse teach the client? Select all that apply.
    1. Sleep with the head of the bed elevated.
    2. Keep a humidifier in the room.
    3. Use caution when performing oral care.
    4. Stay on a full liquid diet until seen by the HCP.
    5. Notify the HCP if developing a cold or fever.

## Meningitis

61. The wife of the client diagnosed with septic meningitis asks the nurse, "I am so scared. What is meningitis?" Which statement would be the most appropriate response by the nurse?
    1. "There is bleeding into his brain causing irritation of the meninges."
    2. "A virus has infected the brain and meninges, causing inflammation."
    3. "This is a bacterial infection of the tissues that cover the brain and spinal cord."
    4. "This is an inflammation of the brain parenchyma caused by a mosquito bite."

62. The public health nurse is giving a lecture on potential outbreaks of infectious meningitis. Which population is most at risk for an outbreak?
    1. Clients recently discharged from the hospital.
    2. Residents of a college dormitory.
    3. Individuals who visit a third world country.
    4. Employees in a high-rise office building.

63. The nurse is assessing the client diagnosed with bacterial meningitis. Which clinical manifestations would support the diagnosis of bacterial meningitis?
    1. Positive Babinski's sign and peripheral paresthesia.
    2. Negative Chvostek's sign and facial tingling.
    3. Positive Kernig's sign and nuchal rigidity.
    4. Negative Trousseau's sign and nystagmus.

64. The nurse is assessing the client diagnosed with meningococcal meningitis. Which assessment data would warrant notifying the HCP?
    1. Purpuric lesions on the face.
    2. Complaints of light hurting the eyes.
    3. Dull, aching, frontal headache.
    4. Not remembering the day of the week.

65. Which type of precautions should the nurse implement for the client diagnosed with septic meningitis?
    1. Standard precautions.
    2. Airborne precautions.
    3. Contact precautions.
    4. Droplet precautions.

66. The nurse is developing a plan of care for a client diagnosed with aseptic meningitis secondary to a brain tumor. Which nursing goal would be most appropriate for the client problem "altered cerebral tissue perfusion"?
    1. The client will be able to complete activities of daily living.
    2. The client will be protected from injury if seizure activity occurs.
    3. The client will be afebrile for 48 hours prior to discharge.
    4. The client will have elastic tissue turgor with ready recoil.

67. The nurse is preparing a client diagnosed with rule-out meningitis for a lumbar puncture. Which interventions should the nurse implement? Select all that apply.
    1. Obtain an informed consent from the client or significant other.
    2. Have the client empty the bladder prior to the procedure.
    3. Place the client in a side-lying position with the back arched.
    4. Instruct the client to breathe rapidly and deeply during the procedure.
    5. Explain to the client what to expect during the procedure.

68. The nurse is caring for a client diagnosed with meningitis. Which collaborative intervention should be included in the plan of care?
    1. Administer antibiotics.
    2. Obtain a sputum culture.
    3. Monitor the pulse oximeter.
    4. Assess intake and output.

69. The client is diagnosed with meningococcal meningitis. Which preventive measure would the nurse expect the health-care provider to order for the significant others in the home?
    1. The *Haemophilus influenzae* vaccine.
    2. Antimicrobial chemoprophylaxis.
    3. A 10-day dose pack of corticosteroids.
    4. A gamma globulin injection.

70. Which statement best describes the scientific rationale for alternating a nonnarcotic antipyretic and a nonsteroidal anti-inflammatory drug (NSAID) every two (2) hours to a female client diagnosed with bacterial meningitis?
    1. This regimen helps to decrease the purulent exudate surrounding the meninges.
    2. These medications will decrease intracranial pressure and brain metabolism.
    3. These medications will increase the client's memory and orientation.
    4. This will help prevent a yeast infection secondary to antibiotic therapy.

71. The client diagnosed with septic meningitis is admitted to the medical floor at noon. Which health-care provider's order would have the highest priority?
    1. Administer intravenous antibiotic.
    2. Obtain the client's lunch tray.
    3. Provide a quite, calm, and dark room.
    4. Weigh the client in hospital attire.

72. The 29-year-old client is admitted to the medical floor diagnosed with meningitis. Which assessment by the nurse has priority?
    1. Assess lung sounds.
    2. Assess the six cardinal fields of gaze.
    3. Assess apical pulse.
    4. Assess level of consciousness.

## Parkinson's Disease

73. The client diagnosed with Parkinson's disease (PD) is being admitted with a fever and patchy infiltrates in the lung fields on the chest x-ray. Which clinical manifestations of PD would explain this assessment data?
    1. Masklike facies and shuffling gait.
    2. Difficulty swallowing and immobility.
    3. Pill rolling of fingers and flat affect.
    4. Lack of arm swing and bradykinesia.

74. The client diagnosed with PD is being discharged on Sinemet, carbidopa/levodopa, an antiparkinsonian drug. Which statement is the scientific rationale for combining these medications?
    1. There will be fewer side effects with this combination than with carbidopa alone.
    2. Dopamine D requires the presence of both of these medications to work.
    3. Carbidopa makes more levodopa available to the brain.
    4. Carbidopa crosses the blood–brain barrier to treat Parkinson's disease.

75. The nurse caring for a client diagnosed with Parkinson's disease writes a problem of "impaired nutrition." Which nursing intervention would be included in the plan of care?
    1. Consult the occupational therapist for adaptive appliances for eating.
    2. Request a low-fat, low-sodium diet from the dietary department.
    3. Provide three meals per day that include nuts and whole-grain breads.
    4. Offer six meals per day with a soft consistency.

76. The nurse and the unlicensed nursing assistant are caring for clients on a medical-surgical unit. Which task should not be assigned to the assistant?
    1. Feed the 69-year-old client diagnosed with Parkinson's disease who is having difficulty swallowing.
    2. Turn and position the 89-year-old client diagnosed with a pressure ulcer secondary to Parkinson's disease.
    3. Assist the 54-year-old client diagnosed with Parkinson's disease with toilet-training activities.
    4. Obtain vital signs on a 72-year-old client diagnosed with pneumonia secondary to Parkinson's disease.

77. The charge nurse is making assignments. Which client should be assigned to the new graduate nurse?
    1. The client diagnosed with aseptic meningitis who is complaining of a headache and the light bothering his eyes.
    2. The client diagnosed with Parkinson's disease who fell during the night and is complaining of difficulty walking.
    3. The client diagnosed with a cerebrovascular accident whose vitals signs are P 60, R 14, and BP 198/68.
    4. The client diagnosed with a brain tumor who has a new complaint of seeing spots before the eyes.

78. The nurse is planning the care for a client diagnosed with Parkinson's disease. Which would be a therapeutic goal of treatment for the disease process?
    1. The client will experience periods of akinesia throughout the day.
    2. The client will take the prescribed medications correctly.
    3. The client will be able to enjoy a family outing with the spouse.
    4. The client will be able to carry out activities of daily living.

79. The nurse researcher is working with clients diagnosed with Parkinson's disease. Which is an example of an experimental therapy?
    1. Sterotactic pallidotomy/thalamotomy.
    2. Dopamine receptor agonist medication.
    3. Physical therapy for muscle strengthening.
    4. Fetal tissue transplantation.

80. The client diagnosed with Parkinson's disease is being discharged. Which statement made by the significant other indicates an understanding of the discharge instructions?
    1. "All of my spouse's emotions will slow down now just like his body movements."
    2. "My spouse may experience hallucinations until the medication starts working."
    3. "I will schedule appointments late in the morning after his morning bath."
    4. "It is fine if we don't follow a strict medication schedule on weekends."

81. The nurse is admitting a client with the diagnosis of Parkinson's disease. Which assessment data support this diagnosis?
    1. Crackles in the upper lung fields and jugular vein distention.
    2. Muscle weakness in the upper extremities and ptosis.
    3. Exaggerated arm swinging and scanning speech.
    4. Masklike facies and a shuffling gait.

82. Which is a common cognitive problem associated with Parkinson's disease?
    1. Emotional lability.
    2. Depression.
    3. Memory deficits.
    4. Paranoia.

83. The nurse is conducting a support group for clients diagnosed with Parkinson's disease and their significant others. Which information regarding psychosocial needs should be included in the discussion?
    1. The client should discuss feelings about being placed on a ventilator.
    2. The client may have rapid mood swings and become easily upset.
    3. "Pill rolling" tremors will become worse when the medication is wearing off.
    4. The client may automatically start to repeat what another person says.

84. The nurse is caring for clients on a medical surgical floor. Which client should be assessed first?
    1. The 65-year-old client diagnosed with seizures who is complaining of a headache that is a 2 on a 1–10 scale.
    2. The 24-year-old client diagnosed with a T-10 spinal cord injury who cannot move his toes.
    3. The 58-year-old client diagnosed with Parkinson's disease who is crying and worried about her facial appearance.
    4. The 62-year-old client diagnosed with a cerebrovascular accident who has a resolving left hemiparesis.

## Substance Abuse

85. The friend of an 18-year-old male client brings the client to the emergency department (ED). The client is unconscious and his breathing is slow and shallow. Which action should the nurse implement first?
    1. Ask the friend what drugs the client has been taking.
    2. Initiate an IV at a keep-open rate.
    3. Call for a ventilator to be brought to the ED.
    4. Apply oxygen at 100% via nasal cannula.

86. The chief executive officer (CEO) of a large manufacturing plant presents to the occupational health clinic with chronic rhinitis and requesting medication. On inspection, the nurse notices holes in the septum that separates the nasal passages. The nurse also notes dilated pupils and tachycardia. The facility has a "No Drug" policy. Which intervention should the nurse implement?
    1. Prepare to complete a drug screen urine test.
    2. Discuss the client's use of illegal drugs.
    3. Notify the client's supervisor about the situation.
    4. Give the client an antihistamine and say nothing.

87. The nurse is working with clients in a substance abuse clinic. Client A tells the nurse that another client, Client B, has "started using again." Which action should the nurse implement?
    1. Tell Client A that you cannot discuss Client B with him.
    2. Find out how Client A got this information.
    3. Inform the HCP that Client B is using again.
    4. Get in touch with Client B and have the client come to the clinic.

88. A 20-year-old female client who tried lysergic acid diethylamide (LSD) as a teen tells the nurse that she has bad dreams that make her want to kill herself. Which is the explanation for this occurrence?
    1. These occurrences are referred to as hold-over reactions to the drug.
    2. These are flashbacks to a time when the client had a "bad trip."
    3. The drug is still in the client's body and causing these reactions.
    4. The client is suicidal and should be on one-to-one precautions.

89. The nurse observes a co-worker acting erratically. The clients assigned to this co-worker don't seem to get relief when pain medications are administered. Which action should the nurse take?
    1. Try to help the co-worker by confronting the co-worker with the nurse's suspicions.
    2. Tell the co-worker that the nurse will give all narcotic medications from now on.
    3. Report the nurse's suspicions to the nurse's supervisor or the facility's peer review.
    4. Do nothing until the nurse can prove the co-worker has been using drugs.

90. The client is diagnosed with Wernicke-Korsakoff syndrome as a result of chronic alcoholism. Which symptoms would the nurse assess?
    1. Insomnia and anxiety.
    2. Visual or auditory hallucinations.
    3. Extreme tremors and agitation.
    4. Ataxia and confabulation.

91. The client diagnosed with delirium tremens when trying to quit drinking cold turkey is admitted to the medical unit. Which medications would the nurse anticipate administering?
    1. Thiamine (vitamin B$_6$) and librium, a benzodiazepine.
    2. Dilantin, an anticonvulsant, and Feosol, an iron preparation.
    3. Methadone, a synthetic narcotic, and Depakote, a mood stabilizer.
    4. Mannitol, an osmotic diuretic, and Ritalin, a stimulant.

92. The client is withdrawing from a heroin addiction. Which interventions should the nurse implement? Select all that apply.
    1. Initiate seizure precautions.
    2. Check vital signs every eight (8) hours.
    3. Place the client in a quiet, calm atmosphere.
    4. Have a consent form signed for HIV testing.
    5. Provide the client with sterile needles.

93. The wife of the client diagnosed with chronic alcoholism tells the nurse, "I have to call his work just about every Monday to let them know he is ill or he will lose his job." Which would be the nurse's best response?
    1. "I am sure that this must be hard for you. Tell me about your concerns."
    2. "You are afraid he will lose his source of income."
    3. "Why would you call in for your husband? Can't he do this?"
    4. "Are you aware that when you do this you are enabling him?"

94. The nurse caring for a client that has been abusing amphetamines writes a problem of "cardiovascular compromise." Which nursing interventions should be implemented?
    1. Monitor the telemetry and vital signs every four (4) hours.
    2. Encourage the client to verbalize the reason for using drugs.
    3. Provide a quiet, calm atmosphere for the client to rest.
    4. Place the client on bed rest and a low-sodium diet.

95. The client diagnosed with substance abuse is being discharged from a drug and alcohol rehabilitation facility. Which information should the nurse teach the client?
    1. Do not go any place where you can be tempted to use again.
    2. It is important that you attend a 12-step meeting regularly.
    3. Now that you are clean, your family will be willing to see you again.
    4. The client should explain to all the client's co-workers what has happened.

96. The nurse is working with clients and their families regarding substance abuse. Which statement is the scientific rationale for teaching the children new coping mechanisms?
    1. The child needs to realize that the parent will be changing behaviors.
    2. The child will need to point out to the parent when the parent is not coping.
    3. Children tend to mimic behaviors of the parents when faced with similar situations.
    4. Children need to feel like they are a part of the parent's recovery.

## Amyotrophic Lateral Sclerosis (ALS or Lou Gehrig's disease)

97. Which diagnostic test is used to confirm the diagnosis of ALS?
    1. Electromyelogram (EMG).
    2. Muscle biopsy.
    3. Serum creatine kinase enzyme (CK).
    4. Pulmonary function test.

98. The client is diagnosed with ALS. Which client problem would be most appropriate for this client?
    1. Disuse syndrome.
    2. Altered body image.
    3. Fluid and electrolyte imbalance.
    4. Alteration in pain.

99. The client is being evaluated to rule out ALS. Which signs/symptoms would the nurse note to confirm the diagnosis?
    1. Muscle atrophy and flaccidity.
    2. Fatigue and malnutrition.
    3. Slurred speech and dysphagia.
    4. Weakness and paralysis.

100. The client diagnosed with ALS asks the nurse, "I know this disease is going to kill me. What will happen to me in the end?" Which statement by the nurse would be most appropriate?
    1. "You are afraid of how you will die?"
    2. "Most people with ALS die of respiratory failure."
    3. "Don't talk like that. You have to stay positive."
    4. "ALS is not a killer. You can live a long life."

101. The client with ALS is admitted to the medical unit with shortness of breath, dyspnea, and respiratory complications. Which intervention should the nurse implement first?
    1. Elevate the head of the bed 30 degrees.
    2. Administer oxygen via nasal cannula.
    3. Assess the client's lung sounds.
    4. Obtain a pulse oximeter reading.

102. The client is to receive a 100-mL intravenous antibiotic over 30 minutes via an intravenous pump. What rate should the nurse set the IV pump? _____

103. The nurse is caring for the following clients on a medical unit. Which client should the nurse assess first?
    1. The client with ALS who is refusing to turn every two (2) hours.
    2. The client with abdominal pain who is complaining of nausea.
    3. The client with pneumonia who has a pulse oximeter reading of 90%.
    4. The client who is complaining about not receiving any pain medication.

104. The client is diagnosed with ALS. As the disease progresses, which intervention should the nurse implement?
    1. Discuss the need to be placed in a long-term care facility.
    2. Explain how to care for a sigmoid colostomy.
    3. Assist the client to prepare an advance directive.
    4. Teach the client how to use a motorized wheelchair.

105. The client is in the terminal stage of ALS. Which intervention should the nurse implement?
    1. Perform passive ROM every two (2) hours.
    2. Maintain a negative nitrogen balance.
    3. Encourage a low-protein, soft-mechanical diet.
    4. Turn the client, have him cough, and deep breathe every shift.

106. The son of a client diagnosed with ALS asks the nurse, "Is there any chance that I could get this disease?" Which statement by the nurse would be most appropriate?
    1. "It must be scary to think you might get this disease."
    2. "No, this disease is not genetic or contagious."
    3. "ALS does have a genetic factor and runs in families."
    4. "If you are exposed to the same virus, you may get the disease."

107. The client with end-stage ALS requires a gastrostomy tube feeding. Which finding would require the nurse to hold a bolus tube feeding?
    1. A residual of 125 mL.
    2. The abdomen is soft.
    3. Three episodes of diarrhea.
    4. The potassium level is 3.4 mEq/L.

108. The client diagnosed with ALS is prescribed an antiglutamate, Riluzole (Rilutek). Which instruction should the nurse discuss with the client?
    1. Take the medication with food.
    2. Do not eat green leafy vegetables.
    3. Use SPF 30 when going out in the sun.
    4. Report any febrile illness.

## Encephalitis

109. When admitting the client into the hospital to rule out encephalitis, the nurse should include which data in the interview that would best assist with the diagnosis? Select all that apply.
    1. Received any recent immunizations.
    2. Recent upper-respiratory tract infections.
    3. An episode of active herpes simplex I.
    4. Recent vacations in the Great Lakes region.
    5. Exposure to soil with fungal spores.

110. The nurse assesses the client admitted with encephalitis; which data would require immediate nursing intervention?
    1. Presence of bilateral facial palsies.
    2. Recurrent temperature of 100.6°F.
    3. Decreased complaint of headache.
    4. Comments that the meal has no taste.

111. The client admitted to the hospital to rule out encephalitis is being prepared for a lumbar puncture. What information should the nurse teach the client post-procedure?
    1. Instruct that all invasive procedures require a written permission.
    2. Explain that this allows analysis of a sample of the cerebrospinal fluid.
    3. Tell the client to increase fluid intake to 300 mL for the next 48 hours.
    4. Discuss that lying supine with the head flat will prevent all hematomas.

112. Which would be an expected outcome for a client diagnosed with encephalitis?
    1. The client will regain as much neurological function as possible.
    2. The client will have no short-term memory loss.
    3. The client will have improved renal function.
    4. The client will apply hydrocortisone cream daily.

113. When caring for the client diagnosed with encephalitis, which intervention should the nurse implement? Select all that apply.
    1. Turn client every two (2) hours.
    2. Encourage the client to increase fluids.
    3. Keep client in the supine position.
    4. Assess for deep vein thrombosis.
    5. Assess for any alterations in elimination.

114. When caring for the client with encephalitis, which intervention should the nurse implement first to determine if the client is deteriorating?
    1. Examine pupil reactions to light.
    2. Assess level of consciousness.
    3. Observe for seizure activity.
    4. Monitor vital signs every shift.

115. The public health department nurse is preparing a lecture on prevention of West Nile virus. What information should the nurse include?
    1. Change water daily in pet dishes and birdbaths.
    2. Wear thick dark clothing when outside to avoid bites.
    3. Apply insect repellent over face and arms only.
    4. Explain that mosquitoes are more prevalent in the morning.

116. Which problem has the highest priority for the client diagnosed with West Nile virus?
    1. Alteration in body temperature.
    2. Altered tissue perfusion.
    3. Fluid volume excess.
    4. Altered skin integrity.

117. When preparing a plan of care for a client diagnosed with West Nile virus, which intervention should the nurse include in this plan?
    1. Monitor respirations frequently.
    2. Refer to dermatologist for treatment of the maculopapular rash.
    3. Treat hypothermia by using ice packs under the client's arms.
    4. Teach the client to report any swollen lymph glands.

118. Which collaborative nursing intervention should the nurse implement while caring for the client with West Nile virus?
    1. Complete neurovascular examinations every eight (8) hours.
    2. Maintain accurate intake and output at the end of each shift.
    3. Assess the client's symptoms to determine if there is improvement.
    4. Administer intravenous fluids while assessing for overload.

119. When caring for the client diagnosed with West Nile virus, which assessment data would require immediate intervention from the nurse?
    1. The vital signs are documented as T 100.2°F, P 80, R 18, and BP 136/78.
    2. The client complains of generalized body aches and pains.
    3. Positive results from the enzyme-linked immunosorbent assay test (ELISA).
    4. The client has become lethargic and difficult to arouse by verbal stimuli.

120. Which rationale explains the transmission of the West Nile virus?
    1. Transmission occurs through exchange of body fluids when sneezing and coughing.
    2. Transmission occurs only through mosquito bites and not between humans.
    3. Transmission can occur from human to human in blood products and breast milk.
    4. Transmission occurs with direct contact from the maculopapular rash drainage.

This section provides the answers for the questions given in the previous section. The correct answer and why it is correct are given in boldface. The reason why each of the other answer options is not the correct or the best answer is also given.

## Cerebrovascular Accident (Stroke)

1. 1. The drug rt-PA may be administered, but a cerebrovascular accident (CVA) must be verified by diagnostic tests prior to administering it. rt-PA helps dissolve a blood clot, and it may be administered if an ischemic CVA is verified, rt-PA would not be given if the client were experiencing a hemorrhagic stroke.
   2. Teaching is important to help prevent another CVA, but it is not the priority intervention on admission to the emergency department. Slurred speech indicates problems that may interfere with teaching.
   3. **A CT scan will determine if the client is having a stroke or has a brain tumor or another neurological disorder. If a CVA is diagnosed, the CT scan can determine if it is a hemorrhagic or ischemic accident and guide treatment.**
   4. The client may be referred for speech deficits and/or swallowing difficulty, but referrals are not priority in the emergency department.

   **TEST-TAKING HINT: When "priority" is used in the stem, all answer options may be appropriate for the client situation, but only one answer is priority. The client must have a documented diagnosis before treatment is started.**

2. 1. A left-sided CVA will result in right-sided motor deficits; hemiparesis is weakness of one half of the body, not just the upper extremity. Apraxia, the inability to perform a previously learned task, is a communication loss, not a motor loss.
   2. **The most common motor dysfunction of a CVA is paralysis of one side of the body, hemiplegia; in this case with a left-sided CVA, the paralysis would affect the right side. Ataxia is an impaired ability to coordinate movement.**
   3. Homonymous hemianopsia (loss of half of the visual field of each eye) and diplopia (double vision) are visual field deficits that a client with a CVA may experience, but they are not motor losses.
   4. Personality disorders occur in clients with a right-sided CVA and are cognitive deficits; hostility is an emotional deficit.

**TEST-TAKING HINT: Be sure to always notice adjectives describing something. In this case, "left-sided" describes the type of CVA. Also be sure to identify exactly what the question is asking—in this case, about "motor loss," which will help rule out many of the possible answers.**

3. 1. **African Americans have twice the rate of CVAs as Caucasians and men have a higher incidence than women; African Americans suffer more extensive damage from a CVA than do people of other cultural groups.**
   2. Females are less likely to have a CVA than males, but advanced age does increase the risk for CVA. The Oriental population has a lower risk, possibly as a result of their relatively high intake of omega-3 fatty acids, antioxidants found in fish.
   3. Caucasians have a lower risk of CVA than do African Americans, Hispanics, and Native Pacific Islanders.
   4. Pregnancy is a minimal risk for having a CVA.

**TEST-TAKING HINT: Note the age of the client if this information is given, but take this information in context with the additional information provided in the question-and-answer possibilities. The 84-year-old may appear to be the best answer but not if the client is a female and Oriental, which rules out this answer for the client most at risk.**

4. 1. Placing a small pillow under the shoulder will prevent the shoulder from adducting toward the chest and developing a contracture.
   2. **The client should be repositioned at least every two (2) hours to prevent contractures, pneumonia, skin breakdown, and other complications of immobility.**
   3. The client should not ignore the paralyzed side, and the nurse must encourage the client to move it as much as possible; a written schedule may assist the client in exercising.
   4. These exercises are recommended, but they must be done at least five (5) times a day for ten (10) minutes to help strengthen the muscles for walking.
   5. The fingers are positioned so that they are barely flexed to help prevent contracture of the hand.

**TEST-TAKING HINT: Be sure to look at the intervals of time for any intervention; note that "every shift" and "three times a day" are not appropriate time intervals for this client.**

**Because this is an all-that-apply question, the test taker must read each answer option and decide if it is correct; one will not eliminate another.**

5. 1. Agnosia is the failure to recognize familiar objects; therefore, observing the client for possible aspiration is not appropriate.
   2. A semi-Fowler's position is appropriate for sleeping, but agnosia is the failure to recognize familiar objects; therefore, this intervention is inappropriate.
   3. Placing suction at the bedside will help if the client has dysphagia (difficulty swallowing), not agnosia, which is failure to recognize familiar objects.
   4. A collaborative intervention is an intervention in which another health-care discipline—in this case, occupational therapy—is used in the care of the client.

   **TEST-TAKING HINT: Be sure to look at what the question is asking and see if the answer can be determined even if some terms are not understood. In this case, note that the question refers to "collaborative intervention." Only choice "4" refers to collaboration with another discipline.**

6. 1. Placing a gait belt prior to ambulating is an appropriate action for safety and would not require the nurse to intervene.
   2. Placing the client in a supine position with the head turned to the side is not a problem position, so the nurse does not need to intervene.
   3. This action is inappropriate and would require intervention by the nurse because pulling on a flaccid shoulder joint could cause shoulder dislocation; the client should be pulled up by placing the arm underneath the back or using a lift sheet.
   4. The client should be encouraged and praised for attempting to perform any activities independently, such as combing hair or brushing teeth.

   **TEST-TAKING HINT: This type of question has three answer possibilities that do not require a nurse to intervene to correct a subordinate. Remember to read every possible answer before deciding on a correct one.**

7. 1. The nurse would anticipate an oral anticoagulant, warfarin (Coumadin), to be prescribed to help prevent thrombi formation in the atria secondary to atrial fibrillation. The thrombi can become embolic and may cause a TIA or CVA (stroke).
   2. Beta blockers slow the heart rate and decrease blood pressure but would not be an anticipated medication to help prevent a TIA secondary to atrial fibrillation.
   3. An anti-hyperuricemic medication is administered for a client experiencing gout and decreases the formation of tophi.
   4. A thrombolytic medication is administered to dissolve a clot, and it may be ordered during the initial presentation for a client with a CVA, but not on discharge.

   **TEST-TAKING HINT: In the stem of this question, there are two disease processes mentioned—atrial fibrillation and TIA. The reader must determine how one process affects the other before answering the question. In this question, the test taker must know that atrial fibrillation predisposes the client to the formation of thrombi and that therefore the nurse should anticipate the health-care provider ordering a medication to prevent clot formation, an anticoagulant.**

8. 1. The rubber mat will stabilize the plate and prevent it from slipping away from the client learning to feed himself, but this does not address generalized weakness.
   2. A long-handled bath sponge will assist the client when showering hard-to-reach areas, but it is not a home modification, nor will it help with generalized weakness.
   3. Clothes with Velcro closures will make dressing easier, but they do not constitute a home modification and do not address generalized weakness.
   4. Raising the toilet seat is modifying the home and addresses the client's weakness in being able to sit down and get up without straining muscles or requiring lifting assistance from the wife.

   **TEST-TAKING HINT: The test taker must read the stem of the question carefully and note that the intervention must be one in which the home is modified in some way. This would eliminate three of the options, leaving the correct answer.**

9. 1. Potential for injury is a physiological problem, not a psychosocial problem.
   2. Expressive aphasia means that the client cannot communicate thoughts but understands what is being communicated; this leads to frustration, anger, depression, and the inability to verbalize needs, which, in turn, causes the client to have a lack of control and feel powerless.

3. A disturbance in thought processes is a cognitive problem; with expressive aphasia the client's thought processes are intact.

4. Sexual dysfunction can have a psychosocial component or a physical component, but it is not related to expressive aphasia.

**TEST-TAKING HINT: The test taker should always make sure that the choice selected as the correct answer matches what the question is asking. The stem has the adjective "psychosocial," so the correct answer must address psychosocial needs.**

10. 1. This glucose level is elevated and could predispose the client to ischemic neurological changes due to blood viscosity, but it is not a risk factor for a hemorrhagic stroke.

2. A carotid bruit predisposes the client to an embolic or ischemic stroke but not to a hemorrhagic stroke.

3. Uncontrolled hypertension is a risk factor for hemorrhagic stroke, which is a ruptured blood vessel inside the cranium.

4. Cancer is not a precursor to developing a hemorrhagic stroke.

**TEST-TAKING HINT: Both "1" and "2" are risk factors for an ischemic or embolic type of stroke. Knowing this, the test taker can rule out these answers as incorrect.**

11. 1. The nurse should not administer any medication to a client without first assessing the cause of the client's complaint or problem.

2. An MRI may be needed, but the nurse must determine the client's neurological status prior to diagnostic tests.

3. Starting an IV is appropriate, but it is not the action the nurse should implement when assessing pain, and 100 mL/hr might be too high a rate for an 85-year-old client.

4. The nurse must complete a neurological assessment to help determine the cause of the headache before taking any further action.

**TEST-TAKING HINT: The test taker should always apply the nursing process when answering questions. If the test taker narrows down the choices to two possible answers, always select the assessment option as the first intervention.**

12. 1. The client is at risk for increased intracranial pressure whenever performing the Valsalva maneuver, which will occur when straining during defecation. Therefore stool softeners would be appropriate.

2. Coughing increases intracranial pressure and is discouraged for any client who has had a craniotomy. The client is encouraged to turn and breathe deeply, but not to cough.

3. Monitoring the neurological status is appropriate for this client, but it should be done much more frequently than every shift.

4. Dopamine is used to increase blood pressure or to maintain renal perfusion, and a BP of 160/90 is too high for this client.

**TEST-TAKING HINT: The test taker should always notice an answer choice has a time frame—every shift, every four (4) hours, or daily. Whether or not the time frame is correct may lead the test taker to the correct answer.**

## Head Injury

13. 1. Awakening the client every two (2) hours allows the identification of headache, dizziness, lethargy, irritability, and anxiety—all signs of post-concussion syndrome—that would warrant the significant other's taking the client back to the emergency department.

2. The nurse should monitor for signs of increased intracranial pressure (ICP), but a layman, the significant other, would not know what these signs and medical terms mean.

3. Hypervigilance, increased alertness and super-awareness of the surroundings, is a sign of amphetamine or cocaine abuse, but it would not be expected in a client with a head injury.

4. The client can eat food as tolerated, but feeding the client every three (3) to four (4) hours does not affect the development of post-concussion syndrome, the signs of which are what should be taught to the significant other.

**TEST-TAKING HINT: Remember to pay close attention to choices that have times (e.g., every two [2] hours, every three [3] to four [4] hours). Also consider the likelihood of the options listed. Would a nurse teach the significant other terms such as increased intracranial pressure or hypervigilance? Probably not, so options "2" and "3" should be eliminated.**

14. 1. The scalp is a very vascular area and a moderate amount of bleeding would be expected.

2. These signs/symptoms—weak pulse, shallow respirations, cool pale skin—indicate increased intracranial pressure from cerebral edema secondary to the fall, and they require immediate attention.

3. This is a normal pupillary response and would not warrant intervention.

4. A headache that resolves with medication is not an emergency situation, and the nurse would

expect the client to have a headache after the fall; a headache not relieved with Tylenol would warrant further investigation.

**TEST-TAKING HINT: The test taker is looking for an answer option that is not normal for the client's situation. Of the answer choices listed, three would be expected and would not warrant a trip to the emergency department.**

15. 1. A client with a head injury must be awakened every two (2) hours to determine alertness; decreasing level of consciousness is the first indicator of increased intracranial pressure.
    2. A diagnostic test, MRI, would be an expected test for a client with left-sided weakness and would not require immediate attention.
    3. The Glasgow Coma Scale is used to determine a client's response to stimuli (eye-opening response, best verbal response, and best motor response) secondary to a neurological problem; scores range from 3 (deep coma) to 15 (intact neurological function). A client with a score of 6 should be assessed first by the nurse.
    4. The nurse would expect a client diagnosed with a CVA (stroke) to have some sequelae of the problem, including the inability to speak.

    **TEST-TAKING HINT: This is a prioritizing question that asks the test taker to determine which client has priority when assessing all four clients. The nurse should assess the client who has abnormal data for the disease process.**

16. 1. This is an oculocephalic test (doll's eyes) that determines brain activity. If the eyes move with the head, it means the brain stem is intact and there is no brain death.
    2. Waveforms on the EEG indicate that there is brain activity.
    3. The cold caloric test, also called the oculo-vestibular test, is a test used to determine if the brain is intact or dead. No eye activity indicates brain death. If the client's eyes moved, that would indicate that the brain stem is intact.
    4. Decorticate posturing after painful stimuli are applied indicates that the brain stem is intact; flaccid paralysis is the worse neurological response when assessing a client with a head injury.

    **TEST-TAKING HINT: The test taker needs to know what the results of the cold caloric test signify—in this case, no eye activity indicates brain death.**

17. 1. Assessing the neurological status is important, but ensuring an airway is priority over assessment.

    2. Monitoring vital signs is important, but maintaining an adequate airway is higher priority.
    3. Initiating an IV access is an intervention the nurse can implement, but it is not the priority intervention.
    4. The most important nursing goal in the management of a client with a head injury is to establish and maintain an adequate airway.

    **TEST-TAKING HINT: If the question asks for a priority intervention, it means that all of the choices would be appropriate for the client but only one intervention is priority. Always apply Maslow's Hierarchy of Needs—an adequate airway is first.**

18. 1. The client in rehabilitation is at risk for the development of deep vein thrombosis; therefore, this is an appropriate medication.
    2. An osmotic diuretic would be ordered in the acute phase to help decrease cerebral edema, but this medication would not be expected to be ordered in a rehabilitation unit.
    3. Clients with head injuries are at risk for post-traumatic seizures; thus an oral anticonvulsant would be administered for seizure prophylaxis.
    4. The client is at risk for a stress ulcer; therefore, an oral proton pump inhibitor would be an appropriate medication.

    **TEST-TAKING HINT: The client is in the rehabilitation unit and therefore must be stable. The use of any intravenous medication should be questioned under those circumstances, even if the test taker is not sure why the medication may be considered.**

19. 1. Purposeless movement indicates that the client's cerebral edema is decreasing. The best motor response is purposeful movement, but purposeless movement indicates an improvement over decorticate movement, which, in turn, is an improvement over decerebrate movement or flaccidity.
    2. Flaccidity would indicate a worsening of the client's condition.
    3. Decerebrate posturing would indicate a worsening of the client's condition.
    4. The eyes respond to light, not painful stimuli, but a 6-mm nonreactive pupil indicates severe neurological deficit.

    **TEST-TAKING HINT: The test taker must have strong assessment skills and know what specific signs/symptoms signify for each of the body systems—in this case, the significance of different stages of posturing/movement in assessing neurological status.**

20. 1. The head of the bed should be elevated no more than 30 degrees to help decrease cerebral edema by gravity.
    2. Stool softeners are initiated to prevent the Valsalva maneuver, which increases intracranial pressure.
    3. Oxygen saturation higher than 93% ensures oxygenation of the brain tissues; decreasing oxygen levels increase cerebral edema.
    4. Noxious stimuli, such as suctioning, increase intracranial pressure and should be avoided.
    5. Mild sedatives will reduce the client's agitation; strong narcotics would not be administered because they decrease the client's level of consciousness.

**TEST-TAKING HINT: In select-all-that apply questions, the test taker should look at each answer option as a separate entity. In "1" the test taker should attempt to get a mental picture of the client's position in the bed. A 60-degree angle is almost upright in the bed. Would any client diagnosed with a head injury be placed this high? The client would be at risk for slumping over because of the inability to control the body position. Nasal suctioning, option "4," which increases intracranial pressure, should also be avoided.**

21. 1. Prior to notifying the HCP the nurse should always make sure that all the needed assessment information is available to discuss with the HCP.
    2. With head injuries, any clear drainage may indicate a cerebrospinal fluid leak; the nurse should not assume the drainage is secondary to allergies and administer an antihistamine.
    3. The presence of glucose in drainage from the nose or ears indicates cerebrospinal fluid and the HCP should be notified immediately once this is determined.
    4. This would be appropriate, but it is not the first intervention. The nurse must determine where the fluid is coming from.

**TEST-TAKING HINT: The question is asking which intervention should be implemented first, and the nurse should always assess the situation before calling the HCP or taking an action.**

22. 1. Assessment is important, but with clients with head injury the nurse must assume spinal cord injury until it is ruled out with x-ray; therefore, stabilizing the spinal cord is priority.
    2. Removing the client from the water is an appropriate intervention, but the nurse must assume spinal cord injury until it is ruled out with x-ray; therefore, stabilizing the spinal cord is priority.
    3. Assessing the client for further injury is appropriate, but the first intervention is to stabilize the spine because the impact was strong enough to render the client unconsciousness.
    4. The nurse should always assume that a client with traumatic head injury may have sustained spinal cord injury. Moving the client could further injure the spinal cord and cause paralysis; therefore, the nurse should stabilize the cervical spinal cord as best as possible prior to removing the client from the water.

**TEST-TAKING HINT: When two possible answers contain the same directive word—in this case, "assess"—the test taker can either rule out these two as incorrect or prioritize between the two assessment responses.**

23. 1. The head of the client's bed should be elevated to help the lungs expand and prevent stasis of secretions that could lead to pneumonia, a complication of immobility.
    2. Active range of motion exercises require that the client participate in the activity. This is not possible because the client is in a coma.
    3. The client is at risk for pressure ulcers and should be turned more frequently than every shift, and research now shows that massaging bony prominences can increase the risk for tissue breakdown.
    4. The nurse should always talk to the client, even if he or she is in a coma, but this will not address the problem of immobility.

**TEST-TAKING HINT: Whenever a client problem is written, interventions must address the specific problem, not the disease. Positioning the client addresses the possibility of immobility complications, whereas "talking to a comatose client" addresses communication deficit and psychosocial needs, not immobility issues.**

24. 1. The client is at risk for seizures and does not process information appropriately. Allowing him to return to his occupation as a forklift operator is a safety risk for him and other employees. Vocational training may be required.
    2. Cognitive pertains to mental processes of comprehension, judgment, memory, and reasoning. Therefore, an appropriate goal would be for the client to stay on task for 10 minutes.
    3. The client's ability to dress self addresses self-care problems, not a cognitive problem.
    4. The client's ability to regain bowel and bladder control does not address cognitive deficits.

**TEST-TAKING HINT: The test taker must note adjectives closely. The question is asking about "cognitive" deficits; therefore the correct answer must address cognition.**

## Spinal Cord Injury

25. 1. The nurse should stabilize the client's neck prior to removal from the car.
    2. The nurse must stabilize the client's neck before doing any further assessment. Most nurses don't carry penlights, and the client's pupil reaction can be determined after stabilization.
    3. The nurse must assume that an unconscious person who has experienced direct trauma to the head may have a head injury and possibly a spinal cord injury. The nurse should stabilize the neck prior to removing the client from the car.
    4. Shaking the patient could cause further damage, possibly leading to paralysis.

    **TEST-TAKING HINT: Remember that in a question asking about which action should be taken first, all of the answers are interventions, but only one should be implemented first. There are very few "always" in the health-care profession, but in this situation, unless the client's car is on fire or under water, stabilizing the client's neck is always priority.**

26. 1. Spinal shock associated with SCI represents a sudden depression of reflex activity below the level of the injury. T-12 is just above the waist; therefore, no reflex activity below the waist would be expected.
    2. Assessment of the movement of the upper extremities would be more appropriate with a higher level injury; an injury in the cervical area might cause an inability to move the upper extremities.
    3. Complaints of a pounding headache are not typical of a T-12 spinal injury.
    4. Hypotension (low blood pressure) and tachycardia (rapid heart rate) are signs of hypovolemic or septic shock, but these do not occur in spinal shock.

    **TEST-TAKING HINT: If the test taker does not have any idea what the answer is, an attempt to relate the anatomical position of keywords in the question stem to words in the answer options is appropriate. In this case, T-12, mentioned in the stem, is around the waist, so answer options involving the anatomy above that level (e.g., the upper extremities) can be eliminated.**

27. 1. Oxygen is administered initially to maintain a high arterial PaO$_2$ because hypoxemia can worsen a neurological deficit to the spinal cord initially, but this client is in the rehabilitation department and thus not in the initial stages of the injury.
    2. Deep vein thrombosis (DVT) is a potential complication of immobility, which can occur because the client cannot move the lower extremities as a result of the L-1 SCI. Low-dose anticoagulation therapy (Lovenox) helps prevent blood from coagulating, thereby preventing DVTs.
    3. The client is unable to move the lower extremities. The nurse should do passive ROM exercises.
    4. A client with a spinal injury at C-4 or above would be dependent on a ventilator for breathing, but a client with an L-1 SCI would not.

    **TEST-TAKING HINT: The test taker should notice any adjectives like "rehabilitation," which should clue the test taker into ruling out oxygen, which is for the acute phase. The test taker should also be very selective if choosing an answer with a definitive word such as "all" (option "1").**

28. 1. Oxygen is administered initially to prevent hypoxemia, which can worsen the spinal cord injury; therefore, the nurse should determine how much oxygen is reaching the periphery.
    2. A C-6 injury would not affect the client's ability to chew and swallow so pureed food is not necessary.
    3. Breathing exercises are supervised by the nurse to increase the strength and endurance of inspiratory muscles, especially those of the diaphragm.
    4. Autonomic dysreflexia occurs during the rehabilitation phase, not the acute phase.
    5. Corticosteroids are administered to decrease inflammation, which will decrease edema, and help prevent edema from ascending up the spinal cord, causing breathing difficulties.

    **TEST-TAKING HINT: The test taker must notice where the client is receiving care, which may be instrumental in being able to rule out incorrect answer options and help in identifying the correct answer. Remember Maslow's Hierarchy of Needs—oxygen and breathing are priority nursing interventions.**

29. 1. Therapeutic communication addresses the client's feelings and attempts to allow the

client to verbalize feelings; the nurse should be a therapeutic listener.
2. This is belittling the client's feelings.
3. The client does not owe the nurse an explanation of his feelings; "why" is never therapeutic.
4. This is advising the client and is not therapeutic.

**TEST-TAKING HINT: When the question requests a therapeutic response, the test taker should select the answer option that has "feelings" in the response.**

30. 1. The machine is very loud and the technician will offer the client earplugs, but hearing difficulty will not affect the MRI.
2. Allergies to dairy products will not affect the MRI.
3. The client does not need to be NPO for this procedure.
4. MRIs are often done in a very confined space; many people who have claustrophobia must be medicated or even rescheduled for the procedure in an open MRI, which is available if needed.

**TEST-TAKING HINT: The nurse must be knowledgeable of diagnostic tests to prepare the client for the tests safely. Be realistic in determining answers—is there any test in which a hearing problem would make the diagnostic test contraindicated?**

31. 1. This action will not address the client's pounding headache and hypertension.
2. Dimming the lights will not help the client's condition.
3. This is an acute emergency caused by exaggerated autonomic responses to stimuli and only occurs after spinal shock has resolved in the client with a spinal cord injury above T-6. The most common cause is a full bladder.
4. The nurse should always assess the client before administering medication.

**TEST-TAKING HINT: The test taker should apply the nursing process when answering questions, and assessing the client comes first, before administering any type of medication.**

32. 1. The halo device is applied by inserting pins into the skull, and the client cannot remove them; the pins should be checked for signs of infection.
2. Reddened areas, especially under the brace, must be reported to the HCP because pressure ulcers can occur when wearing this appliance for an extended period.
3. The vest liner should be changed for hygiene reasons, but the halo part is not removed.

4. The client should be encouraged to ambulate to prevent complications of immobility.

**TEST-TAKING HINT: The test taker would need basic knowledge about a halo device to answer this question easily, but some clues are in the stem. A cervical fracture is in the upper portion of the spine or neck area, and most people understand that a halo is something that surrounds the forehead or higher. So the test taker could get a mental image of a device that must span this area of the body and maintain alignment of the neck. If an HCP attaches pins into the head, then the test taker could assume that they were not to be removed by the client. Redness usually indicates some sort of problem with the skin.**

33. 1. This is not an emergency; therefore, the nurse should not notify the health-care provider.
2. A physiological change in the client requires more than a therapeutic conversation.
3. Increasing the IV rate will not address the cause of the problem.
4. For the first two (2) weeks after an SCI above T-7, the blood pressure tends to be unstable and low; slight elevations of the head of the bed can cause profound hypotension; therefore the nurse should lower the head of the bed immediately.

**TEST-TAKING HINT: The test taker should notice that the only answer option that addresses the "bed" is the correct answer. This does not always help identify the correct answer, but it is a hint that should be used if the test taker has no idea what the correct answer is.**

34. 1. This client has signs/symptoms of a respiratory complication and should be assessed first.
2. This is a psychosocial need and should be addressed, but it does not have priority over a physiological problem.
3. A client with a lower SCI would not be at risk for autonomic dysreflexia; therefore a complaint of headache and feeling hot would not be priority over an airway problem.
4. The client with a T-4 SCI would not be expected to move the lower extremities.

**TEST-TAKING HINT: The nurse should assess the client who is at risk for dying or having some type of complication that requires intervention. Remember Maslow's Hierarchy of Needs in which physiological problems are always priority and airway is the top physiological problem.**

35. 1. The nurse cannot delegate assessment or teaching.

2. Tube feedings should be treated as if they were medications, and this task cannot be delegated.
3. **The assistant can place the client on the bedside commode as part of bowel training; the nurse is responsible for the training but can delegate this task.**
4. Evaluating the client's ability to self-catheterize must be done by the nurse.

**TEST-TAKING HINT: Although each state has its own delegation rules, teaching, assessing, and evaluating are nursing interventions that cannot be delegated to unlicensed personnel.**

36. 1. The ASIA is an appropriate referral for living with this condition, but it does not help find gainful employment after the injury.
2. **The rehabilitation commission of each state will help evaluate and determine if the client can receive training or education for another occupation after injury.**
3. The client is not asking about disability; he is concerned about employment. Therefore the nurse needs to make a referral to the appropriate agency.
4. This does not address the client's concern about gainful employment.

**TEST-TAKING HINT: If the question mentions a specific age for a client, the nurse should consider it when attempting to answer the question. This is a young person who needs to find gainful employment. Remember Erickson's stages of growth and development.**

## Seizures

37. 1. The nurse needs to protect the client from injury. Moving furniture would help ensure that the client would not hit something accidentally, but this is not done first.
2. This is done to help keep the airway patent, but it is not the first intervention in this specific situation.
3. Assessment is important but when the client is having a seizure, the nurse should not touch him or her.
4. **The client should not remain in the chair during a seizure. He should be brought safely to the floor so that he will have room to move the extremities.**

**TEST-TAKING HINT: All of the answer options are possible interventions, so the test taker should go back to the stem of the question and note that the question asks which intervention has priority. "In the chair" is the key to this question because the nurse should always think about safety, and a patient having a seizure is not safe in a chair.**

38. 1. **Head injury is one of the main reasons for epilepsy that can be prevented through occupational safety precautions and highway safety programs.**
2. Sedentary lifestyle is not a cause of epilepsy.
3. Dietary concerns are not a cause of epilepsy.
4. Safety glasses will help prevent eye injuries, but such injuries are not a cause of epilepsy.

**TEST-TAKING HINT: The nurse must be aware of risk factors that cause diseases. If the test taker does not know the correct answer, thinking about which body system the question is asking about may help rule out or rule in some of the answer options. Only "1" and "4" have anything to do with the head, and only helmets on the head are connected with the neurological system.**

39. 1. Anti-seizure drugs, tranquilizers, stimulants, and depressants are withheld before an EEG because they may alter the brain wave patterns.
2. Meals are not withheld because altered blood glucose level can cause changes in brain wave patterns.
3. **The goal is for the client to have a seizure during the EEG. Sleep deprivation, hyperventilating, or flashing lights may induce a seizure.**
4. Electrodes are placed on the client's scalp, but there are no electroshocks or any type of discomfort.

**TEST-TAKING HINT: The test taker should highlight the words "diagnose seizure disorder" in the stem and ask which answer option would possibly cause a seizure.**

40. 1. **Noticing the first thing the client does during a seizure provides information and clues as to the location of the seizure in the brain. It is important to document whether the beginning of the seizure was observed.**
2. Assessment is important, but during the seizure the nurse should not attempt to restrain the head to assess the eyes; muscle contractions are strong, and restraining the client could cause injury.
3. This should be done, but it is not the first intervention when walking into a room where the client is beginning to have a seizure.
4. The client should be protected from onlookers, but the nurse should always address the client first.

**TEST-TAKING HINT: This is a prioritizing question that asks the test taker which intervention to implement first. All four interventions would be appropriate, but only one should be implemented first. If the test taker cannot decide between two choices, always select the**

one that directly affects the client or the condition; privacy is important but helping determine the origin of the seizure is priority.

41. 1. The client is exhausted from the seizure and should be allowed to sleep.
    2. Awakening the client every 30 minutes possibly could induce another seizure as a result of sleep deprivation.
    3. During the postictal (after-seizure) phase, the client is very tired and should be allowed to rest quietly; placing the client on the side will help prevent aspiration and maintain a patent airway.
    4. The client must rest, and asking questions about the seizure will keep the client awake and may induce another seizure as a result of sleep deprivation.

    **TEST-TAKING HINT: Choices "1," "2," and "4" all have something to do with keeping the client awake. This might lead the test taker to choose the option that is different from the other three.**

42. 1. Once the seizure has started, no one should attempt to put anything in the mouth.
    2. The nurse should tell the assistant to stop trying to insert anything in the mouth of the client experiencing a seizure. Broken teeth and injury to the lips and tongue may result from trying to put anything in the clenched jaws of a client having a grand mal seizure.
    3. The primary nurse is responsible for the action of the unlicensed nursing assistant and should stop her from doing anything potentially dangerous to the client. No one should attempt to pry open the jaws that are clenched in a spasm to insert anything.
    4. The primary nurse must correct the action of the assistant immediately, prior to any injury occurring to the client and before notifying the charge nurse.

    **TEST-TAKING HINT: The nurse is responsible for the actions of the unlicensed nursing assistant and must correct the behavior immediately.**

43. 1. Thorough oral hygiene after each meal, gum massage, daily flossing, and regular dental care are essential to prevent or control gingival hyperplasia, which is a common occurrence in clients taking Dilantin.
    2. A serum (venipuncture) Dilantin level is checked monthly at first and then, after a therapeutic level is attained, every six (6) months.
    3. Dilantin does not turn the urine orange.
    4. The use of Dilantin does not ensure that the

client will not have any seizures, and in some instances, the dosage may need to be adjusted or another medication may need to be used.

**TEST-TAKING HINT: The test taker should realize that monitoring blood glucose levels using a glucometer is about the only level that is monitored daily; therefore, "2" in the answer options, which calls for daily monitoring of Dilantin levels, could be eliminated. Remember there are very few absolutes in the health-care field; therefore "4" could be ruled out because "won't have any" is an absolute.**

44. 1. Assessment is an independent nursing action, not a collaborative one.
    2. All clients in the ICD will be placed on telemetry, which does not require an order by another health-care provider or collaboration with one.
    3. Administering an anticonvulsant medication intravenous push requires the nurse to have an order or confer with another member of the health-care team.
    4. Glucocorticoid is a steroid that is not used to treat seizures.

    **TEST-TAKING HINT: The key word in the stem of this question is the adjective "collaborative." The test taker would eliminate the options "1" and "2" because these do not require collaboration with another member of the health-care team and would eliminate "4" because it is not used to treat seizures.**

45. 1. Keeping a seizure and medication chart will be helpful when keeping follow-up appointments with the health-care provider and in identifying activities that may trigger a seizure.
    2. The client should take showers, rather than tub baths, to avoid drowning if a seizure occurs. The nurse should also instruct the client never to swim alone.
    3. Over-the-counter medications may contain ingredients that will interact with anti-seizure medications or, in some cases, as with use of stimulants, possibly cause a seizure.
    4. Most of the anticonvulsant medications have therapeutic serum levels that should be maintained, and regular checks of the serum levels help to ensure the correct level.
    5. A newly diagnosed client would have just been put on medication, which may cause drowsiness. Therefore, the client should avoid activities that require alertness and coordination and should not be driving at all until after the effects of the medication have been evaluated.

**TEST-TAKING HINT:** The test taker must select all interventions that are appropriate for the question. A key word is the adjective "newly."

46. 1. The client with a seizure disorder should avoid stimulants, such as caffeine.
2. The onset of menstruation can cause seizure activity in the female client.
3. Tension states, such as anxiety and frustration, induce seizures in some clients so stress management may be helpful in preventing seizures.
4. Bright flickering lights, television viewing, and some other photic (light) stimulation may cause seizures, but sunlight does not. Wearing dark glasses or covering one eye during potential seizure-stimulating activities may help prevent seizure.

**TEST-TAKING HINT:** Caffeine is a stimulant and its use is not recommended in many disease processes. Menstrual cycle changes are known to affect seizure disorders. Therefore, options "1" and "2" can be eliminated, as can "4" because sunlight does not cause seizures.

47. 1. An aura is a visual, auditory, or olfactory occurrence that takes place prior to a seizure and warns the client a seizure is about to occur. The aura often allows time for the client to lie down on the floor or find a safe place to have the seizure.
2. An aura is not dependent on the client being physically or psychologically exhausted.
3. This is a therapeutic response, reflecting feelings, which is not an appropriate response when answering a client's question.
4. Sleepiness after a seizure is very common, but the aura does not itself cause the sleepiness.

**TEST-TAKING HINT:** If the stem of the question has the client asking a question, then the nurse needs to give factual information, and "3," a therapeutic response, would not be appropriate. Neither would "2" or "4" because the options are worded in such a way as to imply incorrect information.

48. 1. Alzheimer's disease does not lead to seizures.
2. Parkinson's disease does not cause seizures.
3. A CVA (stroke) is the leading cause of seizures in the elderly; increased intracranial pressure associated with the stroke can lead to seizures.
4. Brain atrophy is not associated with seizures.

**TEST-TAKING HINT:** All four answer possibilities are associated with the brain, neurological system, and aging. However, choices "1," "2," and "4" usually occur over time, with the condition gradually getting worse, and thus can be eliminated as a cause of seizures, which are usually sudden.

## Brain Tumors

49. 1. Nervousness is not a symptom of a brain tumor, and brain tumors rarely metastasize outside of the cranium. Brain tumors kill by occupying space and increasing intracranial pressure, but although seizures are not uncommon with brain tumors, seizures are not part of the classic triad of symptoms.
2. The classic triad of symptoms suggesting a brain tumor includes a headache that is dull, unrelenting, and worse in the morning; vomiting unrelated to food intake; and edema of the optic nerve (papilledema), which occurs in 70%–75% of clients diagnosed with brain tumors. Papilledema causes visual disturbances such as decreased visual acuity and diplopia.
3. Hypertension and bradycardia, not hypotension and tachycardia, occur with increased intracranial pressure resulting from pressure on the cerebrum. Tachypnea does not occur with brain tumors.
4. Abrupt loss of motor function occurs with a stroke; diarrhea does not occur with a brain tumor, and the client with a brain tumor does not experience a change in taste.

**TEST-TAKING HINT:** The test taker can rule out "4" because of the symptom of diarrhea, which is a gastrointestinal symptom, not a neurological one. Considering the other three possible choices, the symptom of "headache" would make sense for a client with a brain tumor.

50. 1. A widening pulse pressure and bounding pulse indicate increased intracranial pressure but do not localize the tumor.
2. Diplopia and decreased visual pressure are symptoms indicating papilledema, a general symptom in the majority of all brain tumors.
3. Bradykinesia is slowed movement, a symptom of Parkinson's disease, and scanning speech is symptomatic of multiple sclerosis.
4. Hemiparesis would localize a tumor to a motor area of the brain, and personality changes localize a tumor to the frontal lobe.

**TEST-TAKING HINT:** The test taker could arrive at the correct answer if the test taker realized that specific regions of the brain control motor function and hemiparesis and that other regions are involved in personality changes.

51. 1. This is providing information and is not completely factual. MRIs are loud, but frequently the client will require an IV (an invasive procedure) to be started for a contrast medium to be injected.
    2. This is restating and offering self. Both are therapeutic responses.
    3. This statement is belittling the client's feeling.
    4. This is not dealing with the client's concerns and is passing the buck. The nurse should explore the client's feeling to determine what is concerning the client. The MRI may or may not be the problem. The client may be afraid of the results of the MRI.

**TEST-TAKING HINT: When the question asks the test taker for a therapeutic response, the test taker should choose the response that directly addresses the client's feelings.**

52. 1. There is nothing in the stem that indicates the client has a problem with swallowing, so aspiration precautions are not needed.
    2. Reach to Recovery is an American Cancer Society–sponsored program for clients with breast cancer, but it is not prophylactic.
    3. The client diagnosed with metastatic lesions to the brain is at high risk for seizures.
    4. Teaching about mastectomy care is not prophylactic, and the stem did not indicate whether the client had a mastectomy.

**TEST-TAKING HINT: The test taker should not read into a question—for example, about mastectomy care. The test taker should be careful to read the descriptive words in the stem; in this case "prophylactic" is the key to answering the question correctly.**

53. 1. A social worker is qualified to assist the client with referrals to any agency or personnel that is needed.
    2. The chaplain should be referred if spiritual guidance is required, but the stem did not specify this need.
    3. The HCP also can refer to the social worker, but the nurse can make this referral independently.
    4. The occupational therapist assists with cognitive functioning, activities of daily living (ADL), and modification of the home, but the stem did not define these needs.

**TEST-TAKING HINT: The test taker must decide what each discipline has to offer the client; a social worker has the broadest range of referral capabilities.**

54. 1. Maintaining weight is a nutritional goal.
    2. Competing an advance directive is an end-of-life or psychosocial goal.
    3. Performing activities of daily living is a goal for self-care deficit.
    4. Verbalizing feelings is a psychosocial goal.

**TEST-TAKING HINT: The test taker should read the stem of the question carefully. All of the goals could be appropriate for a client diagnosed with a brain tumor, but only one applies to self-care deficit.**

55. 1. Purposeful movement following painful stimuli would indicate an improvement in the client's condition.
    2. Adducting the upper extremities while internally rotating the lower extremities is decorticate positioning and would indicate that the client's condition had not changed.
    3. Aimless thrashing would indicate an improvement in the client's condition.
    4. The most severe neurological impairment result is flaccidity and no response to stimuli. This indicates that the client's condition has worsened.

**TEST-TAKING HINT: Neurological assessment includes assessing the client for levels of consciousness; the nurse must memorize the stages of neurological progression toward a coma and death.**

56. 1. A transsphenoidal hypophysectomy is done by an incision above the gumline and through the sinuses to reach the sella turcica where the pituitary is located.
    2. The client will be given regular food when awake and able to tolerate food.
    3. Blowing the nose creates increased intracranial pressure and could result in a cerebrospinal fluid leak.
    4. The client will return from surgery with the head of the bed elevated to about 30 degrees; this allows for gravity to assist in draining the cerebrospinal fluid.

**TEST-TAKING HINT: The test taker must know the procedures for specific disease processes to answer this question, but anatomical positioning of the pituitary gland (just above the sinuses) could help to eliminate "1," which calls for a large turban dressing.**

57. 1. A headache after this surgery would be an expected occurrence, not a complication.
    2. An output much larger than the intake could indicate the development of diabetes insipidus. Pressure on the pituitary gland

can result in decreased production of vaso-pressin, the anti-diuretic hormone.

3. A raspy sore throat is common after surgery due to the placement of the endotracheal tube during anesthesia.

4. Dizziness on arising quickly is expected; the client should be taught to rise slowly and call for assistance for safety.

**TEST-TAKING HINT: The test taker could eliminate "1" and "3" as expected occurrences following the surgery and not complications. Option "4" can also be expected.**

58. 1. Making the client NPO (Nothing Per Os) will not help the client to swallow.

2. A low Fowler's position would make it easier for the client to aspirate.

3. The consistency of the food is not an issue; the client will have difficulty swallowing this food as well as regular-consistency food.

4. To decrease the risk of aspiration the client should direct food to the unaffected side of the throat; this helps the client to be able to use the side of the throat that is functioning.

**TEST-TAKING HINT: The test taker should try to visualize the position of the client in the bed. A mostly recumbent position (low Fowler's) would increase the chance of aspiration; thus "2" should be eliminated.**

59. 1. Chemotherapy is systemic therapy that is used extensively in the care of clients diagnosed with cancer. However, most drugs have difficulty in crossing the blood–brain barrier and are not useful in treating brain tumors unless delivered by direct placement into the spinal column or directly to the ventricles of the brain by a device called an Omaya reservoir.

2. The blood–brain barrier is the body's defense mechanism for protecting the brain from chemical effects; in this case, it prevents the chemotherapy from being able to work on the tumor in the brain.

3. Radiation has about the same amount of side effects as chemotherapy, but the effects of radiation tend to last for a much longer time.

4. Some tumors do become resistant to the chemotherapy agents used. When this happens the oncologist switches to different drugs.

**TEST-TAKING HINT: The test taker can eliminate "1" as a possible answer because it states that chemotherapy is used to treat brain tumors, but it does not tell the client why it is**

not being used. Choice "2" is the only one that actually informs the client of a medical reason for not administering chemotherapy for a brain problem.

60. 1. The client should sleep with the head of the bed elevated to promote drainage of the cerebrospinal fluid.

2. Humidified air will prevent drying of the nasal passages.

3. Because the incision for this surgery is just above the gumline, the client should not brush the front teeth. Oral care should be performed using a sponge until the incision has healed.

4. The client can eat a regular diet.

5. The HCP should be notified if the client develops an infection of any kind. A cold with sinus involvement and sneezing places the client at risk for opening the incision and developing a brain infection.

**TEST-TAKING HINT: The test taker could choose option "5" because this is a standard instruction for any surgery. The test taker should look for more than one correct answer in an alternative-type question.**

## Meningitis

61. 1. This is a definition of aseptic meningitis, which refers to irritated meninges from viral or noninfectious sources.

2. This is another example of aseptic meningitis, which refers to irritated meninges from viral or noninfectious sources.

3. Septic meningitis refers to meningitis caused by bacteria; the most common form of bacterial meningitis is caused by the *Neisseria meningitides* bacteria.

4. This is the explanation for encephalitis.

**TEST-TAKING HINT: The nurse should explain the client's diagnosis in laymen's terms when the stem is identifying the significant other as asking the question. Be sure to notice that the adjective "septic" is the key to answering this question, ruling out "1" and "2."**

62. 1. Clients who have been hospitalized are weakened, but they are not at risk for contracting any type of meningitis.

2. Outbreaks of infectious meningitis are most likely to occur in dense community groups such college campuses, jails, and military installations.

3. Third world countries do not pose a risk factor for meningitis. They provide a risk for hepatitis or tuberculosis.
4. Employees in a high-rise building do not live together and they have their own space; therefore they are not at risk for developing meningitis.

**TEST-TAKING HINT: The test taker must remember that the RN-NCLEX tests all areas of nursing so always notice the type of nurse if this is mentioned in the stem. A public health nurse would not be concerned with third world countries.**

63. 1. Babinski's sign is used to assess brain-stem activity, and paresthesia is tingling, which is not a clinical manifestation of bacterial meningitis.
2. Chvostek's sign is used to assess for hypocalcemia, and facial tingling is a sign of hypocalcemia. It is not used to assess for bacterial meningitis.
3. A positive Kernig's sign (client unable to extend leg when lying flat) and nuchal rigidity (stiff neck) are signs of bacterial meningitis, occurring because the meninges surrounding the brain and spinal column are irritated.
4. Trousseau's sign is used to assess for hypocalcemia, and nystagmus is abnormal eye movement. Neither of these is a clinical manifestation of bacterial meningitis.

**TEST-TAKING HINT: If two answer options test for the same thing (Trousseau's and Chvostek's signs), then the test taker can rule out these as possible answers because there cannot be two correct answers in the question, unless the question tells the test taker that it is a select-all-that-apply question.**

64. 1. In clients with meningococcal meningitis, purpuric lesions over the face and extremity are the signs of a fulminating infection that can lead to death within a few hours.
2. Photophobia is a common clinical manifestation of all types of meningitis and would be expected.
3. Inflammation of the meninges results in increased intracranial pressure, which causes a headache. This would be an expected occurrence and would not warrant notifying the HCP.
4. A client not being able to identify the day of the week would not in itself warrant notifying the HCP.

**TEST-TAKING HINT: The stem is asking the nurse to identify which assessment data are abnormal for the disease process and requires an immediate medical intervention to prevent**

the client from experiencing a complication or possible death.

65. 1. Standard precautions are mandated for all clients, but a client with septic meningitis will require more than the standard precautions.
2. Airborne precautions are for contagious organisms that are spread on air currents and require the hospital personnel to wear an ultra-high filtration mask; these precautions would be applied for disease such as tuberculosis.
3. Contact precautions are for contagious organisms that are spread by blood and body fluids such as those that occur with wounds or diarrhea.
4. Droplet precautions are respiratory precautions used for organisms that have a limited span of transmission. Precautions include staying at least four (4) feet way from the client or wearing a standard isolation mask and gloves when coming in close contact with the client. Clients are in isolation for 24 to 48 hours after initiation of antibiotics.

**TEST-TAKING HINT: The test taker must know the types of isolation precautions used for different diseases and note the adjective—septic—in the stem of the question.**

66. 1. This goal is not related to altered cerebral tissue perfusion, but it would be a goal for self-care deficit.
2. A client with a problem of altered cerebral tissue perfusion is at risk for seizure activity secondary to focal areas of cortical irritability; therefore, the client should be on seizure precautions.
3. This would be an appropriate goal for the client who has a problem of infection.
4. This would be an appropriate goal for the client who has a problem of dehydration.

**TEST-TAKING HINT: The goal must be related to the problem—in this case, "altered cerebral tissue perfusion."**

67. 1. A lumbar puncture is an invasive procedure; therefore an informed consent is required.
2. This could be offered for client comfort during the procedure.
3. This position increases the space between the vertebrae, which allows the HCP easier entry into the spinal column.
4. The client is encouraged to relax and breathe normally; hyperventilation may lower an elevated cerebrospinal fluid pressure.
5. The nurse should always explain to the client what is happening prior to and during a procedure.

**TEST-TAKING HINT: This is an alternative-type question, which requires the test taker to select more than one answer option.**

68. 1. A nurse administering antibiotics is a collaborative intervention because the HCP must write an order for the intervention; nurses cannot prescribe medications unless they have additional education and licensure and are NPs with prescriptive authority.
    2. The nurse needs an order to send a culture to the laboratory for payment purposes, but the nurse can obtain a specimen without an order. A sputum specimen is not appropriate for meningitis.
    3. A pulse oximeter measures the amount of oxygen in the periphery and does not require an HCP to order.
    4. Intake and output are independent nursing interventions and do not require an HCP's order.

**TEST-TAKING HINT: The test taker must note adjectives and understand that a collaborative nursing intervention is dependent on another member of the health-care team; an independent nursing intervention does not require collaboration.**

69. 1. This vaccine must be administered prior to exposure to build up an immunity to prevent meningitis resulting from *Haemophilus influenzae*.
    2. Chemoprophylaxis includes administering medication that will prevent infection or eradicate the bacteria and the development of symptoms in people who have been in close proximity to the client. Medications include rifampin (Rifadin), ciprofloxacin (Cipro), and ceftriaxone (Rocephin).
    3. Steroids are used as an adjunct therapy in treatment of clients diagnosed with acute bacterial meningitis. They would not be given as a prophylactic measure to others in the home.
    4. Gamma globulin provides passive immunity to clients who have been exposed to hepatitis. It is not appropriate in this situation.

**TEST-TAKING HINT: The key word in the stem is "preventive." The test taker must pay close attention to the adjectives.**

70. 1. Antibiotics would help decrease the bacterial infection in meningitis, which would cause the exudate. The drugs mentioned in the question would not.
    2. Fever increases cerebral metabolism and intracranial pressure. Therefore, measures are taken to reduce body temperature as soon as possible, and alternating Tylenol and Motrin would be appropriate.
    3. A nonnarcotic anti-pyretic (Tylenol) and an NSAID (Motrin) will not address the client's memory or orientation.
    4. These medications do not prevent or treat a yeast infection.

**TEST-TAKING HINT: The test taker must have a basic knowledge of the disease process and medications that are prescribed to treat a disease. Purulent drainage would require an antibiotic. Therefore, "1" should be eliminated as a possible answer because the question is asking about NSAIDs and a nonnarcotic anti-pyretic (Tylenol).**

71. 1. The antibiotic has the highest priority because failure to treat a bacterial infection can result in shock, systemic sepsis, and death.
    2. The lunch tray is important and may actually arrive prior to the antibiotic, but the priority for the nurse must be the medication.
    3. The client's room should be kept dark because of photophobia, but photophobia is a symptom that is not life threatening.
    4. Knowledge of the client's weight is necessary, but initial antibiotic therapy can be initiated without knowing the client's admission weight.

**TEST-TAKING HINT: The nurse must know how to prioritize care. Which intervention has the potential to avoid a complication related to the disease process? Remember the word priority.**

72. 1. The client's lung sounds should be clear with meningitis, and nothing in the question stem indicates a co-morbid condition. Therefore, assessing lung sounds is not a priority.
    2. The client may experience photophobia and visual disturbances, but assessing the six fields of gaze will not affect the client's condition.
    3. The client's cardiac status is not affected by meningitis. Therefore, the apical pulse would not be priority.
    4. Meningitis directly affects the client's brain. Therefore, assessing the neurological status would have priority for this client.

**TEST-TAKING HINT: The test taker should apply a systemic approach to discerning the priority response. Maslow's Hierarchy of Needs would put "1" as correct, but the disease process of meningitis does not include signs or symptoms of a respiratory component. The next highest priority would be the neurological component, and meningitis definitely is a neurological disease.**

# Parkinson's Disease

**73.** 1. Masklike facies is responsible for lack of expression and is part of motor manifestations of Parkinson's disease but is not related to the symptoms listed. Shuffling is also a motor deficit and does pose a risk for falling, but fever and patchy infiltrates on a chest x-ray do not result from a gait problem. They are manifestations of a pulmonary complication.
2. Difficulty swallowing places the client at risk for aspiration. Immobility predisposes the client to pneumonia. Both clinical manifestations place the client at risk for pulmonary complications.
3. Pill rolling of fingers and flat affect do not have an impact on the development of pulmonary complications.
4. Arm swing and bradykinesia are motor deficits.

**TEST-TAKING HINT: The nurse must recognize the clinical manifestations of a disease and the resulting bodily compromise. In this situation, fever and patchy infiltrates on a chest x-ray indicate a pulmonary complication. Options "1," "3," and "4" focus on motor problems and could be ruled out as too similar. Only "2" includes dissimilar information.**

**74.** 1. Carbidopa is never given alone. Carbidopa is given together with levodopa to help the levodopa cross the blood–brain barrier.
2. Levodopa is a form of dopamine given orally to clients diagnosed with PD.
3. Carbidopa enhances the effects of levodopa by inhibiting decarboxylase in the periphery, thereby making more levodopa available to the central nervous system. Sinemet is the most effective treatment for PD.
4. Carbidopa does not cross the blood–brain barrier.

**TEST-TAKING HINT: The nurse must be knowledgeable of the rationale for administering a medication for a specific disease.**

**75.** 1. Adaptive appliances will not help the client's shaking movements and are not used for clients with Parkinson's disease.
2. Clients with Parkinson's disease are placed on high-calorie, high-protein, soft or liquid diets. Supplemental feedings may also be ordered. If liquids are ordered because of difficulty chewing, then the liquids should be thickened to a honey or pudding consistency.
3. Nuts and whole-grain food would require extensive chewing before swallowing and would not be good for the client. Three large

meals would get cold before the client can consume the meal and one half or more of the food would be wasted.
4. The client's energy levels will not sustain eating for long periods. Offering frequent and easy-to-chew (soft) meals of small proportions is the preferred dietary plan.

**TEST-TAKING HINT: The correct answer for a nursing problem question must address the actual problem.**

**76.** 1. The nurse should not delegate feeding a client that is at risk for complications during feeding. This requires judgment that the assistant is not expected to possess.
2. Unlicensed assistants can turn and position clients with pressure ulcers. The nurse should assist in this at least once during the shift to assess the wound area.
3. The assistant can assist the client to the bathroom every two (2) hours and document the results of the attempt.
4. The assistant can obtain the vital signs on a stable client.

**TEST-TAKING HINT: When reading the answer options in a question in which the nurse is delegating to an unlicensed person, read the stem carefully. Is the question asking what to delegate or what not to delegate? Anything requiring professional judgment should not be delegated.**

**77.** 1. Headache and photophobia are expected clinical manifestations of meningitis. The new graduate could care for this client.
2. This client has had an unusual occurrence (fall) and now has a potential complication (a fracture). The experienced nurse should take care of this client.
3. These vital signs indicate increased intracranial pressure. The more experienced nurse should care for this client.
4. This could indicate a worsening of the tumor. This client is at risk for seizures and herniation of the brain stem. The more experienced nurse should care for this client.

**TEST-TAKING HINT: The test taker should determine if the clinical manifestations are expected as part of the disease process. If they are, a new graduate can care for the client; if they are not expected occurrences, a more experienced nurse should care for the client.**

**78.** 1. Akinesia is lack of movement. The goal in treating PD is to maintain mobility.
2. This could be a goal for a problem of noncom-

pliance with treatment regimen, but not a goal for treating the disease process.

3. This might be a goal for a psychosocial problem of social isolation.

4. **The major goal of treating PD is to maintain the ability to function. Clients diagnosed with PD experience slow, jerky movements and have difficulty performing routine daily tasks.**

**TEST-TAKING HINT: The test taker should match the goal to the problem. A "therapeutic goal" is the key to answering this question.**

79. 1. A stereotactic pallidotomy and/or thalamotomy are surgeries that use CT or MRI scans to localize areas of the brain through electrical stimulation or thermocoagulation of brain cells. These procedures are done when medication has failed to control tremors.

2. Dopamine-receptor agonists are medications that activate the dopamine receptors in the striatum of the brain.

3. Physical therapy is a standard therapy used to improve the quality of life for clients diagnosed with PD.

4. **Fetal tissue transplantation has shown some success in PD, but it is an experimental and highly controversial procedure.**

**TEST-TAKING HINT: The test taker should not overlook the adjective "experimental." This would eliminate at least "3," physical therapy, and "2," which refers to standard dopamine treatment, even if the test taker was not familiar with all of the procedures.**

80. 1. The emotions of a person diagnosed with PD are labile. The client has rapid mood swings and is easily upset.

2. Hallucinations are a sign that the client is experiencing drug toxicity.

3. **Scheduling appointments late in the morning gives the client a chance to complete ADLs without pressure and allows the medications time to give the best benefits.**

4. The client should take the prescribed medications at the same time each day to provide a continuous drug level.

**TEST-TAKING HINT: The test taker could eliminate "2" because hallucinations are never an expected part of legal medication administration.**

81. 1. Crackles and jugular vein distention indicate heart failure, not PD.

2. Upper-extremity weakness and ptosis are clinical manifestations of myasthenia gravis.

3. The client has very little arm swing, and scanning speech is a clinical manifestation of multiple sclerosis.

4. **Masklike facies and a shuffling gait are two clinical manifestations of PD.**

**TEST-TAKING HINT: Option "3" refers to arm swing and speech, both of which are affected by PD. The test taker needs to decide if the adjectives used to describe these activities— "exaggerated" and "scanning"—are appropriate. They are not, but masklike facies and shuffling gait are.**

82. 1. Emotional lability is a psychosocial problem, not a cognitive one.

2. Depression is a psychosocial problem.

3. **Memory deficits are cognitive impairments. The client may also develop a dementia.**

4. Paranoia is a psychosocial problem.

**TEST-TAKING HINT: The test taker must know the definitions of common medical terms. Cognitive refers to mental capacity to function.**

83. 1. This is information that should be discussed when filling out an advance directive form. A ventilator is used to treat a physiological problem.

2. **These are psychosocial manifestations of PD. These should be discussed in the support meeting.**

3. The reduction in the unintentional pill rolling movement of the hands is controlled at times by the medication; this is a physiological problem.

4. Echolalia is a speech deficit in which the client automatically repeats the words or sentences of another person; this is a physiological problem.

**TEST-TAKING HINT: Psychosocial problems should address the client's feelings or interactions with another person.**

84. 1. A headache of 2 on a 1–10 scale is a mild headache.

2. A spinal cord injury at T-10 involves deficits at approximately the waist area. Inability to move the toes would be expected.

3. **Body image is a concern for clients diagnosed with PD. This client is the one client that is not experiencing expected sequelae of the disease.**

4. This client is getting better; resolving indicates an improvement in the client's clinical manifestations.

**TEST-TAKING HINT: At times a psychological problem can have priority. All the physical**

problems are expected and are not life threatening or altering.

## Substance Abuse

85. 1. This should be done so that appropriate care can be provided, but it is not priority action.
    2. This should be done before the client ceases breathing and a cardiac arrest follows, but it is not the first action.
    3. This would be a good step to take to prepare for the worst-case scenario, but it can be done last among these answer options.
    4. Applying oxygen would be the priority action for this client. The client's breathing is slow and shallow. The greater amount of inhaled oxygen, the better the client's prognosis.

    **TEST-TAKING HINT: When the test taker is deciding on a priority, some guidelines should be used. Maslow's Hierarchy of Needs places oxygen at the top of the priority list. In cardiopulmonary resuscitation, airway and breathing are first.**

86. 1. No employee of a facility is above certain rules. In a company with a "No Drugs" policy, this includes the CEO. This client is exhibiting symptoms of cocaine abuse.
    2. The nurse does not have a definitive knowledge that the client is using drugs until a positive drug screen result is obtained. If the nurse is not a trained substance abuse counselor, this intervention would be out of the realm of the nurse's expertise.
    3. The client is the CEO of the facility; only the board of directors or parent company is above this client in supervisory rank.
    4. Giving an antihistamine is prescribing without a license, and the nurse is obligated to intervene in this situation.

    **TEST-TAKING HINT: The title of the client—CEO—eliminates "3." The nurse has noted a potential illegal situation.**

87. 1. The Health Insurance Portability and Accountability Act (HIPAA) requires that a health-care professional not divulge information about one person to an unauthorized person.
    2. This would be discussing Client B and a violation of HIPAA.
    3. The nurse does not know Client B is using drugs so notifying the HCP is not appropriate.
    4. Client B would require an explanation for coming to the clinic, for which, if the nurse

has not violated HIPAA, there is no explanation.

**TEST-TAKING HINT: Nurses are required to practice within the laws of the state and within federal laws. HIPAA is a federal law and applies to all health-care professionals in the United States. Legally the nurse cannot use the information provided by Client A, but morally the nurse might try to identify behavior in Client B that would warrant the nurse's intervention.**

88. 1. These reactions are called "flashbacks."
    2. Flashback reactions occur after the use of hallucinogens in which the client relives a bad episode that occurred while using the drug.
    3. The drug is gone from the body, but the mind-altering effects can occur at any time in the form of memory flashbacks.
    4. The client stated that the dreams are causing her distress. She is asking for help with the dreams, not planning her suicide.

    **TEST-TAKING HINT: The client is 20 years old and took the drug in her teens; drugs do not stay in the body for very long periods. This eliminates "3."**

89. 1. The nurse is not the client's supervisor, and confronting the co-worker about the suspicions could lead to problems if the nurse is not trained to deal with substance abusers.
    2. This is circumventing the problem. The co-worker will find another source of drugs if needed, and it is finding the co-worker guilty without due process.
    3. The co-worker's supervisor or peer review committee should be aware of the nurse's suspicions so that the suspicions can be investigated. This is a client safety and care concern.
    4. The nurse is obligated to report suspicious behavior to protect the clients the co-worker is caring for.

    **TEST-TAKING HINT: The test taker can eliminate "4" on the basis of "do nothing." In this instance, direct confrontation is not recommended, but the nurse must do something—namely, report the suspicions to the supervisor or peer review.**

90. 1. Insomnia and anxiety are symptoms of alcohol withdrawal, not Wernicke-Korsakoff syndrome.
    2. Visual and auditory hallucinations are symptoms of delirium tremens.
    3. Extreme tremors and agitation are symptoms of delirium tremens.

4. Ataxia or lack of coordination and confabulation, making up elaborate stories to explain lapses in memory, are both symptoms of Wernicke-Korsakoff syndrome.

**TEST-TAKING HINT: The test taker can eliminate "2" and "3" if the test taker knows the symptoms of delirium tremens.**

91. 1. Thiamine is given in high doses to decrease the rebound effect on the nervous system as it adjusts to the absence of alcohol, and a benzodiazepine is given in high doses and titrated down over several days for the tranquilizing effect to prevent delirium tremens.
2. The client may have seizures, but valium would control this. The client does not need a long-term anticonvulsant medication (Dilantin), and it is not known that the client needs an iron preparation (Feosol). The vitamin deficiency associated with delirium tremens is lack of thiamine, not iron.
3. Methadone is used for withdrawing clients from heroin, and Depakote can be used as a mood stabilizer in bipolar disorder or as an anticonvulsant.
4. The client does not need a diuretic, and a stimulant would produce an effect opposite to what is desired.

**TEST-TAKING HINT: Option "3" could be eliminated if the test taker knew the treatment for heroin withdrawal, and "4" could be reasoned out because a stimulant would produce an undesired effect.**

92. 1. Chills, sweats, and gooseflesh occur with heroin withdrawal, but seizures do not usually occur, so seizure precautions are not necessary.
2. Vital signs should be taken more frequently, every two (2) to four (4) hours, depending on the client's condition.
3. The client should be in an atmosphere where there is little stimulation. The client will be irritable and fearful.
4. Heroin is administered intravenously. Heroin addicts are at high risk for HIV as a result of shared needles and thus should be tested for HIV.
5. The client is withdrawing from heroin so providing needles is inappropriate. Providing sterile needles to IV drug users is controversial, but it attempts to decrease the incidence of HIV among drug users.

**TEST-TAKING HINT: A select-all-that-apply question will usually have more than one correct answer. One option cannot eliminate another.**

93. 1. This is a therapeutic response. The spouse is not expressing feelings but is stating a fact. The nurse should address the problem.
2. This is a therapeutic response. The spouse is not expressing feelings but is stating a fact. The nurse should address the problem.
3. The spouse is not required to give an explanation to the nurse.
4. The spouse's behavior is enabling the client to continue to drink until he cannot function.

**TEST-TAKING HINT: The stem of the question did not ask for a therapeutic response but did ask for the nurse's best response. The best response is to address the problem.**

94. 1. Telemetry and vital signs would be done to monitor cardiovascular compromise. Amphetamine use causes tachycardia, vasoconstriction, hypertension, and arrhythmias.
2. This might be an intervention for a problem of altered coping.
3. This would be an intervention for a problem of insomnia.
4. These are interventions for heart failure.

**TEST-TAKING HINT: The correct answer must address the problem of cardiovascular compromise, which eliminates "2" and "3."**

95. 1. This is unrealistic. Most restaurants serve some form of alcoholic beverage. It is good advice for the client to try to avoid situations that provide the temptation to use drugs or alcohol again.
2. The client will require a follow-up program such as 12-step meetings if the client is not to relapse.
3. The nurse does not know that this is true.
4. The client should discuss the history with the people the client chooses.

**TEST-TAKING HINT: The test taker must notice descriptive words such as "all" or "do not go anywhere." These words or phrases are absolutes that should cause the test taker to eliminate them.**

96. 1. The child will realize the changed behaviors when and if they happen.
2. This could cause problems between the parent and child.
3. Most coping behaviors are learned from parents and guardians. Children of substance abusers tend to cope with life situations by becoming substance abusers unless taught healthy coping mechanisms.
4. Children can be a part of the parent's recovery, but this is not the rationale for teaching new coping mechanisms.

Neurological

**TEST-TAKING HINT: Most parents do not like to be corrected by their child; this could eliminate " 2. " The correct answer must address a reason for teaching new coping strategies.**

## Amyotrophic Lateral Sclerosis (Lou Gehrig's Disease)

97. 1. EMG is done to differentiate a neuropathy from a myopathy, but it does not confirm ALS.
   2. **Biopsy confirms changes consistent with atrophy and loss of muscle fiber, both characteristic of ALS.**
   3. CK may or may not be elevated in ALS so it cannot confirm the diagnosis of ALS.
   4. This is done as ALS progresses to determine respiratory involvement, but it does not confirm ALS.

   **TEST-TAKING HINT: The test taker must be clear as to what the question is asking. The word "confirm" is the key to answering this question correctly. The test taker would need to know that this disease affects the muscle tissue to correctly identify the answer.**

98. 1. **Disuse syndrome is associated with complications of bed rest. Clients with ALS cannot move and reposition themselves, and they frequently have altered nutritional and hydration status.**
   2. The client does not usually have a change in body image.
   3. ALS is a disease affecting the muscles, not the kidneys or circulatory system.
   4. ALS is not painful.

   **TEST-TAKING HINT: The test taker would have to be knowledgeable about ALS to answer this question. This disease is chronic and debilitating over time and leads to wasting of the muscles.**

99. 1. These signs and symptoms occur during the course of ALS, but they are not early symptoms.
   2. These signs and symptoms will occur as the disease progresses.
   3. These are late signs/symptoms of ALS.
   4. **ALS results from the degeneration and demyelination of motor neurons in the spinal cord, which results in paralysis and weakness of the muscles.**

   **TEST-TAKING HINT: This is an application question in which the test taker must know that ruling out of ALS would result in the answer being early signs/symptoms. The test taker**

could rule out "1" because of atrophy, which is a long-term occurrence; rule out "2" because these symptoms will occur as the disease progresses; and rule out "3" because these are late signs/symptoms.

100. 1. This is a therapeutic response, but the client is asking for specific information.
   2. **About 50% of clients die within two (2) to five (5) years from respiratory failure, aspiration pneumonia, or another infectious process.**
   3. The nurse should allow the client to talk freely about the disease process and should provide educational and emotional support.
   4. This is incorrect information; ALS is a disease that results in death within five (5) years in most cases.

   **TEST-TAKING HINT: When the client is asking for factual information, the nurse should provide accurate and truthful information. This helps foster a trusting client–nurse relationship. Therapeutic response "1" should be used when the client needs to ventilate feelings and is not asking specific questions about the disease process.**

101. 1. Elevating the head of the bed will enhance lung expansion, but it is not the first intervention.
   2. **Oxygen should be given immediately to help alleviate the difficulty breathing. Remember that oxygenation is priority.**
   3. Assessment is the first part of the nursing process and is priority, but assessment will not help the client breathe easier.
   4. This is an appropriate intervention, but obtaining the pulse oximeter reading will not alleviate the client's respiratory distress.

   **TEST-TAKING HINT: The test taker should not automatically select assessment. Make sure that there is not another intervention that will directly help the client, especially if the client is experiencing a life-threatening complication.**

102. 200 mL/hr. This is a basic math question. The IV pump is calculated in mL/hr, so the nurse must double the rate to infuse the IV in 30 minutes.

   **TEST-TAKING HINT: This is a basic calculation that the nurse should be able to make even without a calculator.**

103. 1. Refusing to turn needs to be addressed by the nurse, but it is not priority over a life-threatening condition.

2. Nausea needs to be assessed by the nurse, but it is not priority over an oxygenation problem.

3. **A pulse oximeter reading of less than 93% indicates that the client is experiencing hypoxemia, which is a life-threatening emergency. This client should be assessed first.**

4. The nurse must address the client's complaints, but it is not a priority over a physiological problem.

**TEST-TAKING HINT: The test taker should apply Maslow's Hierarchy of Needs, which is oxygenation. The nurse must know normal parameters for diagnostic tools and laboratory data.**

104. 1. With assistance, the client may be able to stay at home. Therefore, placement in a long-term care facility should not be discussed until the family can no longer care for the client in the home.

2. There is no indication that a client with ALS will need a sigmoid colostomy.

3. **A client with ALS usually dies within five (5) years. Therefore, the nurse should offer the client the opportunity to determine how he wants to die.**

4. ALS affects both upper and lower extremities and leads to a debilitating state, so the client will not be able to transfer into and operate a wheelchair.

**TEST-TAKING HINT: The nurse should always help the client prepare for death in disease processes that are terminal and should discuss advance directives, which include both durable power of attorney for health care and a living will.**

105. 1. **Contractures can develop within a week because extensor muscles are weaker than flexor muscles. If the client cannot perform ROM exercises, then the nurse must do it for him—passive ROM.**

2. The client should maintain a positive nitrogen balance to promote optimal body functioning.

3. Adequate protein is required to maintain osmotic pressure and prevent edema.

4. The client is usually on bed rest in the last stages and should be turned and told to cough and deep breathe more often than every shift.

**TEST-TAKING HINT: Terminal stage is the key word in the stem that should cause the test taker to look for an option addressing immobility issues—option "1." An intervention**

implemented only once in every shift should be eliminated as a possible answer when addressing immobility issues.

106. 1. The child is not sure if he may get ALS so this is not an appropriate response.

2. This is incorrect information.

3. **There is a genetic factor with ALS that is linked to a chromosome 21 defect.**

4. ALS is not caused by a virus. The exact etiology is unknown, but studies indicate that some environmental factors may lead to ALS.

**TEST-TAKING HINT: This question requires knowledge of ALS. There are some questions for which Test-Taking Hints are not available.**

107. 1. **A residual (aspirated gastric contents) of greater than 50 mL to 100 mL indicates that the tube feeding is not being digested and that the feeding should be held.**

2. A soft abdomen is normal; a distended abdomen would be cause to hold the feeding.

3. Diarrhea is a common complication of tube feedings, but it is not a reason to hold the feeding.

4. The potassium level is low and needs intervention, but this would not indicate a need to hold the bolus tube feeding.

**TEST-TAKING HINT: Knowing normal assessment data would lead the test taker to eliminate "2" as a possible correct answer. Diarrhea and hypokalemia would not cause the client to not receive a feeding. Even if the test taker did not know what "residual" means, this would be the best option.**

108. 1. The medication should be given without food at the same time each day.

2. This medication is not affected by green leafy vegetables. (The anticoagulant warfarin [Coumadin] is a well-known medication that is affected by eating green, leafy vegetables.)

3. This medication is not affected by the sun.

4. **The medication can cause blood dyscrasias. Therefore, the client is monitored for liver function, blood count, blood chemistries, and alkaline phosphatase. The client should report any febrile illness. It is the first medication developed to treat ALS.**

**TEST-TAKING HINT: Blood dyscrasias occur with many medications, and this might prompt the test taker to select the correct option. Otherwise, the test taker must be knowledgeable of medication administration.**

## Encephalitis

109. 1. A complication of immunizations for measles, mumps, and rubella can be encephalitis.
    2. Upper respiratory tract illnesses can be a precursor to encephalitis.
    3. The herpes simplex virus, specifically type I, can lead to encephalitis.
    4. Fungal encephalitis is known to occur in certain regions and the nurse should assess for recent trips to areas where these fungal spores exist, but the common areas are the southwest United States and central California.
    5. Exposure to spores does not lead to encephalitis.

    **TEXT-TAKING HINT:** Encephalitis is inflammation of the brain caused by either a hypersensitivity reaction or post-infectious state in which a virus reproduces in the brain. Encephalitis can be a life-threatening disease process. History is vital in the diagnosis.

110. 1. Bilateral facial palsies are a common initial sign and symptom of encephalitis.
    2. Fever is usually one of the first signs and symptoms the client experiences.
    3. A decrease in the client's headache does not indicate that the client's condition is becoming worse and thus does not warrant immediate intervention.
    4. The absence of smell and taste indicates that the cranial nerves may be involved. The client's condition is becoming more serious.

    **TEST-TAKING HINT:** This question requires the test taker to select an option that indicates the disease is progressing and the client is at risk. Option "3" indicates that the client is improving, and options "1" and "2" are common early manifestations of the disease. The only option that reflects cranial nerve involvement, a sign that the client's condition is becoming worse and requires immediate intervention, is "4."

111. 1. A written consent is given for all invasive procedures, but this would reflect care before the lumbar puncture, not after.
    2. This is information that would be shared with the client about the reason the procedure would be done, but not care after.
    3. The nurse should share this information to prevent the severe, throbbing, "spinal headache" caused by the decrease in cerebrospinal fluid.

4. The client should lie with the head of the bed flat for four (4) to eight (8) hours after the lumbar puncture, but this position would not prevent all hematomas.

**TEST-TAKING HINT:** When the test taker is trying to eliminate options, any that have absolute words, such as "all," "never," and "always," are usually wrong and can be eliminated quickly. Rarely is any activity always or never done.

112. 1. Clients diagnosed with encephalitis have neurological deficits while the inflammation is present. The therapeutic plan is to treat the disease process, decrease the edema, and return the client to an optimal level of wellness.
    2. The client may have short-term memory loss from a previous condition.
    3. Renal function is not affected by encephalitis. Only immobility would affect this system.
    4. There is no reason to apply hydrocortisone cream for encephalitis.

    **TEST-TAKING HINT:** The test taker should look at the option that reflects the body system that is involved with the disease. Refer to medical terminology; encephalon means the "brain."

113. 1. Clients with encephalitis should be treated for the disease process and also to prevent complications of immobility. Turning the client will prevent skin breakdown.
    2. Increasing fluids helps prevent urinary tract infections and mobilize secretions in the lungs.
    3. The client would be maintained in a slightly elevated position, semi-Fowler's, for gravity to assist the body in decreasing intracranial pressure.
    4. Immobility causes clients to be at risk for deep vein thrombosis. Therefore, clients with encephalitis should be assessed for deep vein thrombosis.
    5. Immobility causes the gastrointestinal tract to slow, resulting in constipation. Clients can have difficulty emptying their bladders, which can cause retention and urinary tract infections and stones. Assessing these systems can identify problems early.

    **TEST-TAKING HINT:** Each option should be read carefully. If the test taker does not read each one carefully, the test taker could miss important words, such as "supine" in "3," resulting in an incorrect answer.

114. 1. This is an important area to assess for neurological deterioration, but it is not the first indication of increased intracranial pressure.
    2. **This is the most important assessment data. A change in level of consciousness is usually the first sign of neurological deterioration.**
    3. Seizures can occur with inflammation from encephalitis, but their occurrence does not indicate that the client has increased intracranial pressure resulting from a worsening condition.
    4. This is important information to assess, but changes in vital signs are not the first sign and symptom of increased intracranial pressure.

    **TEST-TAKING HINT: The word "first" asks the test taker to prioritize the interventions. Usually all the options are interventions that the nurse should do, but the question implies that the client may be deteriorating. Level of consciousness is the most sensitive indicator of neurological deficit.**

115. 1. **Mosquitoes breed in standing water, even pet dishes and birdbaths. All areas that collect water should be emptied, removed, covered, or turned over. Rain gutters should be cleaned.**
    2. Light-colored, long-sleeved, and loose-fitting clothing should be worn to avoid mosquito bites.
    3. Insect repellent may irritate the eyes, but it should be applied over clothing and on all exposed areas.
    4. Mosquitoes are more prevalent at dusk, dawn, and early evening.

    **TEST-TAKING HINT: Terms such as "only" ("3") should clue the test taker to eliminate that option. Rarely are these absolute terms correct.**

116. 1. An alteration in body temperature in a patient with West Nile virus would not be the highest priority.
    2. **Altered tissue perfusion would be the highest priority because it could be life threatening.**
    3. A problem of fluid volume excess would not apply for the client with West Nile virus. These clients are at risk for fluid volume deficit from nausea, vomiting, and hyperthermia.
    4. A problem with skin integrity could apply to the client with immobility caused by West Nile virus, but it would not be the highest priority problem.

    **TEST-TAKING HINT: When prioritizing client problems oxygenation is the highest priority problem according to Maslow, and tissue perfusion is oxygenation.**

117. 1. Clients with West Nile virus should be continuously assessed for alteration in gas exchanges or patterns.
    2. Nurses do not refer to dermatologists.
    3. Hypothermia is not treated with ice packs, but with warming blankets.
    4. Lymph glands are edematous early in the disease process. There is no reason to teach the client to report this condition.

    **TEST-TAKING HINT: The test taker needs to read words carefully. Prefixes such as "hypo" and "hyper" are important in determining if an option is correct. Even if the test taker did not know if the client is hypothermic or hyperthermic, "hypo" means "less than normal" so hypothermia would not be treated with ice packs. A client with West Nile virus usually has a fever that should be reduced. Thus, a treatment for hypothermia is not needed.**

118. 1. This intervention is independent, not collaborative.
    2. This is an independent nursing intervention.
    3. Assessment is an independent nursing intervention.
    4. **Administering an IV fluid is collaborative because it requires an order from a health-care provider. It does, however, require the nurse to assess the rate, fluid, and site for complications.**

    **TEST-TAKING HINT: When reading test questions, the test taker should pay attention to adjectives. In this question, the word "collaborative" makes all the options incorrect except "4." Collaborative interventions require an order from a health-care provider but the nurse uses judgment and intuition within the scope of practice.**

119. 1. These vital signs are within normal ranges. The temperature is slightly elevated and may require an anti-pyretic but not as an immediate need.
    2. This is a common complaint requiring medication but not immediately.
    3. This test is used to differentiate West Nile virus from encephalitis and would not require immediate intervention. Supportive care is given for West Nile virus. There is no definitive treatment.

4. These assessment data may indicate that the client's condition is deteriorating and requires immediate intervention to prevent complications.

**TEST-TAKING HINT:** **The word "immediate" means that the nurse must recognize and intervene before complications occur. The test taker should eliminate any option that contains normal assessment data.**

120. 1. Transmission does not occur through exposure with sneezed or coughed secretions.
2. The most common transmission of the West Nile Virus to humans is through the bite of the infected mosquito.
3. The West Nile virus can be transmitted through breast milk, blood products, and organ transplants. This is a vector-borne disease. It is transmitted to mosquitoes that bite infected birds. The incubation period is around 15 days.
4. Maculopapular rashes do not drain. Draining is a characteristic of a vesicle.

**TEST-TAKING HINT:** **The test taker should eliminate "2" because of the absolute word "only."**

1. The client is admitted with a diagnosis of trigeminal neuralgia. Which assessment data would the nurse expect to find in this client?
   1. Joint pain of the neck and jaw.
   2. Unconscious grinding of the teeth during sleep.
   3. Sudden severe unilateral facial pain.
   4. Progressive loss of calcium in the nasal septum.

2. The client recently has been diagnosed with trigeminal neuralgia. Which intervention is most important for the nurse to implement with the client?
   1. Assess the client's sense of smell and taste.
   2. Teach the client how to care for the eyes.
   3. Instruct the client to have regular carbamazepine (Tegretol) levels monitored.
   4. Assist the client to identify factors that trigger an attack.

3. The client comes to the clinic and reports a sudden drooping of the left side of the face and complains of pain in that area. The nurse notes that the client cannot wrinkle the forehead or close the left eye. Which condition should the nurse suspect?
   1. Bell's palsy.
   2. Right-sided stroke.
   3. Tetany.
   4. Mononeuropathy.

4. The client comes to the clinic for treatment of a dog bite. Which intervention should the clinic nurse implement first?
   1. Prepare the client for a series of rabies injections.
   2. Notify the local animal control shelter.
   3. Administer a tetanus toxoid in the deltoid.
   4. Determine if the animal has had its vaccinations.

5. The client has glossopharyngeal nerve (cranial nerve IX) paralysis secondary to a stroke. Which referral would be most appropriate for this client?
   1. Hospice nurse.
   2. Speech therapist.
   3. Physical therapist.
   4. Occupational therapist.

6. Which assessment data would make the nurse suspect that the client has amyotrophic lateral sclerosis?
   1. History of a cold or gastrointestinal upset in the last month.
   2. Complaints of double vision and drooping eyelids.
   3. Fatigue, progressive muscle weakness, and twitching.
   4. Loss of sensation below the level of the umbilicus.

7. The client is scheduled for an MRI of the brain to confirm a diagnosis of Creutzfeldt-Jakob disease. Which intervention should the nurse implement prior to the procedure?
   1. Determine if the client has claustrophobia.
   2. Obtain a signed informed consent form.
   3. Determine if the client is allergic to egg yolks.
   4. Start an intravenous line in both hands.

8. Which should be the nurse's first intervention with the client diagnosed with Bell's palsy?
   1. Explain that this disorder will resolve within a month.
   2. Tell the client to apply heat to the involved side of the face.
   3. Encourage the client to eat a soft diet.
   4. Tell the client to protect the affected eye from injury.

9. The client calls the clinic and asks the nurse, "What causes Creutzfeldt-Jakob disease?" Which statement would be the nurse's best response?
   1. "The person must have been exposed to an infected prion."
   2. "It is mad cow disease, and eating contaminated meat is the cause."
   3. "This disease is caused by a virus that is in stagnant water."
   4. "A fungal spore in the lungs infects the brain tissue."

10. The client is diagnosed with Creutzfeldt-Jakob disease. Which referral would be the most appropriate?
    1. Alzheimer's Association.
    2. Creutzfeldt-Jakob Disease Foundation.
    3. Hospice Care.
    4. A neurosurgeon.

11. The client is diagnosed with arboviral encephalitis. Which priority intervention should the nurse implement?
    1. Place the client in strict isolation.
    2. Administer IV antibiotics.
    3. Keep the client in the supine position.
    4. Institute seizure precautions.

12. The client is diagnosed with a brain abscess. Which sign/symptom is the most common?
    1. Projectile vomiting.
    2. Disoriented behavior.
    3. Headaches, worse in the morning.
    4. Petit mal seizure activity.

13. The client diagnosed with a brain abscess has become lethargic and difficult to arouse. Which intervention should the nurse implement first?
    1. Implement seizure precautions.
    2. Assess the client's neurological status.
    3. Close the drapes and darken the room.
    4. Prepare to administer an IV steroid.

14. The client is diagnosed with Huntington's chorea. Which interventions should the nurse implement with the family? Select all that apply.
    1. Refer to Huntington's Chorea Foundation.
    2. Explain the need for the client to wear football padding.
    3. Discuss how to cope with the client's messiness.
    4. Provide three (3) meals a day and no between-meal snacks.
    5. Teach the family how to perform chest percussion.

15. The nurse is discussing psychosocial implications of Huntington's chorea with the child of a client diagnosed with the disease. Which psychosocial intervention should the nurse implement?
    1. Refer the child for genetic counseling as soon as possible.
    2. Teach the child to use a warming tray under the food during meals.
    3. Discuss the importance of not abandoning the parent.
    4. Allow the child to talk about the fear of getting the disease.

16. The client is post-thrombolytic therapy for a stroke. The health-care provider has ordered heparin to be infused at 1000 units per hour. The solution comes 25,000 units of heparin in 500 mL of $D_5W$. At what rate will the nurse set the pump? _____

17. Which finding is considered to be one of the warning signs of developing Alzheimer's disease?
    1. Difficulty performing familiar tasks.
    2. Problems with orientation to date, time, and place.
    3. Having problems focusing on a task.
    4. Atherosclerotic changes in the vessels.

18. Which information should be shared with the client diagnosed with Stage 1 Alzheimer's disease who is prescribed donepezil (Aricept), a cholinesterase inhibitor?
    1. The client must continue taking this medication forever to maintain function.
    2. The drug may delay the progression of the disease, but it does not cure it.
    3. A serum drug level must be obtained monthly to evaluate for toxicity.
    4. If the client develops any muscle aches, the HCP should be notified.

19. The spouse of a recently retired man tells the nurse, "All my husband does is sit around and watch television all day long. He is so irritable and moody. I don't want to be around him." Which action should the nurse implement?
    1. Encourage the wife to leave the client alone.
    2. Tell the wife that he is probably developing Alzheimer's disease.
    3. Recommend that the client see an HCP for an antidepressant medication.
    4. Instruct the wife to buy him some arts and crafts supplies.

20. The nurse in a long-term care facility has noticed a change in the behavior of one of the clients. The client no longer participates in activities and prefers to stay in his room. Which intervention should the nurse implement first?
    1. Insist the client go to the dining room for meals.
    2. Notify the family of the change in behavior.
    3. Determine if the client wants another roommate.
    4. Complete a Geriatric Depression Scale.

21. A family member brings the client to the emergency department reporting that the 78-year-old father has suddenly become very confused and thinks he is living in 1942, that he has to go to war, and that someone is trying to poison him. Which question should the nurse ask the family member?
    1. "Has your father been diagnosed with dementia?"
    2. "What medication has your father taken today?"
    3. "What have you given him that makes him think it's poison?"
    4. "Does your father like to watch old movies on television?"

22. The student nurse asks the nurse, "Why do you ask the client to identify how many fingers you have up when the client hit the front of the head, not the back?" The nurse would base the response on which scientific rationale?
    1. This is part of the routine neurological exam.
    2. This is done to determine if the client has diplopia.
    3. This assesses the amount of brain damage.
    4. This is done to indicate if there is a rebound effect on the brain.

23. The ambulance brings the client with a head injury to the emergency department. The client responds to painful stimuli by muttering and pulling away from the nurse. How would the nurse rate this client on the Glasgow Coma Scale?
    1. 3
    2. 8
    3. 10
    4. 15

## Glasgow Coma Scale

| Eye Opening (E) | Verbal Response (V) | Motor Response (M) |
|---|---|---|
| 4 = Spontaneous | 5 = Normal conversation | 6 = Normal |
| 3 = To voice | 4 = Disoriented conversation | 5 = Localizes to pain |
| 2 = To pain | 3 = Words, but not coherent | 4 = Withdraws to pain |
| 1 = None | 2 = No words...only sounds | 3 = Decorticate posture |
| | 1 = None | 2 = Decerebrate |
| | | 1 = None |
| | | **Total** = **E**+**V**+**M** |

From Teasdale G, Jennett B. Assessment of coma and impaired consciousness. A practical scale. *Lancet* 1974;2:81–84. Reprinted with permission.

24. Which intervention has the highest priority for the client in the emergency department who has been in a motorcycle collision with an automobile and has a fractured left leg?
    1. Assessing the neurological status.
    2. Immobilizing the fractured leg.
    3. Monitoring the client's output.
    4. Starting an 18-gauge saline lock.

25. The nurse writes the nursing diagnosis "altered body temperature related to damaged temperature regulating mechanism" for a client with a head injury. Which would be the most appropriate goal?
    1. Administer acetaminophen (Tylenol) for elevated temperature.
    2. The client's temperature will remain less than 100°F.
    3. Maintain the hypothermia blanket at 99°F for 24 hours.
    4. The basal metabolic temperature will fluctuate no more than two (2) degrees.

26. Which potential pituitary complication should the nurse assess for in the client diagnosed with a traumatic brain injury (TBI)?
    1. Diabetes mellitus type 2 (DM 2).
    2. Seizure activity.
    3. Syndrome of inappropriate antidiuretic hormone (SIADH).
    4. Cushing's disease.

27. The nurse is discussing seizure prevention with a female client who was just diagnosed with epilepsy. Which statement indicates the client needs more teaching?
    1. "I will take calcium supplements daily and drink milk."
    2. "I will see my HCP to have my blood levels drawn regularly."
    3. "I should not drink any type of alcohol while taking the medication."
    4. "I am glad that my periods will not affect my epilepsy."

28. The unlicensed nursing assistant is caring for a client that is having a seizure. Which action by the assistant would warrant immediate intervention by the nurse?
    1. The assistant attempts to insert an oral airway.
    2. The assistant turns the client on the right side.
    3. The assistant has all the side rails padded and up.
    4. The assistant does not leave the client's bedside.

29. The nurse is preparing the male client for an electroencephalogram (EEG). Which intervention should the nurse implement?
    1. Explain that this procedure is not painful.
    2. Premedicate the client with a benzodiazepine drug.
    3. Instruct the client to shave all facial hair.
    4. Tell the client it will cause him to see floaters.

30. Which assessment data indicates that the client with a traumatic brain injury (TBI) exhibiting decorticate posturing on admission is responding effectively to treatment?
    1. The client has flaccid paralysis.
    2. The client has purposeful movement.
    3. The client has decerebrate posturing with painful stimuli.
    4. The client does not move extremities.

31. The intensive care nurse is caring for the client who has had intracranial surgery. Which interventions should the nurse implement? Select all that apply.
    1. Assess for deep vein thrombosis.
    2. Administer intravenous anticoagulant.
    3. Monitor intake and output strictly.
    4. Apply warm compresses to the eyes.
    5. Perform passive range of motion exercises.

32. Which client should the nurse assess first after receiving the shift report?
    1. The client diagnosed with a stroke who has right-sided paralysis.
    2. The client diagnosed with meningitis who complains of photosensitivity.
    3. The client with a brain tumor who has projectile vomiting.
    4. The client with epilepsy who complains of tender gums.

33. The client is reporting neck pain, fever, and a headache. The nurse elicits a positive Kernig's sign. Which diagnostic test procedure should the nurse anticipate the HCP ordering to confirm a diagnosis?
    1. A computed tomography (CT).
    2. Blood cultures times two (2).
    3. Electromyelogram (EMG).
    4. Lumbar puncture (LP).

34. Which behavior is a risk factor for developing and spreading bacterial meningitis?
    1. An upper-respiratory infection.
    2. Unprotected sexual intercourse.
    3. Chronic alcohol consumption.
    4. Use of tobacco products.

35. Which assessment data should the nurse expect to observe for the client diagnosed with Parkinson's disease?
    1. Ascending paralysis and pain.
    2. Masklike facies and pill rolling.
    3. Diplopia and ptosis.
    4. Dysphagia and dysarthria.

36. The client diagnosed with Parkinson's disease is prescribed carbidopa/levodopa (Sinemet). Which intervention should the nurse implement prior to administering the medication?
    1. Discuss how to prevent orthostatic hypotension.
    2. Take the client's apical pulse for one (1) full minute.
    3. Inform the client that this medication is for short-term use.
    4. Tell the client to take the medication on an empty stomach.

37. The client diagnosed with amyotrophic lateral sclerosis (Lou Gehrig's disease) is prescribed medications that require intravenous access. The HCP has ordered a primary intravenous line at a keep vein open (KVO) at 25 mL/hr. The drop factor is 10 gtts/mL. At what rate should the nurse set the IV tubing? _____

38. Which intervention should the nurse take with the client recently diagnosed with amyotrophic lateral sclerosis (Lou Gehrig's disease)?
    1. Discuss a percutaneous gastrostomy tube.
    2. Explain how a fistula is accessed.
    3. Provide an advance directive.
    4. Refer to a physical therapist for leg braces.

39. The public health nurse is discussing St. Louis encephalitis with a group in the community. Which instruction should the nurse provide to help prevent an outbreak?
    1. Yearly vaccinations for the disease.
    2. Advise that the city should spray for mosquitoes.
    3. The use of gloves when gardening.
    4. Not going out at night.

40. The husband of a client who is an alcoholic tells the nurse, "I don't know what to do. I don't know how to deal with my wife's problem." Which response would be most appropriate by the nurse?
    1. "It must be difficult. Maybe you should think about leaving."
    2. "I think you should attend Alcoholics Anonymous."
    3. "I think that Alanon might be very helpful for you."
    4. "You should not enable your wife's alcoholism."

41. The client is brought to the emergency department by the police for public disorderliness. The client reports feeling no pain and is unconcerned that the police have arrested him. The nurse notes the client has epistaxis and nasal congestion. Which substance should the nurse suspect the client has abused?
    1. Marijuana
    2. Heroin.
    3. Ecstasy.
    4. Cocaine.

42. The client with a history of migraine headaches comes to the clinic and reports that a migraine is coming because the client is experiencing bright spots before the eyes. Which phase of migraine headaches is the client experiencing?
    1. Prodrome phase.
    2. Aura phase.
    3. Headache phase.
    4. Recovery phase.

43. The client with a history of migraine headaches comes to the emergency department complaining of a migraine headache. Which collaborative treatment should the nurse anticipate?
    1. Administer an injection of sumatriptan (Imitrex), a triptan.
    2. Prepare for a computed tomography (CT) of the head.
    3. Place the client in a quiet room with the lights off.
    4. Administer propranolol (Inderal), a beta blocker.

44. Which assessment data would make the nurse suspect that the client with a C-7 spinal cord injury is experiencing autonomic dysreflexia?
    1. Abnormal diaphoresis.
    2. A severe throbbing headache.
    3. Sudden loss of motor function.
    4. Spastic skeletal muscle movement.

45. The nurse stops at the scene of a motor vehicle accident and provides emergency first aid at the scene. Which law protects the nurse as a first responder?
    1. The First Aid Law.
    2. Ombudsman Act.
    3. Good Samaritan Act.
    4. First Responder Law.

46. The nurse writes the problem "high risk for impaired skin integrity" for the client with L-5-6 spinal cord injury. Which intervention should the nurse include in the plan of care?
    1. Perform active range of motion exercise.
    2. Massage the legs and trochanters every shift.
    3. Arrange for a Roho cushion in the wheelchair.
    4. Apply petroleum-based lotion to extremities.

47. The nurse is preparing to administer acetaminophen (Tylenol) to a client diagnosed with a stroke who is complaining of a headache. Which intervention should the nurse implement first?
    1. Administer the medication in pudding.
    2. Check the client's armband.
    3. Crush the tablet and dissolve in juice.
    4. Have the client sip some water.

48. Which client would be most at risk for experiencing a stroke?
    1. A 92-year-old client who is an alcoholic.
    2. A 54-year-old client diagnosed with hepatitis.
    3. A 60-year-old client who has a Greenfield filter.
    4. A 68-year-old client with chronic atrial fibrillation.

49. The charge nurse is making client assignments for a neuro-medical floor. Which client should be assigned to the most experienced nurse?
    1. The elderly client who is experiencing a stroke in evolution.
    2. The client diagnosed with a transient ischemic attack 48 hours ago.
    3. The client diagnosed with Guillain-Barré syndrome who complains of leg pain.
    4. The client with Alzheimer's disease who is wandering in the halls.

50. The nurse is assessing a client who is experiencing anosmia on a neurological floor. Which area should the nurse assess for cranial nerve I that is pertinent to anosmia? Select all that apply.

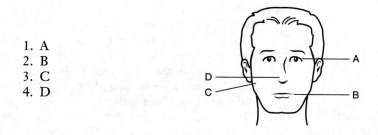

    1. A
    2. B
    3. C
    4. D

51. The nurse arrives at the scene of a motor vehicle accident and the car is leaking gasoline. The client is in the driver's seat of the car complaining of not being able to move the legs. Which actions should the nurse implement? List in order of priority.
    1. Move the client safely out of the car.
    2. Assess the client for other injuries.
    3. Stabilize the client's neck.
    4. Notify the emergency medical system.
    5. Place client in a functional anatomical position.

**1.** 1. Joint pain is usually associated with some type of arthritis.
2. Unconscious grinding of the teeth during sleep is usually associated with temporomandibular joint (TMJ) disorder.
3. Trigeminal neuralgia affects the 5th cranial nerve and is characterized by paroxysms of pain in the area innervated by the three branches of the nerve. The unilateral nature of the pain is an important diagnostic characteristic. The disorder is also known as tic douloureux.
4. The nasal structure is not made up of bone.

**2.** 1. The client's sense of smell and taste are not affected.
2. The cornea is at risk for abrasions because of the twitching, which causes irritation. Therefore, the nurse must teach the client how to care for the eye, but the most important intervention is to prevent the attacks.
3. Tegretol is the treatment of choice for trigeminal neuralgia, but it is not the most important intervention when the client is first diagnosed with this condition.
4. Stimulating specific areas of the face, called trigger zones, many initiate the onset of pain. Therefore, the nurse should help the client identify situations that exacerbate the condition, such as chewing gum, eating, brushing the teeth, or being exposed to a draft of cold air.

**3.** 1. Bell's palsy, called facial paralysis, is a disorder of the 7th cranial nerve (facial nerve) characterized by unilateral paralysis of facial muscles.
2. These are symptoms of a left-sided stroke
3. Tetany is due to low calcium levels. In this disorder, the face twitches when touched; this is known as a positive Chvostek's sign.
4. Mononeuropathy is limited to a singe peripheral nerve and its branches and occurs because the trunk of the nerve is compressed, such as in carpal tunnel syndrome.

**4.** 1. This may be needed if it is determined the dog has not had its shots or if the dog cannot be found, but it is not the first intervention.
2. This is an appropriate action if the client does not know who owns the dog so that the dog can be found and quarantined.
3. If the client has not had a tetanus booster in the last 10 years, one must be administered, but it is usually the last action taken before the client is discharged from the clinic.
4. This is priority because if the dog has had

its vaccinations, the client will not have to undergo a series of very painful injections. The nurse must obtain information about the dog, which is assessment of the situation.

**5.** 1. Clients are referred to hospice when there is a life expectancy of less than six (6) months. This client has difficulty swallowing, which is not life threatening.
2. Speech therapists address the needs of clients who have difficulty with the innervations and musculature of the face and neck.
3. The physical therapist assists the client to ambulate and transfer (e.g., from bed to chair) and with muscle strength training.
4. The occupational therapist focuses on cognitive disability and activities of daily living.

**6.** 1. A history of a cold or gastrointestinal upset in the last month would be assessment data that would make the nurse suspect Guillain-Barré syndrome.
2. Complaints of double vision and drooping eyelids would make the nurse suspect myasthenia gravis.
3. Fatigue, progressive muscle weakness, and twitching are signs of ALS, a progressive neurological disease in which there is a loss of motor neurons. There is no cure, but recently a medication to slow the deterioration of the motor neurons has been found.
4. Loss of sensation would make the nurse suspect some type of spinal cord injury.

**7.** 1. In an MRI, the client is placed in a very narrow tube. If the client is claustrophobic, he or she may need medication or an open MRI may need to be considered.
2. An MRI is not an invasive procedure; therefore, informed consent is not needed.
3. The nurse would need to determine allergies to shellfish or iodine, not to egg yolks.
4. The client will need one saline lock, not two intravenous lines. Often the MRI tech is the person who inserts the IV.

**8.** 1. This is correct information, but it is not priority when discussing Bell's palsy.
2. Heat will help promote comfort and increase blood flow to the muscles, but safety of the client's eye is priority.
3. The client may have difficulty chewing on the affected side so a soft diet should be encouraged, but it not priority teaching.
4. Telling the client to protect the eye is prio-

rity because the eye does not close completely and the blink reflex is diminished, making the eye vulnerable to injury. The client should wear an eye patch at night and wraparound sunglasses or goggles during the day; he or she may also need artificial tears.

9. 1. Would a layperson know what a prion is? This is using medical jargon, which is not the nurse's best response.
   2. **This is the cause of this disease and would be the best response.**
   3. A virus is not the cause of Creutzfeldt-Jakob disease.
   4. Fungal spores do not cause this disease.

10. 1. Creutzfeldt-Jakob disease is not Alzheimer's disease, although the presenting symptoms may mimic Alzheimer's.
    2. There is no foundation for Creutzfeldt-Jakob disease, but if there were, the significant other would be referred to this organization because the disease progresses so rapidly that the client would not get any benefit from the organization.
    3. **This disease is usually fatal within a year, and the symptoms progress rapidly to dementia.**
    4. The nurse does not refer the client to a neurosurgeon and the primary HCP would not refer to a neurosurgeon because there is no surgical or medical treatment for this disease.

11. 1. Arboviral encephalitis is a viral infection transmitted by mosquito bites, and isolation is not required.
    2. Antibiotics are prescribed for bacterial infections, not viral infections. There is no antiviral medication to treat this disease.
    3. Keeping the client supine would increase intracranial pressure, which is a concern when caring for clients with brain diseases.
    4. **Seizure precautions should be instituted because any inflammation of the brain tissue will put the client at risk for seizures.**

12. 1. Vomiting may occur, but it is not projectile and it is not the most common.
    2. Disoriented behavior may occur, but it is not the most common.
    3. **The most common and prevailing symptom of a brain abscess is a headache that is worse in the morning because of increased intracranial pressure as a result of lying flat (gravity).**
    4. The client with a brain abscess may have seizure activity, but it is usually tonic-clonic (grand mal) and it is not the most common.

13. 1. This is an appropriate intervention, but it is not the first.
    2. **Remember, assessment is the first step of the nursing process and should be implemented first whenever there is a change in the client's behavior.**
    3. This helps prevent stimulation that could initiate a seizure, but it is not the first intervention.
    4. Steroids may be administered to clients with brain abscesses to decrease inflammation, but assessment is the first intervention.

14. 1. **Foundations offer the family and client information about the disease, support groups, and up-to-date information on current research.**
    2. **The use of padding will help prevent injury from the constant movement that occurs with this disease.**
    3. **The constant movement causes the client to be messy when eating, dressing, or performing activities of daily living.**
    4. **The constant movements expend more calories; therefore, the client should have three meals plus between-meal snacks.**
    5. The client is at risk for choking; therefore, teaching the Heimlich maneuver is appropriate, but teaching chest compression is not.

15. 1. Referring the client is not a psychosocial intervention. The gene that determines if a client has Huntington's chorea has been identified, and genetic counseling could rule out or confirm that the client's child will develop Huntington's chorea.
    2. This is an appropriate intervention, but it is not a psychosocial intervention. (Read the stem closely.)
    3. This is placing a lot of responsibility on the child concerning the parent's debilitating, chronic, and devastating disease. The client may need to be in a long-term care facility, and the child should not feel guilty if this is necessary.
    4. **The child will develop this disease if he or she inherited the gene. It can be frightening to watch a parent progress through this disease and understand that they too will get it.**

16. **20 mL/hr.** To arrive at the answer, the test taker must divide 25,000 units by 500 mL = 50 units in 1 mL. Divide 1000 units by 50 units = 20 mL/hr.

17. 1. The client may experience minor difficulty in work or social activities but has adequate cognitive ability to hide the loss and continue to function independently.
    2. **Disorientation to time and place is a warning sign.**

3. Not being able to focus on a task is more likely a sign of attention deficit/hyperactivity disorder.

4. Atherosclerotic changes are not warning signs of Alzheimer's disease. Amyloid protein plaques do appear to have something to do with the disease, but they are not found until autopsy.

18. 1. This is not a true statement. The client will be no longer be prescribed this medication as the disease progresses and it becomes ineffective.

2. **This medication does not cure Alzheimer's, and at some point it will become ineffective as the disease progresses.**

3. There is no monthly drug level to be monitored. Toxicity includes jaundice and gastrointestinal distress.

4. Muscle aches are an adverse effect of the lipid-lowering medications, not of Aricept.

19. 1. If the wife could leave the client alone, she would not be sharing her concerns with the nurse. The nurse needs to address the wife's concerns as well as the husband's.

2. This is not the typical signs/symptoms of stage 1 Alzheimer's disease.

3. **This behavior indicates the client is depressed and should be treated with antidepressants. A major lifestyle change has occurred and he may need short-term medication therapy, depending on how the client adjusts to retirement.**

4. The client may not want to participate in arts and crafts.

20. 1. The nurse cannot insist that the client do anything. The nurse can encourage, but remember, this is the client's home.

2. The family may need to be notified, but the nurse should first assess what is happening that is causing this change in behavior.

3. There is nothing that indicates the client is unhappy with the roommate. In fact, the client wants to stay in the room, which does not indicate a need for a room change.

4. **A change in behavior may indicate depression. The Geriatric Depression Scale measures satisfaction with life's accomplishment. The elderly should be in Erikson's generativity versus stagnation stage of life.**

21. 1. Dementia involves behavior changes that are irreversible and occur over time. Delirium, however, occurs suddenly (as in this man's symptom onset), is caused by an acute event, and is reversible.

2. **Drug toxicity and interactions are common causes of delirium in the elderly.**

3. This is blaming the family member for the client's paranoid ideation.

4. Watching old movies on television will not cause delirium.

22. 1. This is part of the neurological exam, but this is not the scientific rationale for why it is done. The nurse must understand what is being assessed to interpret the data.

2. Diplopia, double vision, is a sign of head injury, but it is not the scientific rationale.

3. The procedure does assess for brain damage but does not explain why.

4. **When the client hits the front of the head, there is a rebound effect known as "coup-contrecoup" in which the brain hits the back of the skull. The occipital lobe is in the back of the head and an injury to it may be manifested by seeing double.**

23. 1. A score of 3 is the lowest score and indicates deep coma and impending brain death.

2. **A score of 8 indicates severe increased intracranial pressure, but with appropriate care the client may survive. The nurse would rate the client at an 8: 1 for opening the eyes; 3 for verbal response; and 4 for motor response.**

3. A score of 10 indicates moderate increased intracranial pressure.

4. A score of 15 is the highest score a client can receive, indicating normal function.

24. 1. **Assessment is the first step in the nursing process, and a client with a motorcycle accident must be assessed for a head injury.**

2. Neurological assessment is priority over a fractured leg.

3. The client's urinary output is not priority over assessment.

4. An 18-gauge IV access should be started in case the client has to go to surgery, but it is not priority over an assessment.

25. 1. Administering acetaminophen is an intervention, which is not a goal.

2. **This is an appropriate goal. It addresses the client, addresses the problem (temperature elevation), and is measurable.**

3. Maintaining the blanket temperature is a nursing intervention, which should eliminate this as a possible answer.

4. The basal metabolic temperature is evaluated for a woman trying to get pregnant; it helps indicate ovulation.

26. 1. Diabetes mellitus type 2 is a pancreatic disease that has nothing to do with the pituitary gland or head injury.

2. Seizure activity is a possible complication of traumatic brain injury (TBI), but it is not a pituitary complication.

3. The pituitary gland produces vasopressin, the antidiuretic hormone (ADH), and any injury that causes increased intracranial pressure will exert pressure on the pituitary gland and can cause the syndrome of inappropriate antidiuretic hormone (SIADH).

4. Cushing's disease is caused by an excess production of glucocorticoids and mineralocorticoids from the adrenal gland.

27. 1. Because of bone loss associated with long-term use of anticonvulsants, the client should increase calcium intake to reduce the risk of osteoporosis.

2. Anticonvulsant medications have a narrow range of therapeutic value and the levels should be checked regularly.

3. Alcohol interferes with anticonvulsant medication and should be avoided.

4. Women with epilepsy note an increase in the frequency of seizures during menses. This is thought to be linked to the increase in sex hormones that alter the excitability of the neurons in the brain.

28. 1. The nurse must intervene to stop the assistant because the client's jaws are clenched. Attempting to insert anything into the mouth could cause injury to the client or to the assistant.

2. Side-lying positions help to prevent aspiration and are an appropriate intervention.

3. The client's safety is priority, and this will help protect the client from injury.

4. Staying with the client is an appropriate behavior that would not warrant intervention by the nurse.

29. 1. This procedure is not painful, although electrodes are attached to the scalp. The client will need to wash the hair after the procedure.

2. Anti-anxiety medication would make the client drowsy and could cause a false EEG reading.

3. There is no reason for facial hair to be shaved.

4. This procedure measures the electrical conductivity in the brain and does not cause the client to see floaters (spots before eyes). Flashing bright lights may be used in an attempt to evoke a seizure.

30. 1. Flaccid paralysis indicates a worsening of the increased intracranial pressure.

2. Purposeful movement indicates the client is getting better and is responding to the treatment.

3. Decerebrate positioning indicates a worsening of the increased intracranial pressure.

4. This is the same as flaccid paralysis and indi-

cates a worsening of the increased intracranial pressure.

31. 1. Assessing for deep vein thrombosis, which is a complication of immobility, would be appropriate for this client.

2. Anticoagulants may cause bleeding; therefore the client who has had surgery would not be prescribed this medication.

3. Monitoring of intake and output helps to detect possible complications of the pituitary gland, which include diabetes insipidus and syndrome of inappropriate antidiuretic hormone (SIADH).

4. The nurse should apply cool compresses to alleviate periocular edema.

5. The nurse does not want the client to be active and possibly increase intracranial pressure; therefore, the nurse should perform passive range of motion for the client.

32. 1. Paralysis is an expected occurrence with a client who has had a stroke.

2. Photosensitivity is an expected sign of meningitis.

3. Projectile vomiting indicates that the increased intracranial pressure is exerting pressure on the vomiting center of the brain.

4. Tender gums could be secondary to medication given for epilepsy. The client may need to see a dentist, but this client does not need to be assessed first.

33. 1. The symptoms and a positive Kernig's sign suggest meningitis, but a CT scan is not diagnostic of meningitis.

2. Blood cultures determine septicemia or infections of the bloodstream, not meningitis.

3. An electromyogram (EMG) evaluates electrical conductivity through the muscle.

4. The client's symptoms, along with a positive Kernig's sign, should make the nurse suspect meningitis. The definitive diagnostic test for meningitis is a lumbar puncture to retrieve cerebrospinal fluid for culture.

34. 1. An upper-respiratory infection (URI) is not a behavior. The question asked which behavior was a risk factor so this option can be ruled out. However, a URI is a risk factor for developing and spreading bacterial meningitis because of increased droplet production.

2. Unprotected sexual intercourse is a risk factor for sexually transmitted diseases (STDs), but not for meningitis.

3. Chronic alcohol consumption can cause pancreatitis or hepatitis but not meningitis.

4. Tobacco use increases respiratory secre-

tions and droplet production and thus is a risk factor for developing and spreading bacterial meningitis.

35. 1. The spread of pain and paralysis are signs/symptoms of Guillain-Barré syndrome.
    2. **Masklike facies and pill rolling are signs/symptoms of Parkinson's disease, along with cog wheeling, postural instability, and stooped and shuffling gait.**
    3. Diplopia and ptosis are signs/symptoms of myasthenia gravis.
    4. Dysphagia and dysarthria are signs/symptoms of myasthenia gravis.

36. 1. **Because carbidopa/levodopa has been linked to hypotension, teaching a client given the medication ways to help prevent a drop in blood pressure when standing—orthostatic hypotension—decreases the risks associated with hypotension and falling.**
    2. The medication will not cause the heart rate to change so taking the client's apical pulse for one (1) minute is not priority.
    3. This medication is prescribed for the client the rest of his or her life unless the medication stops working or the client experiences adverse side effects.
    4. The medication should be administered with food to help prevent gastrointestinal distress.

37. **4 gtts/min.** The nurse must know the formula for regulating IV drips: the amount to infuse (25 mL/hr) times the drop factor (10 gtts/mL) divided by the minutes. Thus, $25 \times 10 = 250 \div 60 = 4.11$ or 4 gtts.

38. 1. The client was diagnosed recently and at some point may need a percutaneous gastrostomy tube (PEG) tube, but it is too early for this discussion.
    2. A fistula is used for hemodialysis, and ALS does not cause renal dysfunction.
    3. **It is never too early to discuss advance directives with a client diagnosed with a terminal illness.**
    4. A client with ALS does not have leg braces as part of the therapeutic regimen.

39. 1. There is no vaccine for preventing encephalitis.
    2. **Mosquitoes are the vectors that spread the disease, and spraying to kill mosquito larvae will help prevent an outbreak in the community.**
    3. Gloves will not protect a person from being bitten by a mosquito.
    4. Mosquitoes are more prevalent at night, but

this is an unrealistic intervention and will not help prevent an outbreak.

40. 1. This advice might be appropriate at some point from a professional counselor but not from the nurse.
    2. Alcoholics Anonymous is the support group that alcoholics—in this case, the wife, not the husband—should attend.
    3. **Alanon is the support group for significant others of alcoholics. Al-A-Teen is for teenaged children of alcoholics.**
    4. This statement is making a judgment that is not given in the stem and is not applicable to all husbands of alcoholic wives.

41. 1. Symptoms of marijuana use are apathy, delayed time, and not wanting to eat.
    2. Heroin symptoms include pupil changes and respiratory depression.
    3. Ecstasy is a hallucinogen that is an "upper."
    4. **Disorderly behavior and the symptoms of epistaxis and nasal congestion would make the nurse suspect cocaine abuse.**

42. 1. The prodrome phase occurs hours to days before the migraine headache.
    2. **This is the aura phase, which is characterized by focal neurological symptoms.**
    3. The headache phase occurs when vasodilation occurs in the brain, along with a decline in serotonin levels, causing a throbbing headache.
    4. The recovery phase is when the pain begins to gradually subside.

43. 1. **Sumatriptan is a medication of choice for migraine headaches. It vasoconstricts blood vessels and reduces inflammation. The nurse administering the medication is part of a collaborative effort because the nurse must act on the order or prescription of a physician or other health-care provider who has prescriptive authority.**
    2. This is a collaborative intervention, but it is not routinely ordered because the client reports having a history of migraine headaches.
    3. This is an appropriate independent nursing intervention.
    4. Propranolol is not used for acute migraine headaches; it is prescribed for long-term prophylaxis of migraines so the nurse should not anticipate its use in this situation,

44. 1. Sweating is not a sign of autonomic dysreflexia.
    2. **A throbbing headache is the classic sign of autonomic dysreflexia, which is caused by a stimulus such as a full bladder.**
    3. Sudden loss of motor function occurs with the

original injury. Autonomic dysreflexia does not occur until spinal shock has resolved; it usually occurs in the rehabilitation phase.

4. Spastic skeletal muscle movement could be secondary to the reflex arch in lower motor neuron injuries.

45. 1. There is no such law known as the First Aid Law.
2. The Ombudsman Act addresses many areas, such as advance directives, elderly advocacy, and several other areas.
3. **The Good Samaritan Act protects the nurse from judgment against them when in an emergency situation in which the nurse is not receiving compensation for the skills and expertise rendered. The nurse is held to a different standard than a layman; the nurse must act as any reasonable and prudent nurse would in the same situation.**
4. There is no such law known as the First Responder Law.

46. 1. A patient with an L-5-6 spinal cord injury is paralyzed and cannot perform active ROM exercises.
2. Massaging bony prominences can cause trauma to the underlying blood vessels and will increase the risk for skin breakdown.
3. **The nurse must realize that the client is at risk for skin breakdown even when sitting in the chair. A Roho cushion is an air-filled cushion that provides reduced pressure on the ischium.**
4. Lotion will not prevent skin breakdown and should be water based, not petroleum based.

47. 1. The medication can be administered in pudding, but it is not the first intervention.
2. The arm band should be checked but not before determining if the client can swallow.
3. Tylenol comes in liquid form, and the nurse should request this before crushing a very bitter tablet.
4. **Asking the client to sip some water assesses the client's ability to swallow, which is priority when placing anything in the mouth of the client who has had a stroke.**

48. 1. An alcoholic is not at risk for having a stroke anymore than someone in the general population.
2. A client with hepatitis is not at risk for having a stroke anymore than someone in the general population.
3. A Greenfield filter is positioned in the inferior vena cava to prevent an embolism resulting from deep vein thrombosis; these filters prevent strokes and pulmonary emboli.
4. **A client with atrial fibrillation is at high risk to have a stroke and is usually given oral anticoagulants to prevent a stroke.**

49. 1. **This client is experiencing a progressing stroke, is at risk for dying, and should be cared for by the most experienced nurse.**
2. A TIA by definition lasts less than 24 hours so this client should be stable at this time.
3. Pain is expected in clients with Guillain-Barré, and symptoms are on the lower half of the body, which does not affect the airway. Therefore, a less experienced nurse could care for this client.
4. The charge nurse could delegate much of the care of this client to a UAP.

50. 1. The eyes, indicated by A, would be assessed if checking cranial nerves II, III, IV, or VI.
2. The tongue located in the mouth, indicated by B, would be assessed if checking cranial nerves IX, X, or XII.
3. The cheek, indicated by C, would be assessed if checking for cranial nerve V, the trigeminal nerve.
4. **Anosmia, the loss of the sense of smell, would require the nurse to assess for cranial nerve I, the olfactory nerve, indicated by D.**

51. In order of priority: 3, 2, 1, 5, 4.
3. **Stabilizing the client's neck is priority action to prevent further injury to the client, and it must be done prior to moving the client.**
2. **The nurse should assess for any other injuries prior to moving the client from the vehicle.**
1. **Because the vehicle is leaking fuel and there is potential for an explosion or fire, the client should be moved to an area of safety.**
5. **Placing the client in a functional anatomical position is an attempt to prevent further spinal cord injury.**
4. **Because the vehicle is leaking fuel, the priority is to remove the client and then obtain emergency medical assistance.**

# 3

# Cardiac Disorders

*If you have knowledge, let others light their candles in it.*—Margaret Fuller

Heart disease is the leading cause of death in the United States. A nurse must have a thorough knowledge of the signs/symptoms of cardiac disorders and of what to expect in assessing and treating clients with heart-related problems.

## KEYWORDS

atelectasis
buccal
cardiac tamponade
crackles
dyspnea
dysrhythmia
eupnea
exacerbation
intermittent claudication
nocturia
orthostatic hypotension
paresthesia
petechiae
pulse oximeter
pulsus paradoxus
pyrosis
splinter hemorrhages
telemetry

## ABBREVIATIONS

Activities Of Daily Living (ADLs)
Angiotensin-Converting Enzyme (ACE)
Basal Metabolic Panel (BMP)
Blood Pressure (BP)
Blood Urea Nitrogen (BUN)
B-Type Natriuretic Peptide (BNP)
Capillary Refill Time (CRT)
Cardiopulmonary Resuscitation (CPR)
Chest X-Ray (CXR)
Chronic Obstructive Pulmonary Disease (COPD)
Congestive Heart Failure (CHF)
Coronary Artery Disease (CAD)
Dyspnea on Exertion (DOE)
Electrocardiogram (ECG)
Endotracheal (ET)
Health-Care Provider (HCP)
Implantable Cardioverter Defibrillator (ICD)
International Normalized Ratio (INR)
Intravenous Push (IVP)
Jugular Vein Distention (JVD)
Myocardial Infarction (MI)
Nonsteroidal Anti-Inflammtory Drugs (NSAIDs)
Nothing By Mouth (NPO)
Partial Thromboplastin Time (PTT)
Percutaneous Transluminal Angioplasty (PTCA)
Premature Ventricular Contraction (PVC)
Pulmonary Embolus (PE)
Rule Out (R/O)
Ventilation Perfusion (V/Q)
White Blood Cells (WBC)

## Congestive Heart Failure

1. The client is admitted to the telemetry unit diagnosed with acute exacerbation of congestive heart failure (CHF). Which signs/symptoms would the nurse expect to find when assessing this client?
   1. Apical pulse rate of 110 and 4+ pitting edema of feet.
   2. Thick white sputum and crackles that clear with cough.
   3. The client sleeping with no pillow and eupnea.
   4. Radial pulse rate of 90 and capillary refill time <3 seconds.

2. The nurse is developing a nursing care plan for a client diagnosed with congestive heart failure. A nursing diagnosis of "decreased cardiac output related to inability of the heart to pump effectively" is written. Which short-term goal would be best for the client? The client will:
   1. Be able to ambulate in the hall by date of discharge.
   2. Have an audible S1 and S2 with no S3 heard by end of shift.
   3. Turn, cough, and deep breathe every two (2) hours.
   4. Have a pulse oximeter reading of 98% by day two (2) of care.

3. The nurse is developing a discharge-teaching plan for the client diagnosed with congestive heart failure. Which intervention should be included in the plan? Select all that apply.
   1. Notify health-care provider of a weight gain of more than one (1) pound in a week.
   2. Teach client how to count the radial pulse when taking digoxin, a cardiac glycoside.
   3. Instruct client to remove the saltshaker from the dinner table.
   4. Encourage client to monitor urine output for change in color to become dark.
   5. Discuss the importance of taking the loop diuretic furosemide at bedtime.

4. The nurse enters the room of the client diagnosed with congestive heart failure. The client is lying in bed gasping for breath, is cool and clammy, and has buccal cyanosis. Which intervention would the nurse implement first?
   1. Sponge the client's forehead.
   2. Obtain a pulse oximetry reading.
   3. Take the client's vital signs.
   4. Assist the client to a sitting position.

5. The nurse is assessing the client diagnosed with congestive heart failure. Which signs/symptoms would indicate that the medical treatment has been effective?
   1. The client's peripheral pitting edema has gone from 3+ to 4+.
   2. The client is able to take the radial pulse accurately.
   3. The client is able to perform activities of daily living without dyspnea.
   4. The client has minimal jugular vein distention.

6. The nurse is assessing the client diagnosed with congestive heart failure. Which laboratory data would indicate that the client is in severe congestive heart failure?
   1. An elevated B-type natriuretic peptide (BNP).
   2. An elevated creatine kinase (CK-MB).
   3. A positive D-dimer.
   4. A positive ventilation-perfusion (V/Q) scan.

7. The health-care provider has ordered an angiotensin-converting enzyme (ACE) inhibitor for the client diagnosed with congestive heart failure. Which discharge instructions should the nurse include?
   1. Instruct the client to take a cough suppressant if a cough develops.
   2. Teach the client how to prevent orthostatic hypotension.
   3. Encourage the client to eat bananas to increase potassium level.
   4. Explain the importance of taking medication with food.

8. The nurse on the telemetry unit has just received the A.M. shift report. Which client should the nurse assess first?
   1. The client diagnosed with myocardial infarction who has an audible S3 heart sound.
   2. The client diagnosed with congestive heart failure who has 4+ sacral pitting edema.
   3. The client diagnosed with pneumonia who has a pulse oximeter reading of 94%.
   4. The client with chronic renal failure who has an elevated creatinine level.

9. The nurse and an unlicensed nursing assistant are caring for four clients on a telemetry unit. Which nursing task would be best for the nurse delegate to the unlicensed nursing assistant?
   1. Assist the client to go down to the smoking area for a cigarette.
   2. Transport the client to the Intensive Care Unit via a stretcher.
   3. Provide the client going home discharge-teaching instructions.
   4. Help position the client who is having a portable x-ray done.

10. The charge nurse is making shift assignments for the medical floor. Which client should be assigned to the most experienced registered nurse?
    1. The client diagnosed with congestive heart failure who is being discharged in the morning.
    2. The client who is having frequent incontinent liquid bowel movements and vomiting.
    3. The client with an apical pulse rate of 116, a respiratory rate of 26, and a blood pressure of 94/62.
    4. The client who is complaining of chest pain with inspiration and a nonproductive cough.

11. The client diagnosed with congestive heart failure is complaining of leg cramps at night. Which nursing interventions should be implemented?
    1. Check the client for peripheral edema and make sure the client takes a diuretic early in the day.
    2. Monitor the client's potassium level and assess the client's intake of bananas and orange juice.
    3. Determine if the client has gained weight and instruct the client to keep the legs elevated.
    4. Instruct the client to ambulate frequently and perform calf-muscle stretching exercises daily.

12. The nurse has written an outcome goal "demonstrates tolerance for increased activity" for a client diagnosed with congestive heart failure. Which intervention should the nurse implement to assist the client to achieve this outcome?
    1. Measure intake and output.
    2. Provide two (2)-g sodium diet.
    3. Weigh client daily.
    4. Plan for frequent rest periods.

## Angina/Myocardial Infarction

13. Which cardiac enzyme would the nurse expect to elevate first in a client diagnosed with a myocardial infarction?
    1. Creatine phosphokinase (CPK-MB).
    2. Lactate dehydrogenase (LDH).
    3. Troponin.
    4. White blood cells (WBC).

14. Along with persistent, crushing chest pain, which signs/symptoms would make the nurse suspect that the client is experiencing a myocardial infarction?
    1. Mid-epigastric pain and pyrosis.
    2. Diaphoresis and cool clammy skin.
    3. Intermittent claudication and pallor.
    4. Jugular vein distention and dependent edema.

15. The client diagnosed with rule-out myocardial infarction is experiencing chest pain while walking to the bathroom. Which action should the nurse implement first?
    1. Administer sublingual nitroglycerin.
    2. Obtain a STAT electrocardiogram.
    3. Have the client sit down immediately.
    4. Assess the client's vital signs.

16. The nurse is caring for a client diagnosed with a myocardial infarction who is experiencing chest pain. Which interventions should the nurse implement? Select all that apply.
    1. Administer morphine intramuscularly.
    2. Administer an aspirin orally.
    3. Apply oxygen via a nasal cannula.
    4. Place the client in a supine position.
    5. Administer nitroglycerin subcutaneously.

17. The client is diagnosed with a myocardial infarction. Which referral would be most appropriate for the client?
    1. Social worker.
    2. Physical therapy.
    3. Cardiac rehabilitation.
    4. Occupational therapist.

18. The client is one (1) day postoperative coronary artery bypass surgery. The client complains of chest pain. Which intervention should the nurse implement first?
    1. Medicate the client with intravenous morphine.
    2. Assess the client's chest dressing and vital signs.
    3. Encourage the client to turn from side to side.
    4. Check the client's telemetry monitor.

19. The client diagnosed with a myocardial infarction is six (6) hours post–right femoral percutaneous transluminal angioplasty (PTCA), also known as balloon surgery. Which assessment data would require immediate intervention by the nurse?
    1. The client is keeping the affected extremity straight.
    2. The pressure dressing to the right femoral area is intact.
    3. The client is complaining of numbness in the right foot.
    4. The client's right pedal pulse is 3+ and bounding.

20. The intensive care department nurse is assessing the client who is 12 hours post-myocardial infarction. The nurse assesses a S3 heart sound. Which intervention should the nurse implement?
    1. Notify the health-care provider immediately.
    2. Elevate the head of the client's bed.
    3. Document this as a normal and expected finding.
    4. Administer morphine intravenously.

21. The nurse is administering a calcium channel blocker to the client diagnosed with a myocardial infarction. Which assessment data would cause the nurse to question administering this medication?
    1. The client's apical pulse is 64.
    2. The client's calcium level is elevated.
    3. The client's telemetry shows occasional PVCs.
    4. The client's blood pressure is 90/62.

22. The client diagnosed with a myocardial infarction is on bed rest. The unlicensed nursing assistant is encouraging the client to move the legs. Which action should the nurse implement?
    1. Instruct the assistant to stop encouraging the leg movements.
    2. Report this behavior to the charge nurse as soon as possible.
    3. Praise the nursing assistant for encouraging the client to move legs.
    4. Take no action concerning the nursing assistant's behavior.

23. The client diagnosed with a myocardial infarction asks the nurse, "Why do I have to rest and take it easy? My chest doesn't hurt anymore." Which statement would be the nurse's best response?
    1. "Your heart is damaged and needs about four (4) to six (6) weeks to heal."
    2. "There is necrotic myocardial tissue that puts you at risk for dysrhythmias."
    3. "Your doctor has ordered bed rest. Therefore, you must stay in the bed."
    4. "Just because your chest doesn't hurt anymore doesn't mean you are out of danger."

24. The client has just returned from a cardiac catheterization. Which assessment data would warrant immediate intervention from the nurse?
    1. The client's BP is 110/70 and pulse is 90.
    2. The client groin dressing is dry and intact.
    3. The client refuses to keep the leg straight.
    4. The client denies any numbness and tingling.

## Coronary Artery Disease

25. The male client is diagnosed with coronary artery disease (CAD) and is prescribed sublingual nitroglycerin. Which statement indicates the client needs more teaching?
    1. "I should keep the tablets in the dark colored bottle they came in."
    2. "If the tablets do not burn under my tongue, they are not effective."
    3. "I should keep the bottle with me in my pocket at all times."
    4. "If my chest pain is not gone with one tablet, I will go to the ER."

26. The client with coronary artery disease asks the nurse, "Why do I get chest pain?" Which statement would be the most appropriate response by the nurse?
    1. "Chest pain is caused by decreased oxygen to the heart muscle."
    2. "There is ischemia to the myocardium as a result of hypoxemia."
    3. "The heart muscle is unable to pump effectively to perfuse the body."
    4. "Chest pain occurs when the lungs cannot adequately oxygenate the blood."

27. The client is scheduled for a right femoral cardiac catheterization. Which nursing intervention should the nurse implement after the procedure?
    1. Perform passive range of motion exercises.
    2. Assess the client's neurovascular status.
    3. Keep the client in high-Fowler's position.
    4. Assess the gag reflex prior to feeding the client.

28. The nurse is preparing to administer a beta blocker to the client diagnosed with coronary artery disease. Which assessment data would cause the nurse to question administering the medication?
    1. The client has a BP of 110/70.
    2. The client has an apical pulse of 56.
    3. The client is complaining of a headache.
    4. The client's potassium level is 4.5 mEq/L.

29. Which intervention should the nurse implement when administering a loop diuretic to a client diagnosed with coronary artery disease?
    1. Assess the client's radial pulse.
    2. Assess the client's serum potassium level.
    3. Assess the client's glucometer reading.
    4. Assess the client's pulse oximeter reading.

30. Which client teaching should the nurse implement for the client diagnosed with coronary artery disease? Select all that apply.
    1. Encourage a low-fat, low-cholesterol diet.
    2. Instruct client to walk 30 minutes a day.
    3. Decrease the salt intake to 2 g a day.
    4. Refer to counselor for stress reduction techniques.
    5. Increase fiber in the diet.

31. The elderly client has coronary artery disease. Which question should the nurse ask the client during the client teaching?
    1. "Do you have a daily bowel movement?"
    2. "Do you get yearly chest x-rays?"
    3. "Are you sexually active?"
    4. "Have you had any weight change?"

32. The nurse is discussing the importance of exercise with the client diagnosed with coronary artery disease. Which intervention should the nurse implement?
    1. Perform isometric exercises daily.
    2. Walk for 15 minutes three (3) times a week.
    3. Do not walk if it is less than 40°F.
    4. Wear open-toed shoes when ambulating.

33. The nurse is discussing angina with a client who is diagnosed with coronary artery disease. Which action should the client take first when experiencing angina?
    1. Put a nitroglycerin tablet under the tongue.
    2. Stop the activity immediately and rest.
    3. Document when and what activity caused angina.
    4. Notify the health-care provider immediately.

34. The client with coronary artery disease is prescribed a Holter monitor. Which intervention should the nurse implement?
    1. Instruct client to keep a diary of activity, especially when having chest pain.
    2. Discuss the need to remove Holter monitor during A.M. care and showering.
    3. Explain that all medications should be withheld while wearing a Holter monitor.
    4. Teach the client the importance of decreasing activity while wearing the monitor.

35. Which statement by the client diagnosed with coronary artery disease indicates that the client understands the discharge teaching concerning diet?
    1. "I will not eat more than six (6) eggs a week."
    2. "I should bake or grill any meats I eat."
    3. "I will drink eight (8) ounces of whole milk a day."
    4. "I should not eat any type of pork products."

36. The charge nurse is making assignments for clients on a cardiac unit. Which client should the charge nurse assign to a new graduate nurse?
    1. The 44-year-old client diagnosed with a myocardial infarction.
    2. The 65-year-old client admitted with unstable angina.
    3. The 75-year-old client scheduled for a cardiac catheterization.
    4. The 50-year-old client complaining of chest pain.

## Valvular Heart Disease

37. A client is being seen in the clinic to R/O mitral valve stenosis. Which assessment data would be most significant?
    1. The client complains of shortness of breath when walking.
    2. The client has jugular vein distention and 3+ pedal edema.
    3. The client complains of chest pain after eating a large meal.
    4. The client's liver is enlarged and the abdomen is edematous.

38. Which assessment data would the nurse expect to auscultate in the client diagnosed with mitral valve insufficiency?
    1. A loud S1, S2 split, and a mitral opening snap.
    2. A holosystolic murmur heard best at cardiac apex.
    3. A mid-systolic ejection click or murmur heard at the base.
    4. A high-pitched sound heard at the 3rd left intercostal space.

39. The client has just received a mechanical valve replacement. Which behavior by the client indicates the client needs more teaching?
    1. The client takes prophylactic antibiotics.
    2. The client uses a soft-bristle toothbrush.
    3. The client takes an enteric-coated aspirin daily.
    4. The client alternates rest with activity.

40. The nurse is teaching a class on valve replacements. Which statement identifies a disadvantage of having a biologic tissue valve replacement?
    1. The client must take lifetime anticoagulant therapy.
    2. The client's infections are easier to treat.
    3. There is a low incidence of thromboembolism.
    4. The valve has to be replaced frequently.

41. The nurse is preparing to administer warfarin (Coumadin), an oral anticoagulant, to a client with a mechanical valve replacement. The client's International Normalized Ratio (INR) is 2.7. Which action should the nurse implement?
    1. Administer the medication as ordered.
    2. Prepare to administer vitamin K (AquaMephyton).
    3. Hold the medication and notify the HCP.
    4. Assess the client for abnormal bleeding.

42. Which signs/symptoms should the nurse assess in any client who has a long-term valvular heart disease? Select all that apply.
    1. Paroxysmal nocturnal dyspnea.
    2. Orthopnea.
    3. Cough.
    4. Pericardial friction rub.
    5. Pulsus paradoxus.

43. The client is being evaluated for valvular heart disease. Which information would be most significant?
    1. The client has a history of coronary artery disease.
    2. There is a family history of valvular heart disease.
    3. The client has a history of smoking for ten (10) years.
    4. The client has a history of rheumatic heart disease.

44. The client who has just had a percutaneous balloon valvuloplasty is in the recovery room. Which intervention should the recovery room nurse implement?
    1. Assess the client's chest tube output.
    2. Monitor the client's chest dressing.
    3. Evaluate the client's endotracheal (ET) lip line.
    4. Keep the client's affected leg straight.

45. The client with a mechanical valve replacement asks the nurse, "Why do I have to take antibiotics before getting my teeth cleaned?" Which response by the nurse is most appropriate?
    1. "You are at risk of developing an infection in your heart."
    2. "Your teeth will not bleed as much if you have antibiotics."
    3. "This procedure may cause your valve to malfunction."
    4. "Antibiotics will prevent vegetative growth on your valves."

46. The client had open-heart surgery to replace the mitral valve. Which intervention should the intensive care unit nurse implement?
    1. Restrict the client's fluids as ordered.
    2. Keep the client in the supine position.
    3. Maintain oxygen saturation at 90%.
    4. Monitor the total parenteral nutrition.

47. Which client would the nurse suspect of having a mitral valve prolapse?
    1. A 60-year-old female with congestive heart failure.
    2. A 23-year-old male with Marfan syndrome.
    3. An 80-year-old male with atrial fibrillation.
    4. A 33-year-old female with Down syndrome.

48. The charge nurse is making shift assignments. Which client would be most appropriate for the charge nurse to assign to a new graduate that just completed orientation to the medical floor?
    1. The client admitted for diagnostic tests to rule out valvular heart disease.
    2. The client three (3) days post-myocardial infarction who is being discharged tomorrow.
    3. The client exhibiting supraventricular tachycardia (SVT) on telemetry.
    4. The client diagnosed with atrial fibrillation who has an INR of five (5).

## Dysrhythmias and Conduction Problems

49. The telemetry nurse is unable to read the telemetry monitor at the nurse's station. Which intervention should the telemetry nurse implement first?
    1. Go to the client's room to check the client.
    2. Instruct the primary nurse to assess the client.
    3. Contact the client on the client call system.
    4. Request the nursing assistant to take the crash cart to the client's room.

50. The client shows ventricular fibrillation on the telemetry at the nurse's station. Which action should the telemetry nurse implement first?
    1. Administer epinephrine IVP.
    2. Prepare to defibrillate the client.
    3. Call a STAT code.
    4. Start cardiopulmonary resuscitation.

51. The client is experiencing multifocal premature ventricular contractions. Which anti-dysrhythmic medication would the nurse expect the health-care provider to order for this client?
    1. Lidocaine.
    2. Atropine.
    3. Digoxin.
    4. Adenosine.

52. The client is exhibiting sinus bradycardia, is complaining of syncope and weakness, and has a BP of 98/60. Which collaborative treatment should the nurse anticipate being implemented?
    1. Administer a thrombolytic medication.
    2. Assess the client's cardiovascular status.
    3. Prepare for an insertion of a pacemaker.
    4. Obtain a permit for synchronized cardioversion.

53. Which intervention should the nurse implement when defibrillating a client who is in ventricular fibrillation?
    1. Defibrillate the client at 50, 100, and 200 joules.
    2. Do not remove the oxygen source during defibrillation.
    3. Place petroleum jelly on the defibrillator pads.
    4. Shout "all clear" prior to defibrillating the client.

54. The client has chronic atrial fibrillation. Which discharge teaching should the nurse discuss with the client?
    1. Instruct the client to use a soft-bristle toothbrush.
    2. Discuss the importance of getting a monthly partial thromboplastin time (PTT).
    3. Teach the client about signs of pacemaker malfunction.
    4. Explain to the client the procedure for synchronized cardioversion.

55. The client is exhibiting ventricular tachycardia. Which intervention should the nurse implement first?
    1. Administer lidocaine, an antidysrhythmic, IVP.
    2. Prepare to defibrillate the client at 200 joules.
    3. Assess the client's apical pulse and blood pressure.
    4. Start basic cardiopulmonary resuscitation.

56. The client is in complete heart block. Which intervention should the nurse implement first?
    1. Prepare to insert a pacemaker.
    2. Administer atropine, an antidysrhythmic.
    3. Obtain a STAT electrocardiogram (ECG).
    4. Notify the health-care provider.

57. The client is in ventricular fibrillation. Which interventions should the nurse implement? Select all that apply.
    1. Start cardiopulmonary resuscitation.
    2. Prepare to administer the antidysrhythmic adenosine IVP.
    3. Prepare to defibrillate the client.
    4. Bring the crash cart to the bedside.
    5. Prepare to administer the antidysrhythmic amiodarone IVP.

58. The client that is one (1)-day postoperative coronary artery bypass surgery is exhibiting sinus tachycardia. Which intervention should the nurse implement?
    1. Assess the apical heart rate for one (1) full minute.
    2. Notify the client's cardiac surgeon.
    3. Prepare the client for synchronized cardioversion.
    4. Determine if the client is having pain.

59. The client's telemetry reading shows a P-wave before each QRS complex and the rate is 78. Which action should the nurse implement?
    1. Document this as normal sinus rhythm.
    2. Request a 12-lead electrocardiogram.
    3. Prepare to administer the cardiotonic digoxin po.
    4. Assess the client's cardiac enzymes.

60. Which client problem has priority for the client with a cardiac dysrhythmia?
    1. Alteration in comfort.
    2. Decreased cardiac output.
    3. Impaired gas exchange.
    4. Activity intolerance.

## Inflammatory Cardiac Disorders

61. The client is diagnosed with pericarditis. Which are the most common signs/symptoms the nurse would expect to find when assessing the client?
    1. Pulsus paradoxus.
    2. Complaints of fatigue and arthralgias.
    3. Petechiae and splinter hemorrhages.
    4. Increased chest pain with inspiration.

62. The client is diagnosed with acute pericarditis. Which sign/symptom warrants immediate attention by the nurse?
    1. Muffled heart sounds.
    2. Nondistended jugular veins.
    3. Bounding peripheral pulses.
    4. Pericardial friction rub.

63. The client is admitted to the medical unit to rule out carditis. Which question should the nurse ask the client during the admission interview to support this diagnosis?
    1. "Have you had a sore throat in the last month?"
    2. "Did you have rheumatic fever as a child?"
    3. "Do you have a family history of carditis?"
    4. "What over-the-counter (OTC) medications do you take?"

64. The client with pericarditis is prescribed a nonsteroidal anti-inflammatory drug (NSAID). Which teaching instruction should the nurse discuss with the client?
    1. Explain the importance of tapering off the medication.
    2. Discuss that the medication will make the client drowsy.
    3. Instruct the client to take the medication with food.
    4. Tell the client to take the medication when the pain level is around "8."

65. The client diagnosed with pericarditis is complaining of increased pain. Which intervention should the nurse implement first?
    1. Administer oxygen via nasal cannula.
    2. Evaluate the client's urinary output.
    3. Assess the client for cardiac complications.
    4. Encourage the client to use the incentive spirometer.

66. The client diagnosed with pericarditis is experiencing cardiac tamponade. Which collaborative intervention should the nurse anticipate for this client?
    1. Prepare for a pericardiocentesis.
    2. Request STAT cardiac enzymes.
    3. Perform a 12-lead electrocardiogram.
    4. Assess the client's heart and lung sounds.

67. The female client is diagnosed with rheumatic fever and prescribed penicillin, an antibiotic. Which statement indicates the client needs more teaching concerning the discharge teaching?
    1. "I must take all the prescribed antibiotics."
    2. "I may get a vaginal yeast infection with penicillin."
    3. "I will have no problems as long as I take my medication."
    4. "My throat culture was positive for a streptococcal infection."

68. Which potential complication should the nurse assess for in the client with infective endocarditis who has embolization of vegetative lesions from the mitral valve?
    1. Pulmonary embolus.
    2. Decreased urine output.
    3. Hemoptysis.
    4. Deep vein thrombosis.

69. Which nursing diagnosis would be priority for the client diagnosed with myocarditis?
    1. Anxiety related to possible long-term complications.
    2. High risk for injury related to antibiotic therapy.
    3. Increased cardiac output related to valve regurgitation.
    4. Activity intolerance related to impaired cardiac muscle function.

70. The client diagnosed with pericarditis is being discharged home. Which intervention should the nurse include in the discharge teaching?
    1. Be sure to allow for uninterrupted rest and sleep.
    2. Refer client to outpatient occupational therapy.
    3. Maintain oxygen via nasal cannula at two (2) L/min.
    4. Discuss upcoming valve replacement surgery.

71. The client has just had a pericardiocentesis. Which interventions should the nurse implement? Select all that apply.
    1. Monitor vital signs every 15 minutes for the first hour.
    2. Assess the client's heart and lung sounds.
    3. Record the amount of fluid removed as output.
    4. Evaluate the client's cardiac rhythm.
    5. Keep the client in the supine position.

72. The client with infective endocarditis is admitted to the medical department. Which health-care provider's order should be implemented first?
    1. Administer intravenous antibiotic.
    2. Obtain blood cultures times two (2).
    3. Schedule an echocardiogram.
    4. Encourage bed rest with bathroom privileges.

## Congestive Heart Failure

1. 1. The client with CHF would exhibit tachycardia (apical pulse rate of 110), dependent edema, fatigue, third heart sounds, lung congestion, and change in mental status.
   2. The client with CHF usually has pink frothy sputum and crackles that do not clear with coughing.
   3. The client with CHF would report sleeping on at least two pillows, if not sleeping in an upright position, and labored breathing, not eupnea, which means normal breathing.
   4. In a client diagnosed with heart failure, the apical pulse, not the radial pulse, is the best place to assess the cardiac status.

   **TEST-TAKING HINT:** In answer option "3," the word "no" is an absolute term, and usually absolutes, such as "no," "never," "always," and "only," are incorrect because there is no room for any other possible answer. If the test taker is looking for abnormal data, then exclude the options that have normal values in them such as eupnea, pulse rate of 90, and capillary refill time (CRT) <3 seconds.

2. 1. Ambulating in the hall by day of discharge would be a more appropriate goal for an activity-intolerance nursing diagnosis.
   2. Audible S1 and S2 sounds are normal for a heart with adequate output. An audible S3 sound might indicate left ventricular failure that could be life threatening.
   3. This is a nursing intervention, not a short-term goal, for this client.
   4. A pulse oximeter reading would be a goal for impaired gas exchange, not for cardiac output.

   **TEST-TAKING HINT:** When reading a nursing diagnosis or problem, the test taker must be sure that the answer selected addresses the problem. An answer option may be appropriate care for the disease process but not fit with the problem or etiology. Remember that when given an etiology in a nursing diagnosis the answer will be doing something to the problem (etiology). In this question the test taker should look for an answer that addresses the ability of the heart to pump blood.

3. 1. The client should notify the HCP of weight gain of more than two (2) or three (3) pounds in one (1) day.
   2. The client should not take digoxin if radial pulse is less than 60.
   3. The client should be on a low-sodium diet to prevent water retention.
   4. The color of the urine should not change to a dark color; if anything, it might become lighter and the amount will increase with diuretics.
   5. Instruct client to take the diuretic in the morning to prevent nocturia.

   **TEST-TAKING HINT:** This is an alternative-type question—in this case, "select all that apply." If the test taker missed this statement, it is possible to jump at the first correct answer. This is one reason that it is imperative to read all options before deciding on the correct one. This could be a clue to reread the question for clarity. Another hint that this is an alternative question is the number of options. The other questions have four potential answers; this one has five. Numbers in an answer option are always important. Is 1 enough pounds to indicate a problem that should be brought to the attention of the health-care provider?

4. 1. Sponging the client's forehead would be appropriate, but it is not the first intervention.
   2. Obtaining a pulse oximeter reading would be appropriate, but it is not the first intervention.
   3. Taking the vital signs would be appropriate, but it is not the first intervention.
   4. The nurse must first put the client in a sitting position to decrease the workload of the heart by decreasing venous return and maximizing lung expansion. Then, the nurse could take vital signs and check the pulse oximeter and then sponge the client's forehead.

   **TEST-TAKING HINT:** In a question that asks the nurse to set priorities, all the answer options can be appropriate actions by the nurse for a given situation. The test taker should apply some guidelines or principles, such as Maslow's Hierarchy, to determine what will give the client the most immediate assistance.

5. 1. Pitting edema from 3+ to 4+ indicates a worsening of the CHF.
   2. The client's ability to take the radial pulse would evaluate teaching, not medical treatment.
   3. Being able to perform activities of daily living (ADLs) without shortness of breath (dyspnea) would indicate the client's condition is improving. The client's heart is a more effective pump and can oxygenate the body better without increasing fluid in the lungs.
   4. Any jugular vein distention indicates that the right side of the heart is failing, which would not indicate effective medical treatment.

   **TEST-TAKING HINT:** When asked to determine whether treatment is effective, the test taker

Cardiac

must know the signs and symptoms of the disease being treated. An improvement in the signs and symptoms indicates effective treatment.

6. 1. BNP is a specific diagnostic test. Levels higher than normal indicate congestive heart failure, with the higher the number, the more severe the CHF.
   2. An elevated CK-MB would indicate a myocardial infarction, not severe CHF. CK-MB is an isoenzyme.
   3. A positive D-dimer would indicate a pulmonary embolus.
   4. A positive ventilation-perfusion (V/Q) scan (ratio) would indicate a pulmonary embolus.

   **TEST-TAKING HINT: This question requires the test taker to discriminate between CHF, MI, and PE. If unsure of the answer of this type of question, the test taker should eliminate any answer options that the test taker knows are wrong. For example, the test taker may not know about pulmonary embolus but might know that CK-MB data are used to monitor MI and be able to eliminate "2" as a possibility. Then, there is a 1:3 chance of getting the correct answer.**

7. 1. If a cough develops, the client should notify the health-care provider because this is an adverse reaction and the HCP will discontinue the medication.
   2. **Orthostatic hypotension may occur with ACE inhibitors as a result of vasodilation. Therefore, the nurse should instruct the client to rise slowly and sit on the side of the bed until equilibrium is restored.**
   3. ACE inhibitors may cause the client to retain potassium; therefore, the client should not increase potassium intake.
   4. An ACE inhibitor should be taken one (1) hour before meals or two (2) hours after a meal to increase absorption of the medication.

   **TEST-TAKING HINT: If the test taker knows that an ACE inhibitor is also given for hypertension, then looking at answer options referring to hypotension would be appropriate.**

8. 1. **An S3 heart sound indicates left ventricular failure, and the nurse must assess this client first because it is an emergency situation.**
   2. The nurse would expect a client with CHF to have sacral edema of 4+; the client with an S3 would be in a more life-threatening situation.
   3. A pulse oximeter reading of greater than 93% is considered normal.

4. An elevated creatinine level is expected in a client diagnosed with chronic renal failure.

**TEST-TAKING HINT: Because the nurse will be assessing each client, the test taker must determine which client is a priority. A general guideline for this type of question is for the test taker to ask "Is this within normal limits?" or "Is this expected for the disease process?" If the answer is yes to either question, then the test taker can eliminate these options and look for abnormal data that would make that client a priority.**

9. 1. Allowing the unlicensed assistive personnel (UAP) to take a client down to smoke is not cost effective and is not supportive of the medical treatment regimen that discourages smoking.
   2. The client going to the ICU would be unstable, and the nurse should not delegate to an UAP any nursing task that involves an unstable client.
   3. The nurse cannot delegate teaching.
   4. **The UAP can assist the x-ray technician in positioning the client for the portable x-ray. This does not require judgment.**

   **TEST-TAKING HINT: The test taker must be knowledgeable about the individual state's Nursing Practice Act regarding what a nurse may delegate to unlicensed assistive personnel. Generally, the answer options that require higher level of knowledge or ability are reserved for licensed staff.**

10. 1. This client is stable because discharge is scheduled for the following day. Therefore, this client does not need to be assigned to the most experienced registered nurse.
    2. This client requires more custodial nursing care than care from the most experienced registered nurse. Therefore the charge nurse could assign a less experienced nurse to this client.
    3. **This client is exhibiting signs/symptoms of shock, which makes this client the most unstable. An experienced nurse should care for this client.**
    4. These complaints usually indicate muscular or pleuritic chest pain; cardiac chest pain does not fluctuate with inspiration. This client does not require the care of an experienced nurse as much as does the client with signs of shock.

    **TEST-TAKING HINT: When deciding on an answer for this type of question, the test taker should reason as to which client is stable and which has a potentially higher level of need.**

11. 1. The client with peripheral edema will experience calf tightness but would not have leg

cramping, which is the result of low potassium levels. The timing of the diuretic will not change the side effect of leg cramping resulting from low potassium levels.

2. **The most probable cause of the leg cramping is potassium excretion as a result of diuretic medication. Bananas and orange juice are foods that are high in potassium.**

3. Weight gain is monitored in clients with CHF and elevating the legs would decrease peripheral edema by increasing the rate of return to the central circulation, but these interventions would not help with leg cramps.

4. Ambulating frequently and performing leg stretching exercises will not be effective in alleviating the leg cramps.

**TEST-TAKING HINT: The timing "at night" in this question was not important in answering the question, but it could have made the test taker jump at option "1." Be sure to read all answer options before deciding on an answer. Answering this question correctly requires knowledge of the side effects of treatments used for CHF.**

12. 1. Measuring the intake and output is an appropriate intervention to implement for a client with CHF, but it does not address getting the client to tolerate activity.

2. Dietary sodium is restricted in clients with CHF, but this is an intervention for decreasing fluid volume, not for increasing tolerance for activity.

3. Daily weighing monitors fluid volume status, not activity tolerance.

4. **Scheduling activities and rest periods allows the client to participate in his or her own care and addresses the desired outcome.**

**TEST-TAKING HINT: With questions involving nursing diagnoses or goals and outcomes, the test taker should realize that all activities referred to in the answer options may be appropriate for the disease but may not be specific for the desired outcome.**

## Angina/Myocardial Infarction

13. 1. CPK-MB elevates in 12 to 24 hours.
2. LDH elevates in 24 to 36 hours.
3. **Troponin is the enzyme that elevates within 1 to 2 hours.**
4. WBC elevates as a result of necrotic tissue, but this is not a cardiac enzyme.

**TEST-TAKING HINT: The test taker should be aware of the words "cardiac enzyme," which**

would eliminate "d" as a possible answer. The word in the stem is "first." This is a knowledge-based question.

14. 1. Mid-epigastric pain would support a diagnosis of peptic ulcer disease; pyrosis is belching.

2. **Sweating is a systemic reaction to the MI. The body vasoconstricts to shunt blood from the periphery to the trunk of the body; this, in turn, leads to cold, clammy skin.**

3. Intermittent claudication is leg pain secondary to decreased oxygen to the muscle, and pallor is paleness of the skin as a result of decreased blood supply. Neither is an early sign of MI.

4. Jugular vein distension (JVD) and dependent edema are signs/symptoms of congestive heart failure, not of MI.

**TEST-TAKING HINT: The stem already addresses chest pain; therefore, the test taker could eliminate answer option "1" as a possible answer. Intermittent claudication, "3," is the classic sign of arterial occlusive disease, and JVD is very specific to congestive heart failure. The nurse must be able to identify at least two or three signs/symptoms of disease processes.**

15. 1. The nurse must assume the chest pain is secondary to decreased oxygen to the myocardium and administer a sublingual nitroglycerin, which is a coronary vasodilator, but this is not the first action.

2. An ECG should be ordered, but it is not the first intervention.

3. **Stopping all activity will decrease the need of the myocardium for oxygen and may help decrease the chest pain.**

4. Assessment is often the first nursing intervention, but when the client has chest pain and a possible MI, the nurse must first take care of the client. Taking vital signs would not help relieve chest pain.

**TEST-TAKING HINT: Whenever the test taker wants to select an assessment intervention, be sure to think about whether that intervention will help the client, especially if the client is experiencing pain. Do not automatically select the answer option that is assessment.**

16. 1. Morphine should be administered intravenously, not intramuscularly.

2. **Aspirin is an antiplatelet medication and should be administered orally.**

3. **Oxygen will help decrease myocardial ischemia, thereby decreasing pain.**

4. **The supine position will increase respiratory effort, which will increase myocardial oxygen consumption; the client should be in a semi-Fowler's position.**

5. Nitroglycerin, a coronary vasodilator, is administered sublingually, not subcutaneously.

**TEST-TAKING HINT:** This is an alternate-type question that requires the test taker to select all options that are applicable. The test taker must correctly identify all correct answers to receive credit for a correct answer; no partial credit is given. Remember to read the question carefully—it is not meant to be tricky.

17. 1. The social worker addresses financial concerns or referrals after discharge, which is not indicated for this client.
    2. Physical therapy addresses gait problems, lower-extremity strength building, and assisting with transfer, which is not required for this client.
    3. Cardiac rehabilitation is the most appropriate referral. The client can start rehabilitation in the hospital and then attend an outpatient cardiac rehabilitation, which includes progressive exercise, diet teaching, and classes on modifying risk factors.
    4. Occupational therapy addresses the client in regaining activities of daily living and covers mainly fine motor activities.

**TEST-TAKING HINT:** The test taker must be familiar with the responsibilities of the other members of the health-care team. If the test taker had no idea which would be the most appropriate referral, the word "cardiac," which means "heart," should help the test taker in deciding that this is the most sensible option because the client had a myocardial infarction, a heart attack.

18. 1. The nurse should medicate the client as needed, but it is not the first intervention.
    2. The nurse must always assess the client to determine if the chest pain that is occurring is expected postoperatively or if it is a complication of the surgery.
    3. Turning will help decrease complications from immobility, such as pneumonia, but it will not help relieve the client's pain.
    4. The nurse, not a machine, should always take care of the client.

**TEST-TAKING HINT:** The stem asks the nurse to identify the first intervention that should be implemented. Therefore, the test taker should apply the nursing process and select an assessment intervention. Both options "2" and "4" involve assessment, but the nurse should always assess the client, not a machine or diagnostic test.

19. 1. After PTCA, the client must keep the right leg straight for at least six (6) to eight (8) hours to prevent any arterial bleeding from the insertion site in the right femoral artery.
    2. A pressure dressing is applied to the insertion site to help prevent arterial bleeding.
    3. Any neurovascular assessment data that are abnormal require intervention by the nurse; numbness may indicate decreased blood supply to the right foot.
    4. A bounding pedal pulse indicates that adequate circulation is getting to the right foot; therefore, this would not require immediate intervention.

**TEST-TAKING HINT:** This question requires the test taker to identify abnormal, unexpected, or life-threatening data. The nurse must know that a PTCA is performed by placing a catheter in the femoral artery and that internal or external bleeding is the most common complication.

20. 1. An S3 indicates left ventricular failure and should be reported to the health-care provider. It is a potential life-threatening complication of a myocardial infarction.
    2. Elevating the head of the bed will not do anything to help a failing heart.
    3. This is not a normal finding; it indicates heart failure.
    4. Morphine is administered for chest pain, not for heart failure, which is suggested by the S3 sound.

**TEST-TAKING HINT:** There are some situations in which the nurse must notify the health-care provider, and the test taker should not automatically eliminate this as a possible correct answer. The test taker must decide if any of the other three options will help correct a life-threatening complication. Normal assessment concepts should help identify the correct option. The normal heart sounds are S1, S2 "lub-dub," S3 is abnormal.

21. 1. The apical pulse is within normal limits—60 to 100 beats per minute.
    2. The serum calcium level is not monitored when calcium channel blockers are given.
    3. Occasional PVCs would not warrant immediate intervention prior to administering this medication.
    4. The client's blood pressure is low, and a calcium channel blocker would cause the blood pressure to bottom out.

**TEST-TAKING HINT:** The test taker must know when to question administering medications. The test taker is trying to select an option that, if the medication is administered, would cause serious harm to the client.

22. 1. Leg movement is an appropriate action, and the assistant should not be told to stop encouraging it.
    2. This behavior is not unsafe or dangerous and should not be reported to the charge nurse.
    3. The nurse should praise and encourage assistants to participate in the client's care. Clients on bed rest are at risk for deep vein thrombosis, and moving the legs will help prevent that.
    4. The nurse should praise subordinates for appropriate behavior, especially when it is helping to prevent life-threatening complications.

    TEST-TAKING HINT: This is a management question. The test taker must know the chain of command and when to report behavior. The test taker could eliminate "1" and "2" when acknowledging that moving legs is a safe activity for the client. When having to choose between "3" and "4" the test taker should select doing something positive, instead of taking no action. This is a management concept.

23. 1. The heart tissue is dead, stress or activity may cause heart failure, and it does take about six (6) weeks for scar tissue to form.
    2. The nurse should talk to the client in layman's terms, not medical terms. Medical terminology is a foreign language to most clients.
    3. This is not answering the client's question. The nurse should take any opportunity to teach the client.
    4. This is a condescending response, and telling the client that he or she is not out of danger is not an appropriate response.

    TEST-TAKING HINT: When attempting to answer a client's question, the nurse should provide factual information in simple, understandable terms. The test taker should select the answer option that provides this type of information.

24. 1. These vital signs are within normal limits and would not require any immediate intervention.
    2. The groin dressing should be dry and intact.
    3. If the client bends the leg, it could cause the insertion site to bleed. This is arterial blood and the client could bleed to death very quickly, so this requires immediate intervention.
    4. The nurse must check the neurovascular assessment, and paresthesia would warrant immediate intervention, but no numbness and tingling is a good sign.

    TEST-TAKING HINT: "Warrants immediate intervention" means the nurse should proba-

bly notify the health-care provider or do something independently because a complication may occur. Therefore, the test taker must select an answer option that is abnormal or unsafe. In the data listed, there are three normal findings and one abnormal finding.

## Coronary Artery Disease

25. 1. If the tablets are not kept in a dark bottle, they will lose their potency.
    2. The tablets should burn or sting when put under the tongue.
    3. The client should keep the tablets with him in case of chest pain.
    4. The client should take one tablet every five (5) minutes and, if no relief occurs after the third tablet, have someone drive him to the emergency department or call 911.

    TEST-TAKING HINT: This question is an "except" question, requiring the test taker to identify which statement indicates the client doesn't understand the teaching. Sometimes the test taker could restate the question and think which statement indicates the client understands the teaching.

26. 1. This is a correct statement presented in layman's terms. When the coronary arteries cannot supply adequate oxygen to the heart muscle, there is chest pain.
    2. This is the explanation in medical terms that should not be used when explaining medical conditions to a client.
    3. This explains congestive heart failure but does not explain why chest pain occurs.
    4. Respiratory compromise occurs when the lungs cannot oxygenate the blood, such as occurs with altered level of consciousness, cyanosis, and increased respiratory rate.

    TEST-TAKING HINT: The nurse must select the option that best explains the facts in terms a client who does not have medical training can understand.

27. 1. The client's right leg should be kept straight to prevent arterial bleeding from the femoral insertion site for the catheter used to perform the catheterization.
    2. The nurse must make sure that blood is circulating to the right leg so the client should be assessed for pulses, paresthesia, paralysis, coldness, and pallor.
    3. The head of the bed should be elevated no more than 10 degrees. The client should be kept on bed rest, flat with the affected extrem-

ity straight, to help decrease the chance of femoral artery bleeding.

4. The gag reflex is assessed if a scope is inserted down the trachea (bronchoscopy) or esophagus (endoscopy) because the throat is numbed when inserting the scope. A catheter is inserted in the femoral or brachial artery when performing a cardiac catheterization.

**TEST-TAKING HINT: The nurse should apply the nursing process when determining the correct answer. Therefore either "2" or "4" could possibly be the correct answer. The test taker then should apply anatomy concepts—where is the left femoral artery? Neurovascular assessment is performed on extremities.**

28. 1. This blood pressure is normal and the nurse would administer the medication.
2. A beta blocker decreases sympathetic stimulation to the heart, thereby decreasing the heart rate. An apical rate less than 60 indicates lower-than-normal heart rate and should make the nurse question administering this medication because it will further decrease the heart rate.
3. A headache will not affect administering the medication to the client.
4. The potassium level is within normal limits, but it is usually not monitored prior to administering a beta blocker.

**TEST-TAKING HINT: If the test taker does not know when to question the use of a certain medication, evaluate the options to determine if any options include abnormal data based on normal parameters. This would make the test taker select "2" because the normal apical pulse on an adult is 60 to 100.**

29. 1. The nurse should always assess the apical pulse, but the pulse is not affected by a loop diuretic.
2. Loop diuretics cause potassium to be lost in the urine output. Therefore, the nurse should assess the client's potassium level, and if the client is hypokalemic, the nurse should question administering this medication.
3. The glucometer provides a glucose level, which is not affected by a loop diuretic.
4. The pulse oximeter reading evaluates peripheral oxygenation and is not affected by a loop diuretic.

**TEST-TAKING HINT: Knowing that diuretics increase urine output would lead the test taker to eliminate glucose level and oxygenation ("3" and "4"). In very few instances does the**

nurse assess the radial pulse; the apical pulse is assessed.

30. 1. A low-fat, low-cholesterol diet will help decrease the buildup of atherosclerosis in the arteries.
2. Walking will help increase collateral circulation.
3. Salt should be restricted in the diet of a client with hypertension, not coronary artery disease.
4. Stress reduction is encouraged for clients with CAD because this helps prevent excess stress on the heart muscle.
5. Increasing fiber in the diet will help remove cholesterol via the gastrointestinal system.

**TEST-TAKING HINT: This is an alternate-type question where the test taker must select all interventions that are applicable to the situation. Coronary artery disease is a common disease and the nurse must be knowledgeable about ways to modify risk factors.**

31. 1. Bowel movements are important, but they are not pertinent to coronary artery disease.
2. Chest x-rays are usually done for respiratory problems, not for coronary artery disease.
3. Sexual activity is a risk factor for angina resulting from coronary artery disease. The client's being elderly should not affect the nurse's assessment of the client's concerns about sexual activity.
4. Weight change is not significant in a client with coronary artery disease.

**TEST-TAKING HINT: Remember if the client is described with an adjective such as "elderly," this may be the key to selecting the correct answer. The nurse must not be judgmental about the elderly, especially about issues concerning sexual activity.**

32. 1. Isometric exercises are weight lifting–type exercises. A client with CAD should perform isotonic exercises, which increase muscle tone, not isometric exercises.
2. The client should walk at least 30 minutes a day to increase collateral circulation.
3. When it is cold outside, vasoconstriction occurs, and this will decrease oxygen to the heart muscle. Therefore, the client should not exercise when it is cold outside.
4. The client should wear good supportive tennis shoes when ambulating, not sandals or other open-toed shoes.

**TEST-TAKING HINT: The test taker should be aware of adjectives such as "isometric," which makes answer option "1" incorrect, and "open-toed," which makes "4" incorrect.**

Cardiac

33. 1. The client should take the coronary vasodilator nitroglycerin sublingually, but it is not the first intervention.
2. **Stopping the activity decreases the heart's need for oxygen and may help decrease the angina, chest pain.**
3. The client should keep a diary of when angina occurs, what activity causes it, and how many tablets are taken before chest pain is relieved.
4. If the chest pain (angina) is not relieved with three (3) nitroglycerin tablets, the client should call 911 or have someone take him to the emergency department. Notifying the HCP may take too long.

**TEST-TAKING HINT: The question is asking which action the client should take first. This implies that more than one of the answer options could be appropriate for the chest pain, but that only one is done first. The test taker should select the answer that will help the client directly and quickly—and that is stopping the activity.**

34. 1. The Holter monitor is a 24-hour electrocardiogram, and the client must keep an accurate record of activity so that the health-care provider can compare the ECG recordings with different levels of activity.
2. The Holter monitor should not be removed for any reason.
3. All medications should be taken as prescribed.
4. The client should perform all activity as usual while wearing the Holter monitor so the HCP can get an accurate account of heart function during a 24-hour period.

**TEST-TAKING HINT: In some instances, the test taker must be knowledgeable about diagnostic test and there are no Test-Taking Hints. The test taker might eliminate "3" by realizing that, unless the client is NPO for a test or surgery, medications are usually taken.**

35. 1. According to the American Heart Association, the client should not eat more than 3 eggs a week, especially the egg yolk.
2. **The American Heart Association recommends a low-fat, low-cholesterol diet for a client with coronary artery disease. The client should avoid any fried foods, especially meats, and bake, boil, or grill any meat.**
3. The client should drink low-fat milk, not whole milk.
4. Pork products (bacon, sausage, ham) are high in sodium, which is prohibited in a low-salt diet, not a low-cholesterol, low-fat diet.

**TEST-TAKING HINT: The test taker must be knowledgeable of prescribed diets for specific**

disease processes. **This is mainly memorizing facts. There is no test-taking hint to help eliminate any of the options.**

36. 1. This client is at high risk for complications related to necrotic myocardial tissue and will need extensive teaching, so this client should not be assigned to a new graduate.
2. Unstable angina means this client is at risk for life-threatening complications and should not be assigned to a new graduate.
3. **A new graduate should be able to complete a pre-procedure checklist and get this client to the catheterization lab.**
4. Chest pain means this client could be having a myocardial infarction and should not be assigned to a new graduate.

**TEST-TAKING HINT: "New graduate" is the key to answering this question correctly. What type of client should be assigned to an inexperienced nurse? The test taker should not assign the new graduate a client who is unstable or at risk for a life-threatening complication.**

## Valvular Heart Disease

37. 1. Dyspnea on exertion (DOE) is typically the earliest manifestation of mitral valve stenosis.
2. Jugular vein distension (JVD) and 3+ pedal edema are signs/symptoms of right-sided heart failure and indicate worsening of the mitral valve stenosis. These signs would not be expected in a client with early manifestations of mitral valve stenosis.
3. Chest pain rarely occurs with mitral valve stenosis.
4. An enlarged liver and edematous abdomen are late signs of right-sided heart failure that can occur with long-term untreated mitral valve stenosis.

**TEST-TAKING HINT: Whenever the test taker reads "rule out," the test taker should look for data that would not indicate a severe condition of the body system that is affected. Chest pain, JVD, and pedal edema are late signs of heart problems.**

38. 1. This would be expected with mitral valve stenosis.
2. **The murmur associated with mitral valve insufficiency is loud, high-pitched, rumbling, and holosystolic (occurring throughout systole) and is heard best at the cardiac apex.**
3. This would be expected with mitral valve prolapse.

4. This would be expected with aortic regurgitation.

**TEST-TAKING HINT: This is a knowledge-based question and there is no test-taking hint to help the test taker rule out distracters.**

39. 1. Prophylactic antibiotics before invasive procedures prevent infectious endocarditis.
2. The client is undergoing anticoagulant therapy and should use a soft-bristle toothbrush to help prevent gum trauma and bleeding.
3. Aspirin and nonsteroidal anti-inflammatory drugs (NSAIDs) interfere with clotting and may potentiate the effects of the anticoagulant therapy, which the client with a mechanical valve will be prescribed. Therefore, the client should not take aspirin daily.
4. The client should alternate rest with activity to prevent fatigue to help decrease the workload of the heart.

**TEST-TAKING HINT: The stem asks the test taker to identify which behavior means the client does not understand the teaching. Therefore, the test taker should select the distracter that does not agree with the condition. There is not any condition that would not recommend alternating rest with activity.**

40. 1. An advantage of having a biologic valve replacement is that no anticoagulant therapy is needed. Anticoagulant therapy is needed with a mechanical valve replacement.
2. This is an advantage of having a biologic valve replacement; infections are harder to treat in clients with mechanical valve replacement.
3. This is an advantage of having a biologic valve replacement; there is a high incidence of thromboembolism in clients with mechanical valve replacement.
4. **Biologic valves deteriorate and need to be replaced frequently; this is a disadvantage of them. Mechanical valves do not deteriorate and do not have to be replaced often.**

**TEST-TAKING HINT: This is an "except" question. The test taker might reverse the question and ask, "Which is an advantage of a biologic valve?"—which might make answering the question easier.**

41. 1. The therapeutic range for most clients' INR is 2–3, but for a client with a mechanical valve replacement it is 2–3.5. The medication should be given as ordered and not withheld.
2. Vitamin K is the antidote for an overdose of warfarin, but 2.7 is within therapeutic range.
3. This laboratory result is within the therapeutic range, INR 2–3, and the medication does not need to be withheld.

4. There is no need for the nurse to assess for bleeding because 2.7 is within therapeutic range.

**TEST-TAKING HINT: The test taker has to know the therapeutic range for INR to be able to answer this question correctly. The test taker should keep a list of normal and therapeutic laboratory values that must be remembered.**

42. 1. Paroxysmal nocturnal dyspnea is a sudden attack of respiratory distress usually occurring at night because of the reclining position and occurs in valvular disorders.
2. This is an abnormal condition in which a client must sit or stand to breathe comfortably and occurs in valvular disorders.
3. Coughing occurs when the client with long-term valvular disease has difficulty breathing when walking or performing any type of activity.
4. Pericardial friction rub is a sound auscultated in clients with pericarditis, not valvular heart disease.
5. Pulsus paradoxus is a marked decrease in amplitude during inspiration. It is a sign of cardiac tamponade, not valvular heart disease.

**TEST-TAKING HINT: The test taker should notice that answer options "1," "2," and "3" are all signs/symptoms that have something to do with the lungs. It would be a good choice to select these three as correct answers. They are similar in description.**

43. 1. An acute myocardial infarction can damage heart valves, causing tearing, ischemia, or damage to heart muscles that affects valve leaflet function, but coronary heart disease does not cause valvular heart disease.
2. Valvular heart disease does not show a genetic etiology.
3. Smoking can cause coronary artery disease, but it does not cause valvular heart disease.
4. **Rheumatic heart disease is the most common cause of valvular heart disease.**

**TEST-TAKING HINT: The test taker could rule out option "1" because of knowledge of anatomy: Coronary artery disease has to do with blood supply to heart muscle, whereas the valves are a part of the anatomy of the heart.**

44. 1. Percutaneous balloon valvuloplasty is not an open-heart surgery; therefore, the chest will not be open and the client will not have a chest tube.
2. This is not an open-heart surgery; therefore, the client will not have a chest dressing.
3. The endotracheal (ET) tube is inserted if the client is on a ventilator, and this surgery does not require putting the client on a ventilator.

4. In this invasive procedure, performed in a cardiac catheterization laboratory, the client has a catheter inserted into the femoral artery. Therefore, the client must keep the leg straight to prevent hemorrhaging at the insertion site.

**TEST-TAKING HINT: If the test taker knows that the word percutaneous means via the skin, then the answer options "1" and "2" could be eliminated as possible correct answers.**

45. 1. The client is at risk for developing endocarditis and should take prophylactic antibiotics before any invasive procedure.
    2. Antibiotics have nothing to do with how much the teeth bleed during a cleaning.
    3. Teeth cleaning will not cause the valve to malfunction.
    4. Vegetation develops on valves secondary to bacteria that cause endocarditis, but the client will not understand vegetative growth on the valves; therefore, this is not the most appropriate answer.

**TEST-TAKING HINT: The test taker should select an option that answers the client's question in the easiest and most understandable terms, not in medical jargon. This would cause the test taker to eliminate "4" as a possible correct answer. The test taker should know antibiotics do not affect bleeding and so can eliminate "2."**

46. 1. Fluid intake may be restricted to reduce the cardiac workload and pressures within the heart and pulmonary circuit.
    2. The head of the bed should be elevated to help improve alveolar ventilation.
    3. Oxygen saturation should be no less than 93%; 90% indicates an arterial oxygen saturation of around 60 (normal is 80–100)
    4. Total parenteral nutrition would not be prescribed for a client with mitral valve replacement. It is ordered for clients with malnutrition, gastrointestinal disorders, or conditions in which increased calories are needed, such as burns.

**TEST-TAKING HINT: A client with a heart or lung problem should never have the head of the bed in a flat (supine) position; therefore, "2" should be eliminated as a possible correct answer. The test taker must know normal values for monitoring techniques such as pulse oximeters and keep a list of normal values.**

47. 1. Congestive heart failure does not predispose the female client to having a mitral valve prolapse.
    2. Clients with Marfan syndrome have life-threatening cardiovascular problems, in-

cluding mitral valve prolapse, progressive dilation of the aortic valve ring, and weakness of the arterial walls, and they usually do not live past the age of 40 because of dissection and rupture of the aorta.
    3. Atrial fibrillation does not predispose a client to mitral valve prolapse.
    4. A client with Down syndrome may have congenital heart anomalies but not mitral valve prolapse.

**TEST-TAKING HINT: The test taker could eliminate "1" and "3" based on knowledge that these are commonly occurring cardiovascular problems and the nurse should know that possible complications of these problems do not include mitral valve prolapse.**

48. 1. This client requires teaching and an understanding of the pre-procedure interventions for diagnostic tests; therefore a more experienced nurse should be assigned to this client.
    2. Because this client is being discharged, it would be an appropriate assignment for the new graduate.
    3. Supraventricular tachycardia (SVT) is not life threatening, but the client requires intravenous medication and close monitoring and therefore should be assigned to a more experienced nurse.
    4. A client with atrial fibrillation is usually taking the anticoagulant warfarin (Coumadin) and the therapeutic INR is 2–3. An INR of 5 is high and the client is at risk for bleeding.

**TEST-TAKING HINT: The test taker must realize that a new graduate must be assigned the least critical client, remember teaching is a primary responsibility of the nurse; physical care is not always the criteria that should be used when making client assignments.**

## Dysrhythmias and Conduction Problems

49. 1. The telemetry nurse should not leave the monitors unattended at any time.
    2. The telemetry nurse must have someone go assess the client, but this is not the first intervention.
    3. If the client answers the call light and is not experiencing chest pain, then there is probably a monitor artifact, which is not a life-threatening emergency. After talking with the client, send a nurse to the room to check the monitor.
    4. The crash cart should be taken to a room when the client is experiencing a code.

**TEST-TAKING HINT:** When the test taker sees the word "first," he/she must realize that more than one answer option may be a possible intervention but that only one should be implemented first. The test taker should try to determine which intervention directly affects the client.

50. 1. There are many interventions that should be implemented prior to administering medication.
    2. The treatment of choice for ventricular fibrillation is defibrillation, but it is not the first action.
    3. The nurse must call a code that activates the crash cart being brought to the room and a team of health-care providers that will care for the client according to an established protocol.
    4. The first person at the bedside should start cardiopulmonary resuscitation (CPR), but the telemetry nurse should call a code so that all necessary equipment and personnel are at the bedside.

**TEST-TAKING HINT:** The test taker must realize that ventricular fibrillation is life threatening and immediate action must be implemented. Remember that when the question asks "first," all options could be appropriate interventions, but only one should be implemented first.

51. 1. Lidocaine suppresses ventricular ectopy and is the drug of choice for ventricular dysrhythmias.
    2. Atropine decreases vagal stimulation and is the drug of choice for asystole.
    3. Digoxin slows heart rate and increases cardiac contractility and is the drug of choice for atrial fibrillation.
    4. Adenosine is the drug of choice for supraventricular tachycardia.

**TEST-TAKING HINT:** This is a knowledge-based question and the test taker must know the answer. The nurse must know what medications treat specific dysrhythmias.

52. 1. A thrombolytic medication is administered for a client experiencing a myocardial infarction.
    2. Assessment is an independent nursing action, not a collaborative treatment.
    3. The client is symptomatic and will require a pacemaker.
    4. Synchronized cardioversion is used for ventricular tachycardia with a pulse or atrial fibrillation.

**TEST-TAKING HINT:** The key to answering this question is the adjective "collaborative," which means requires obtaining a health-care provider's order or working with another member of the health-care team. This would cause the test taker to eliminate "2" as a possible correct answer.

53. 1. The client should be defibrillated at 200, 300, and 360 joules.
    2. The oxygen source should be removed to prevent any type of spark during defibrillation.
    3. The nurse should use defibrillator pads or defibrillator gel to prevent any type of skin burns while defibrillating the client.
    4. If any member of the health-care team is touching the client or the bed during defibrillation, that person could possibly be shocked. Therefore, the nurse should shout "all clear."

**TEST-TAKING HINT:** The test taker should always consider the safety of the client and the health-care team. Options "2" and "3" put the client at risk for injury during defibrillation.

54. 1. A client with chronic atrial fibrillation will be taking an anticoagulant to help prevent clot formation. Therefore, the client is at risk for bleeding and should be instructed to use a soft-bristle toothbrush.
    2. The client will need a monthly INR to determine the therapeutic level for the anticoagulant warfarin (Coumadin); PTT levels are monitored for heparin.
    3. A client with symptomatic sinus bradycardia, not a client with atrial fibrillation, may need a pacemaker.
    4. Synchronized cardioversion may be prescribed for new-onset atrial fibrillation but not for chronic atrial fibrillation.

**TEST-TAKING HINT:** The key to answering this question is the adjective "chronic." The test taker must know that HCPs prescribe anticoagulant therapy for clients with chronic atrial fibrillation.

55. 1. Lidocaine is the drug of choice for ventricular tachycardia, but it is not the first intervention.
    2. Defibrillation may be needed, but it is not the first intervention.
    3. The nurse must assess the apical pulse and blood pressure to determine if the client is in cardiac arrest and then treat as ventricular defibrillation. If the client's heart is beating, the nurse would then administer lidocaine.
    4. CPR is only performed on a client who is not breathing and does not have a pulse. The nurse must establish if this is occurring first, prior to taking any other action.

**TEST-TAKING HINT:** When the stem asks the test taker to select the first intervention, all answer options could be plausible interventions, but only one is implemented first. The test taker should use the nursing process to answer the question and select the intervention that addresses assessment, which is the first step in the nursing process.

56. 1. A pacemaker will have to be inserted, but it is not the first intervention.
    2. Atropine will decrease vagal stimulation and increase the heart rate. Therefore, it is the first intervention.
    3. A STAT ECG may be done, but the telemetry reading shows complete heart block, which is a life-threatening dysrhythmia and must be treated.
    4. The HCP will need to be notified but not prior to administering a medication. The test taker must assume the nurse has the order to administer medication. Many telemetry departments have standing protocols.

**TEST-TAKING HINT:** The test taker must select the intervention that should be implemented first and will directly affect the dysrhythmia. Medication is the first intervention, and then pacemaker insertion. The test taker should not eliminate an option because he/she thinks there is not an order by a health-care provider.

57. 1. Ventricular fibrillation indicates the client does not have a heartbeat. Therefore CPR should be instituted.
    2. Adenosine, an antidysrhythmic, is the drug of choice for supraventricular tachycardia, not for ventricular fibrillation.
    3. Defibrillation is the treatment of choice for ventricular fibrillation.
    4. The crash cart has the defibrillator and is used when performing advanced cardiopulmonary resuscitation.
    5. Amiodarone is an antidysrhythmic that is used in ventricular dysrhythmias.

**TEST-TAKING HINT:** This is an alternate-type question that requires the test taker to possibly select more that one option. To receive credit, the test taker must select all correct options; partial credit is not given for these type questions.

58. 1. The telemetry reading is accurate, and there is no need for the client to assess the client heart rate.
    2. There is no reason to notify the surgeon for a client exhibiting sinus tachycardia.
    3. Synchronized cardioversion is prescribed for clients in acute atrial fibrillation or ventricular fibrillation with a pulse.
    4. Sinus tachycardia means the sino-atrial node is the pacemaker, but the rate is greater than 100 because of pain, anxiety, or fever. The nurse must determine the cause and treat appropriately. There is no specific medication for sinus tachycardia.

**TEST-TAKING HINT:** The test taker must use the nursing process to determine the correct option and select an option that addresses assessment, the first step of the nursing process. Because both "1" and "4" address assessment, the test taker must determine which option is more appropriate. How will taking the apical pulse help treat sinus tachycardia? Determining the cause for sinus tachycardia is the most appropriate intervention.

59. 1. The P-wave represents atrial contraction, and the QRS complex represents ventricular contraction—a normal telemetry reading. A rate between 60 and 100 indicates normal sinus rhythm. Therefore, the nurse should document this as normal sinus rhythm and not take any action.
    2. A 12-lead ECG should be requested for chest pain or abnormal dysrhythmias.
    3. Digoxin is used to treat atrial fibrillation.
    4. Cardiac enzymes are monitored to determine if the client has had a myocardial infarction. Nothing in the stem indicates the client has had an MI.

**TEST-TAKING HINT:** The test taker must know normal sinus rhythm and there are no Test-Taking Hints to help eliminate incorrect options. The test taker should not automatically select assessment as the correct answer, but if the test taker had no idea of the answer, remember assessment of laboratory data is not the same as assessing the client.

60. 1. Not every cardiac dysrhythmia causes alteration in comfort; angina is caused by decreased oxygen to the myocardium.
    2. Any abnormal electrical activity of the heart causes decreased cardiac output.
    3. Impaired gas exchange is the result of pulmonary complications, not cardiac dysrhythmias.
    4. Not all clients with cardiac dysrhythmias have activity intolerance.

**TEST-TAKING HINT:** Answer option "2" has the word "cardiac," which refers to the heart. Therefore, even if the test taker had no idea what the correct answer was, this would be an appropriate option. The test taker should use medical terminology to help identify the correct option.

## Inflammatory Cardiac Disorders

61. 1. Pulsus paradoxus is the hallmark of cardiac tamponade; a paradoxical pulse is markedly decreased in amplitude during inspiration.
    2. Fatigue and arthralgias are nonspecific signs/symptoms that usually occur with myocarditis.
    3. Petechiae on the trunk, conjunctiva, and mucous membranes and hemorrhagic streaks under the fingernails or toenails occur with endocarditis.
    4. **Chest pain is the most common symptom of pericarditis, usually has an abrupt onset, and is aggravated by respiratory movements (deep inspiration, coughing), changes in body position, and swallowing.**

    **TEST-TAKING HINT: The test taker who has no idea what the answer is should apply the test-taking strategy of asking which body system is affected. In this case, it is the cardiac system, specifically the outside of the heart. The test taker should select the option that has something to do with the heart, which is either "1" or "4."**

62. 1. **Acute pericardial effusion interferes with normal cardiac filling and pumping, causing venous congestion and decreased cardiac output. Muffled heart sounds, indicative of acute pericarditis, must be reported to the health-care provider.**
    2. Distended, not nondistended, jugular veins would warrant immediate intervention.
    3. Decreasing quality of peripheral pulses, not bounding peripheral pulses, would warrant immediate intervention.
    4. A pericardial friction rub is a classic symptom of acute pericarditis, but it would not warrant immediate intervention.

    **TEST-TAKING HINT: The test taker must understand what the question is asking. "Warrants" is a word that should make the test taker think that the correct answer will be something "bad," so the test taker should look for abnormal data; this would cause the test taker to eliminate "2" and "3."**

63. 1. A sore throat in the last month would not support the diagnosis of carditis.
    2. **Rheumatic fever, a systemic inflammatory disease caused by an abnormal immune response to pharyngeal infection by group A beta-hemolytic streptococci, causes carditis in about 50% of the people.**

3. Carditis is not a genetic or congenital disease process.
4. This is an appropriate question to ask any client, but OTC medications do not cause carditis.

**TEST-TAKING HINT: This is a knowledge-based question, but the test taker could eliminate "4" realizing this is a question to ask any client, and the stem asks which question will support the diagnosis of carditis.**

64. 1. Steroids, such as prednisone, not NSAIDs, must be tapered off to prevent adrenal insufficiency.
    2. NSAIDs will not make clients drowsy.
    3. **NSAIDs must be taken with food, milk, or antacids to help decrease gastric distress. NSAIDs reduce fever, inflammation, and pericardial pain.**
    4. NSAIDs should be taken regularly around the clock to help decrease inflammation, which, in turn, will decrease pain.

    **TEST-TAKING HINT: The test taker must remember that NSAIDs and steroids cause gastric distress to the point of causing peptic ulcer disease. These medications are administered for a variety of conditions and diseases.**

65. 1. Oxygen may be needed, but it is not the first intervention.
    2. This would be appropriate to determine if the urine output is at least 30 mL/hr, but it is not the first intervention.
    3. **The nurse must assess the client to determine if the pain is expected pain secondary to pericarditis or if the pain is indicative of a complication that requires intervention from the health-care provider.**
    4. Using the incentive spirometer will increase the client's alveolar ventilation and help prevent atelectasis, but it is not the first intervention.

    **TEST-TAKING HINT: The test taker must apply the nursing process when determining the correct answer and select the option that addresses the first step in the nursing process—assessment.**

66. 1. **A pericardiocentesis removes fluid from the pericardial sac and is the emergency treatment for cardiac tamponade.**
    2. Cardiac enzymes may be slightly elevated because of the inflammatory process, but evaluation of these would not be ordered to treat or evaluate cardiac tamponade.
    3. A 12-lead ECG would not help treat the medical emergency of cardiac tamponade.
    4. Assessment by the nurse is not collaborative; it is an independent nursing action.

**TEST-TAKING HINT: Collaborative means another member of the health-care team must order or participate in the intervention. Therefore "4" could be deleted as a possible correct answer.**

67. 1. The full course of antibiotics must be taken to help ensure complete destruction of streptococcal infection.
  2. Antibiotics kill bacteria but also destroy normal body flora in the vagina, bowel, and mouth, leading to a superinfection.
  3. Even with antibiotic treatment for rheumatic fever, the client may experience bacterial endocarditis in later years and should know this may occur.
  4. A throat culture is taken to diagnose group A beta hemolytic streptococcus and is positive in 25%–40% of clients with acute rheumatic fever.

**TEST-TAKING HINT: The question is asking the test taker to identify which statement indicates the client does not understand the teaching; this is an "except" question. The test taker can ask which statement indicates the teaching is effective and choose the one option that is not appropriate.**

68. 1. Pulmonary embolus would occur with an embolization of vegetative lesions from the tricuspid valve on the right side of the heart.
  2. Bacteria enter the bloodstream from invasive procedures and sterile platelet-fibrin vegetation forms on heart valves. The mitral valve is on the left side of the heart and, if the vegetation breaks off, it will go through the left ventricle into the systemic circulation and may lodge in the brain, kidneys, or peripheral tissues.
  3. Coughing up blood (hemoptysis) occurs when the vegetation breaks off the tricuspid valve in the right side of the heart and enters the pulmonary artery.
  4. Deep vein thrombosis is a complication of immobility, not of a vegetative embolus from the left side of the heart.

**TEST-TAKING HINT: If the test taker does not know the answer, knowledge of anatomy may help determine the answer. The mitral valve is on the left side of the heart and any emboli would not enter the lung first, thereby eliminating "1" and "3" as possible correct answers.**

69. 1. Anxiety is a psychosocial nursing diagnosis, which is not a priority over a physiological nursing diagnosis.
  2. Antibiotic therapy does not result in injury to the client.

3. Myocarditis does not result in valve damage (endocarditis does), and there would be decreased, not increased, cardiac output.
  4. Activity intolerance is priority for the client with myocarditis, an inflammation of the heart muscle. Nursing care is aimed at decreasing myocardial work and maintaining cardiac output.

**TEST-TAKING HINT: If the test taker has no idea which is the correct answer, then "myo," which refers to muscle, and "card," which refers to the heart, should lead the test taker to the only option, which has both muscle and heart in it, option "4."**

70. 1. Uninterrupted rest and sleep help decrease the workload of the heart and help ensure the restoration of physical and emotional health.
  2. Occupational therapy addresses activities of daily living. The client should be referred to physical therapy to develop a realistic and progressive plan of activity.
  3. The client with pericarditis is not usually prescribed oxygen and 2 L/min is a low dose of oxygen that is prescribed for a client with chronic obstructive pulmonary disease (COPD).
  4. Endocarditis, not pericarditis, may lead to surgery for valve replacement.

**TEST-TAKING HINT: A concept that the test taker must remember with any client being discharged from the hospital should be to alternate rest with activity to avoid problems associated with immobility. If the test taker does not know the answer to a question, using basic concepts is the best option.**

71. 1. The nurse should monitor the vital signs for any client who has just undergone surgery.
  2. A pericardiocentesis involves entering the pericardial sac. Assessing heart and lung sounds involves entering the pericardial sac and allows assessment for cardiac failure.
  3. The pericardial fluid is documented as output.
  4. Evaluating the client's cardiac rhythm allows the nurse to assess for cardiac failure, which is a complication of pericardial centesis.
  5. The client should be in the semi-Fowler's position, not in a flat position, which increases the workload of the heart.

**TEST-TAKING HINT: This is an alternate-type question that requires the test taker to select possibly more than one option as a correct answer.**

**72.** 1. The nurse must obtain blood cultures prior to administering antibiotics.
2. **Blood cultures must be done before administering antibiotics so that an adequate number of organisms can be obtained to culture and identify.**
3. An echocardiogram allows visualization of vegetations and evaluation of valve function. However, antibiotic therapy is priority before diagnostic tests, and blood cultures must be obtained before administering medication.

4. Bed rest should be implemented, but the first intervention should be obtaining blood cultures so that antibiotic therapy can be started as soon as possible.

**TEST-TAKING HINT: The test taker must identify the first HCP's order to be implemented. Infective should indicate that this is an infection, which requires antibiotics, but the nurse should always assess for allergies and obtain cultures prior to administering any antibiotic.**

1. Which population is at a higher risk for dying from a myocardial infarction?
   1. Caucasian males.
   2. Hispanic females.
   3. Asian males.
   4. African American females.

2. Which pre-procedure information should be taught to the female client having an exercise stress test in the morning?
   1. Wear open-toed shoes to the stress test.
   2. Inform the client not to wear a bra.
   3. Do not eat anything for four (4) hours.
   4. Take the beta blocker one (1) hour before the test.

3. Which intervention should the nurse implement with the client diagnosed with dilated cardiomyopathy?
   1. Keep the client in the supine position with the legs elevated.
   2. Discuss a heart transplant, which is the definitive treatment.
   3. Prepare the client for coronary artery bypass graft.
   4. Teach the client to take a calcium-channel blocker in the morning.

4. Which medical client problem should the nurse include in the plan of care for a client diagnosed with cardiomyopathy?
   1. Heart failure.
   2. Activity intolerance.
   3. Powerlessness.
   4. Anticipatory grieving.

5. The client has an implantable cardioverter defibrillator (ICD). Which discharge instructions should the nurse teach the client?
   1. Do not lift or carry more than 23 kg.
   2. Have someone drive the car for the rest of your life.
   3. Carry the cell phone on the opposite side of the ICD.
   4. Avoid using the microwave oven in the home.

6. To what area should the nurse place the stethoscope to best auscultate the apical pulse?

   1. A
   2. B
   3. C
   4. D

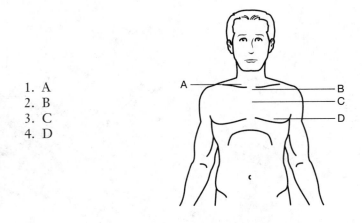

7. The telemetry nurse notes a peaked T-wave for the client diagnosed with congestive heart failure. Which laboratory data should the nurse assess?
   1. CPK-M2.
   2. Troponin.
   3. BNP (beta-type natriuretic peptide).
   4. Potassium.

Cardiac

8. The client comes to the emergency department saying, "I am having a heart attack." Which question is most pertinent when assessing the client?
   1. "Can you describe your chest pain?"
   2. "What were you doing when the pain started?"
   3. "Did you have a high-fat meal today?"
   4. "Does the pain get worse when you lie down?"

9. The client with coronary artery disease is prescribed transdermal nitroglycerin, a coronary vasodilator. Which behavior indicates the client understands the discharge teaching concerning this medication?
   1. The client places the medication under the tongue.
   2. The client removes the old patch before placing the new.
   3. The client applies the patch to a hairy area.
   4. The client changes the patch every 36 hours.

10. Which client would most likely be misdiagnosed for having a myocardial infarction?
    1. A 55-year-old Caucasian male with crushing chest pain and diaphoresis.
    2. A 60-year-old Native American male with an elevated troponin level.
    3. A 40-year-old Hispanic female with a normal electrocardiogram.
    4. An 80-year-old Peruvian female with a normal CPK-MB at 12 hours.

11. Which meal would indicate the client understands the discharge teaching concerning the recommended diet for coronary artery disease?
    1. Baked fish, steamed broccoli, and garden salad.
    2. Enchilada dinner with fried rice and refried beans.
    3. Tuna salad sandwich on white bread and whole milk.
    4. Fried chicken, mashed potatoes, and gravy.

12. The unlicensed nursing assistant comes and tells the primary nurse that the client diagnosed with coronary artery disease is having chest pain. Which action should the nurse take first?
    1. Tell the assistant to go take the client's vital signs.
    2. Ask the assistant to have the telemetry nurse read the strip.
    3. Notify the client's health-care provider.
    4. Go to the room and assess the client's chest pain.

13. Which interventions should the nurse discuss with the client diagnosed with coronary artery disease? Select all that apply.
    1. Instruct the client to stop smoking.
    2. Encourage the client to exercise three (3) days a week.
    3. Teach about coronary vasodilators.
    4. Prepare client for a carotid endarterectomy.
    5. Eat foods high in monosaturated fats.

14. Which laboratory data confirm the diagnosis of congestive heart failure?
    1. Chest x-ray (CXR).
    2. Liver function tests.
    3. Blood urea nitrogen (BUN).
    4. Beta-type natriuretic peptide (BNP).

15. What is the priority problem in the client diagnosed with congestive heart failure?
    1. Fluid volume overload.
    2. Decreased cardiac output.
    3. Activity intolerance.
    4. Knowledge deficit.

16. Which data would cause the nurse to question administering digoxin to a client diagnosed with congestive heart failure?
    1. The potassium level is 3.2 mEq/L.
    2. The digoxin level is 1.2 mcg/mL.
    3. The client's apical pulse is 64.
    4. The client denies yellow haze.

17. The nurse is caring for clients on a cardiac floor. Which client should the nurse assess first?
    1. The client with three (3) unifocal PVCs in a minute.
    2. The client diagnosed with coronary artery disease that wants to ambulate.
    3. The client diagnosed with mitral valve prolapse with an audible S3.
    4. The client diagnosed with pericarditis that is in normal sinus rhythm.

18. The nurse is told in report that the client has aortic stenosis. Which anatomical position should the nurse auscultate to assess the murmur?
    1. Second intercostal space, right sternal notch.
    2. Erb's point.
    3. Second intercostal space, left sternal notch.
    4. Fourth intercostal space, left sternal border.

19. The nurse is caring for a client who goes into ventricular tachycardia. Which intervention should the nurse implement first?
    1. Call a code immediately.
    2. Assess the client for a pulse.
    3. Begin chest compressions.
    4. Continue to monitor the client.

20. The nurse is assisting with a synchronized cardioversion on a client in atrial fibrillation. When the machine is activated, there is a pause. What action should the nurse take?
    1. Wait until the machine discharges.
    2. Shout "all clear" and don't touch the bed.
    3. Make sure the client is all right.
    4. Increase the joules and redischarge.

21. The client is diagnosed with pericarditis. When assessing the client, the nurse is unable to auscultate a friction rub. Which action should the nurse implement?
    1. Notify the health-care provider.
    2. Document that the pericarditis has resolved.
    3. Ask the client to lean forward and listen again.
    4. Prepare to insert a unilateral chest tube.

22. The nurse assessing the client with pericardial effusion at 1600 notes the apical pulse is 72 and the BP is 138/94. At 1800, the client has neck vein distention, the apical pulse is 70, and the BP is 106/94. Which action would the nurse implement first?
    1. Stay with the client and use a calm voice.
    2. Notify the health-care provider immediately.
    3. Place the client left lateral recumbent.
    4. Administer morphine intravenous push slowly.

23. The client is admitted to the emergency department, and the nurse suspects a cardiac problem. Which assessment interventions should the nurse implement? Select all that apply.
    1. Obtain a mid-stream urine specimen.
    2. Attach telemetry monitor to the client.
    3. Start a saline lock in the right arm.
    4. Draw a basic metabolic panel (BMP).
    5. Request an order for a STAT 12-lead ECG.

24. The client is three (3) hours post-myocardial infarction. Which data would warrant immediate intervention by the nurse?
    1. Bilateral peripheral pulses two (2) +.
    2. The pulse oximeter reading is 96%.
    3. The urine output is 240 mL in the last four (4) hours.
    4. Cool, clammy, diaphoretic skin.

25. The nurse is transcribing the doctor's orders for a client with congestive heart failure. The order reads 2.5 mg of Lanoxin daily. Which action should the nurse implement?
    1. Discuss the order with the health-care provider.
    2. Take the client's apical pulse rate before administering.
    3. Check the client's potassium level before giving the medication.
    4. Determine if a digoxin level has been drawn.

26. The nurse is teaching basic cardiopulmonary resuscitation (CPR) to individuals in the community. Which is the order of basic CPR? List in order of performance.
    1. Perform head tilt chin lift.
    2. Give two (2) rescue breaths.
    3. Look, listen, and feel for breathing.
    4. Begin cardiac compressions.
    5. Shake and shout.

1. 1. Caucasian males have a high rate of coronary artery disease, but they do not delay seeking health care as long as some other ethnic groups. The average delay time is five (5) hours.
   2. Hispanic females are at higher risk for diabetes than for dying from a myocardial infarction.
   3. Asian males have fewer cardiovascular events, which is attributed to their diet, which is high in fiber and omega-3 fatty acids.
   4. **African American females are 35% more likely to die from coronary artery disease than any other population. This population has significantly higher rates of hypertension and it occurs at a younger age. The higher risk of death from an MI is also attributed to a delay in seeking emergency care—an average of 11 hours.**

2. 1. The client should wear firm-fitting, solid athletic shoes.
   2. The client should wear a bra to provide adequate support during the exercise.
   3. **NPO decreases the chance of aspiration in case of emergency. In addition, if the client has just had a meal, the blood supply will be shunted to the stomach for digestion and away from the heart, perhaps leading to an inaccurate test result.**
   4. A beta blocker is not taken prior to the stress test because it will decrease the pulse rate and blood pressure by direct parasympathetic stimulation to the heart.

3. 1. Most clients with dilated cardiomyopathy prefer to sit up with their legs in dependent position. This position causes pooling of blood in the periphery and reduces preload.
   2. **Without a heart transplant, this client will end up in end-stage heart failure. A transplant is the only treatment for a client with dilated cardiomyopathy.**
   3. A bypass is the treatment of choice for a client with occluded coronary arteries.
   4. Calcium-channel blockers are contraindicated in clients with dilated cardiomyopathy because they interfere with the contractility of the heart.

4. 1. **Medical client problems indicate the nurse and the physician must collaborate to care for the client; the client must have medications for heart failure.**
   2. The nurse can instruct the client to pace activities and can teach about rest versus activity without a physician's order.
   3. This is a psychosocial client problem that does not require a physician's order to effectively care for the client.

4. Anticipatory grieving involves the nurse addressing issues that will occur based on the knowledge of the poor prognosis of this disease.

5. 1. Clients should not lift more than 5–10 pounds because it puts a strain on the heart, 23 kg is more than 50 pounds.
   2. There may be driving restrictions, but the client should be able to drive independently.
   3. **Cell phones may interfere with the functioning of the ICD if they are placed too close to it.**
   4. Microwave ovens should not cause problems with the ICD.

6. 1. This is the best place to auscultate the aortic valve, the second intercostal right sternal notch.
   2. This is the best place to auscultate the pulmonic valve, the second intercostal space left sternal notch.
   3. This is the best place to auscultate the tricuspid valve, the third intercostal space left sternal border.
   4. **The best place to auscultate the apical pulse is over the mitral valve area, which is the fifth intercostal space midclavicular line.**

7. 1. CPK-MB is assessed to determine if the client has had a myocardial infarction. The electrical activity of the heart will not be affected by elevation of this enzyme.
   2. Troponin is assessed to determine if the client has had a myocardial infarction. The electrical activity of the heart will not be affected by elevation of this enzyme.
   3. BNP is elevated in clients with congestive heart failure, but it does not affect the electrical activity of the heart.
   4. **Hyperkalemia will cause a peaked T-wave; therefore, the nurse should check this laboratory data.**

8. 1. **The chest pain for an MI usually is described as an elephant sitting on the chest or a belt squeezing the substernal mid-chest, often radiating to the jaw or left arm.**
   2. This helps to identify if it is angina (resulting from activity) or MI (not necessarily brought on by activity).
   3. Learning about a client's intake of a high-fat meal would help the nurse to identify a gallbladder attack.
   4. This is a question that the nurse might ask the client with reflux esophagitis.

9. 1. The client does not understand how to apply this medication; it is placed on the skin, not under the tongue.

2. This behavior indicates the client understands the discharge teaching.
3. The patch needs to be in a nonhairy place so that it makes good contact with the skin.
4. The patch should be changed every 12 or 24 hours but never every two (2) hours. It takes two (2) hours for the patch to warm up and begin delivering the optimum dose of medication.

10. 1. Crushing pain and sweating are classic signs of an MI and should not be misdiagnosed.
2. An elevated troponin level is a benchmark in diagnosing an MI and should not be misdiagnosed.
3. **The clients who are misdiagnosed concerning MIs usually present with atypical symptoms. They tend to be female, be younger than 55 years old, be members of a minority group, and have normal electrocardiograms.**
4. CPK-MB may not elevate until up to 24 hours after onset of chest pain.

11. 1. **The recommended diet for CAD is low fat, low cholesterol, and high fiber. The diet described is a diet that is low in fat and cholesterol.**
2. This is a diet very high in fat and cholesterol.
3. The word "salad" implies something has been mixed with the tuna, usually mayonnaise, which is high in fat, but even if the test taker did not know this, white bread is low in fiber and whole milk is high in fat.
4. Meats should be baked, broiled, or grilled—not fried. Gravy is high in fat.

12. 1. The client with CAD who is having chest pain is unstable and requires further judgment to determine appropriate actions to take, and the assistant does not have that knowledge.
2. The assistant could go ask the telemetry nurse, but this is not the first action.
3. The client's HCP may need to be notified, but this is not the first intervention.
4. **Assessment is the first step in the nursing process and should be implemented first; chest pain is priority.**

13. 1. **Smoking is the one risk factor that must be stopped totally; there is no compromise.**
2. **Exercising helps develop collateral circulation and decrease anxiety; it also helps clients to lose weight.**
3. **Clients with coronary artery disease are usually prescribed nitroglycerin, which is the treatment of choice for angina.**
4. Carotid endarterectomy is a procedure to

remove atherosclerotic plaque from the carotid arteries, not the coronary arteries.
5. The client should eat polyunsaturated fats, not monosaturated fats, to help decrease atherosclerosis.

14. 1. The CXR will show an enlarged heart, but it is not used to confirm the diagnosis of congestive heart failure.
2. Liver function tests may be ordered to evaluate the effects of heart failure on the liver, but they do not confirm the diagnosis.
3. The BUN is elevated in heart failure, dehydration, and renal failure, but it is not used to confirm congestive heart failure.
4. **BNP is a hormone released by the heart muscle in response to changes in blood volume and is used to diagnose and grade heart failure.**

15. 1. Fluid volume overload is a problem in clients with congestive heart failure, but it is not priority because if the cardiac output is improved, then the kidneys are perfused, which leads to elimination of excess fluid from the body.
2. **Decreased cardiac output is responsible for all the signs/symptoms associated with CHF and eventually causes death, which is why it is the priority problem.**
3. Activity intolerance alters quality of life, but it is not life threatening.
4. Knowledge deficit is important, but it is not priority over a physiological problem.

16. 1. **This potassium level is below normal levels; hypokalemia can potentiate digoxin toxicity and lead to cardiac dysrhythmias.**
2. This digoxin level is within therapeutic range, 0.5 to 2.0 mcg/mL.
3. The nurse would question the medication if the apical pulse were less than 60.
4. Yellow haze is a sign of digoxin toxicity.

17. 1. Three (3) unifocal PVCs in a minute is not life threatening.
2. The client wanting to ambulate is not a priority over a client with a physiological problem.
3. **An audible S3 indicates the client is developing left-sided heart failure and needs to be assessed immediately.**
4. A client in normal sinus rhythm will not be priority over someone with a potentially life-threatening situation.

18. 1. **The second intercostal space, right sternal notch, is the area on the chest where the aorta can best be heard opening and closing.**
2. Erb's point allows the nurse to hear the opening and closing of the tricuspid valve.

3. The second intercostal space, left sternal notch, is the area on the chest where the pulmonic valve can best be heard opening and closing.

4. The fourth intercostal space, left sternal border, is another area on the chest that can assess the tricuspid valve.

19. 1. The nurse should call a code if the client does not have vital signs.

2. **The nurse must first determine if the client has a pulse. Pulseless ventricular tachycardia is treated as ventricular fibrillation. Stable ventricular tachycardia is treated with medications.**

3. Chest compression is only done if the client is not breathing and has no pulse.

4. Ventricular tachycardia is a potentially life-threatening dysrhythmia and needs to be treated immediately.

20. 1. **Cardioversion involves the delivery of a timed electrical current. The electrical impulse discharges during ventricular depolarization and therefore there might be a short delay. The nurse should wait until it discharges.**

2. Calling "all clear" and not touching the bed should be done prior to discharging the electrical current.

3. A pause is an expected event, and asking if the client is all right may worry the client unnecessarily.

4. Increasing joules and redischarging is implemented during defibrillation, not during synchronized cardioversion.

21. 1. These assessment data are not life threatening and do not warrant notifying the HCP.

2. The nurse should attempt to hear the friction rub in multiple ways before documenting that it is not heard. The nurse does not determine if pericarditis has resolved.

3. **Having the client lean forward and to the left uses gravity to force the heart nearer to the chest wall, which allows the friction rub to be heard.**

4. Chest tubes are not the treatment of choice for not hearing a friction rub.

22. 1. **This is a medical emergency; the nurse should stay with the client, keep him calm, and call the nurses' station to notify the health-care provider. Cardiac output declines with each contraction as the pericardial sac constricts the myocardium.**

2. The client's signs/symptoms would make the nurse suspect cardiac tamponade, a medical emergency. The pulse pressure is narrowing, and the client is experiencing severe rising central venous pressure exhibited by neck vein distention. Notifying the health-care provider is important, but the nurse should stay with the client first.

3. A left lateral recumbent position is used when administering enemas.

4. Morphine would be given to a client with pain from myocardial infarction; it is not a treatment option for cardiac tamponade.

23. 1. A mid-stream urine specimen is ordered for a client with a possible urinary tract infection, not for a client with cardiac problems.

2. **Any time a nurse suspects cardiac problems, the electrical conductivity of the heart should be assessed.**

3. **Emergency medications for heart problems are primarily administered intravenously, so starting a saline lock in the right arm is appropriate.**

4. This serum blood test is not specific to assess cardiac problems. A BMP evaluates potassium, sodium, glucose, and more.

5. **A 12-lead ECG evaluates the electrical conductivity of the heart from all planes.**

24. 1. This pulse indicates the heart is pumping adequately. Normal pulses should be 2+ to 3+.

2. A pulse oximeter reading of greater than 93% indicates the heart is perfusing the periphery.

3. An output of 30 mL/hr indicates the heart is perfusing the kidneys adequately.

4. **Cold, clammy skin is an indicator of cardiogenic shock, which is a complication of MI and warrants immediate intervention.**

25. 1. **This dosage is 10 times the normal dose for a client with CHF. This dose is potentially lethal.**

2. No other action can be taken because of the incorrect dose.

3. No other action can be taken because of the incorrect dose.

4. No other action can be taken because of the incorrect dose.

26. In the order of performance: 5, 1, 3, 2, 4

5. **The first step in CPR is to determine if the client is unresponsive.**

1. **The rescuer performs the head tilt chin lift maneuver to open the client's airway.**

3. **The next action must be to determine if the client is breathing.**

2. **If the rescuer determines the client is not breathing, then two (2) rescue breaths should be given.**

4. **After determining that the client has no pulse, the rescuer begins compression.**

# Peripheral Vascular Disorders

**4**

Peripheral vascular disorders (PVDs) are very common disorders, affecting many people in the United States. Among the most common of these are hypertension, atherosclerosis, arterial occlusive disease, abdominal aortic aneurysms (AAA), deep vein thrombosis (DVT), and venous insufficiency. These disorders cause pain and an interruption of activities and sometimes lead to life-threatening complications.

## KEYWORDS

bruit
dehiscence
dependent position
Doppler device
evisceration
intermittent claudication
neuropathy
petechiae
sequential compression device
thrill

## ABBREVIATIONS

Abdominal Aortic Aneurysm (AAA)
Angiotensin-Converting Enzyme (ACE)
Blood Pressure (BP)
Blood Urea Nitrogen (BUN)
Capillary Refill Time (CRT)
Congestive Heart Failure (CHF)
Coronary Artery Disease (CAD)
Deep Vein Thrombosis (DVT)
Electrocardiogram (ECG)
Guillain-Barré (GB) Syndrome
Health-Care Provider (HCP)
High-Density Lipoprotein (HDL)
International Normalized Rate (INR)
Intravenous (IV)
Low-Density Lipoprotein (LDL)
Low Molecular Weight Heparin (LMWH)
Nothing By Mouth (NPO)
Partial Thromboplastin Time (PTT)
Peripheral Vascular Disease (PVD)
Physical Therapy (PT)
Prothrombin Time (PT)
Range Of Motion (ROM)
When Required, As Needed (PRN)

### Arterial Hypertension

1. The 66-year-old male client has his blood pressure (BP) checked at a health fair. The B/P is 168/98. Which action should the nurse implement first?
   1. Recommend that the client have his blood pressure checked in one (1) month.
   2. Instruct the client to see his health-care provider as soon as possible.
   3. Discuss the importance of eating a low-salt, low-fat, low-cholesterol diet.
   4. Explain that this B/P is within the normal range for an elderly person.

2. The nurse is teaching the client recently diagnosed with essential hypertension. Which instruction should the nurse provide when discussing exercise?
   1. Walk at least 30 minutes a day on flat surfaces.
   2. Perform light weight lifting three (3) times a week.
   3. Recommend high-level aerobics daily.
   4. Encourage the client to swim laps once a week.

3. The health-care provider prescribes an ACE inhibitor for the client diagnosed with essential hypertension. Which statement is the most appropriate rationale for administering this medication?
   1. ACE inhibitors prevent the beta-receptor stimulation in the heart.
   2. This medication blocks the alpha receptors in the vascular smooth muscle.
   3. ACE inhibitors prevent vasoconstriction and sodium and water retention.
   4. ACE inhibitors decrease blood pressure by relaxing vascular smooth muscle.

4. The nurse is administering a beta blocker to the client diagnosed with essential hypertension. Which intervention should the nurse implement?
   1. Notify the health-care provider if the potassium level is 3.8 mEq.
   2. Question administering the medication if the blood pressure is <90/60 mmHg.
   3. Do not administer the medication if the client's radial pulse is >100.
   4. Monitor the client's blood pressure while he or she is lying, standing, and sitting.

5. The male client diagnosed with essential hypertension has been prescribed an alpha-adrenergic blocker. Which intervention should the nurse discuss with the client?
   1. Eat at least one (1) banana a day to help increase the potassium level.
   2. Explain that impotence is an expected side effect of the medication.
   3. Take the medication on an empty stomach to increase absorption.
   4. Change position slowly when going from lying to sitting position.

6. The nurse just received the A.M. shift report. Which client should the nurse assess first?
   1. The client diagnosed with coronary artery disease who has a BP of 170/100.
   2. The client diagnosed with deep vein thrombosis who is complaining of chest pain.
   3. The client diagnosed with pneumonia who has a pulse oximeter reading of 98%.
   4. The client diagnosed with ulcerative colitis who has nonbloody diarrhea.

7. The client diagnosed with essential hypertension asks the nurse, "Why do I have high blood pressure?" Which response by the nurse would be most appropriate?
   1. "You probably have some type of kidney disease that causes the high BP."
   2. "More than likely you have had a diet high in salt, fat, and cholesterol."
   3. "There is no specific cause for hypertension, but there are many known risk factors."
   4. "You are concerned that you have high blood pressure. Let's sit down and talk."

8. The nurse is teaching the Dietary Approaches to Stop Hypertension (DASH) diet to a client diagnosed with essential hypertension. Which statement indicates that the client understands the client teaching concerning the DASH diet?
   1. "I should eat at least four (4) to five (5) servings of vegetables a day."
   2. "I should eat meat that has a lot of white streaks in it."
   3. "I should drink no more than two (2) glasses of whole milk a day."
   4. "I should decrease my grain intake to no more than twice a week."

9. The client diagnosed with essential hypertension is taking a loop diuretic daily. Which assessment data would require immediate intervention by the nurse?
   1. The telemetry reads normal sinus rhythm.
   2. The client has a weight gain of 2 kg within 1–2 days.
   3. The client's blood pressure is 148/92.
   4. The client's serum potassium level is 4.5 mEq.

10. The client diagnosed with essential hypertension asks the nurse, "I don't know why the doctor is worried about my blood pressure. I feel just great." Which statement by the nurse would be the most appropriate response?
    1. "Damage can be occurring to your heart and kidneys even if you feel great."
    2. "Unless you have a headache your blood pressure is probably within normal limits."
    3. "When is the last time you saw your doctor? Does he know you are feeling great?"
    4. "Your blood pressure reflects how well your heart is working."

11. The intensive care department nurse is calculating the total intake for a client diagnosed with hypertensive crisis. The client has received 880 mL of D5W, IVPB of 100 mL of 0.9% NS, 8 ounces of water, 4 ounces of milk, and 6 ounces of chicken broth. The client has had a urinary output of 1480 mL. What is the total intake for this client?_____

12. The nurse is teaching a class on arterial essential hypertension. Which modifiable risk factors would the nurse include when preparing this presentation?
    1. Include information on retinopathy and nephropathy.
    2. Discuss sedentary lifestyle and smoking cessation.
    3. Include discussions on family history and gender.
    4. Provide information on a low-fiber and high-salt diet.

## Arterial Occlusive Disease

13. The client comes to the clinic complaining of muscle cramping and pain in both legs when walking for short periods of time. Which medical term would the nurse document in the client's record?
    1. Peripheral vascular disease (PVD).
    2. Intermittent claudication.
    3. Deep vein thrombosis (DVT).
    4. Dependent rubor.

14. Which instruction should be included when a client diagnosed with peripheral arterial disease is being discharged?
    1. Encourage the client to use a heating pad on lower extremities.
    2. Demonstrate to the client the correct way to apply elastic support hose.
    3. Instruct the client to walk daily for at least 30 minutes.
    4. Tell the client to check both feet for red areas at least once a week.

15. The nurse is teaching the client diagnosed with arterial occlusive disease. Which interventions should the nurse include in the teaching? Select all that apply.
    1. Wash legs and feet daily in warm water.
    2. Apply moisturizing cream to feet.
    3. Buy shoes in the morning hours only.
    4. Do not wear any type of knee stocking.
    5. Wear clean white cotton socks.

16. Which assessment data would warrant immediate intervention in the client diagnosed with arterial occlusive disease?
    1. The client has 2+ pedal pulses.
    2. The client is able to move the toes.
    3. The client has numbness and tingling.
    4. The client's feet are red when standing.

Vascular

Vascular

17. Which client problem would be priority in a client diagnosed with arterial occlusive disease who is admitted to the hospital with a foot ulcer?
    1. Impaired skin integrity.
    2. Activity intolerance.
    3. Ineffective health maintenance.
    4. Risk for peripheral neuropathy.

18. The client diagnosed with arterial occlusive disease is one (1) day post-operative right femoral popliteal bypass. Which intervention should the nurse implement?
    1. Keep the right leg in the dependent position.
    2. Apply sequential compression devices to lower extremities.
    3. Monitor the client's pedal pulses every shift.
    4. Assess the client's leg dressing every four (4) hours.

19. The nurse is unable to assess a pedal pulse in the client diagnosed with arterial occlusive disease. Which intervention should the nurse implement first?
    1. Complete a neurovascular assessment.
    2. Use the Doppler device.
    3. Instruct the client to hang the feet off the side of the bed.
    4. Wrap the legs in a blanket.

20. The wife of a client with arterial occlusive disease tells the nurse, "My husband says he is having rest pain. What does that mean?" Which statement by the nurse would be most appropriate?
    1. "It describes the type of pain he has when he stops walking."
    2. "His legs are deprived of oxygen during periods of inactivity."
    3. "You are concerned that your husband is having rest pain."
    4. "This term is used to support that his condition is getting better."

21. The nurse is assessing the client diagnosed with long-term arterial occlusive disease. Which assessment data support the diagnosis?
    1. Hairless skin on the legs.
    2. Brittle, flaky toe nails.
    3. Petechiae on the soles of feet.
    4. Nonpitting ankle edema.

22. The health-care provider ordered a femoral angiogram for the client diagnosed with arterial occlusive disease. Which intervention should the nurse implement?
    1. Explain that this procedure will be done at the bedside.
    2. Discuss with the client that he or she will be on bed rest with bathroom privileges.
    3. Inform the client that no intravenous access will be needed.
    4. Inform the client that fluids will be increased after the procedure.

23. Which medication should the nurse expect the health-care provider to order for a client diagnosed with arterial occlusive disease?
    1. An anticoagulant medication.
    2. An antihypertensive medication.
    3. An antiplatelet medication.
    4. A muscle relaxant.

24. The nurse and an unlicensed nursing assistant are caring for a 64-year-old client who is four (4) hours post-operative bilateral femoral–popliteal bypass surgery. Which nursing task should be delegated to the unlicensed nursing assistant?
    1. Monitor the continuous passive motion machine.
    2. Assist the client to the bedside commode.
    3. Feed the client the evening meal.
    4. Elevate the foot of the client's bed.

## Atherosclerosis

25. The nurse is teaching a class on coronary artery disease. Which modifiable risk factors should the nurse discuss when teaching about atherosclerosis?
    1. Stress.
    2. Age.
    3. Gender.
    4. Family history.

26. The client asks the nurse, "My doctor just told me that atherosclerosis is why my legs hurt when I walk. What does that mean?" Which response by the nurse would be the best response?
    1. "The muscle fibers and endothelial lining of your arteries have become thickened."
    2. "The next time you see your HCP ask what atherosclerosis means."
    3. "The valves in the veins of your legs are incompetent so your legs hurt."
    4. "You have a hardening of your arteries that decreases the oxygen to your legs."

27. The client diagnosed with peripheral vascular disease is overweight, has smoked two (2) packs of cigarettes a day for 20 years, and sits behind a desk all day. What is the strongest factor in the development of atherosclerotic lesions?
    1. Being overweight.
    2. Sedentary lifestyle.
    3. High-fat, high-cholesterol diet.
    4. Smoking cigarettes.

28. The client tells the nurse that his cholesterol level is 240 mg/dL. Which action should the nurse implement?
    1. Praise the client for having a normal cholesterol level.
    2. Explain that the client needs to lower the cholesterol level.
    3. Discuss dietary changes that could help increase the level.
    4. Allow the client to ventilate feelings about the blood test result.

29. The nurse is discussing the pathophysiology of atherosclerosis with a client who has a normal high-density lipoprotein (HDL) level. Which information should the nurse discuss with the client concerning HDL?
    1. A normal HDL is good because it has a protective action in the body.
    2. HDL lipoprotein level measures the free fatty acids and glycerol in the blood.
    3. HDLs are the primary transporters of cholesterol into the cell.
    4. The client needs to decrease the amount of cholesterol and fat in the diet.

30. Which assessment data would cause the nurse to suspect the client has atherosclerosis?
    1. Change in bowel movements.
    2. Complaints of a headache.
    3. Intermittent claudication.
    4. Venous stasis ulcers.

31. The nurse is teaching a class on atherosclerosis. Which statement describes the scientific rationale as to why diabetes is a risk factor for developing atherosclerosis?
    1. Glucose combines with carbon monoxide, instead of with oxygen, and this leads to oxygen deprivation of tissues.
    2. Diabetes stimulates the sympathetic nervous system, resulting in peripheral constriction that increases the development of atherosclerosis.
    3. Diabetes speeds the atherosclerotic process by thickening the basement membrane of both large and small vessels.
    4. The increased glucose combines with the hemoglobin, which causes deposits of plaque in the lining of the vessels.

Vascular

32. The nurse is discussing the importance of exercising with a client who is diagnosed with CAD. Which statement best describes the scientific rationale for encouraging 30 minutes of walking daily to help prevent complications of atherosclerosis?
    1. Exercise promotes the development of collateral circulation.
    2. Isometric exercises help develop the client's muscle mass.
    3. Daily exercise helps prevent plaque from developing in the vessel.
    4. Isotonic exercises promote the transport of glucose into the cell.

33. The HCP prescribes an HMG-COA reductase inhibitor (statin) medication to a client with CAD. Which should the nurse teach the client about this medication?
    1. Take this medication on an empty stomach.
    2. This medication should be taken in the evening.
    3. Do not be concerned if muscle pain occurs.
    4. Check your cholesterol level daily.

34. The nurse knows the client understands the teaching concerning a low-fat, low-cholesterol diet when the client selects which meal?
    1. Fried fish, garlic mashed potatoes, and iced tea.
    2. Ham and cheese on white bread and whole milk.
    3. Baked chicken, baked potato, and skim milk.
    4. A hamburger, French fries, and carbonated beverage.

35. Which interventions should the nurse discuss with the client diagnosed with atherosclerosis? Select all that apply.
    1. Include significant other in the discussion.
    2. Stop smoking or using any type of tobacco products.
    3. Maintain a sedentary lifestyle as much as possible.
    4. Avoid stressful situations.
    5. Daily isometric exercises are important.

36. The nurse is caring for clients on a telemetry floor. Which nursing task would be most appropriate to delegate to an unlicensed nursing assistant?
    1. Teach the client how to perform a Glucometer check.
    2. Assist feeding the client diagnosed with congestive heart failure.
    3. Check the cholesterol level for the client diagnosed with atherosclerosis.
    4. Assist the nurse to check the unit of blood at the client's bedside.

## Abdominal Aortic Aneurysm

37. Which assessment data would support the diagnosis of abdominal aortic aneurysm (AAA)?
    1. Shortness of breath.
    2. Abdominal bruit.
    3. Ripping abdominal pain.
    4. Decreased urinary output.

38. Which medical treatment would be prescribed for the client with an AAA less than 3 cm?
    1. Ultrasound every six (6) months.
    2. Intravenous pyelogram yearly.
    3. Assessment of abdominal girth monthly.
    4. Repair of abdominal aortic aneurysm.

39. Which client would be most likely to develop an abdominal aortic aneurysm?
    1. A 45-year-old female with a history of osteoporosis.
    2. An 80-year-old female with congestive heart failure.
    3. A 69-year-old male with peripheral vascular disease.
    4. A 30-year-old male with a genetic predisposition to AAA.

40. The client is diagnosed with an abdominal aortic aneurysm. Which statement would the nurse expect the client to make during the admission assessment?
    1. "I have stomach pain every time I eat a big, heavy meal."
    2. "I don't have any abdominal pain or any type of problems."
    3. "I have periodic episodes of constipation and then diarrhea."
    4. "I belch a lot, especially when I lay down after eating."

41. The client is admitted for surgical repair of an 8-cm abdominal aortic aneurysm. Which sign/symptom would make the nurse suspect the client has an expanding AAA?
    1. Complaints of low back pain.
    2. Weakened radial pulses.
    3. Decreased urine output.
    4. Increased abdominal girth.

42. The client is one (1) day post-operative abdominal aortic aneurysm repair. Which information from the unlicensed nursing assistant would require immediate intervention from the nurse?
    1. The client refuses to turn from the back to the side.
    2. The client's urinary output is 90 mL in six (6) hours.
    3. The client wants to sit on the side of the bed.
    4. The client's vital signs are T 98, P 90, R 18, and BP 130/70.

43. The client had an abdominal aortic aneurysm repair two (2) days ago. Which intervention should the nurse implement first?
    1. Assess the client's bowel sounds.
    2. Administer an IV prophylactic antibiotic.
    3. Encourage the client to splint the incision.
    4. Ambulate the client in the room with assistance.

44. Which health-care provider's order should the nurse question in a client diagnosed with an expanding abdominal aortic aneurysm who is scheduled for surgery in the morning?
    1. Type and cross-match for two (2) units of blood.
    2. Tap water enema until clear fecal return.
    3. Bed rest with bathroom privileges.
    4. Keep NPO after midnight.

45. The client is diagnosed with a small abdominal aortic aneurysm. Which interventions should be included in the discharge teaching? Select all that apply.
    1. Tell the client to exercise three (3) times a week for 30 minutes.
    2. Encourage the client to eat a low-fat, low-cholesterol diet.
    3. Instruct the client to decrease tobacco use.
    4. Discuss with the client the importance of losing weight.
    5. Teach the client to wear a truss at all times.

46. Which assessment data would require immediate intervention by the nurse for the client who is six (6) hours post-operative abdominal aortic aneurysm repair?
    1. Absent bilateral pedal pulses.
    2. Complaints of pain at the site of the incision.
    3. Distended, tender abdomen.
    4. An elevated temperature of 100°F.

47. The nurse is discussing discharge teaching with the client who is three (3) days post-operative abdominal aortic aneurysm repair. Which discharge instructions should the nurse include when teaching the client?
    1. Notify HCP of any redness or irritation of incision.
    2. Do not lift anything more than 20 pounds.
    3. Inform client that there may be pain not relieved with pain medication.
    4. Stress the importance of having daily bowel movements.

48. On which area would the nurse place the bell of the stethoscope when assessing the client with an abdominal aortic aneurysm?

1. A
2. B
3. C
4. D

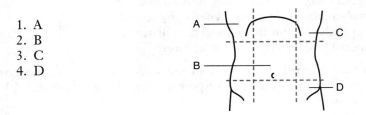

## Deep Vein Thrombosis

49. The nurse is discharging a client diagnosed with DVT from the hospital. Which discharge instructions should be provided to the client?
    1. Have the PTT levels checked weekly until therapeutic range is achieved.
    2. Staying at home is best, but if traveling, airplanes are better than automobiles.
    3. Avoid green leafy vegetables and notify the HCP of red or brown urine.
    4. Wear knee stockings with an elastic band around the top.

50. The nurse is caring for clients on a surgical floor. Which client should be assessed first?
    1. The client who is four (4) day post-operative abdominal surgery and is complaining of left calf pain when ambulating.
    2. The client who is one (1) day post-operative hernia repair who has just been able to void 550 mL of clear amber urine.
    3. The client who is five (5) day post-operative open cholecystectomy who has a T tube and is being discharged.
    4. The client who is 16 hours post–abdominal hysterectomy and is complaining of abdominal pain and is expelling flatus.

51. The male client is diagnosed with Guillain Barré syndrome (GB) and is in the intensive care unit on a ventilator. Which cardiovascular rationale explains implementing passive range of motion (ROM) exercises?
    1. Passive ROM will prevent contractures from developing.
    2. The client will feel better if he is able to exercise and stretch his muscles.
    3. Range of motion exercises will help alleviate the pain associated with GB.
    4. They help to prevent DVTs by movement of the blood through the veins.

52. The nurse and an unlicensed nursing assistant are bathing a bedfast client. Which action by the assistant warrants immediate intervention?
    1. The assistant closes the door and cubicle curtain before undressing the client.
    2. The assistant begins to massage and rub lotion into the client's calf.
    3. The assistant tests the temperature of the water with the wrist before starting.
    4. The assistant collects all the linens and supplies and brings them to the room.

53. The client diagnosed with a DVT is placed on a medical unit. Which nursing interventions should be implemented? Select all that apply.
    1. Place sequential compression devices on both legs.
    2. Instruct the client to stay in bed and not ambulate.
    3. Encourage fluids and a diet high in roughage.
    4. Monitor IV site every shift and PRN.
    5. Assess Homans' sign every 24 hours.

54. The nurse is caring for a client receiving heparin sodium via constant infusion. The heparin protocol reads to increase the IV rate by 100 units/hour if the PTT is less than 50 seconds. The current PTT level is 46 seconds. The heparin comes in 500 mL of D5W with 25,000 units of heparin added. The current rate on the IV pump is 18 mL per hour. At what rate should the nurse set the pump?_____

55. Which assessment data would warrant immediate intervention by the nurse?
    1. The client diagnosed with DVT who complains of pain on inspiration.
    2. The immobile client has refused to turn for the last three (3) hours.
    3. The client who has had an open cholecystectomy does not want to breathe deeply.
    4. The client who has had an inguinal hernia repair who must void before discharge.

56. The client diagnosed with a DVT is on a heparin (an anticoagulant) drip at 1400 units per hour, and Coumadin (warfarin sodium; also an anticoagulant) 5 mg twice a day. Which intervention should the nurse implement first?
    1. Check the PTT and PT/INR.
    2. Check with the HCP to see which drug should be discontinued.
    3. Administer both medications.
    4. Discontinue the heparin because the client is receiving Coumadin.

57. Which actions should the surgical scrub nurse take to prevent from personally developing a DVT?
    1. Keep the legs in a dependent position and stand as still as possible.
    2. Flex the leg muscles and change the leg positions frequently.
    3. Wear white socks and shoes that have a wedge heel.
    4. Ask the surgeon to allow the nurse to take a break midway through each surgery.

58. The client receiving low molecular weight heparin (LMWH) subcutaneously to prevent DVT following hip replacement surgery complains to the nurse that there are small purple hemorrhaged areas on the upper abdomen. Which action should the nurse implement?
    1. Notify the HCP immediately.
    2. Check the client's PTT level.
    3. Explain that this results from the medication.
    4. Assess the client's vital signs.

59. The home health nurse is admitting a client diagnosed with a DVT. Which action by the client warrants immediate intervention by the nurse?
    1. The client takes a stool softener every day at dinnertime.
    2. The client is wearing a medic alert bracelet.
    3. The client takes vitamin E over-the-counter medications.
    4. The client has purchased a new recliner that will elevate the legs.

60. The client is being admitted with Coumadin (warfarin), an anticoagulant, toxicity. Which laboratory data should the nurse monitor?
    1. Blood urea nitrogen levels (BUN).
    2. Bilirubin levels.
    3. International Normalized Ratio (INR).
    4. Partial thromboplastin time (PTT).

## Peripheral Venous Disease

61. The nurse is teaching a class on venous insufficiency. The nurse would identify which condition as the most serious complication of chronic venous insufficiency?
    1. Arterial thrombosis.
    2. Deep vein thrombosis.
    3. Venous ulcerations.
    4. Varicose veins.

62. Which assessment data would support that the client has a venous stasis ulcer?
    1. Superficial pink open area on the medial part of the ankle.
    2. A deep pale open area over the top side of the foot.
    3. A reddened blistered area on the heel of the foot.
    4. A necrotic gangrenous area on the dorsal side of the foot.

63. The client is employed in a job that requires extensive standing. Which intervention should the nurse include when discussing how to prevent varicose veins?
    1. Wear low-heeled, comfortable shoes.
    2. Wear white, clean, cotton socks.
    3. Move the legs back and forth often.
    4. Wear graduated compression hose.

64. The client with varicose veins asks the nurse, "What caused me to have these?" Which statement by the nurse would be most appropriate?
    1. "You have incompetent valves in your legs."
    2. "Your legs have decreased oxygen to the muscle."
    3. "There is an obstruction in the saphenous vein."
    4. "Your blood is thick and can't circulate properly."

65. The nurse is caring for the client with chronic venous insufficiency. Which statement indicates that the client understands the discharge teaching?
    1. "I shouldn't cross my legs for more than 15 minutes."
    2. "I need to elevate the foot of my bed while sleeping."
    3. "I should take a baby aspirin every day with food."
    4. "I should increase my fluid intake to 3000 mL a day."

66. The unlicensed nursing assistant is caring for the client diagnosed with chronic venous insufficiency. Which action would warrant immediate intervention from the nurse?
    1. Applying compression stockings before going to bed.
    2. Taking the client's blood pressure manually.
    3. Assisting the client by opening the milk on the tray.
    4. Calculating the client's shift intake and output.

67. The 80-year-old client is being discharged home after having surgery to debride a chronic venous ulcer on the right ankle. Which referral would be most appropriate for the client?
    1. Occupational therapist.
    2. Social worker.
    3. Physical therapist.
    4. Cardiac rehabilitation.

68. Which assessment data would the nurse expect to find in the client diagnosed with chronic venous insufficiency?
    1. Decreased pedal pulses.
    2. Cool skin temperature.
    3. Intermittent claudication.
    4. Brown discolored skin.

69. Which client would be most at risk for developing varicose veins?
    1. A Caucasian female who is a nurse.
    2. An African American male who is a bus driver.
    3. An Asian female with no children.
    4. An elderly male with diabetes.

70. The client with varicose veins is six (6) hours post-operative vein ligation. Which nursing intervention should the nurse implement first?
    1. Assist the client to dangle the legs off the side of the bed.
    2. Assess and maintain pressure bandages on the affected leg.
    3. Apply a sequential compression device to the affected leg.
    4. Administer the prescribed prophylactic intravenous antibiotic.

71. The nurse has just received the A.M. shift report. Which client would the nurse assess first?
    1. The client with a venous stasis ulcer who is complaining of pain.
    2. The client with varicose veins who has dull aching muscle cramps.
    3. The client with arterial occlusive disease who cannot move the foot.
    4. The client with deep vein thrombosis who has a positive Homans' sign.

72. The nurse is completing a neurovascular assessment on the client with chronic venous insufficiency. What should be included in this assessment? Select all that apply.
    1. Assess for paresthesia.
    2. Assess for pedal pulses.
    3. Assess for paralysis.
    4. Assess for pallor.
    5. Assess for paresthesia.

## Arterial Hypertension

1. 1. This BP is elevated and the client should have his BP checked frequently but not before seeking medical treatment.
   2. The diastolic blood pressure should be less than 85 according to the American Heart Association; therefore, this client should see the health-care provider.
   3. Teaching is important, but the nurse must first make sure the client sees the health-care provider for a thorough checkup and antihypertensive medication prescription. Diet alone should not be recommended by the nurse.
   4. This is not the normal range for an elderly person's blood pressure; the diastolic should be less than 85 mmHg.

   **TEST-TAKING HINT: Remember the question asks which action should be implemented first. Therefore, there is more than one answer that is appropriate but the first should be the one that directly affects the client.**

2. 1. Walking 30 to 45 minutes a day will help in reducing blood pressure, weight, and stress and will increase a feeling of overall well-being.
   2. Isometric exercises (such as weight lifting) should be discouraged because performing them can raise the systolic blood pressure.
   3. The client should walk, cycle, jog, or swim daily; high-level aerobics may increase the client's blood pressure.
   4. Swimming laps is recommended, but it should be daily, not once a week.

   **TEST-TAKING HINT: Remember to look at the frequency of interventions; it makes a difference when selecting the correct answers.**

3. 1. Beta-adrenergic blocking agents, not ACE inhibitors, prevent the beta-receptor stimulation in the heart, which decreases heart rate and cardiac output.
   2. Alpha-adrenergic blockers, not ACE inhibitors, block alpha receptors in the vascular smooth muscle, which decreases vasomotor tone and vasoconstriction.
   3. Angiotensin-converting enzyme (ACE) inhibitors prevent the conversion of angiotensin I to angiotensin II, and this, in turn, prevents vasoconstriction and sodium and water retention.
   4. Vasodilators, not ACE inhibitors, reduce blood pressure by relaxing vascular smooth muscle, especially in the arterioles.

**TEST-TAKING HINT: The test taker needs to understand how the major classifications of medications work to answer this question.**

4. 1. The potassium level is within normal limits (3.5–5.5 mEq/L), and it is not usually checked prior to administering beta blockers.
   2. The nurse should question administering the beta blocker if the B/P is low because this medication will cause the blood pressure to drop even lower, leading to hypotension.
   3. The nurse would not administer the medication if the apical (not radial) pulse were less than 60 beats per minute.
   4. The nurse needs to assess the blood pressure only once prior to administering the medication (not take all three blood pressures prior to administering the medication).

   **TEST-TAKING HINT: Be sure to read the entire question and all the answer options and note the specific numbers that are identified. The test taker must know normal laboratory data and assessment findings.**

5. 1. The potassium level is not affected by an alpha-adrenergic blocker.
   2. Impotence is a major cause of noncompliance with taking prescribed medications for hypertension in male clients. The noncompliance should be reported to the HCP immediately so the medication can be changed.
   3. The medication can be taken on an empty or a full stomach, depending on whether the client becomes nauseated after taking the medication.
   4. Orthostatic hypotension may occur when the blood pressure is decreasing and may lead to dizziness and light-headedness so the client should change position slowly.

   **TEST-TAKING HINT: The test taker should understand the side effects of medications. The test taker who does not know the answer may realize that hypertension is being treated and that hypotension is the opposite of hypertension and might be a complication of treating hypertension. Only option "4" refers to hypotension, providing advice on how to avoid orthostatic hypotension.**

6. 1. This blood pressure is elevated, but it is not life threatening.
   2. The chest pain could be a pulmonary embolus secondary to deep vein thrombosis and requires immediate intervention by the nurse.

Vascular

3. A pulse oximeter reading of greater than 93% is within normal limits.
4. Nonbloody diarrhea is an expected sign of ulcerative colitis and would not require immediate intervention by the nurse.

**TEST-TAKING HINT: The nurse should assess the client who has abnormal assessment data or a life-threatening condition first when determining which client is priority.**

7. 1. Kidney disease leads to secondary hypertension; secondary hypertension is elevated blood pressure resulting from an identifiable underlying process.
2. A high-salt, high-fat, high-cholesterol diet is a risk factor for essential hypertension, but it is not the only cause; therefore this would be an incorrect answer.
3. There is no known cause for essential hypertension, but many factors, both modifiable (obesity, smoking, diet) and nonmodifiable (family history, age, gender) are risk factors for essential hypertension.
4. This is a therapeutic reply that is inappropriate because the client needs facts.

**TEST-TAKING HINT: When clients request information, the exchange should not address emotions. Just facts should be given. Therefore, option "4" can be eliminated as a correct answer.**

8. 1. The DASH diet has proved beneficial in lowering blood pressure. It recommends eating a diet high in vegetables and fruits.
2. The DASH diet recommends two (2) or fewer servings of lean meats, which have very little white streaks; the white streaks indicate the meat is high in fat.
3. The DASH diet recommends two (2) to three (3) servings of nonfat or low-fat milk, not whole milk.
4. The DASH diet recommends seven (7) to eight (8) servings of grain a day.

**TEST-TAKING HINT: The test taker is looking for correct information about the DASH diet. A recommended diet for hypertension would limit fatty meats and whole milk.**

9. 1. Normal sinus rhythm indicates that the client's heart is working normally.
2. Rapid weight gain—for example, 2 kg in 1–2 days—indicates that the loop diuretic is not working effectively; 2 kg equals 4.4 lbs; 1 L of fluid weighs 1 kg.
3. This blood pressure is not life-threateningly high and does not require immediate intervention.

4. Loop diuretics cause an increase in potassium excretion in the urine; therefore, the potassium level should be assessed, but 4.5 mEq/L is within normal limits (3.5 to 5.5 mEq/L).

**TEST-TAKING HINT: The phrase "requires immediate intervention" should make the test taker think that the correct answer will be abnormal assessment data, data that require medical intervention or is life threatening.**

10. 1. Even if the client feels great, the blood pressure can be elevated, causing damage to the heart, kidney, and blood vessels.
2. A headache may indicate an elevated blood pressure, but the client with essential hypertension can be asymptomatic and still have a very high blood pressure reading.
3. This response does not answer the client's question as to why the doctor is worried about the client's blood pressure.
4. The blood pressure does not necessarily reflect how well the heart is working. Many other diagnostic tests assess how well the heart is working, including an electrocardiogram (ECG), an ultrasound, or a chest x-ray.

**TEST-TAKING HINT: The test taker should select the option that provides the client with correct information in a nonthreatening, nonjudgmental approach.**

11. **1520 mL total intake.** The urinary output is not used in this calculation. The nurse must add up both intravenous fluids and oral fluids to obtain the total intake for this client; 880 + 100 = 980 IV fluids; (1 ounce = 30 mL) 8 ounces × 30 mL = 240 mL, 4 ounces × 30 mL = 120 mL, 6 ounces × 30 mL = 180 mL; 240 + 120 + 180 = 540 oral fluids. Total intake is 980 + 540 = 1520.

**TEST-TAKING HINT: The reader must know the conversion equivalents before performing any type of math problems. The key to this answer is 1 ounce = 30 mL.**

12. 1. Retinopathy and nephropathy are complications of uncontrolled hypertension, not modifiable risk factors.
2. Sedentary lifestyle is discouraged in clients with hypertension, and daily isotonic exercises are recommended. Smoking increases the atherosclerotic process in vessels; causes vasoconstriction of vessels; and adheres to hemoglobin, decreasing oxygen levels.
3. Family history and gender are nonmodifiable risk factors. The question is asking for information on modifiable risk factors.

4. A low-salt diet is recommended because increased salt intake causes water retention, which increases the workload of the heart. A high-fiber diet is recommended because it helps decrease cholesterol levels.

**TEST-TAKING HINT: Remember to look at the adjectives. The stem of the question is asking about "modifiable risk factors."**

## Arterial Occlusive Disease

13. 1. PVD is a broad term that encompasses both venous and arterial peripheral problems of the lower extremities.
    2. This is the classic symptom of arterial occlusive disease.
    3. This is characterized by calf tenderness, calf edema, and positive Homans' sign.
    4. This term is a sign of arterial occlusive disease, the legs are pale when elevated but are dark red when in the dependent position.

**TEST-TAKING HINT: The test taker could eliminate "1" and "3" as possible answers if the words "medical term" were noted. Both "1" and "3" are disease processes not medical terms.**

14. 1. External heating devices are avoided to reduce the risk of burns.
    2. Elastic support hose reduce the circulation to the skin and are avoided.
    3. Walking promotes the development of collateral circulation to ischemic tissue and slows the process of atherosclerosis.
    4. The feet must be checked daily not weekly.

**TEST-TAKING HINT: The test taker must note the adjective "week" in "4," which could eliminate this distracter as a possible answer.**

15. 1. Cold water causes vasoconstriction and hot water may burn the client's feet; therefore, warm tepid water should be recommended.
    2. Moisturizing prevents drying of the feet.
    3. Shoes should be purchased in the afternoon when the feet are the largest.
    4. This will further decrease circulation to the legs.
    5. Colored socks have dye and dirty socks may cause foot irritation that may lead to breaks in the skin.

**TEST-TAKING HINT: The test taker must select all appropriate interventions; "3" could be eliminated as a correct answer because of "only," which is an absolute word. There are very few absolutes in health care.**

16. 1. These are normal pedal pulses and would not require any intervention.
    2. Moving the toes is a good sign in a client with arterial occlusive disease.
    3. Numbness and tingling are paresthesia, which is a sign of a severely decreased blood supply to the lower extremities.
    4. Reddened extremities are expected secondary to increased blood supply when the legs are in the dependent position.

**TEST-TAKING HINT: "Warrants immediate intervention," indicates that the test taker must select the distracter that is abnormal, unexpected, or life-threatening for the client's disease process. Sometimes if the test taker flips the question and thinks which assessment data are normal for the disease process, it is easier to identify the correct answer.**

17. 1. The client has a foot ulcer, therefore the protective lining of the body—the skin—has been impaired.
    2. This is an appropriate problem but would not take priority over impaired skin integrity.
    3. The client needs teaching but it does not take priority over a physiological problem.
    4. The client has peripheral neuropathy, not a risk for; this is the primary pathological change in a client with arterial occlusive disease.

**TEST-TAKING HINT: Remember Maslow's Hierarchy of Needs and physiological needs are priority.**

18. 1. The right leg should be elevated to decrease edema not flat or hanging off the side of the bed (dependent).
    2. The left foot could have a sequential compression device to prevent deep vein thrombosis, but it should not be on the leg with an operative incision site.
    3. The client is one (1) day post-operative and the pedal pulses must be assessed more than once every eight (8) or twelve (12) hours.
    4. The leg dressing needs to be assessed for hemorrhaging or signs of infection.

**TEST-TAKING HINT: The test taker must be observant of time "one (1) day postoperative" and doing an intervention every "shift" should cause the test taker to eliminate this distracter. The test taker must know terms used to describe positioning such as dependent, prone, and supine.**

19. 1. An absent pulse is not uncommon in a client diagnosed with arterial occlusive disease, but the nurse must ensure that the

feet can be moved and are warm, which indicates adequate blood supply to the feet.

2. To identify the location of the pulse the nurse should use a Doppler device to amplify the sound, but it is not the first intervention.

3. This position will increase blood flow and may help the nurse palpate the pulse, but it is not the first intervention.

4. Cold can cause vasoconstriction and decrease the ability to palpate the pulse, and warming will dilate the arteries helping the nurse find the pedal pulse, but it is not the first intervention.

**TEST-TAKING HINT: The stem asks the nurse to identify the first intervention and the test taker should apply the nursing process and implement an assessment intervention.**

20. 1. The pain stops when the client quits walking, therefore it is not rest pain.

2. Rest pain indicates a worsening of the arterial occlusive disease; the muscles of the legs are not getting enough oxygen when the client is resting to prevent muscle ischemia.

3. This is a therapeutic response and does not answer the wife's question.

4. Rest indicates that the arterial occlusive disease is getting worse.

**TEST-TAKING HINT: The nurse should answer questions with factual information, therefore "3" could be eliminated as a possible answer. Pain usually does not indicate that a condition is getting better, which would cause the test taker to eliminate distracter "4."**

21. 1. The decreased oxygen over time causes the loss of hair on top of feet and ascends both legs.

2. The toenails are usually thickened due to hypoxemia.

3. Petechiae are tiny purple or red spots that appear on the skin as a result of minute hemorrhages within the dermal layer, this does not occur with arterial occlusive disease.

4. There may be edema but it is usually pitting, non-pitting edema resolves with elevation but not with arterial occlusive disease.

**TEST-TAKING HINT: The test taker should apply the pathophysiological concept that arterial blood supplies oxygen and nutrients and if the hair cannot get nutrients it will not grow.**

22. 1. This procedure will be done in a cath lab or special room, not at the bedside because machines are used to visualize the extent of the arterial occlusion.

2. The client will have to keep the leg straight for

at least six (6) hours after the procedure to prevent bleeding from the femoral artery.

3. An intravenous contrast medium is injected and vessels are visualized using fluoroscopy and x-rays.

4. Fluids will help flush the contrast dye out of the body and help prevent kidney damage.

**TEST-TAKING HINT: The nurse must be knowledgeable of diagnostic tests but if not the test taker could dissect the word, "angio" means vessel, which could help eliminate "3" as a possible answer because some type of dye would have to be used to visualize a vessel. Adjectives should be noted—anything done in the femoral artery would require pressure at the site to prevent bleeding—this information could help the test taker to eliminate "2" as a possible answer. Very few diagnostic tests are done at the bedside.**

23. 1. An anticoagulant medication is prescribed for venous problems, such as deep vein thrombosis.

2. Arterial occlusive disease is caused by atherosclerosis, which may cause hypertension along with arterial occlusive disease, but antihypertensive medications are not prescribed for this disease.

3. Anti-platelet medications inhibit platelet aggregations in the arterial blood, such as aspirin or clopidogrel (Plavix).

4. A muscles relaxant will not help the leg pain since the origin of pain is decreased oxygen to the muscle.

**TEST-TAKING HINT: The test taker should apply the knowledge learned in anatomy and physiology class; platelets are part of the arterial blood, therefore this would be an excellent selection if the test taker did not have any idea about the answer.**

24. 1. A continuous passive motion machine is used for a client with a total knee replacement, not for this type of surgery.

2. The client will be on bed rest at four (4) hours after the surgery. Remember the client had bilateral surgery on the legs.

3. There is nothing in the stem that would indicate the client could not feed himself. The nurse should encourage independence as much as possible.

4. After the surgery, the client's legs will be elevated to help decrease edema. The surgery has corrected the decreased blood supply to the lower legs.

**TEST-TAKING HINT: A concept that is applicable to surgery is decreasing edema and extremity**

Vascular

surgeries usually include elevating the affected extremity. **The test taker must apply basic concepts when answering questions.**

## Atherosclerosis

25. 1. A modifiable risk factor is a risk factor that can possibly be altered by modifying or changing behavior, such as developing new ways to deal with stress.
    2. The client cannot do anything about getting older so it cannot be modified.
    3. Gender is a risk factor that cannot be changed.
    4. Having a family history of coronary artery disease predisposes the client to a higher risk, but this cannot be changed by the client.

**TEST-TAKING HINT: The test taker needs to key in on adjectives when reading the stem of a question. The word "modifiable" should cause the test taker to select "stress" because it is the only answer option referring to something that can be changed or modified.**

26. 1. The nurse should assume the client is a layperson and should not explain disease processes using medical terminology.
    2. This is passing the buck; the nurse should have the knowledge to answer this question.
    3. Atherosclerosis involves the arteries, not veins.
    4. This response explains in plain terms why the client's legs hurt from atherosclerosis.

**TEST-TAKING HINT: If the test taker knows medical terminology, "3" could be eliminated because "athero" means "arteries," not veins. The test taker should be very cautious when choosing an option that asks the health-care provider to answers questions that nurses should be able to answer.**

27. 1. Being overweight is not a risk factor for atherosclerotic lesions, but it does indicate that the client does not eat a healthy diet or exercise as needed.
    2. Lack of exercise is a risk factor, but it is not the strongest.
    3. Although the stem did not explicitly identify diet, the nurse should assume that a client who is obese would not eat a low-fat, low-cholesterol diet.
    4. Tobacco use is the strongest factor in the development of atherosclerotic lesions. Nicotine decreases blood flow to the extremities and increases heart rate and blood pressure. It also increases the risk of clot formation by increasing the aggregation of platelets.

**TEST-TAKING HINT: The test taker should look at the answer options closely to determine if any are similar. This will help eliminate two options—"1" and "3"—as possible answers. An unhealthy diet will cause the client to be overweight.**

28. 1. The cholesterol level should be less than 200 mg/dL.
    2. The client needs to be taught ways to lower the cholesterol level.
    3. The client should be taught a low-fat, low-cholesterol diet to help lower the cholesterol level.
    4. The nurse needs to discuss facts concerning the cholesterol level and teach the client. A therapeutic conversation would not be appropriate.

**TEST-TAKING HINT: The nurse needs to know normal laboratory test findings. If the test taker is not aware of normal cholesterol levels, he or she could only guess the answer to the question.**

29. 1. A normal HDL level is good because HDL transports cholesterol away from the tissues and cells of the arterial wall to the liver for excretion. This helps decrease the development of atherosclerosis.
    2. The normal HDL level was the result of a test measuring high-density lipoproteins, not free fatty acids and glycerol in the blood, which are measured by the serum triglyceride level. Triglycerides are a source of energy.
    3. Low-density lipoproteins (LDLs), not HDLs, are the primary transporters of cholesterol into the cell. They have the harmful effect of depositing cholesterol into the walls of the arterial vessels.
    4. A normal HDL is good and the client does not need to change the diet.

**TEST-TAKING HINT: If the test taker has no idea what the correct answer is, look at the specific words in the answer options. Normal lab data would probably be good for the client; therefore "1" would be a probable correct answer.**

30. 1. A change in bowel movements may indicate cancer but not atherosclerosis.
    2. A headache is not a sign/symptom of atherosclerosis.
    3. Intermittent claudication is a sign of generalized atherosclerosis and is a marker of atherosclerosis.
    4. Atherosclerosis indicates arterial involvement, not venous involvement.

**TEST-TAKING HINT: Knowledge of medical terminology—in this case, knowing that "atherosclerosis" refers to arteries—would**

allow the test taker to rule out all of the answer options, except "3," even if the test taker does not know what intermittent claudication means.

31. 1. Glucose does not combine with carbon monoxide.
    2. Vasoconstriction is not a risk factor for developing atherosclerosis.
    3. This is the scientific rationale why diabetes mellitus is a modifiable risk factor for atherosclerosis.
    4. When glucose combines with the hemoglobin in a laboratory test called glycosylated hemoglobin, the result can determine the client's average glucose level over the past three (3) months.

    **TEST-TAKING HINT:** The nurse must understand the reason "why," or the scientific rationale, for teaching in addition to nursing interventions. This is critical thinking.

32. 1. Collateral circulation is the development of blood supply around narrowed arteries; it helps prevent complications of atherosclerosis, including myocardial infarction, cerebrovascular accidents, and peripheral vascular disease. Exercise promotes the development of collateral circulation.
    2. Isometric (weight-lifting) exercises help develop muscle mass, but this type of exercise does not help decrease complications of atherosclerosis.
    3. A low-fat, low-cholesterol diet may help decrease the plaque formation, but exercise will not do this.
    4. Isotonic exercises, such as walking and swimming, promote the movement of glucose across the cell membrane, but this is not why such exercises are recommended for prevention of atherosclerotic complications.

    **TEST-TAKING HINT:** The test taker must understand what the stem of the question is asking and note the words "the complications of atherosclerosis." Isometric, which refers to "muscle" (remember "m"), and "isotonic," which refers to "tone" (remember "t"), exercises do not directly help prevent the complications of atherosclerosis, so options "2" and "4" can be eliminated.

33. 1. A statin medication can be taken with food or on an empty stomach.
    2. Statin medications should be taken in the evening for best results because the enzyme that destroys cholesterol works best in the evening and the medication enhances this process.

    3. Cholesterol-reducing medications can cause serious liver problems, and if a client has muscle pain, it is an adverse effect that should be reported to the HCP.
    4. The cholesterol level is checked every few months, not on a daily basis.

    **TEST-TAKING HINT:** The test taker must be aware of adjectives such as "daily." Cholesterol is not monitored daily, so "4" can be eliminated. There are only a few medications taken on an empty stomach; most medications can and should be administered with food to help prevent gastric irritation.

34. 1. Fried foods are high in fat and cholesterol.
    2. White bread is not high in fiber; wheat bread should be recommended because it is high in fiber. Whole milk is high in fat; skim milk should be used.
    3. Baked, broiled, or grilled meats are recommended; a plain baked potato is appropriate; and skim milk is low in fat—so this meal is appropriate for a low-fat, low-cholesterol diet.
    4. Hamburger meat is high in fat, French fries are usually cooked in oil (which is high in fat), and carbonated beverages are high in calories.

    **TEST-TAKING HINT:** The nurse must be aware of special diets, and a low-fat, low-cholesterol diet is often prescribed for clients with atherosclerosis. Remember baked, broiled, and grilled meats are lower in fat and cholesterol than fried meats.

35. 1. Adherence to lifestyle modifications is enhanced when the client receives support from significant others.
    2. Tobacco use is the most significant modifiable risk factor that contributes to the development of atherosclerosis.
    3. A sedentary lifestyle should be discouraged; daily walking or swimming is encouraged.
    4. This is an unrealistic intervention. The nurse needs to help the client learn ways to deal with stressful situations, not avoid the situations.
    5. Isometric exercises are weight-lifting exercises, which should be discouraged; isotonic exercises, such as walking or swimming, are encouraged.

    **TEST-TAKING HINT:** This type of alternate question requires the test taker to select all answer options that apply. Some interventions are universal to all teaching, such as including significant others. Be careful with words such as "avoid."

36. 1. Teaching cannot be delegated to a nursing assistant.

2. The nursing assistant can feed a client.

3. The nursing assistant cannot assess the client and does not have the education to interpret laboratory data.

4. A unit of blood must be checked by two (2) registered nurses at the bedside.

TEST-TAKING HINT: Many states have rules concerning what tasks can be delegated to unlicensed nursing assistants, but even those states that don't have delegation rules agree that teaching, assessing, evaluating, and medication administration cannot be delegated to unlicensed assistive personnel.

## Abdominal Aortic Aneurysm

37. 1. Shortness of breath indicates a respiratory problem or possible a thoracic aneurysm, not an AAA.

2. A systolic bruit over the abdomen is a diagnostic indication of an AAA.

3. Ripping or tearing pain indicates a dissecting aneurysm.

4. Urine output is not diagnostic of an AAA.

TEST-TAKING HINT: The test taker who has no idea of the answer should note that two of the answer options—"2" and "3"—have the word "abdominal" and choose between them, ruling out "1" and "4," both of which refer to other systems of the body (respiratory and urinary).

38. 1. When the aneurysm is small (<5–6 cm) an abdominal sonogram will be done every six (6) months until the aneurysm reaches a size at which surgery to prevent rupture is of more benefit than possible complications of an abdominal aortic aneurysm repair.

2. An intravenous pyelogram evaluates the kidney.

3. The abdomen will not distend as the AAA enlarges.

4. This AAA is too small to perform surgery to remove.

TEST-TAKING HINT: The AAA less than 3 cm should make the test taker assume that surgery is not an option; therefore "4" could be ruled out as a correct answer. "Pyelo" means "kidney" so "2" could be ruled out. The term "medical treatment" in the stem of the question should cause the test taker to rule out abdominal girth.

39. 1. AAAs affect males four (4) times more often than women.

2. AAAs affect males four (4) times more often than women.

3. The most common cause of AAA is atherosclerosis (which is the cause of peripheral

vascular disease); it occurs in men four (4) times more often than women and primarily in Caucasians.

4. AAAs occur most often in elderly men and there is no genetic predisposition.

TEST-TAKING HINT: If the test taker knew that AAA and peripheral vascular disease both occur with atherosclerosis, it might possibly lead to the selection of "3" as the correct answer.

40. 1. This statement would not make the nurse suspect an AAA.

2. Only about two-fifths of clients with AAA have symptoms; the remainder are asymptomatic.

3. Periodic episodes of constipation and diarrhea may indicate colon cancer but do not support a diagnosis of AAA.

4. Belching does not support a diagnosis of AAA, but it could possibly indicate gastroesophageal reflux or a hiatal hernia.

TEST-TAKING HINT: The test taker must remember that not all disease processes or conditions have signs/symptoms. The test taker should attempt to determine what disease processes the other answer options are describing.

41. 1. Low back pain is present because of the pressure of the aneurysm on the lumbar nerves; this is a serious symptom, usually indicating that the aneurysm is expanding rapidly and about to rupture.

2. If any pulses were affected, it would be the pedal pulses, not the radial pulses.

3. Decreased urine output would not indicate an expanding AAA, but decreased urine output may occur when the AAA ruptures, causing hypovolemia.

4. The abdominal girth would not increase for an expanding AAA, but it might increase with a ruptured AAA.

TEST-TAKING HINT: If the test taker knows the anatomical position of the abdominal aorta and understands the term "expanding," it may lead the test taker to select low back pain as the correct answer.

42. 1. The nurse needs to intervene, but it does not require immediate intervention.

2. The client must have 30 mL urinary output every hour. Clients who are post-operative AAA are at high risk for renal failure because of the anatomical location of the AAA near the renal arteries.

3. The client can sit on the bed the first day post-operation; this is, in fact, encouraged.

4. These vital signs would not warrant immediate intervention by the nurse.

**TEST-TAKING HINT: A basic concept that the test taker should remember is that any urine output less than 30 mL per hour should be cause for investigation.**

43. 1. Assessment is the first part of the nursing process and is the first intervention the nurse should implement.
    2. Administering an antibiotic is an appropriate intervention, but it is not priority over assessment.
    3. The client should splint the incision when coughing and deep breathing to help decrease the pain, but this intervention is not priority over assessment.
    4. Ambulating the client as soon as possible is an appropriate intervention to help decrease complications from immobility, but it is not priority over assessment.

**TEST-TAKING HINT: If the test taker has difficulty in determining the first intervention, always rely on the nursing process and select the assessment intervention if the intervention is appropriate for the disease process or condition.**

44. 1. The client is at risk for bleeding; therefore, this order would not be questioned.
    2. **Increased pressure in the abdomen secondary to a tap water enema could cause the AAA to rupture.**
    3. The client should be able to ambulate to the bathroom without any problems.
    4. Clients are NPO prior to surgery to help prevent aspiration or problems from general anesthesia.

**TEST-TAKING HINT: Expanding AAA should cause the test taker to realize that no additional pressure should be placed on the AAA and that, therefore, selecting "2" would be the most appropriate answer. Options "1," "3," and "4" would be appropriate for a client scheduled for an AAA repair or most types of surgeries. Remember basic concepts.**

45. 1. The most common cause of AAA is atherosclerosis, so teaching should address this area.
    2. A low-fat, low-cholesterol diet will help decrease development of atherosclerosis.
    3. The client should not decrease tobacco use—he or she must quit totally. Smoking is the one modifiable risk factor that is not negotiable.
    4. Losing weight will help decrease the pressure on the AAA and will help address decreasing the cholesterol level.

5. A truss is worn by a client with a hernia, not an AAA.

**TEST-TAKING HINT: Select-all-that-apply questions are an alternate type question that requires the nurse to select all interventions that are applicable to the question. The RN-NCLEX does not give partial credit; the test taker must select all appropriate answers to receive full credit for the question.**

46. 1. **Any neurovascular abnormality in the client's lower extremities indicates the graft is occluded or possibly bleeding and requires immediate intervention by the nurse.**
    2. The nurse would expect the client to have incisional pain six (6) hours after surgery, so this is not priority over a complication.
    3. The nurse would expect the client to have a distended, nontender abdomen as a result of post-operative edema.
    4. A slightly elevated temperature would not be uncommon in a client who has had surgery.

**TEST-TAKING HINT: Any time the test taker has an answer option that has the word "absent" in it, the test taker should determine if this is normal for any client and, if not, then should select it as the correct answer because the stem is asking which information warrants immediate intervention.**

47. 1. **Redness or irritation of the incision indicates infection and should be reported immediately to the HCP.**
    2. The client should not lift anything heavier than five (5) pounds because it may cause dehiscence or evisceration of the bowel.
    3. The pain medication should keep the client comfortable; if it doesn't, the client should call the HCP.
    4. Some clients do not have daily bowel movements, but the nurse should instruct the client not to get constipated, which will increase pressure on the incision.

**TEST-TAKING HINT: The test taker should use basic concepts to answers questions. Signs/symptoms of incisional infection or systemic infection should always be reported to the HCP. Remember, do not eliminate an option as a possible answer just because the test taker thinks it is too easy an answer.**

48. 1. Organs in the right upper quadrant include the liver and gallbladder.
    2. **The aorta transverses the abdomen in the midline position and that is the best location to hear an abdominal bruit. The bell should be placed midline above the umbilicus to best auscultate an abdominal bruit.**

Vascular

3. Organs in the left upper quadrant include the stomach, pancreas, and spleen.
4. Organs in the left lower quadrant are the colon and ovaries in females.

**TEST-TAKING HINT: There may be questions on the RN-NCLEX that require the test taker to point to a specific area. The test taker must know correct anatomical positions for body parts and organs.**

## Deep Vein Thrombosis

49. 1. The client will be taking an oral anticoagulant, warfarin (Coumadin). Prothrombin time (PT) and International Normalized ratio (INR) levels, not partial thromboplastin time (PTT), are monitored when this medication is taken. The client should be in therapeutic range before discharge. The HCP will determine how often to monitor the levels, usually in two (2) to three (3) weeks and then at three (3) to six (6) month intervals.
2. The client is not restricted to the home. The client should not take part in any activity that does not allow frequent active and passive leg exercises. In an airplane the client should be instructed to drink plenty of fluids, move the legs up and down, and flex the muscles. If in an automobile, the client should take frequent breaks to walk around.
3. **Green leafy vegetables contain vitamin K, which is the antidote for warfarin. These foods will interfere with the action of warfarin. Red or brown urine may indicate bleeding.**
4. The client should be instructed to wear stockings that do not constrict any area of the leg.

**TEST-TAKING HINT: The test taker must know laboratory data for specific medications. INR and PT are monitored for oral anticoagulants. Remember: "PT boats go to war" (warfarin). PTT monitors heparin (tt is like an H for heparin).**

50. 1. **A complication of immobility after surgery is developing a DVT. This client with left calf pain should be assessed for a DVT.**
2. This is an expected finding.
3. Clients who require an open cholecystectomy frequently are discharged with a T tube. This client needs to know how to care for the tube before leaving, but this is not a priority over a possible surgical complication.
4. This is expected for this client.

**TEST-TAKING HINT: In priority setting questions, the test taker must decide if the infor-**

mation in the answer option is expected or abnormal for the situation. Based on this, "2," "3," and "4" can be eliminated.

51. 1. Passive range of motion exercises are recommended to prevent contracture formation and muscle atrophy, but this is a musculoskeletal complication, not a cardiovascular one.
2. If the client is on a ventilator, then the paralysis associated with GB has moved up the spinal column to include the muscles of respiration. Passive range of motion exercises are done by the staff; the client will not be able to do active ROM.
3. Range of motion exercises will not alleviate the pain of GB.
4. **One reason for performing range of motion exercises is to assist the blood vessels in the return of blood to the heart, preventing DVT.**

**TEST-TAKING HINT: The question is asking for a cardiovascular reason for range of motion exercises. Options "1," "2," and "3" do not have any cardiovascular component. Only "4" discusses veins and blood.**

52. 1. This protects the client's privacy.
2. **The assistant could dislodge a blood clot in the leg when massaging the calf. The assistant can apply lotion gently, being sure not to massage the leg.**
3. Testing the temperature of the water prevents scalding the client with water that is too hot or making the client uncomfortable with water that is too cold.
4. Collecting supplies needed before beginning the bath is using time wisely and avoids interrupting the bath to go and get items needed.

**TEST-TAKING HINT: This is an "except" question, so all options except one will be actions that should be encouraged. The test taker should not jump to the first option and choose it as the correct answer.**

53. 1. Sequential compression devices provide gentle compression of the legs to prevent DVT, but they are not used to treat DVT because the compressions could cause the clot to break loose.
2. **Clients should be on bed rest for five (5) to seven (7) days after diagnosis to allow time for the clot to adhere to the vein wall, thereby preventing embolization.**
3. **Bed rest and limited activity predispose the client to constipation. Fluids and diets high in fiber will help prevent constipation. Fluids will also help provide adequate fluid volume in the vasculature.**

Vascular

4. The client will be administered a heparin IV drip, which should be monitored.
5. Homans' sign is done to determine if a DVT is present. This client has already been diagnosed with a DVT. Manipulating the leg to determine Homans' sign could dislodge the clot.

**TEST-TAKING HINT: Two (2) of the answer options are used to determine if a DVT is present or to prevent one. The test taker should not become confused about treatment and prevention or early diagnosis.**

54. **20 mL/hour.** To determine the rate, the test taker must first determine how many units are in each mL of fluid; 25,000 divided by 500 = 50 units of heparin in each mL of fluid, and 50 divided into 100 = 2, and 2 + 18 = 20.

**TEST-TAKING HINT: This math question is worked in several steps, but every step is simple addition, multiplication, or division.**

55. 1. A potentially life-threatening complication of DVT is a pulmonary embolus, which causes chest pain. The nurse should determine if the client has "thrown" a pulmonary embolus.
2. An immobile client should be turned at least every two (2) hours, but a pressure area is not life threatening.
3. This is expected in a client who has a large upper abdominal incision. It hurts to breathe deeply. The nurse should address this but has some time. The life-threatening complication is priority.
4. Clients who have had inguinal hernia repair often have difficulty voiding afterward. This is expected.

**TEST-TAKING HINT: The test taker should determine which option contains information that is a potentially life-threatening situation. This is the priority client.**

56. 1. The nurse should check the laboratory values pertaining to the medications before administering the medications.
2. The client will be administered an oral medication while still receiving a heparin drip to allow time for the client to achieve a therapeutic level of the oral medication before discontinuing the heparin. The effects of oral medications take three (3) to five (5) days to become therapeutic.
3. The laboratory values should be noted before administering the medications.
4. The heparin will be continued for three (3) to five (5) days before being discontinued.

**TEST-TAKING HINT: Knowing the actions of each medication, as well as the laboratory tests that monitor the safe range of dosing, is important. Remember, assessment is first. Assess blood levels and then administer the medication.**

57. 1. Keeping the legs dependent and standing still will promote the development of a DVT.
2. Flexing the leg muscles and changing positions assist the blood to return to the heart and move out of the peripheral vessels.
3. The nurse should wear support stockings, not socks, and change the types of shoes worn from day to day, varying the type of heels.
4. This is not in the client's best interest.

**TEST-TAKING HINT: The test taker can eliminate option "4" by imagining the reaction of the HCP if this were done. The adverbs "dependent" and "still" make "1" wrong.**

58. 1. This occurs from the administration of the low molecular weight heparin and is not a reason to notify the HCP.
2. A therapeutic range will not be achieved with LMWH, and PTT levels are usually not done.
3. This is not hemorrhaging, and the client should be reassured that this is a side effect of the medication.
4. Assessing the vital signs will not provide any pertinent information to help answer the client's question.

**TEST-TAKING HINT: Before selecting "Notify the HCP," the test taker should ask, "What will the HCP do with this information? What can the HCP order or do to help the purple hemorrhaged areas?" This would cause the test taker to eliminate "1" as a possible answer.**

59. 1. There is nothing that contraindicates the use of a stool softener, and use of one may be recommended if the client is prone to constipation and hard stool that could cause some bleeding from hemorrhoids.
2. A medic alert bracelet notifies any emergency HCP of the client's condition and medications.
3. Vitamin E can affect the action of warfarin. The nurse should explain to the client that these and other medications could potentiate the action of warfarin.
4. This would be recommended for the client if the footrest does not restrict blood flow in the calves.

**TEST-TAKING HINT: The test taker can eliminate "1" by realizing that a stool softener would not cause a problem and could help with an unrelated problem. Medic alert bracelets**

Vascular

are frequently recommended for many clients with certain diseases and conditions.

60. 1. BUN lab tests are measurements of renal functioning.
    2. Bilirubin is a liver function test.
    3. PT/INR is a test to monitor warfarin (Coumadin) action in the body.
    4. PTT levels monitor heparin activity.

**TEST-TAKING HINT:** The test taker should devise some sort of memory-jogging mnemonic or aid to remember which lab test monitors for which condition. Try "PT boats go to war," so PT monitors warfarin.

## Peripheral Venous Disease

61. 1. Venous insufficiency is a venous problem, not an arterial problem.
    2. Deep vein thrombosis is not a complication of chronic venous insufficiency, but it may be a cause.
    3. Venous ulcerations are the most serious complication of chronic venous insufficiency. It is very difficult for these ulcerations to heal, and often clients must be seen in wound care clinics for treatment.
    4. Varicose veins may lead to chronic venous insufficiency, but they are not a complication.

**TEST-TAKING HINT:** The test taker must use knowledge of anatomy, which would eliminate "1" because "venous" and "arterial" refer to different parts of the vascular system. The test taker must key in on the most serious complication to select the correct answer.

62. 1. The medial part of the ankle usually ulcerates because of edema that leads to stasis, which, in turn, causes the skin to break down.
    2. A deep, pale, open area over the top side of the foot describes an arterial ulcer.
    3. A reddened blistered area on the heel describes a blister that may result from wearing shoes that are too tight or that rub on the heel.
    4. Gangrene does not usually occur with venous problems; it occurs with arterial ulcers.

**TEST-TAKING HINT:** There are some questions that require the test taker to be knowledgeable of the disease process.

63. 1. Low-heeled comfortable shoes should be recommended to help decrease foot pain, but they will not help prevent varicose veins.
    2. Wearing white, clean socks will help prevent irritation to the feet.
    3. Moving the legs back and forth often may help

prevent deep vein thrombosis, but it will not prevent varicose veins.
    4. Graduated compression hose help decrease edema and increase the circulation back to the heart; this helps prevent varicose veins.

**TEST-TAKING HINT:** Options "1" and "2" could be eliminated as possible answers if the test taker knows that the varicose veins are in the leg because "1" and "2" are addressing the feet.

64. 1. Varicose veins are irregular, tortuous veins with incompetent valves that do not allow the venous blood to ascend the saphenous vein.
    2. Decreased oxygen to the muscle occurs with arterial occlusive disease.
    3. This is the explanation for a deep vein thrombosis.
    4. Thick, poorly circulating blood could be an explanation for diabetic neuropathy.

**TEST-TAKING HINT:** Knowing that veins have valves and arteries might help the test taker select the correct answer. The test taker should use knowledge of anatomy and physiology to determine the answer.

65. 1. The client should not cross legs at all because this further impedes the blood from ascending the saphenous vein.
    2. Elevating the foot of the bed while sleeping helps the venous blood return to the heart and decreases pressure in the lower extremity.
    3. Antiplatelet therapy is for arterial blood, not venous blood.
    4. Fluid intake will not help prevent or improve chronic venous insufficiency.

**TEST-TAKING HINT:** Knowing about the venous and arterial blood system will help the test taker eliminate or identify the correct answer. Venous blood goes back to the heart, so elevating the feet will help return it. Options "3" and "4" do not have anything to do with the extremities.

66. 1. Research shows that removing the compression stockings while the client is in bed promotes perfusion of the subcutaneous tissue. The foot of the bed should be elevated.
    2. The assistant can take the blood pressure with a machine or manually; therefore, the nurse would not need to intervene.
    3. The assistant can help the client with meals as long as the client is stable.
    4. The assistant can calculate the intake and output, but the nurse must evaluate the data to determine if they are normal for the client.

TEST-TAKING HINT: This is a backward "except" question. Flipping the question and asking which actions would be appropriate for the assistant to implement might make it easier for the test taker to answer the question.

67. 1. The occupational therapist assists the client with activities of daily living skills, such as eating, bathing, or brushing teeth.
    2. The social worker would assess the client to determine if home health care services or financial interventions were appropriate for the client. The client is elderly, immobility is a concern, and wound care must be a concern when the client is discharged home.
    3. The physical therapist addresses gait training and transferring.
    4. Cardiac rehabilitation helps clients who have had myocardial infarctions, cardiac bypass surgery, or congestive heart failure recover.

TEST-TAKING HINT: The test taker must be aware of the responsibilities of other members of the health-care team. "Discharge" is the key word in the stem. The test taker should select an answer that will help the client in the home.

68. 1. Pedal pulses are normal in venous insufficiency, but pulses are decreased or absent in arterial insufficiency.
    2. The skin is warm in venous insufficiency; the skin is cool in arterial insufficiency.
    3. Intermittent claudication, pain that occurs when walking, is a symptom of arterial insufficiency.
    4. Chronic venous insufficiency leads to chronic edema that, in turn, causes a brownish pigmentation to the skin.

TEST-TAKING HINT: The test taker could apply anatomical concepts to eliminate both "1" and "2" because it is the arteries that have pulses and control the temperature of the skin.

69. 1. Varicose veins are more common in white females in occupations that involve prolonged standing.
    2. Driving a bus does not require prolonged standing, which is a risk factor for developing varicose veins.
    3. Studies suggest that the increased risk for varicose veins is common and may be the result of venous stasis during pregnancy.
    4. Diabetes may lead to diabetic neuropathy and arterial occlusive disease, but it does not lead to varicose veins.

TEST-TAKING HINT: The test taker must know that prolonged standing is a risk factor for

varicose veins and identify which occupations include being on the feet most of the time.

70. 1. Because the saphenous vein is removed during vein ligation, standing and sitting are prohibited during the initial recovery period to prevent increased pressure in the lower extremities.
    2. Pressure bandages are applied for up to six (6) weeks after vein ligation to help prevent bleeding and to help venous return from the lower extremities when in the standing or sitting position.
    3. Sequential compression devices are used to help prevent deep vein thrombosis.
    4. Antibiotics would be ordered prophylactically for surgery, but it is not the first intervention.

TEST-TAKING HINT: When the question asks the test taker to implement the first intervention, two or more of the answer options could be possible interventions, but only one is implemented first. Apply the nursing process and select the intervention that addresses assessment, which is the first part of the nursing process.

71. 1. The client with a venous stasis ulcer should have pain, so this would be expected.
    2. Dull, aching muscle cramps are expected with varicose veins.
    3. The inability to move the foot means that a severe neurovascular compromise has occurred, and the nurse should assess this client first.
    4. A positive Homans' sign is expected in a client diagnosed with deep vein thrombosis.

TEST-TAKING HINT: The nurse should assess the client who is experiencing an abnormal, unexpected, or life-threatening complication of the disease process. Do not automatically select the client with pain; pain in many instances is not life threatening or unexpected.

72. 1. The nurse should determine if the client has any numbness or tingling.
    2. The nurse should determine if the client has pulses, the presence of which indicates there is no circulatory compromise.
    3. The nurse should determine if the client can move the feet and legs.
    4. The nurse should determine if the client's feet are pink or pale.
    5. The nurse should assess the feet to determine if they are cold or warm.

TEST-TAKING HINT: These five (5) assessment interventions along with assessing for pain are known as the 6s, which is the neurovascular assessment.

1. Which client behavior would be a causative factor for developing Buerger's disease (thromboangiitis obliterans)?
   1. Drinking alcohol daily.
   2. Eating a high-fat diet.
   3. Chewing tobacco.
   4. Inhaling gasoline fumes.

2. Which signs/symptoms would the nurse expect to find when assessing a client diagnosed with subclavian steal syndrome?
   1. Complaints of arm tiredness with exertion.
   2. Complaints of shortness of breath while resting.
   3. Jugular vein distention when sitting at a 35-degree angle.
   4. Dilated blood vessels above the nipple line.

3. Which question should the nurse ask the male client diagnosed with aorto-iliac disease during the admission interview?
   1. "Do you have trouble sitting for long periods of time?"
   2. "How often do you have a bowel movement and urinate?"
   3. "When you lie down do you feel throbbing in your abdomen?"
   4. "Have you experienced any problems having sexual intercourse?"

4. The client is four (4) hours post-operative abdominal aortic aneurysm repair. Which nursing intervention should be implemented for this client?
   1. Assist the client to ambulate.
   2. Assess the client's bilateral pedal pulses.
   3. Maintain continuous IV heparin drip.
   4. Provide a clear liquid diet to the client.

5. Which referral would be most appropriate for the client diagnosed with thoracic outlet syndrome?
   1. The physical therapist.
   2. The thoracic surgeon.
   3. The occupational therapist.
   4. The social worker.

6. Which instruction should the nurse discuss with the client diagnosed with Raynaud's phenomenon?
   1. Explain exacerbations will not occur in the summer.
   2. Use nicotine gum to help quit smoking.
   3. Wear extra warm clothing during cold exposure.
   4. Avoid prolonged exposure to direct sunlight.

7. The client diagnosed with diabetes mellitus type 2 is admitted to the hospital with cellulitis of the right foot secondary to an insect bite. Which intervention should the nurse implement first?
   1. Administer intravenous antibiotics.
   2. Apply warm moist packs every two (2) hours.
   3. Elevate the right foot on two (2) pillows.
   4. Teach the client about skin and foot care.

8. Which discharge instruction should the nurse discuss with the client to prevent recurrent episodes of cellulitis?
   1. Soak your feet daily in Epsom salts for 20 minutes.
   2. Wear thick white socks when working in the yard.
   3. Use a mosquito repellant when going outside.
   4. Inspect the foot between the toes for cracks in the skin.

9. Which discharge instruction should the nurse teach the client diagnosed with varicose veins who has received sclerotherapy?
   1. Walk 15 to 20 minutes three (3) times a day.
   2. Keep the legs in the dependent position when sitting.
   3. Remove compression bandages before going to bed.
   4. Perform Berger-Allen exercises four (4) times a day.

10. The nurse is teaching the client with peripheral vascular disease. Which interventions should the nurse discuss with the client? Select all that apply.
    1. Wash your feet in antimicrobial soap.
    2. Wear comfortable, well-fitting shoes.
    3. Cut your toenails in an arch.
    4. Keep the area between the toes dry.
    5. Use a heating pad when feet are cold.

11. The unlicensed nursing assistant is applying elastic compression stockings to the client. Which action by the assistant would warrant immediate intervention by the nurse?
    1. The assistant is putting the stockings on while the client is in the chair.
    2. The assistant inserted two (2) fingers under the proximal end of the stocking.
    3. The assistant elevated the feet while lying down prior to putting on the stockings.
    4. The assistant made sure the toes were warm after putting the stockings on.

12. The nurse is administering a beta blocker to the client diagnosed with essential hypertension. Which data would cause the nurse to question administering the medication?
    1. The client's BP is 110/70.
    2. The client's potassium level is 3.4 mEq/L.
    3. The client has a barky cough.
    4. The client's apical pulse is 56.

13. The client diagnosed with acute deep vein thrombosis is receiving a continuous heparin drip, an intravenous anticoagulant. The health-care provider orders warfarin (Coumadin), an oral anticoagulant. Which action should the nurse take?
    1. Discontinue the heparin drip prior to initiating the Coumadin.
    2. Check the client's INR prior to beginning Coumadin.
    3. Clarify the order with the health-care provider as soon as possible.
    4. Administer the Coumadin along with the heparin drip as ordered.

14. The nurse is caring for the client on strict bed rest. Which intervention is priority when caring for this client?
    1. Encourage the client to drink liquids.
    2. Perform active range of motion exercises.
    3. Elevate the head of the bed to 45 degrees.
    4. Provide a high-fiber diet to the client.

15. The nurse is caring for clients on a medical floor. Which client will the nurse assess first?
    1. The client with an abdominal aortic aneurysm who is constipated.
    2. The client on bed rest who ambulated to the bathroom.
    3. The client with essential hypertension who has epistaxis and a headache.
    4. The client with arterial occlusive disease who has a decreased pedal pulse.

16. The client with peripheral venous disease is scheduled to go to the whirlpool for a dressing change. Which is the nurse's priority intervention?
    1. Escort the client to the physical therapy department.
    2. Medicate the client 30 minutes before going to whirlpool.
    3. Obtain the sterile dressing supplies for the client.
    4. Assist the client to the bathroom prior to the treatment.

Vascular

17. The client is receiving prophylactic low molecular weight heparin. There is no PT/PTT, INR on the client's chart since admission three (3) days ago. Which action should the nurse implement?
    1. Administer the medication as ordered.
    2. Notify the health-care provider immediately.
    3. Obtain a PT/PTT, INR prior to administering.
    4. Hold the medication until the HCP makes rounds.

18. The client diagnosed with atherosclerosis asks the nurse, "I have heard of atherosclerosis for many years but I never really knew what it meant. Am I going to die?" Which statement would be the nurse's best response?
    1. "This disease process will not kill you, so don't worry."
    2. "The blood supply to your brain is being cut off."
    3. "It is what caused you to have your high blood pressure."
    4. "Atherosclerosis is a buildup of plaque in your arteries."

19. Which signs/symptoms would the nurse expect to find in the female client diagnosed with Marfan's syndrome?
    1. Xerostomia, dry eyes, and complaints of a dry vagina.
    2. A triad of arthritis, conjunctivitis, and urethritis.
    3. Very tall stature and long bones in the hands and feet.
    4. Spinal deformities of the vertebral column and malaise.

20. The nurse is preparing to administer 7.5 mg of an oral anticoagulant. The medication available is 5 mg per tablet. How many tablets should the nurse administer?_____

21. Which dietary selection indicates the client with essential hypertension understands the discharge teaching?
    1. Fried pork chops, a loaded baked potato, and coffee.
    2. Spaghetti and meatballs, garlic bread, and iced tea.
    3. Baked ham, macaroni and cheese, and milk.
    4. Broiled fish, steamed broccoli, and garden salad.

22. The client diagnosed with Buerger's disease (thromboangiitis obliterans) asks the nurse, "What is the worse thing that could happen if I don't quit smoking? I love my cigarettes." Which statement is the nurse's best response?
    1. "You are concerned about quitting smoking. Let's sit down and talk about it."
    2. "Many clients end up having to have an amputation, especially a leg."
    3. "If you are worried about quitting, you should attend Smokenders."
    4. "Your coronary arteries could block and cause a heart attack."

23. The client diagnosed with subclavian steal syndrome has undergone surgery. Which assessment data would warrant immediate intervention by the nurse?
    1. The client's pedal pulse on the left leg is absent.
    2. The client complains of numbness in the right hand.
    3. The client's brachial pulse is strong and bounding.
    4. The client's capillary refill time (CRT) is <three (3) seconds.

24. The client with a left-sided mastectomy is diagnosed with elephantiasis of the left arm. Which signs/symptoms should the nurse expect to assess?
    1. Edematous arm from axillary area to fingertips.
    2. Painful edematous reddened lower forearm.
    3. Tented skin turgor over the entire left arm.
    4. Nipple retraction and *peau d'orange* skin.

Vascular

25. The client is four (4) hours post-operative femoral–popliteal bypass surgery. Which pulse would be best for the nurse to assess for complications related to an occluded vessel?
    1. A
    2. B
    3. C
    4. D

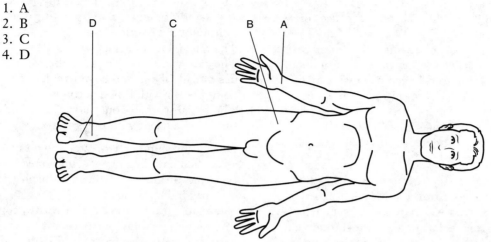

26. The client admitted with a diagnosis of pneumonia complains of tenderness and pain in the left calf, and the nurse assesses a positive Homans' sign. Which interventions should the nurse implement? List in order of priority.
    1. Notify the health-care provider.
    2. Initiate an intravenous line.
    3. Monitor the client's PTT.
    4. Administer a continuous heparin infusion.
    5. Instruct the client not to get out of the bed.

Vascular

1.  1. Drinking alcohol daily is not a cause of Buerger's disease.
    2. Eating a high-fat diet is not a cause of Buerger's disease.
    3. **Heavy smoking or chewing tobacco is a causative or aggravating factor for Buerger's disease. Cessation of tobacco use may cause cessation of the disease process in some clients.**
    4. Inhaling gasoline fumes is not a cause of Buerger's disease; however, this can cause neurological damage.

2.  1. **Subclavian steal syndrome occurs in the upper extremities from a subclavian artery occlusion or stenosis, which causes arm tiredness, paresthesia, and exercise-induced pain in the forearm when the arms are elevated. This is also known as upper-extremity arterial occlusive disease.**
    2. Shortness of breath could be a sign of a variety of diseases, including congestive heart failure, pneumonia, or chronic obstructive pulmonary disease.
    3. Jugular vein distension could indicate congestive heart failure.
    4. Dilated vessels above the nipple line are a sign of superior vena cava syndrome, an oncologic emergency.

3.  1. The client would not experience problems sitting; walking causes the pain.
    2. The client does not have elimination dysfunction.
    3. This would indicate an abdominal aortic aneurysm but not an aortoiliac problem.
    4. **Aortoiliac disease is caused by atherosclerosis of the aortoiliac arch, which causes pain in the lower back and buttocks and impotence in men.**

4.  1. At four (4) hours post-operative the client would not be able to ambulate and would be in the intensive care unit. The client usually ambulates the first day post-operative.
    2. **A neurovascular assessment is priority to make sure the graft is perfusing the lower extremities.**
    3. Intravenous anticoagulant therapy would cause the client to bleed post-operatively. Prophylactic anticoagulant therapy may be ordered to help prevent deep vein thrombosis.
    4. The client will be NPO and have a nasogastric tube for at least 24 hours.

5.  1. **Thoracic outlet syndrome is a compression of the subclavian artery at the thoracic outlet by an anatomical structure such as a rib or muscle. Physical therapy, exercises, and avoiding aggravating positions are recommended treatment.**
    2. The nurse does not refer to a surgeon.
    3. The occupational therapist helps with activities of daily living and cognitive disorders that do not occur with this syndrome.
    4. The social worker would not need to be consulted for a client with this syndrome.

6.  1. During the summer a sweater should be available when entering an air-conditioned room.
    2. Nicotine of any type causes vasoconstriction and may induce attacks.
    3. **Raynaud's phenomenon is a form of intermittent arteriolar vasoconstriction that results in coldness, pain, and pallor of fingertips or toes; therefore the client should keep warm to prevent vasoconstriction of the extremities.**
    4. Sunlight does not cause an exacerbation of this disease.

7.  1. This would be an appropriate intervention but not before elevating the foot.
    2. Warm, moist packs cause necessary dilatation, but it is not the first intervention.
    3. **Elevating the foot above the heart will decrease edema and thereby help decrease the pain. It is the easiest and first intervention for the nurse to implement.**
    4. Educating the client is important, but it is not the first intervention. The client will be hospitalized for seven (7) to fourteen (14) days.

8.  1. Soaking the feet will not help prevent cellulitis; salt would be drying to the tissue, causing cracks that may lead to cellulitis.
    2. Thick white socks do not prevent cellulitis.
    3. Mosquito repellant would help to prevent encephalitis but not cellulitis.
    4. **The key to preventing cellulitis is identifying the sites of bacterial entry. The most commonly overlooked areas are the cracks and fissures that occur between the toes.**

9.  1. **After sclerotherapy clients are taught to perform walking activities to maintain blood flow in the leg and enhance dilution of the sclerosing agent.**
    2. The legs should be elevated to decrease edema. The legs should not be below the level of the heart, which is the dependent position.
    3. The compression bandages should be kept on at all times for at least five (5) days or when the

health-care provider removes them for the first time.

4. These exercises are recommended for clients with arterial occlusive disease, not a venous disease.

10. 1. Antimicrobial soap is harsh and can dry the skin; the client should use mild soap and room-temperature water.

   2. **Shoes must be comfortable to prevent blisters or ulcerations of the feet.**

   3. The toenails should be cut straight across; cutting in an arch increases the risk for ingrown toenails.

   4. **Moisture between the toes increases fungal growth, leading to skin breakdown.**

   5. The client with PVD has decreased sensation in the feet and should not use a heating pad.

11. 1. **Stockings should be applied after the legs have been elevated for a period of time when the amount of blood in the leg vein is at its lowest; therefore, the nurse should intervene when the assistant is putting them on while the client is in the chair.**

   2. The top of the stocking should not be tight; being able to insert two (2) fingers indicates it is not too tight.

   3. This is the correct way to apply stockings.

   4. Warm toes mean the stockings are not too tight and that there is adequate circulation.

12. 1. This BP indicates the medication is effective and in the desired range, and the nurse should not question administering the medication.

   2. This potassium level is low, but a beta blocker does not affect the potassium level.

   3. A barky cough is associated with an ACE inhibitor, not a beta blocker.

   4. **The beta blocker decreases sympathetic stimulation to the beta cells of the heart. Therefore, the nurse should question administering the medication if the apical pulse is less than 60 beats per minute.**

13. 1. This is an inappropriate intervention.

   2. The INR is checked to determine if the medication is within therapeutic range, not prior to administering the first dose.

   3. The order does not need to be clarified.

   4. **It will require several days for the Coumadin to reach therapeutic levels; the client will continue receiving the heparin drip until the therapeutic range can be attained.**

14. 1. Fluids will help prevent dehydration and renal calculi, but it is not the priority nursing intervention.

2. **Preventing deep vein thrombosis is the priority nursing intervention because the client is on strict bed rest; ROM exercises should be done every four (4) hours.**

3. Elevating the head of the bed will not help prevent immobility complications.

4. High-fiber diets will help prevent constipation, but it is not priority.

15. 1. This is not priority unless the client is actively having a bowel movement and is performing the Valsalva maneuver.

   2. This client needs to be addressed and orders need to be clarified, but this is not priority.

   3. **A bloody nose and a headache indicate the client is experiencing very high blood pressure and should be assessed first because of a possible myocardial infarction or stroke.**

   4. A decreased pedal pulse is expected in this client.

16. 1. The physical therapy department comes and gets the client; if not, the nursing assistant should escort the client to physical therapy.

   2. **The client's pain is priority, and the nurse should premedicate prior to treatment.**

   3. The physical therapy department will have the supplies for dressing the wound.

   4. This could be done, but it is not priority for the nurse.

17. 1. **Subcutaneous heparin will not achieve a therapeutic level because of the short half-life of the medication; therefore the nurse should administer the medication.**

   2. There is no need to notify the HCP.

   3. There is no need to monitor these lab tests.

   4. There is no need to notify the HCP.

18. 1. This is not a true statement. Atherosclerosis causes strokes, heart attacks, and hypertension, which are all possibly lethal diseases.

   2. This may occur, but it does not answer the client's question.

   3. This may occur, but it does not answer the client's question.

   4. **A buildup of plaque in the arteries is occurring in the body when the client has atherosclerosis.**

19. 1. Xerostomia, dry eyes, and dry vagina are symptoms of Sjögren's syndrome.

   2. A triad of arthritis, conjunctivitis, and urethritis are symptoms of Reiter's syndrome.

   3. **Clients with Marfan's syndrome are very tall and have long bones in the hands and feet. They also have abnormalities of the cardiovascular system resulting in valvular**

problems and aneurysms, which are the leading cause of death during the late 20s.
4. Spinal deformities and malaise are symptoms of ankylosing spondylitis.

20. 1.5 tablets. The nurse must score one tablet and administer one and a half tablets to ensure that the correct dose is administered.

21. 1. Fried foods have a lot of grease, a loaded bake potato is high in fat, and coffee has caffeine. This is a high-calorie, high-sodium diet that is not recommended.
2. Spaghetti is high in carbohydrates, meat is high in fat, garlic bread is high in carbohydrates, and iced tea has caffeine.
3. Ham is cured meat and is high in sodium, but many clients do not realize this; cheese and milk are high in sodium.
4. **The client should be eating a low-fat, low-cholesterol, low-sodium diet. This meal reflects this diet.**

22. 1. This is a therapeutic response and does not answer the client's question.
2. **Smoking aggravates Buerger's disease. Aggravated or severe Buerger's disease can lead to arterial occlusion caused by superficial thrombophlebitis causing poor wound healing and poor circulation. This can lead to the need for amputation.**
3. This is an appropriate referral, but it does not answer the question.
4. Buerger's disease affects the arteries and veins of the upper and lower extremities, but it does not affect the coronary arteries.

23. 1. Subclavian steal syndrome affects the upper extremities only.
2. **Subclavian steal syndrome occurs in the upper extremities from a subclavian artery occlusion or stenosis; therefore, any abnormal neurovascular assessment would warrant intervention.**

3. This is a normal finding and would not warrant immediate intervention.
4. These are normal findings and would not warrant immediate intervention.

24. 1. **Elephantiasis is obstruction of the lymphatic vessels that causes chronic fibrosis, thickening of the subcutaneous tissue, and hypertrophy of the skin; this condition causes chronic edema of the extremity that recedes only slightly with elevation.**
2. This may be cellulitis.
3. This may indicate dehydration of the tissue.
4. Nipple retraction and *peau d'orange* skin would be an indication of late-stage breast cancer.

25. 1. An absent radial pulse would not indicate a complication of a lower-extremity surgery.
2. The femoral pulse would be an appropriate pulse to assess, but it is not the best because the nurse needs to determine if the blood is getting to the most distal area of the leg.
3. The popliteal pulse would be an appropriate pulse to assess, but it is not the best because the nurse needs to determine if the blood is getting to the most distal area of the leg.
4. **The pedal pulse is the best pulse to assess because it indicates if there is adequate circulation to the most distal site of the extremity. The bypass extends from the mid-thigh to the mid-calf area.**

26. In order of priority: 5, 1, 2, 4, 3
5. **The nurse should suspect a deep vein thrombosis and should not allow the client to get out of the bed.**
1. **This is a medical emergency and the HCP should be notified as soon as possible.**
2. **The client needs an intravenous line so that IV heparin can be administered.**
4. **The treatment for DVT is to prevent further coagulation until the clot dissolves.**
3. **The client's PTT is monitored when receiving heparin therapy.**

# Hematological Disorders

**5**

Hematological disorders include a broad range of blood dyscrasias, which may be hereditary or have an unknown etiology; some may be fatal, and some clients may live a normal life. Among the most serious blood disorders—types of cancer—are leukemia and lymphoma. Others include bleeding disorders, both hereditary (hemophilia and von Willebrand's disease) and nonhereditary (thrombocytopenia purpura); clotting disorders (disseminated intravascular coagulation); and anemias characterized by abnormal red blood cells (sickle cell anemia, thalassemia). The nurse must know the signs/symptoms of these disorders, what is expected with the disorder, and when immediate intervention is necessary. The questions and answers that follow cover these topics.

## KEYWORDS

angiogram
apoptosis
autologous
epistaxis
hemarthrosis
hematemesis
hematoma
hematuria
leukocytosis
leukopenia
melena
menorrhagia
neutropenia
pancytopenia
placenta previa
purpura

## ABBREVIATIONS

Absolute Neutrophil Count (ANC)
Activities of Daily Living (ADL)
Acute Respiratory Distress Syndrome (ARDS)
American Cancer Society (ACS)
Arterial Blood Gases (ABG)
Arterial Partial Pressure of Oxygen ($Pao_2$)
As Needed (PRN)
Capillary Refill Time (CRT)
Chronic Lymphocytic Leukemia (CLL)
Complete Blood Count (CBC)
Continuous Passive Motion (CPM)
Disseminated Intravascular Coagulation (DIC)
End-Stage Renal Disease (ESRD)
Gastrointestinal Tract (GI)
Health-Care Provider (HCP)
Hematocrit (Hct)
Hemoglobin (Hb)
Hemoglobin and Hematocrit (H&H)
Human Leukocyte Antigen (HLA)
Idiopathic Thrombocytopenia Purpura (ITP)
Immediately (STAT)
Intramuscular (IM)
Intravenous (IV)
Intravenous Push (IVP)
Medication Administration Record (MAR)
Nonsteroidal Anti-Inflammatory Drug (NSAID)
Over-The-Counter (OTC)
Packed Red Blood Cell (PRBC)
Partial Pressure of Carbon Dioxide ($Pco_2$)
Partial Thromboplastin Time (PTT)
Post-Anesthesia Care Unit (PACU)
Prothrombin Time (PT)
Red Blood Cell (RBC)
Sickle Cell Anemia (SCA)
Unlicensed Assistive Personnel (UAP)
White Blood Cell (WBC)

### Leukemia

1. The nurse is caring for clients on an oncology unit. Which neutropenia precautions should be implemented?
   1. Hold all venipuncture sites for at least five (5) minutes.
   2. Limit fresh fruits and flowers.
   3. Place all clients in reverse isolation.
   4. Have the client use a soft-bristle toothbrush.

2. The nurse is assessing a client diagnosed with acute myeloid leukemia. Which assessment data support this diagnosis?
   1. Fever and infections.
   2. Nausea and vomiting.
   3. Excessive energy and high platelet counts.
   4. Cervical lymph node enlargement and positive acid-fast bacillus.

3. The client diagnosed with leukemia has central nervous system involvement. Which instructions should the nurse teach?
   1. Sleep with the head of the bed elevated to prevent increased intracranial pressure.
   2. Take an analgesic medication for pain only when the pain becomes severe.
   3. Explain that radiation therapy to the head may result in permanent hair loss.
   4. Discuss end-of-life decisions prior to cognitive deterioration.

4. The client diagnosed with leukemia is scheduled for a bone marrow transplant. Which interventions should be implemented to prepare the client for this procedure? Select all that apply.
   1. Administer high-dose chemotherapy.
   2. Teach the client about autologous transfusions.
   3. Have the family members' HLA typed
   4. Monitor the complete blood cell count daily.
   5. Provide central line care per protocol.

5. The client is diagnosed with chronic lymphocytic leukemia (CLL) after routine laboratory tests during a yearly physical. Which is the scientific rationale for the random nature of discovering the illness?
   1. CCL is not serious, and clients die from other causes first.
   2. There are no symptoms with this form of leukemia.
   3. This is a childhood illness and is self-limiting.
   4. In early stages of CLL the client may be asymptomatic.

6. The client diagnosed with leukemia is being admitted for an induction course of chemotherapy. Which laboratory values indicate a diagnosis of leukemia?
   1. A left shift in the white blood cell count differential.
   2. A large number of WBCs that decreases after the administration of antibiotics.
   3. An abnormally low hemoglobin (Hgb) and hematocrit (Hct) level.
   4. Red blood cells that are larger than normal.

7. Which medication is contraindicated for a client diagnosed with leukemia?
   1. Bactrim, a sulfa antibiotic.
   2. Morphine, a narcotic analgesic.
   3. Epogen, a biologic response modifier.
   4. Gleevec, a genetic blocking agent.

8. The laboratory results for a male client diagnosed with leukemia include RBC count 2.1 mm $\times$ $10^6$, WBC 150 mm $\times$ $10^3$, platelets 22 $\times$ $10^3$, K+ 3.8 mEq/L, Na+ 139mEq/L. Based on these results, which interventions should the nurse teach the client?
   1. Encourage the client to eat foods high in iron.
   2. Instruct the client to use an electric razor when shaving.
   3. Discuss the importance of limiting sodium in the diet.
   4. Instruct the family to limit visits to once a week.

9. The nurse writes a nursing problem of "altered nutrition" for a client diagnosed with leukemia who has received a treatment regimen of chemotherapy and radiation. Which nursing intervention should be implemented?
    1. Administer an antidiarrheal medication prior to meals.
    2. Monitor the client's serum albumin levels.
    3. Assess for signs and symptoms of infection.
    4. Provide skin care to irradiated areas,

10. The nurse and licensed practical nurse (LPN) are caring for clients on an oncology floor. Which client should not be assigned to the LPN?
    1. The client newly diagnosed with chronic lymphocytic leukemia.
    2. The client who is four (4) hours post-procedure bone marrow biopsy.
    3. The client who received two (2) units of PRBCs on the previous shift.
    4. The client who is receiving multiple intravenous piggyback medications.

11. The nurse is completing a care plan for a client diagnosed with leukemia. Which independent problem should be addressed?
    1. Infection.
    2. Anemia.
    3. Nutrition.
    4. Grieving.

12. The nurse is caring for a client diagnosed with acute myeloid leukemia. Which assessment data warrant immediate intervention?
    1. T 99°, P 102, R 22, and BP 132/68.
    2. Hyperplasia of the gums.
    3. Weakness and fatigue.
    4. Pain in the left upper quadrant.

## Lymphoma

13. The client diagnosed with non-Hodgkin's lymphoma is scheduled for a lymphangiogram. Which information should the nurse teach?
    1. The scan will identify any malignancy in the vascular system.
    2. Radiopaque dye will be injected between the toes.
    3. The test will be done similar to a cardiac angiogram.
    4. The test will be completed in about five (5) minutes.

14. The client asks the nurse, "They say I have cancer. How can they tell if I have Hodgkin's disease from a biopsy?" The nurse's answer is based on which scientific rationale?
    1. Biopsies are nuclear medicine scans that can detect cancer.
    2. A biopsy is a laboratory test that detects cancer cells.
    3. It determines which kind of cancer the client has.
    4. The HCP takes a small piece out of the tumor and looks at the cells.

15. The nurse is admitting a client with rule-out Hodgkin's lymphoma. When the nurse assesses the client, which data would support this diagnosis?
    1. Night sweats and fever without "chills."
    2. Edematous lymph nodes in the groin.
    3. Malaise and complaints of an upset stomach.
    4. Pain in the neck area after a fatty meal.

16. Which client is at the highest risk for developing a lymphoma?
    1. The client diagnosed with chronic lung disease who is taking a steroid.
    2. The client diagnosed with breast cancer who has extensive lymph involvement.
    3. The client who received a kidney transplant several years ago.
    4. The client who has had ureteral stent placements for a neurogenic bladder.

17. The female client recently diagnosed with Hodgkin's lymphoma asks the nurse about her prognosis. Which is the nurse's best response?
    1. Survival for Hodgkin's disease is relatively good with standard therapy.
    2. Survival depends on becoming involved in an investigational therapy program.
    3. Survival is poor, with more than 50% of clients dying within six (6) months.
    4. Survival is fine for primary Hodgkin's, but secondary cancers occur within a year.

18. The nurse writes the problem of "grieving" for a client diagnosed with non-Hodgkin's lymphoma. Which collaborative intervention should be included in the plan of care?
    1. Encourage the client to talk about feelings of loss.
    2. Arrange for the family to plan a memorable outing.
    3. Refer the client to the American Cancer Society's (ACS) Dialogue group.
    4. Have the chaplain visit with the client.

19. Which test is considered diagnostic for Hodgkin's lymphoma?
    1. A magnetic resonance image (MRI) of the chest.
    2. A computed tomography (CT) scan of the cervical area.
    3. An erythrocyte sedimentation rate (ESR).
    4. A biopsy of the cervical lymph nodes.

20. Which client should be assigned to the experienced medical-surgical nurse who is in the first week of orientation to the oncology floor?
    1. The client diagnosed with non-Hodgkin's lymphoma who is having daily radiation treatments.
    2. The client diagnosed with Hodgkin's disease who is receiving combination chemotherapy.
    3. The client diagnosed with leukemia who has petechiae covering both anterior and posterior body surfaces.
    4. The client diagnosed with diffuse histolytic lymphoma who is to receive two (2) units of packed red blood cells.

21. Which information about reproduction should be taught to the 27-year-old female client diagnosed with Hodgkin's disease?
    1. The client's reproductive ability will be the same after treatment is completed.
    2. The client should practice birth control for at least two (2) years following therapy.
    3. All clients become sterile from the therapy and should plan to adopt.
    4. The therapy will temporarily interfere with the client's menstrual cycle.

22. Which clinical manifestation of Stage I non-Hodgkin's lymphoma would the nurse expect to find when assessing the client?
    1. Enlarged lymph tissue anywhere in the body.
    2. Tender left upper quadrant.
    3. No symptom in this stage.
    4. Elevated B cell lymphocytes on the CBC.

23. The nurse and an unlicensed assistive personnel (UAP) are caring for clients in a bone marrow transplant unit. Which nursing task should the nurse delegate?
    1. Take the hourly vital signs on a client receiving blood transfusions.
    2. Monitor the infusion of antineoplastic medications.
    3. Transcribe the doctor's orders onto the Medication Administration Record (MAR).
    4. Determine the client's response to the therapy.

24. The 33-year-old client diagnosed with Stage IV Hodgkin's lymphoma is at the five (5)-year remission mark. Which information should the nurse teach the client?
    1. Instruct the client to continue scheduled screenings for cancer.
    2. Discuss the need for follow-up appointments every five (5) years.
    3. Teach the client that the cancer risk is now the same as for the general population.
    4. Have the client talk with the family about funeral arrangements.

## Anemia

25. The nurse is admitting a 24-year-old African American female client with a diagnosis of rule-out anemia. The client has a history of gastric bypass surgery for obesity four (4) years ago. Current assessment findings include height 5′5″; weight 75 kg; P 110, R 27, and BP 104/66; pale mucous membranes and dyspnea on exertion. Which type of anemia would the nurse suspect the client has developed?
    1. Vitamin $B_{12}$ deficiency.
    2. Folic acid deficiency.
    3. Iron deficiency.
    4. Sickle cell anemia.

26. The client diagnosed with menorrhagia complains to the nurse of feeling listless and tired all the time. Which scientific rationale would explain why these symptoms occur?
    1. The pain associated with the menorrhagia does not allow the client to rest.
    2. The client's symptoms are unrelated to the diagnosis of menorrhagia.
    3. The client probably has been exposed to a virus that causes chronic fatigue.
    4. Menorrhagia has caused the client to have decreased levels of hemoglobin.

27. The nurse writes a diagnosis of altered tissue perfusion for a client diagnosed with anemia. Which interventions should be included in the plan of care? Select all that apply.
    1. Monitor the client's Hb and Hct.
    2. Move the client to a room near the nurse's desk.
    3. Limit the client's dietary intake of green vegetables.
    4. Assess the client for numbness and tingling.
    5. Allow for rest periods during the day for the client.

28. The client diagnosed with iron-deficiency anemia is prescribed ferrous gluconate orally. Which should the nurse teach the client?
    1. Take Imodium, an antidiarrheal, OTC for diarrhea.
    2. Limit exercise for several weeks until a tolerance is achieved.
    3. The stools may be very dark, and this can mask blood.
    4. Eat only red meats and organ meats for protein.

29. The nurse and unlicensed nursing assistant are caring for clients on a medical unit. Which task should the nurse delegate to the unlicensed nursing assistant?
    1. Check on the bowel movements of a client diagnosed with melena.
    2. Take the vitals signs of a client who received blood the day before.
    3. Evaluate the dietary intake of a client who has been noncompliant with eating.
    4. Shave the client diagnosed with severe hemolytic anemia.

30. The client is diagnosed with congestive heart failure and anemia. The HCP ordered a transfusion of two (2) units of packed red blood cells. The unit has 250 mL of red blood cells plus 45 mL of additive. At what rate should the nurse set the IV pump to infuse each unit of packed red blood cells?_____

31. The client is being admitted with folic acid–deficiency anemia. Which would be the most appropriate referral?
    1. Alcoholic Anonymous.
    2. Leukemia Society of America.
    3. A hematologist.
    4. A social worker.

32. The charge nurse is making assignments on a medical floor. Which client should be assigned to the most experienced nurse?
    1. The client diagnosed with iron-deficiency anemia who is prescribed iron supplements.
    2. The client diagnosed with pernicious anemia who is receiving vitamin B$_{12}$ intramuscularly (IM).
    3. The client diagnosed with aplastic anemia who has developed pancytopenia.
    4. The client diagnosed with renal disease who has a deficiency of erythropoietin.

33. The client diagnosed with anemia begins to complain of dyspnea when ambulating in the hall. Which intervention should the nurse implement first?
    1. Apply oxygen via nasal cannula.
    2. Get a wheelchair for the client.
    3. Assess the client's lung fields.
    4. Assist the client when ambulating in the hall.

34. The nurse is transcribing the HCP's order for an iron supplement on the MAR. At which time should the nurse schedule the daily dose?
    1. 0900.
    2. 1000.
    3. 1200.
    4. 1630.

35. The nurse is discharging a client diagnosed with anemia. Which discharge instruction should the nurse teach?
    1. Take the prescribed iron until it is completely gone.
    2. Monitor pulse and blood pressure at a local pharmacy weekly.
    3. Have a complete blood count checked at the HCP's office.
    4. Perform isometric exercise three (3) times a week.

36. The nurse writes a client problem of "activity intolerance" for a client diagnosed with anemia. Which intervention should the nurse implement?
    1. Pace activities according to tolerance.
    2. Provide supplements high in iron and vitamins.
    3. Administer packed red blood cells.
    4. Monitor vital signs every four (4) hours.

## Bleeding Disorders

37. The charge nurse in the intensive care unit is making client assignments. Which client should the charge nurse assign to the graduate nurse who has just finished the three (3)-month orientation?
    1. The client with an abdominal peritoneal resection who has a colostomy.
    2. The client diagnosed with pneumonia who has acute respiratory distress syndrome.
    3. The client with a head injury developing disseminated intravascular coagulation.
    4. The client admitted with a gunshot wound who has an H&H of 7 and 22.

38. Which client would be most at risk for developing disseminated intravascular coagulation (DIC)?
    1. A 35-year-old pregnant client with placenta previa.
    2. A 42-year-old client with a pulmonary embolus.
    3. A 60-year-old client receiving hemodialysis three (3) days a week.
    4. A 78-year-old client diagnosed with septicemia.

39. The client admitted with full-thickness burns may be developing DIC. Which signs/symptoms would support the diagnosis of DIC?
    1. Oozing blood from the IV catheter site.
    2. Sudden onset of chest pain and frothy sputum.
    3. Foul smelling, concentrated urine.
    4. A reddened, inflamed central line catheter site.

40. Which laboratory result would the nurse expect in the client diagnosed with DIC?
    1. A decreased prothrombin time (PT).
    2. A low fibrinogen level.
    3. An increased platelet count.
    4. An increased white blood cell count.

41. Which collaborative treatment would the nurse anticipate for the client diagnosed with DIC?
    1. Administer oral anticoagulants.
    2. Prepare for plasmapheresis.
    3. Administer frozen plasma.
    4. Calculate the intake and output.

42. The unlicensed nursing assistant asks the primary nurse, "How does someone get hemophilia A?" Which statement would be the primary nurse's best response?
    1. "It is an inherited x-linked recessive disorder."
    2. "There is a deficiency of the clotting factor VIII."
    3. "The person is born with hemophilia A."
    4. "The mother carries the gene and gives it to the son."

43. Which sign/symptom should the nurse expect to assess in the client diagnosed with hemophilia A?
    1. Epistaxis.
    2. Petechiae.
    3. Subcutaneous emphysema.
    4. Intermittent claudication.

44. Which situation might cause the nurse to think that the client has von Willebrand's disease?
    1. The client has had unexplained episodes of hematemesis.
    2. The client has microscopic blood in the urine.
    3. The client has prolonged bleeding following surgery.
    4. The female client developed abruptio placentae.

45. The client with hemophilia A is experiencing hemarthrosis. Which intervention should the nurse recommend to the client?
    1. Alternate aspirin and acetaminophen to help with the pain.
    2. Apply cold packs for 24–48 hours to the affected area.
    3. Perform active range of motion exercise on the extremity.
    4. Put the affected extremity in the dependent position.

46. Which sign would the nurse expect to assess in the client diagnosed with idiopathic thrombocytopenia purpura (ITP)?
    1. Petechiae on the anterior chest, arms, and neck.
    2. Capillary refill of less than three (3) seconds.
    3. An enlarged spleen.
    4. Pulse oximeter reading of 95%.

47. The nurse is caring for the following clients. Which client should the nurse assess first?
    1. The client whose partial thromboplastin time (PTT) is 38 seconds.
    2. The client's whose hemoglobin is 14 gm/dL and hematocrit is 45%.
    3. The client's whose platelet count is 75,000 per milliliter of blood.
    4. The client's whose red blood cell count is $48 \times 10^6$ mm.

48. Which nursing interventions should the nurse implement when caring for a client diagnosed with hemophilia A? Select all that apply.
    1. Instruct the client to use a razor blade to shave.
    2. Avoid administering enemas to the client.
    3. Encourage participation in noncontact sports.
    4. Teach the client how to apply direct pressure if bleeding occurs.
    5. Explain the importance of not flossing gums.

## Blood Transfusions

49. The client has a hematocrit of 22.3% and a hemoglobin of 7.7 mg/dL. The HCP has ordered two (2) units of packed red blood cells to be transfused. Which interventions should the nurse implement? Select all that apply.
    1. Obtain a signed consent.
    2. Initiate a 22-gauge IV.
    3. Assess the client's lungs.
    4. Check for allergies.
    5. Hang a keep-open IV of D5W.

50. The client is admitted to the emergency department after a motor-vehicle accident. The nurse notes profuse bleeding from a right-sided abdominal injury. Which intervention should the nurse implement first?
    1. Type and cross-match for red blood cells immediately (STAT).
    2. Initiate an IV with a #18-gauge needle and hang NS.
    3. Have the client sign a consent for an exploratory laparotomy.
    4. Notify the significant other of the client's admission.

51. The nurse is working in a blood bank facility procuring units of blood from donors. Which client would not be a candidate to donate blood?
    1. The client who had wisdom teeth removed a week ago.
    2. The nursing student who received a measles immunization 2 months ago.
    3. The mother with a six (6)-week-old newborn.
    4. The client who developed an allergy to aspirin in childhood.

52. The client with O+ blood is in need of an emergency transfusion but the lab does not have any O+ blood available. Which potential unit of blood could be given to the client?
    1. The O− unit.
    2. The A+ unit.
    3. The B+ unit.
    4. Any Rh+ unit.

53. The client is scheduled to have a total hip replacement in two (2) months and has chosen to prepare for autologous transfusions. Which medication would the nurse administer to prepare the client?
    1. Prednisone, a glucocorticoid.
    2. Zithromax, an antibiotic.
    3. Ativan, a tranquilizer.
    4. Epogen, a biologic response modifier.

54. The client undergoing knee replacement surgery has a "cell-saver" apparatus attached to the knee when he arrives in the post-anesthesia care unit (PACU). Which intervention should the nurse implement to care for this drainage system?
    1. Infuse the drainage into the client when a prescribed amount fills the chamber.
    2. Attach an hourly drainage collection bag to the unit and discard the drainage.
    3. Replace the unit with a continuous passive motion unit and start it on low.
    4. Have another nurse verify the unit number prior to reinfusing the blood.

55. Which statement is the scientific rationale for infusing a unit of blood in less than four (4) hours?
    1. The blood will coagulate if left out of the refrigerator for longer than four (4) hours.
    2. The blood has the potential for bacterial growth if allowed to infuse longer.
    3. The blood components begin to break down after four (4) hours.
    4. The blood will not be affected; this is a laboratory procedure.

56. The HCP orders two (2) units of blood to be administered over eight (8) hours each for a client diagnosed with heart failure. Which intervention(s) should the nurse take?
    1. Call the HCP to question the order because blood must infuse within four (4) hours.
    2. Retrieve the blood from the laboratory and run each unit at an eight (8)-hour rate.
    3. Notify the lab to split each unit into half units and infuse each half for four (4) hours.
    4. Infuse each unit for four (4) hours, the maximum rate for a unit of blood.

57. The client receiving a unit of PRBCs begins to chill and develops hives. Which action should be the nurse's first response?
    1. Notify the laboratory and health-care provider.
    2. Administer the histamine-1 blocker, Benadryl, IV.
    3. Assess the client for further complications.
    4. Stop the transfusion and change the tubing at the hub.

58. The nurse and unlicensed nursing assistant are caring for clients on an oncology floor. Which nursing task would be delegated to the unlicensed nursing assistant?
    1. Assess the urine output on a client who has had a blood transfusion reaction.
    2. Take the first 15 minutes of vital signs on a client receiving a unit of PRBCs.
    3. Auscultate the lung sounds of a client prior to a transfusion.
    4. Assist a client who received ten (10) units of platelets in brushing teeth.

59. The nurse is caring for clients on a medical floor. After the shift report, which client should be assessed first?
    1. The client who is two-thirds of the way through a blood transfusion and has had no complaints of dyspnea or hives.
    2. The client diagnosed with leukemia who has a hematocrit of 18% and petechiae covering the body.
    3. The client with peptic ulcer disease who called over the intercom to say that he is vomiting blood.
    4. The client diagnosed with Crohn's disease who is complaining of perineal discomfort.

60. The client received two (2) units of packed red blood cells of 250 mL with 63 mL of preservative each during the shift. There was 240 mL of saline remaining in the 500-mL bag when the nurse discarded the blood tubing. How many milliliters of fluid should be documented on the intake and output record?_____

## Sickle Cell Anemia

61. The student nurse asks the nurse, "What is sickle cell anemia?" Which statement by the nurse would be the best answer to the student's question?
    1. "There is some written material at the desk that will explain the disease."
    2. "It is a congenital disease of the blood in which the blood does not clot."
    3. "The client has decreased synovial fluid that causes joint pain."
    4. "The blood becomes thick when the client is deprived of oxygen."

62. The client's nephew has just been diagnosed with sickle cell anemia. The client asks the nurse, "How did my nephew get this disease?" Which statement would be the best response by the nurse?
    1. "Sickle cell anemia is an inherited autosomal recessive disease."
    2. "He was born with it and both his parents were carriers of the disease."
    3. "At this time, the cause of sickle cell anemia is unknown."
    4. "Your sister was exposed to a virus while she was pregnant."

63. The client diagnosed with sickle cell anemia comes to the emergency department complaining of joint pain throughout the body. The oral temperature is 102.4°F and the pulse oximeter reading is 91%. Which action should the emergency room nurse implement first?
    1. Request arterial blood gases STAT.
    2. Administer oxygen via nasal cannula.
    3. Start an IV with an 18-gauge Angiocath.
    4. Prepare to administer analgesics as ordered.

64. The client diagnosed with sickle cell anemia is experiencing with a vasoocclusive sickle cell crisis secondary to an infection. Which medical treatment should the nurse anticipate the HCP ordering for the client?
    1. Administer meperidine (Demerol) intravenously.
    2. Admit the client to a private room and keep in reverse isolation.
    3. Infuse D5W 0.33% NS at 150 mL/hr via pump.
    4. Insert a 22-French Foley catheter with a urimeter.

65. The nurse is assessing an African American client diagnosed with sickle cell crisis. Which assessment data is most pertinent when assessing for cyanosis in clients with dark skin?
    1. Assess the client's oral mucosa.
    2. Assess the client's metatarsals.
    3. Assess the client's capillary refill time.
    4. Assess the sclera of the client's eyes.

66. The client is diagnosed with sickle cell crisis. The nurse is calculating the client's intake and output (I&O) for the shift. The client had 20 ounces of water, eight (8) ounces of apple juice, three (3) cartons of milk with four (4) ounces each, 1800 mL of IV for the last 12 hours, and a urinary output of 1200. What is the client's total intake for this shift? _____

67. The nurse is caring for the female client recovering from a sickle cell crisis. The client tells the nurse that her family is planning a trip this summer to Yellowstone National Park. Which response would be best for the nurse?
    1. "That sounds like a wonderful trip to take this summer."
    2. "Have you talked to your doctor about taking the trip?"
    3. "You really should not take a trip to areas with high altitudes."
    4. "Why do you want to go to Yellowstone National Park?"

68. Which is a potential complication that occurs specifically to a male client diagnosed with sickle cell anemia during a sickle cell crisis?
    1. Chest syndrome.
    2. Compartment syndrome.
    3. Priapism.
    4. Hypertensive crisis.

69. The nurse is completing discharge teaching for the client diagnosed with a sickle cell crisis. The nurse recommends the client getting the flu and pneumonia vaccines. The client asks, "Why should I take those shots? I hate shots." Which statement by the nurse is the best response?
    1. "These vaccines promote health in clients with chronic illnesses."
    2. "You are susceptible to infections. These shots may help prevent a crisis."
    3. "The vaccines will help your blood from sickling secondary to viruses."
    4. "The doctor wanted to make sure that I discussed the vaccines with you."

70. The client diagnosed with sickle cell anemia asks the nurse, "Should I join the Sickle Cell Foundation? I received some information from the Sickle Cell Foundation. What kind of group is it?" Which statement is the best response by the nurse?
    1. "It is a foundation that deals primarily with research for a cure for SCA."
    2. "It provides information on the disease and on support groups in this area."
    3. "I recommend joining any organization that will help deal with your disease."
    4. "The foundation arranges for families that have children with sickle cell to meet."

71. Which sign/symptom will the nurse expect to assess in the client diagnosed with a vasoocclusive sickle cell crisis?
    1. Lordosis.
    2. Epistaxis.
    3. Hematuria.
    4. Petechiae.

72. The male client with sickle cell anemia comes to the emergency room with a temperature of 101.4°F and tells the nurse that he is having a sickle cell crisis. Which diagnostic test should the nurse anticipate the emergency room doctor ordering for the client?
    1. Spinal tap.
    2. Hemoglobin electrophoresis.
    3. Sickle-turbidity test (Sickledex).
    4. Blood cultures.

## Leukemia

1. 1. This would be done for thrombocytopenia (low platelets), not neutropenia (low white blood cells).
   2. Fresh fruits and flowers may carry bacteria or insects on the skin of the fruit or dirt on the flowers and leaves, so they are restricted around clients with low white blood cell counts.
   3. Clients with severe neutropenia may be placed in reverse isolation, but not all clients with neutropenia will be placed in reverse isolation. Clients are at a greater risk for infecting themselves from endogenous fungi and bacteria than from being exposed to noninfectious individuals.
   4. This is an intervention for thrombocytopenia.

   **TEST-TAKING HINT: The test taker must match the problem with the answer option. Options "1" and "4" would probably be implemented for the client with a bleeding disorder. Option "3" has the word "all" in it, which would make the test taker not select this option.**

2. 1. Fever and infection are hallmark symptoms of leukemia. They occur because the bone marrow is unable to produce white blood cells of the number and maturity needed to fight infection.
   2. Nausea and vomiting are symptoms related to the treatment of cancer but not to the diagnosis of leukemia.
   3. The clients are frequently fatigued and have low platelet counts. The platelet count is low as a result of the inability of the bone marrow to produce the needed cells. In some forms of leukemia, the bone marrow is not producing cells at all, and in others, the bone marrow is stuck producing tens of thousands of immature cells.
   4. Cervical lymph node enlargement is associated with Hodgkin's lymphoma, and positive acid-fast bacillus is diagnostic for tuberculosis.

   **TEST-TAKING HINT: Option "3" could be eliminated because of the excessive energy. Illness normally drains energy reserves; it does not increase them.**

3. 1. Sleeping with the head of the bed elevated might relieve some intracranial pressure, but it will not prevent intracranial pressure from occurring.
   2. Analgesic medications for clients with cancer are given on a scheduled basis with a fast-acting analgesic administered PRN for breakthrough pain.
   3. Radiation therapy to the head and scalp area is the treatment of choice for central nervous system involvement of any cancer. Radiation therapy has longer-lasting side effects than chemotherapy. If the radiation therapy destroys the hair follicle, the hair will not grow back.
   4. Cognitive deterioration does not usually occur.

   **TEST-TAKING HINT: The test taker must be aware of the treatments used for the disease processes to answer this question but might eliminate "2" because it violates basic principles of pain management.**

4. 1. All of the bone marrow cells must be destroyed prior to "implanting" the healthy bone marrow. High-dose chemotherapy and full-body irradiation therapy are used to accomplish this.
   2. Autologous transfusions are infusions from the client himself. This client has a cancer involving blood tissue. To reinfuse the client's own tissues would be to purposefully give the client cancer cells.
   3. The best bone marrow donor comes from an identical twin; next best comes from a sibling who matches. The most complications occur from a matched unrelated donor (MUD). The client's body recognizes the marrow as foreign and tries to reject it, resulting in graft-versus-host disease (GVHD).
   4. The CBC must be monitored daily to assess for infections, anemia, and thrombocytopenia.
   5. Clients will have at lest one multiple-line central venous access. These clients are seriously ill and require multiple transfusions and antibiotics.

   **TEST-TAKING HINT: If the test taker knows the definition of autologous, then "2" could be eliminated.**

5. 1. All types of leukemia are serious and can cause death. The chronic types of leukemia are more insidious in the onset of symptoms and can have a slower progression of the disease. Chronic types of leukemia are more common in the adult population.
   2. The symptoms may have a slower onset, but anemia causing fatigue and weakness and thrombocytopenia causing bleeding can be present (usually in the later stages of the disease). Organ enlargement from infiltration may be present, and the "2" symptoms of fever, night sweats, and weight loss may also be present.

Hematological

3. This disease is usually found in adults.
4. In this form of leukemia the cells seem to escape apoptosis (programmed cell death), which results in many thousands of mature cells clogging the body. Because the cells are mature, the client may be asymptomatic in the early stages.

**TEST-TAKING HINT: The test taker can eliminate option "1" on the basis of "not serious"; common sense lets the test taker know this is not true.**

6. 1. A left shift indicates that immature white blood cells are being produced and released into the circulating blood volume. This should be investigated for the malignant process of leukemia.
2. Leukocytosis (elevated WBC) is normal in the presence of an infection, but it should decrease as the infection clears.
3. A low hemoglobin and hematocrit level indicates anemia and can be caused by a number of factors. Anemia does occur in leukemia, but it is not diagnostic for leukemia.
4. Red blood cells larger than normal occur in macrocytic anemias (vitamin $B_{12}$ and folic acid deficiency). They are not characteristic of leukemia.

**TEST-TAKING HINT: The test taker should recognize elevated WBCs that resolve with antibiotics as an infection. Option "3" is not specific enough to be the correct answer.**

7. 1. Because of the ineffective or nonexistent WBCs (segmented neutrophils) characteristic of leukemia, the body cannot fight infections, and antibiotics are given to treat infections.
2. Leukemic infiltrations into the organs or the central nervous system cause pain. Morphine is the drug of choice for most clients with cancer.
3. Epogen is a biologic response modifier that stimulates the bone marrow to produce red blood cells. The bone marrow is the area of malignancy in leukemia. Stimulating the bone marrow would be generally ineffective for the desired results and would have the potential to stimulate malignant growth.
4. Gleevec is a drug that specifically works in leukemic cells to block the expression of the BCR-ABL protein, preventing the cells from growing and dividing.

**TEST-TAKING HINT: If the test taker was not familiar with the drug mentioned in "4," then it would not be a good choice. Options "1" and "2" are common drugs and should not be chosen as the answer unless the test taker knows for sure that they are contraindicated.**

8. 1. The anemia that occurs in leukemia is not related to iron deficiency, and eating foods high in iron will not help.
2. The platelet count of $22 \times 10^3$ indicates a platelet count of 22,000. The definition of thrombocytopenia is a count less than 100,000. This client is at risk for bleeding. Bleeding precautions include decreasing the risk by using soft-bristle toothbrushes and electric razors and holding all venipuncture sites for a minimum of five (5) minutes.
3. The sodium level is within normal limits. The client is encouraged to eat whatever the client wants to eat unless some other disease process limits food choices.
4. The client is at risk for infection, but unless the family or significant others are ill they should be encouraged to visit whenever possible.

**TEST-TAKING HINT: The test taker could eliminate "3" on the basis of a normal laboratory values. The RBC, WBC, and platelet values are all not in normal range. The correct answer option must address one of these values.**

9. 1. The nurse should administer an antiemetic prior to meals, not an antidiarrheal medication.
2. Serum albumin is a measure of the protein content in the blood that is derived from the foods eaten; albumin monitors nutritional status.
3. Assessment of the nutritional status is indicated for this problem, not assessment of the signs and symptoms of infections.
4. This addresses an altered skin-integrity problem.

**TEST-TAKING HINT: The stem of the question asks for interventions for "altered nutrition." Assessment is the first step of the nursing process, but option "3" is not assessing nutrition.**

10. 1. The newly diagnosed client will need to be taught about the disease and about treatment options. The registered nurse cannot delegate teaching to a an LPN.
2. This client is postprocedure and could be cared for by the LPN.
3. This client has received the blood products; this client requires routine monitoring, which the LPN could perform.
4. The LPN can administer antibiotic medications.

**TEST-TAKING HINT: The nurse cannot assign assessment, teaching, or evaluation. The clients in options "2," "3," and "4" are stable or have expected situations.**

Hematological

11. 1. Treating infections, which require HCP orders for cultures and antibiotics, is a collaborative problem.
    2. The treatment of anemia is a collaborative problem.
    3. The provision of adequate nutrition requires collaboration between the nurse, HCP, and dietitian.
    4. Grieving is an independent problem, and the nurse can assess and treat this problem with or without collaboration.

    **TEST-TAKING HINT: The stem of the question asks for an independent intervention. If the test taker understands the problem and the treatment needs, options "1," "2," and "3" can be eliminated.**

12. 1. These vital signs are not alarming. The vital signs are slightly elevated and indicate monitoring at intervals, but they do not indicate an immediate need.
    2. Hyperplasia of the gums is a symptom of myeloid leukemia, but it is not an emergency.
    3. Weakness and fatigue are symptoms of the disease and are expected.
    4. Pain is expected, but it is a priority, and pain control measures should be implemented.

    **TEST-TAKING HINT: If all the answer options contain expected events, the test taker must decide which is priority—and pain is a priority need.**

## Lymphoma

13. 1. The scan detects abnormalities in the lymphatic system, not the vascular system.
    2. Dye is injected between the toes of both feet and then scans are performed in a few hours, at 24 hours, and then possibly once a day for several days.
    3. Cardiac angiograms are performed through the femoral or brachial arteries and are completed in one session.
    4. The test takes 30 minutes to one (1) hour and then is repeated at intervals.

    **TEST-TAKING HINT: The test taker must be aware of diagnostic tests used to diagnose specific diseases. Options "1" and "3" could be eliminated because of the words "vascular" and "cardiac"; these words pertain to the cardiovascular system, not the lymphatic system.**

14. 1. Biopsies are surgical procedures requiring needle aspiration or excision of the area; they are not nuclear medicine scans.

2. The biopsy specimen is sent to the pathology lab for the pathologist to determine the type of cell. "Laboratory test" refers to tests of body fluids performed by a laboratory technician.
3. A biopsy is used to determine if the client has cancer and, if so, what kind. However, this response does not answer the client's question.
4. A biopsy is the removal of cells from a mass and examination of the tissue under a microscope to determine if the cells are cancerous. Reed-Sternberg cells are diagnostic for Hodgkin's disease. If these cells are not found in the biopsy, the HCP can rebiopsy to make sure the specimen provided the needed sample or, depending on involvement of the tissue, diagnose a non-Hodgkin's lymphoma.

**TEST-TAKING HINT: Option "1" can be eliminated if the test taker knows what the word "biopsy" means. Option "3" does not answer the question and can be eliminated for this reason.**

15. 1. Clients in late stages of Hodgkin's disease experience drenching diaphoresis, especially at night; fever without chills; and unintentional weight loss. Early-stage disease is indicated by a painless enlargement of a lymph node on one side of the neck (cervical area). Pruritus is also a common symptom.
    2. Lymph node enlargement with Hodgkin's disease is in the neck area.
    3. Malaise and stomach complaints are not associated with Hodgkin's disease.
    4. Pain in the neck area at the site of the cancer occurs in some clients after the ingestion of alcohol. The cause for this is unknown.

    **TEST-TAKING HINT: The test taker must notice the descriptive words, such as "groin" and "fatty," to decide if these options could be correct.**

16. 1. Long-term steroid use suppresses the immune system and has many side effects, but it is not the highest risk for the development of lymphoma.
    2. This client would be considered to be in late-stage breast disease. Cancers are described by the original cancerous tissue. This client has breast cancer that has metastasized to the lymph system.
    3. Clients who have received a transplant must take immunosuppressive medications to prevent rejection of the organ. This immunosuppression blocks the immune system from protecting the body against

cancers and other diseases. There is a high incidence of lymphoma among transplant recipients.

4. A neurogenic bladder is a benign disease; stent placement would not put a client at risk for cancer.

**TEST-TAKING HINT: To answer this question the test taker must be aware of the function of the immune system in the body and of the treatments of the disease processes.**

17. 1. Up to 90% of clients responds well to standard treatment with chemotherapy and radiation therapy, and those that relapse usually respond to a change of chemotherapy medications. Survival depends on the individual client and the stage of disease at diagnosis.
2. Investigational therapy regimens would not be recommended for clients initially diagnosed with Hodgkin's because of the expected prognosis with standard therapy.
3. Clients usually achieve a significantly longer survival rate than six (6) months. Many clients survive to develop long-term secondary complications.
4. Secondary cancers can occur as long as 20 years after a remission of the Hodgkin's disease has occurred.

**TEST-TAKING HINT: The test taker must have a basic knowledge of the disease process but could rule out "2" on the basis of the word "investigational."**

18. 1. Encouraging the client to talk about his or her feelings is an independent nursing intervention.
2. Discussing activities that will make pleasant memories and planning a family outing improve the client's quality of life and assists the family in the grieving process after the client dies, but this is an independent nursing intervention.
3. Nurses can and do refer clients diagnosed with cancer to the American Cancer Society–sponsored groups independently. Dialogue is a group support meeting that focuses on dealing with the feelings associated with a cancer diagnosis.
4. Collaborative interventions involve other departments of the health-care facility. A chaplain is a referral that can be made, and the two disciplines should work together to provide the needed interventions.

**TEST-TAKING HINT: The stem of the question asks for a collaborative intervention, which means that another health-care discipline must be involved. Options "1," "2," and "3"**

are all interventions that the nurse can do without another discipline being involved.

19. 1. An MRI of the chest area will determine numerous disease entities, but it cannot determine the specific morphology of Reed-Sternberg cells, which are diagnostic for Hodgkin's disease.
2. A CT scan will show tumor masses in the area, but it is not capable of pathological diagnosis.
3. ESR lab tests are sometimes used to monitor the progress of the treatment of Hodgkin's disease, but ESR levels can be elevated in several disease processes.
4. Cancers of all types are definitively diagnosed through biopsy procedures. The pathologist must identify Reed-Sternberg cells for a diagnosis of Hodgkin's disease.

**TEST-TAKING HINT: The test taker can eliminate the first three (3) answer options on the basis that these tests give general information on multiple diseases. A biopsy procedure of the involved tissues is the only procedure that provides a definitive diagnosis.**

20. 1. This client is receiving treatments that can have life-threatening side effects; the nurse is not experienced with this type of client.
2. Chemotherapy is administered only by nurses who have received training in chemotherapy medications and their effects on the body and are aware of necessary safety precautions; this nurse is in the first week of orientation.
3. This is expected in a client with leukemia, but it indicates a severely low platelet count; a nurse with more experience should care for this client.
4. This client is receiving blood. The nurse with experience on a medical-surgical floor should be able to administer blood and blood products.

**TEST-TAKING HINT: The key to this question is the fact that, although the nurse is an experienced medical-surgical nurse, the nurse is not experienced in oncology. The client who could receive a treatment on a medical-surgical floor should be assigned to the nurse.**

21. 1. This is a false promise. Many clients undergo premature menopause as a result of the cancer therapy.
2. The client should be taught to practice birth control during treatment and for at least two (2) years after treatment has ceased. The therapies used to treat the cancer can cause cancer. Antineoplastic medications are carcinogenic, and radiation therapy has proved to be a precursor to

Hematological

leukemia. A developing fetus would be subjected to the internal conditions of the mother.

3. Some clients—but not all—do become sterile. The client must understand the risks of therapy, but the nurse should give a realistic picture of what the client can expect. It is correct procedure to tell the client that the nurse does not know the absolute outcome of therapy. This is the ethical principle of veracity.

4. The therapy may interfere with the client's menses, but it may be temporary.

**TEST-TAKING HINT:** Option "3" can be eliminated on the basis that it says "all" clients; if the test taker can think of one case where "all" does not apply, then the option is incorrect.

22. 1. Enlarged lymph tissue would occur in stage III or IV Hodgkin's lymphoma.
    2. A tender left upper quadrant would indicate spleen infiltration and occur at a later stage.
    3. Stage I lymphoma presents with no symptoms; for this reason, clients are usually not diagnosed until the later stages of lymphoma.
    4. B cell lymphocytes are the usual lymphocytes that are involved in the development of lymphoma, but a serum blood test must be done specifically to detect B cells. They are not tested on a CBC.

**TEST-TAKING HINT:** Most cancers are staged from 0 to IV. Stage 0 is micro-invasive and stage I is minimally invasive, progressing to stage IV, which is large tumor load or distant disease. If the test taker noted the stage "I," then choosing the option that presented with the least amount of known disease, "3," would be a good choice.

23. 1. After the first 15 minutes during which the client tolerates the blood transfusion, it is appropriate to ask the unlicensed nursing assistant to take the vital signs as long as the assistant has been given specific parameters for the vital signs. Any vital sign outside the normal parameters must have an intervention by the nurse.
    2. Antineoplastic medication infusions must be monitored by a chemotherapy-certified, competent nurse.
    3. This is the responsibility of the ward secretary or the nurse, not the unlicensed nursing assistant.
    4. This represents the evaluation portion of the nursing process and cannot be delegated.

**TEST-TAKING HINT:** The test taker must decide what is within the realm of duties of an unli-

censed nursing assistant. Three (3) of the options have the assistant doing some action with medications. This could eliminate all of these. Option "1" did not say monitor or evaluate or decide on a nursing action; this option only says the assistant can take vital signs on a client who is presumably stable because the infusion has been going long enough to reach the hourly time span.

24. 1. The five (5)-year mark is a time for celebration for clients diagnosed with cancer, but the therapies can cause secondary malignancies and there may be a genetic predisposition for the client to develop cancer. The client should continue to be tested regularly.
    2. Follow-up appointments should be at least yearly.
    3. The client's risk for developing cancer has increased as a result of the therapies undergone for the lymphoma.
    4. This client is in remission, and death is not imminent.

**TEST-TAKING HINT:** The test taker should look at the time frames in the answer options. It would be unusual for a client to be told to have a checkup every five (5) years. Option "4" can be eliminated by the stem, which clearly indicates that the client is progressing well at the five (5)-year remission mark.

## Anemia

25. 1. The rugae in the stomach produce intrinsic factor, which allows the body to use vitamin $B_{12}$ from the foods eaten. Gastric bypass surgery reduces the amount of rugae drastically. Clients develop pernicious anemia (vitamin $B_{12}$ deficiency). Other symptoms of anemia include dizziness and the tachycardia and dyspnea listed in the stem.
    2. Folic acid deficiency is usually associated with chronic alcohol intake.
    3. Iron deficiency is the result of chronic blood loss or inadequate dietary intake of iron.
    4. Sickle cell anemia is associated with African Americans, but the symptoms and history indicate a different anemia.

**TEST-TAKING HINT:** The question did not give a lifetime history of anemia, which would be associated with sickle cell disease. The stem related a history of obesity and surgery. The test taker should look for an answer related to intake of vitamins and minerals. A review of the anatomy of the stomach is the key to the question.

26. 1. Menorrhagia (excessive blood loss during menses) does not cause pain. Fibroids or other factors that cause the menorrhagia may cause pain, but rest or sleep is not responsible for the listlessness or fatigue.
    2. The symptoms are the direct result of the excessive blood loss.
    3. Some viruses do cause a chronic fatigue syndrome, but there is a direct cause and effect from the menorrhagia.
    4. Menorrhagia is excessive blood loss during menses. If the blood loss is severe, then the client will not have the blood's oxygen-carrying capacity needed for daily activities. The most frequent symptom and complication of anemia is fatigue. It frequently has the greatest impact on the client's ability to function and quality of life.

    **TEST-TAKING HINT: Three (3) of the answer options have the word menorrhagia in them, but "3" detours from the subject to talk about viruses; this could eliminate it as a consideration. This question requires the test taker to understand medical terminology—in this case, what menorrhagia means—and then decide what results from that process in the body.**

27. 1. The nurse should monitor the hemoglobin and hematocrit in all clients diagnosed with anemia.
    2. Because decreased oxygenation levels to the brain can cause the client to become confused, a room where the client can be observed frequently—near the nurse's desk—is a safety issue.
    3. The client should include leafy green vegetables in the diet. These are high in iron.
    4. Numbness and tingling may occur in anemia as a result of neurological involvement.
    5. Fatigue is the number-one presenting symptom of anemia.

    **TEST-TAKING HINT: This is an alternative question requiring the test taker to select multiple correct answers. The test taker could eliminate "3" because the only clients told to limit green leafy vegetables are those receiving Coumadin, an oral anticoagulant.**

28. 1. Iron is constipating; an antidiarrheal is contraindicated for this drug.
    2. Iron can cause gastrointestinal distress and tolerance to it is built up gradually; exercise has nothing to do with tolerating iron.
    3. The stool will be a dark green–black and

can mask the appearance of blood in the stool.
    4. The client should eat a well-balanced diet high in iron, vitamins, and protein. Fowl and fish are encouraged.

    **TEST-TAKING HINT: The test taker could eliminate "4" as a possible answer because of the absolute word "only." Health-care professionals usually encourage the client to limit red and organ meats.**

29. 1. The nurse should evaluate the stools of a client diagnosed with melena (dark, tarry stools indicate blood) as part of the ongoing assessment.
    2. The unlicensed nursing assistant can take the vital signs of a client who is stable; this client received the blood the day before.
    3. Evaluation is the nurse's responsibility; the nurse should know exactly what the client is eating.
    4. A client with severe hemolytic anemia would have pancytopenia and is at risk for bleeding.

    **TEST-TAKING HINT: Melena indicates a problem with the bowel movements and would indicate a need for nursing judgment. A nurse cannot delegate judgment decisions.**

30. <u>74 mL/hour.</u> Pumps are set at an hourly rate. The client in congestive heart failure should receive blood at the slowest possible rate to prevent the client from further complications of fluid volume overload. Each unit of blood must be infused within four (4) hours of initiation of the infusion.

    250 mL + 45 mL = 295 ml
    <u>295 mL ÷ 4</u> = 73 3/4 mL/hour, which rounded is 74 mL/hour

    **TEST-TAKING HINT: The test taker must think about the disease process and the normal requirement for administering blood to arrive at the correct answer.**

31. 1. Most clients diagnosed with folic acid anemia have developed the anemia from chronic alcohol abuse. Alcohol consumption increases the use of folates, and the alcoholic diet is usually deficient in folic acid. A referral to Alcoholics Anonymous would be appropriate.
    2. There is no connection between folic acid deficiency and leukemia, therefore this referral would not be appropriate.
    3. A hematologist may see the client, but nurses usually don't make this kind of referral; the HCP would make this referral if the HCP felt incapable of caring for the client.
    4. The social worker is not the most appropriate referral.

Hematological

**TEST-TAKING HINT: The stem asks the test taker to decide which referral is most appropriate. Option "4" might be appropriate for a number of different clients, but nothing in the stem indicates a specific need for social services. The test taker must decide which could be a possible cause of folic acid deficiency anemia.**

32. 1. Any nurse should be able to administer iron supplements, which are oral iron preparations.
    2. Any nurse should be able to give an intramuscular medication.
    3. Pancytopenia is a situation that develops in clients diagnosed with aplastic anemia because the bone marrow is not able to produce cells of any kind. The client has anemia, thrombocytopenia, and leukopenia. This client could develop an infection or hemorrhage, go into congestive heart failure, or have a number of other complications develop. This client needs the most experienced nurse.
    4. A deficiency of erythropoietin is common in clients diagnosed with renal disease. The current treatment for this is to administer erythropoietin, a biologic response modifier, subcutaneously or, if the anemia is severe enough, a blood transfusion.

**TEST-TAKING HINT: The test taker could eliminate options "1" and "2" because of the words " most experienced nurse" in the stem.**

33. 1. The client may need oxygen, but getting the client a wheelchair and getting the client back to bed is priority.
    2. The client is experiencing dyspnea on exertion, which is common for clients with anemia. The client needs a wheelchair to limit the exertion.
    3. The problem with this client is not a pulmonary one; it is a lack of hemoglobin.
    4. Even if the nurse helps the client ambulate, the client still will not have the needed oxygen for the tissues.

**TEST-TAKING HINT: The test taker should ask, "What is causing the distress and what will alleviate the distress the fastest?" The distress is caused by exertion and it is occurring in the hallway. The most expedient intervention is to have the client stop the activity that is causing the distress; a chair will accomplish this, but the client should be returned to the room so it needs to be a wheelchair.**

34. 1. The usual medication dosing time for daily medications is 0900, but this is only an hour after the breakfast meal. Iron absorption is reduced when taken with food.

2. This is approximately two (2) hours after breakfast and is the correct dosing time for iron to achieve the best effects. Iron preparations should be administered one (1) hour before a meal or two (2) hours after a meal. Iron can cause gastrointestinal upset, but if administered with a meal, absorption can be diminished by as much as 50%.
3. This is the usual time that health-care facilities serve lunch.
4. This time would be very close to the evening meal and would decrease the absorption of the iron.

**TEST-TAKING HINT: The test taker could eliminate "3" and "4" if the test taker realized that both of these times are very close to meal times, so, with this in common, food must pose a problem for the medication.**

35. 1. This is an instruction for antibiotics, not iron. The client will take iron for an indefinite period.
    2. Pulse is indirectly affected by anemia when the body attempts to compensate for the lack of oxygen supply, but this is an indirect measure, and blood pressure is not monitored for anemia.
    3. The client should have a complete blood count regularly to determine the status of the anemia.
    4. Isometric exercises are bodybuilding exercises, and the client should not be exerting himself or herself in this manner.

**TEST-TAKING HINT: The test taker could eliminate "1" because this applies to antibiotics and "4" because it is isometric exercise.**

36. 1. The client's problem is activity intolerance, and pacing activities directly affect the diagnosis.
    2. This is an appropriate intervention for iron or vitamin deficiency, but it is not for activity intolerance.
    3. This may be done, but not specifically for the diagnosis.
    4. This would not help activity intolerance.

**TEST-TAKING HINT: The test taker should read the stem closely and choose only interventions that directly affect an activity. The word "activity" is in the diagnosis and in the correct answer. When an answer option matches with the stem, it is a good choice.**

## Bleeding Disorders

37. 1. This is a major surgery but has a predictable course with no complications identi-

fied in the stem, and a colostomy is expected with this type of surgery. The graduate nurse could be assigned this client.

2. Acute respiratory distress syndrome (ARDS) is a potentially life-threatening complication and should be assigned to a more experienced nurse.

3. Disseminated intravascular coagulation (DIC) is life threatening. The client is unstable and should be assigned to a more experienced nurse.

4. This client is experiencing hypovolemia, which means hemorrhaging and potential emergency surgery; therefore, this client should be assigned to a more experienced nurse.

**TEST-TAKING HINT: The test taker must think about what type of client a new graduate should be assigned. The least critical client is the correct choice.**

38. 1. DIC is a complication in many obstetric problems, including septic abortion, abruptio placentae, amniotic fluid embolus, and retained dead fetus, but it is not a complication of placenta previa.

2. A client with a fat embolus is at risk for DIC, but a client with a pulmonary embolus is not.

3. Hemodialysis is not a risk factor for developing DIC.

4. DIC is a clinical syndrome that develops as a complication of a wide variety of other disorders, with sepsis being the most common cause of DIC.

**TEST-TAKING HINT: The test taker could eliminate "3" if the test taker knew that DIC is a complication of another disorder. Age is not a risk factor for developing DIC.**

39. 1. The signs/symptoms of DIC result from clotting and bleeding, ranging from oozing blood to bleeding from every body orifice and into the tissues.

2. Chest pain and frothy sputum may indicate a pulmonary embolus.

3. Foul smelling, concentrated urine may indicate dehydration or urinary tract infection.

4. A reddened, inflamed central line catheter site indicates a possible infection.

**TEST-TAKING HINT: If the test taker realized that coagulation deals with blood, then the only answer option that addresses any type of bleeding is "1."**

40. 1. The prothrombin time (PT), along with the partial thromboplastin time (PTT) and thrombin time, are prolonged or increased in a client with DIC.

2. The fibrinogen level helps predict bleeding

in DIC. As it becomes lower, the risk of bleeding increases.

3. The platelet count is decreased in DIC. The platelets are used up because clotting and bleeding are occurring simultaneously.

4. White blood cell counts increase as a result of infection, not from DIC.

**TEST-TAKING HINT: An understanding of bleeding may help the test taker rule out "3" and "4" because platelets are needed for clotting, so an increased platelet count would not cause bleeding, and WBCs are associated with infection. If the test taker thinks about oral anticoagulant therapy and remembers that PT is prolonged with bleeding, it might lead to eliminating "1" as a possible correct answer.**

41. 1. Heparin, a parenteral anticoagulant, is administered to interfere with the clotting cascade and may prevent further clotting factor consumption as a result of uncontrolled bleeding, but its use is controversial. Oral anticoagulants are not administered.

2. Plasmapheresis involves the removal of plasma from withdrawn blood by centrifugation, reconstituting it in an isotonic solution, and then reinfusing the solution back into the body, but it is not a treatment for DIC.

3. Fresh frozen plasma and platelet concentrates are administered to restore clotting factors and platelets.

4. Calculating the intake and output is adding up how much oral and intravenous fluids went into the client and how much fluid came out of the client. It does not require an HCP's order and thus is not a collaborative treatment.

**TEST-TAKING HINT: Collaborative means another health-care discipline must order or perform the intervention. A test-taking hint that may help with unit examinations, but not with the RN-NCLEX, is if the test taker has studied the assigned content and has never heard of a word in the answer options, the test taker should not select that answer—in this case, perhaps the word "plasmapheresis."**

42. 1. This is a true statement, but it is medical jargon explaining how someone gets hemophilia A and so is not the best response.

2. This is a true statement, but it refers to the pathophysiology of hemophilia A and does not explain how someone gets the disease.

3. This is a true statement, but it does not answer the question of how someone gets it.

4. This is a true statement and explains exactly how someone gets hemophilia A: the mother passes it to the son.

**TEST-TAKING HINT: When the stem has the word "best" in it, then all four answer options could be correct and, in this case, statements that the nurse could reply, but only one answer option is best. The test taker needs to evaluate the stem and identify adjectives that may help select the best option; in this case, a UAP is asking the question and a direct answer without using medical jargon should be given.**

43. 1. Nosebleeds along with hemarthrosis, cutaneous hematoma formation, bleeding gums, hematemesis, occult blood, and hematuria are all signs/symptoms of hemophilia.
    2. Petechiae are tiny purple or red spots that appear on the skin as a result of minute hemorrhages within the dermal or submucosal layers, but they are not signs of hemophilia.
    3. Subcutaneous emphysema is air under the skin, which may occur with chest tube or tracheostomy insertion.
    4. Intermittent claudication is severe leg pain that occurs from decreased oxygenation to the leg muscles.

**TEST-TAKING HINT: If the test taker knows that hemophilia is a bleeding disorder, the test taker should eliminate any answer options that don't address bleeding—in this case, options "3" and "4."**

44. 1. Vomiting blood is not a situation that would indicate the client has von Willebrand's disease.
    2. Microscopic blood in the urine is not a sign of von Willebrand's disease.
    3. von Willebrand's disease is a type of hemophilia. The most common hereditary bleeding disorder, it is caused by a deficiency in von Willebrand's (vW) factor and is often diagnosed after prolonged bleeding following surgery or dental extraction.
    4. Abruptio placentae is not a situation that might cause von Willebrand's disease.

**TEST-TAKING HINT: The test taker must be knowledgeable about vW factor to be able to answer this question. Risk factors or situations are facts that need to be memorized.**

45. 1. The client should avoid prescription and over-the-counter drugs containing aspirin because these drugs may have an antiplatelet effect, leading to bleeding.
    2. Hemarthrosis is bleeding into the joint. Applying ice to the area can cause vasoconstriction, which can help decrease bleeding.
    3. The joint should be immobilized for 24–48 hours after the bleeding starts.

4. Dependent position is putting the extremity below the level of the heart; the extremity should be elevated if possible.

**TEST-TAKING HINT: If the test taker does not know the answer, the test taker could apply medical terminology; in this case, the terminology contains "hema," which refers to "blood." A basic concept with bleeding is that cold causes vasoconstriction; therefore "2" would be a good choice to select.**

46. 1. ITP is due to bleeding from small vessels and mucous membranes. Petechiae, tiny purple or red spots that appear on the skin as a result of minute hemorrhages within the dermal or submucosal layers, and purpura, hemorrhaging into the tissue beneath the skin and mucous membranes, are the first signs of ITP.
    2. A capillary refill time (CRT) less than three (3) seconds is a normal assessment finding and would not indicate ITP.
    3. A splenectomy is the treatment of choice if glucocorticosteroid therapy does not treat the ITP, but the spleen is not enlarged.
    4. ITP causes bleeding, but it does not affect the oxygen that gets to the periphery.

**TEST-TAKING HINT: Knowing medical terminology—in this case, that "thrombo" refers to "platelets"—the test taker could conclude that an answer option that includes something about bleeding would be the most appropriate selection for the correct answer. Options "2" and "4" could be eliminated as possible answers based on the knowledge that these are normal values.**

47. 1. A range for the normal PTT is 32–39 seconds.
    2. These are normal hemoglobin/hematocrit levels for either a male or female client.
    3. A platelet count of less than 100,000 per milliliter of blood indicates thrombocytopenia.
    4. This is a normal red blood cell count.

**TEST-TAKING HINT: The test taker must be knowledgeable of normal laboratory values. The test taker should write these normal values on a 3 × 5 card, carry it with them, and memorize the values.**

48. 1. The client should use an electric razor, which minimizes the opportunity to develop superficial cuts that may result in bleeding.
    2. Enemas, rectal thermometers, and intramuscular injections can pose a risk of tissue and vascular trauma that can precipitate bleeding.

3. Even minor trauma can lead to serious bleeding episodes; safer activities such as swimming or golf should be recommended.
4. Direct pressure occludes bleeding vessels.
5. There is no reason why the client can't floss the teeth.

**TEST-TAKING HINT:** This type of question requires the test taker to select all interventions that apply. Bleeding is the priority concern with hemophilia A so all interventions should be based around activities that can potentially cause bleeding and ways to treat bleeding.

## Blood Transfusions

49. 1. The client must give permission to receive blood or blood products because of the nature of potential complications.
2. Most blood products require at least a 20-gauge IV because of the size of the cells. RBCs are best infused through an 18-gauge IV. If unable to achieve cannulation with an 18-gauge, a 20 is the smallest acceptable IV. Smaller IVs damage the cell walls of the RBCs and reduce the life expectancy of the RBCs.
3. Because infusing IV fluids can cause a fluid volume overload, the nurse must assess for congestive heart failure. Assessing the lungs includes auscultating for crackles and other signs of left-sided heart failure. Assessing the client for jugular vein distention, peripheral edema, and liver engorgement indicates right-sided failure.
4. Checking for allergies is important prior to administering any medication. Some medications are administered prior to blood administration.
5. A keep-open IV of 0.9% saline would be hung. D5W causes red blood cells to hemolyze in the tubing.

**TEST-TAKING HINT:** This is an alternative type question. These type of questions can appear anywhere on the RN-NCLEX examination. Each answer option must be evaluated on its own merit. One will not rule out another. Assessing is the first step of the nursing process. Unless the test taker is absolutely sure that an option is wrong, the test taker could select an option based on "assessing," such as "3" and "4." Ethically speaking, informed consent should always be given for any procedure unless an emergency life-or-death situation exists. The other options require knowledge of blood and blood product administration.

50. 1. This should be done, but the client requires the IV first. This client is at risk for shock.
2. The first action in a situation in which the nurse suspects the client has a fluid volume loss is to replace the volume as quickly as possible.
3. The client will probably need to have surgery to correct the source of the bleeding, but stabilizing the client with fluid resuscitation is first.
4. This is the last thing on this list in order of priority.

**TEST-TAKING HINT:** The question requires the test taker to decide which of the actions comes first. Only one of the options actually has the nurse treating the client. The test taker must not read into a question—for example, that consent is needed to send a client to surgery to correct the problem so that could be first. Only one answer option has the potential to stabilize the client.

51. 1. Oral surgeries are associated with transient bacteremia, and the client cannot donate for 72 hours after an oral surgery.
2. The client cannot donate blood following rubella immunizations for one (1) month.
3. The client cannot donate blood for 6 months after a pregnancy because of the nutritional demands on the mother.
4. Recent allergic reactions prevent donation because passive transference of hypersensitivity can occur. This client has an allergy that developed during childhood.

**TEST-TAKING HINT:** All of the answer options have a given time period, and these time frames make each option correct or incorrect. The test taker must pay particular attention whenever an option contains time frames. Is it long enough or too frequently?

52. 1. O− (O negative) blood is considered the universal donor because it does not contain the antigens A, B, or Rh. (AB+ is considered the universal recipient because a person with this blood type has all the antigens on the blood).
2. A+ blood contains the antigen A that the client will react to, causing the development of antibodies. The unit being Rh+ is compatible with the client.
3. B+ blood contains the antigen B that the client will react to, causing the development of antibodies. The unit being Rh+ is compatible with the client.
4. This client does not have antigens A or B on the blood. Administration of these types would cause an antigen/antibody reaction within the

client's body, resulting in massive hemolysis of the client's blood and death.

**TEST-TAKING HINT: This is a knowledge-based question that requires memorization of the particular facts regarding blood typing. Three of the possible answer options have a positive (+) Rh factor; only one has a negative (−) Rh factor.**

53. 1. A steroid could delay healing time after the surgery and has no effect on the production of red blood cells.
    2. An antibiotic does not increase the production of red blood cells. Orthopedic surgeries frequently involve blood loss. The client is wishing to donate blood to himself (autologous).
    3. Tranquilizers do not affect the production of red blood cells.
    4. Epogen or Procrit are forms of erythropoietin, the substance in the body that stimulates the bone marrow to produce red blood cells. A client may be prescribed iron preparations to prevent depletion of iron stores and erythropoietin to increase RBC production. A unit of blood can be withdrawn once a week beginning at 6 weeks prior to surgery. No phlebotomy will be done within 72 hours of surgery.

**TEST-TAKING HINT: The test taker should examine the key words "autologous" and "transfusion." If the test taker did not know the meaning of the word autologous, "auto" as a prefix refers to "self," such as an autobiography is one's own story. Pairing "self" with transfusion then should make the test taker look for an option that would directly affect the production of blood cells.**

54. 1. A cell saver is a device to catch the blood lost during orthopedic surgeries to reinfuse into the client, rather than giving the client donor blood products. The cells are washed with saline and reinfused through a filter into the client. The salvaged cells cannot be stored and must be used within four (4) hours or discarded because of bacterial growth.
    2. The cell saver has a measuring device; an hourly drainage bag is part of a urinary drainage system. A cell saver is a sterile system that should not be broken until ready to disconnect for reinfusion.
    3. The post-anesthesia care unit nurse would not replace the cell saver; it is inserted into the surgical wound. A continuous passive motion (CPM) machine can be attached on the outside of the bandage and started if the surgeon so

orders, but this has nothing to do with the blood.
    4. The blood has not been cross-matched so there is not a cross-match number.

**TEST-TAKING HINT: The test taker could discard option "4" if the test taker realized that the laboratory is not involved with this blood at all. The test taker must have basic knowledge of surgical care.**

55. 1. Blood will coagulate if left out for an extended period, but blood is stored with a preservative that prevents this and prolongs the life of the blood.
    2. Blood is a medium for bacterial growth, and any bacteria contaminating the unit will begin to grow if left outside of a controlled refrigerated temperature for longer than four (4) hours, placing the client at risk for septicemia.
    3. Blood components are stable and do not break down at four (4) hours.
    4. These are standard nursing and laboratory procedures to prevent the complication of septicemia.

**TEST-TAKING HINT: The test taker must know the rationale behind nursing interventions to be able to answer this question.**

56. 1. The HCP has written an appropriate order for this client who has heart failure and does not need to be called to verify the order before the nurse implements it.
    2. Blood or blood components have a specified amount of infusion time, and this is not eight (8) hours. The time constraints are for the protection of the client.
    3. The correct procedure for administering a unit of blood over eight (8) hours is to have the unit split into halves. Each half unit is treated as a new unit and checked accordingly. This slower administration allows the compromised client, such as one with heart failure, to assimilate the extra fluid volume.
    4. This rate has all ready been determined by the HCP to be unsafe for this client.

**TEST-TAKING HINT: The key to this question is the time frame of eight (8) hours and the client's diagnosis of heart failure. Basic knowledge of heart failure allows the test taker to realize that fluid volume is the problem. Only one option addresses administering a smaller volume at a time.**

57. 1. This should be done but after preventing any more of the PRBCs from infusing.

2. Benadryl may be administered to reduce the severity of the transfusion reaction, but it is not first.

3. The nurse should assess the client, but in this case the nurse has all the assessment data needed to stop the transfusion.

4. The priority in this situation is to prevent a further reaction if possible. Stopping the transfusion and changing the fluid out at the hub will prevent any more of the transfusion from entering the client's bloodstream.

**TEST-TAKING HINT: In a question that requires the test taker to determine a priority action, the test taker must decide what will have the most impact on the client. Option "4" does this. All the options are interventions that should be taken, but only one will be first.**

58. 1. Unlicensed nursing assistants cannot assess. The nurse cannot delegate assessment.

2. The likelihood of a reaction is the greatest during the first 15 minutes of a transfusion. The nurse should never leave the client until after this time. The nurse should take and assess the vital signs during this time.

3. Auscultation of the lung sounds and administering blood based on this information are the nurse's responsibility. Any action requiring nursing judgment cannot be delegated.

4. The unlicensed nursing assistant can assist a client to brush the teeth. Instructions about using soft-bristle toothbrushes and the need to report to the nurse any pink or bleeding should be given prior to delegating the procedure.

**TEST-TAKING HINT: The test taker must be aware of delegation guidelines. The nurse cannot delegate assessment or any intervention requiring nursing judgment. Options "1," "2," and "3" require judgment and cannot be delegated to an unlicensed assistant.**

59. 1. The likelihood of a client who has already received more than half of the blood product having a transfusion reaction is slim. The first 15 minutes have passed and to this point the client is tolerating the blood.

2. Clients diagnosed with leukemia have a cancer involving blood cell production. These are expected findings in a client diagnosed with leukemia.

3. This client has a potential for hemorrhage and is reporting blood in the vomitus. This client should be assessed first.

4. Crohn's disease involves frequent diarrhea stools, leading to perineal irritation and skin excoriation. This is expected and not life threatening. Clients "1," "2," and "3" should be seen before this client.

**TEST-TAKING HINT: In a prioritizing question, the test taker should be able to rank in order which client to see first, second, third, and fourth. Expected but not immediately life-threatening situations are seen after a situation in which the client has a life-threatening problem.**

60. 886 mL of fluid has infused.
250 mL + 63 mL = 313 mL per unit.
313 + 313 = 626 ml.
500 mL of saline − 240 mL remaining = 260 mL infused
626 mL + 260 mL = 886 mL of fluid infused.

**TEST-TAKING HINT: This problem has several steps but only requires basic addition and subtraction. The test taker should use the pull-down calculator on the computer to check the answer or doublecheck the answer to make sure that simple mistakes are not made.**

## Sickle Cell Anemia

61. 1. Offering the nursing student written material is appropriate, but the nurse's best statement would be to answer the student's question.

2. The problem in sickle cell anemia is that the blood does clot inappropriately when there is a decrease in oxygenation.

3. This is a true statement but it is not the best response because it is not answering the nursing student's question.

4. Sickle cell anemia is a disorder of the red blood cells characterized by abnormally shaped red cells that sickle or clump together, leading to oxygen deprivation and resulting in crisis and severe pain.

**TEST-TAKING HINT: When answering a question the test taker should really close the eyes and answer the question exactly how he or she would answer in the clinical setting. Most nurses would answer the student's question and not offer written material.**

62. 1. This is the etiology for sickle cell anemia (SCA), but a layperson would not understand this explanation.

2. This explains the etiology in terms that a layperson could understand. When both parents are carriers of the disease, each pregnancy has a 25% chance of producing a child who has sickle cell anemia.

3. The cause of SCA is known, and genetic counseling can explain it to the prospective parent.
4. A virus does not cause sickle cell anemia.

**TEST-TAKING HINT:** When discussing disease processes with laypersons the nurse should explain the facts in terms that the client can understand. Would a layperson know what autosomal recessive means? The test taker should consider terminology when selecting an answer.

63. 1. The health-care provider could order STAT ABGs, but caring directly for the client is always the first priority.
2. A pulse oximeter reading of less than 93% indicates hypoxia, which warrants oxygen administration.
3. The nurse should start an 18-gauge IV catheter angiocatheter because the client may need blood, but this is not the nurse's first intervention.
4. The medication will be administered intravenously, so the IV will have to be started before administering the medication.

**TEST-TAKING HINT:** If the test taker can eliminate two (2) options and cannot decide between the other two (2), the test taker should apply a rule such as Maslow's Hierarchy of Needs and select the intervention that addresses oxygenation or airway.

64. 1. Demerol is no longer recommended for long-term pain management because the accumulative effect of normeperidine can cause seizures.
2. The client does not need to be in reverse isolation because other people will not affect the crisis.
3. Increased intravenous fluid reduces the viscosity of blood, thereby preventing further sickling as a result of dehydration.
4. The client needs to be receiving intake and output monitoring, but there is no reason to insert a Foley catheter.

**TEST-TAKING HINT:** The test taker would have to know that sickling is caused by decreased oxygen or dehydration to know this answer. Possibly looking at the word infection and increasing fluids may help the test taker select this option.

65. 1. To assess for cyanosis (blueness) in individuals with dark skin, the oral mucosa and conjunctiva should be assessed because cyanosis cannot be assessed in the lips or fingertips.
2. Metatarsals are the fingers, which should not be assessed for cyanosis.

3. Capillary refill time is not a reliable indicator for cyanosis in individuals with dark skin.
4. The nurse should assess the conjunctiva for paleness, indicating hypoxemia; the sclera is assessed for jaundice.

**TEST-TAKING HINT:** The test taker must realize that assessing different nationalities or races requires different assessment techniques and data. Knowing anatomical terms would rule out "2" and "3" because capillary refill is evaluated in the fingers as well as toes.

66. 3000 mL. The key is knowing that 1 ounce is equal to 30 mL. Then, 20 ounces (20 × 30) = 600 mL, 8 ounces (8 × 30) = 240 mL, 4 ounces (4 × 30) = 120 × 3 cartons = 360 mL for a total of 600 + 240 + 360 = 1200 mL of oral fluids. That, plus 1800 mL of IV, makes the total intake for this shift 3000 mL.

67. 1. Whenever an opportunity presents itself, the nurse should teach the client about his or her condition. This client should not go to areas that have decreased oxygen such as Yellowstone National Park, which is at high altitudes.
2. This is passing the buck. The nurse can respond to this comment.
3. High altitudes have decreased oxygen, which could lead to a sickle cell crisis.
4. It is none of the nurse's business why the client wants to go to Yellowstone National Park. The client's safety comes first and the nurse needs to teach the client.

**TEST-TAKING HINT:** Even if the test taker did not know the answer to this question, the only answer option that does any teaching is "3," which would be the best choice. Yellowstone National Park, because of its altitude, has something to do with the answer.

68. 1. Chest syndrome refers to chest pain; fever; and dry, hacking cough with or without preexisting pneumonia and is not a fatal complication. It can occur in either gender.
2. Compartment syndrome is a complication of a cast that has been applied too tightly or to a fracture in which there is edema in a muscle compartment.
3. This is a term that means painful and constant penile erection that can occur in male clients with SCA during a sickle cell crisis.
4. A hypertensive crisis is potentially fatal, but it is not a complication of SCA. The client with sickle cell anemia usually has cardiomegaly or systolic murmurs; both genders have this.

**TEST-TAKING HINT:** This is a knowledge-based question, but if the test taker realized that

Hematological

priapism could only occur with males this might help the test taker select "3" as a correct answer. Whenever there is a gender for the client, it usually has something to do with the correct answer.

69. 1. Health promotion is important in clients with chronic illnesses, but the best answer should address the client's specific disease process, not chronic illnesses in general.
2. An individual with SCA has a reduction in splenic activity from infarcts occurring during crises. This situation progresses to the spleen no longer being able to function and this increases the client's susceptibility to infection.
3. These vaccines do nothing to prevent sickling of the blood cells.
4. Teaching the client is an independent nursing intervention and does not need to rely on the HCP to designate what should be taught to the client.

**TEST-TAKING HINT:** Vaccines are recommended to clients with chronic problems to help prevent the flu and pneumonia. The test taker should see if a widely accepted concept could help answer the question and not get caught up in the client's disease process.

70. 1. Research and a search for a cure are not the missions of the Sickle Cell Foundation.
2. **The Foundation's mission is to provide information about the disease and about support groups in the area. This information helps decrease the client's and significant others' feelings of frustration and helplessness.**
3. The nurse should not force personal thoughts on the client. The nurse should provide information and let the client make his or her own decision. This empowers the client.
4. The nurse can arrange for families to meet, but this is not the mission of the foundation.

**TEST-TAKING HINT:** The nurse should know about organizations for specific disease pro-

cesses in the geographic area, but most organizations provide information on the disease process and support groups.

71. 1. Skeletal deformities, such as lordosis or kyphosis, are common. They are secondary to chronic vasoocclusive crisis, not an acute crisis.
2. A bloody nose is not an expected finding in a client diagnosed with an acute vasoocclusive crisis.
3. **Vasoocclusive crisis, the most frequent crisis, is characterized by organ infarction, which will result in bloody urine secondary to kidney infarction.**
4. Petechiae are small pinpoint blood spots on the skin, but they are not signs/symptoms of a vasoocclusive crisis.

**TEST-TAKING HINT:** Understanding medical terminology of assessment data is an important part of being able to answer RN-NCLEX questions. These terms can help eliminate or select an answer option.

72. 1. A spinal tap is a test used to diagnose meningitis.
2. Hemoglobin electrophoresis is a test used to help diagnose sickle cell anemia; it is the "finger-printing" of the protein, which detects homozygous and heterozygous forms of the disease.
3. The Sickledex test is a screening test commonly used to screen for sickle cell anemia. It is performed by a finger stick with results in three (3) minutes.
4. **The elevated temperature is the first sign of bacteremia. Bacteremia leads to a sickle cell crisis. Therefore, the bacteria must be identified so the appropriate antibiotics can be prescribed to treat the infection. Blood cultures assist in determining the type and source of infection so that it can be treated appropriately.**

**TEST-TAKING HINT:** The client's temperature in the stem is the key to selecting blood cultures as the correct answer.

Hematological

1. The client is diagnosed with severe iron-deficiency anemia. Which statement is the scientific rationale regarding oral replacement therapy?
   1. Iron supplements are well tolerated without side effects.
   2. There is no benefit from oral preparations; the best route is IV.
   3. Oral iron preparations cause diarrhea if not taken with food.
   4. Very little of the iron supplement will be absorbed by the body.

2. The client's lab values are RBC 5.5 mm ($10^6$), WBC 8.9 mm ($10^3$), and platelets 189 mm ($10^3$). Which intervention should the nurse implement?
   1. Prepare to administer packed red blood cells.
   2. Continue to monitor the client.
   3. Request an order for Neupogen, a biologic response modifier.
   4. Institute bleeding precautions.

3. The client diagnosed with anemia is admitted to the emergency department with dyspnea, cool pale skin, and diaphoresis. Which assessment data warrant immediate intervention?
   1. The vital signs are T 98.6° F, P 116, R 28, and BP 88/62.
   2. The client is allergic to multiple antibiotic medications.
   3. The client has a history of receiving chemotherapy.
   4. ABGs are pH 7.35, $PCO_2$ 44, $HCO_3$ 22, $PaO_2$ 92.

4. The client diagnosed with anemia has an Hgb of 6.1 g/dL. Which complication should the nurse assess for?
   1. Decreased pulmonary functioning.
   2. Impaired muscle functioning.
   3. Congestive heart failure.
   4. Altered gastric secretions.

5. The nurse writes a diagnosis of "activity intolerance" for a client diagnosed with anemia. Which intervention should the nurse implement?
   1. Encourage isometric exercises.
   2. Assist the client with ADLs.
   3. Provide a high-protein diet.
   4. Refer to the physical therapist.

6. The client diagnosed with cancer has been undergoing systemic treatments and has red blood cell deficiency. Which signs and symptoms should the nurse teach the client to manage?
   1. Nausea associated with cancer treatment.
   2. Shortness of breath and fatigue.
   3. Controlling mucositis and diarrhea.
   4. The emotional aspects of having cancer.

7. The nurse is assisting the HCP with a bone marrow biopsy. Which intervention post-procedure has priority?
   1. Apply pressure to site for five (5) to ten (10) minutes.
   2. Medicate for pain with morphine slow IVP.
   3. Maintain head of bed in a high Fowler's position.
   4. Apply oxygen via nasal cannula at 5 LPM.

8. The client diagnosed with end-stage renal disease (ESRD) has developed anemia. Which would the nurse anticipate the HCP prescribing for this client?
   1. Place the client in reverse isolation.
   2. Discontinue treatments until blood count improves.
   3. Monitor CBC daily to assess for bleeding.
   4. Give client erythropoietin, a biologic response modifier.

9. The nurse is planning the care of a client diagnosed with aplastic anemia. Which interventions should be taught to the client? Select all that apply.
    1. Avoid alcohol.
    2. Pace activities.
    3. Stop smoking.
    4. Eat a balanced diet.
    5. Use a safety razor.

10. The nurse is caring for a client in a sickle cell crisis. Which is the pain regimen of choice to relieve the pain?
    1. Frequent aspirin (acetylsalicylic acid) and a nonnarcotic analgesic.
    2. Motrin (ibuprofen), an NSAID, PRN.
    3. Demerol (meperidine), a narcotic analgesic, every four (4) hours.
    4. Morphine, a narcotic analgesic, every two (2) to three (3) hours PRN.

11. The client is diagnosed with hereditary spherocytosis. Which treatment/procedure would the nurse prepare the client to receive?
    1. Bone marrow transplant.
    2. Splenectomy.
    3. Frequent blood transfusions.
    4. Liver biopsy.

12. Which is the primary goal of care for a client diagnosed with sickle cell anemia?
    1. The client will call the HCP if feeling ill.
    2. The client will be compliant with medical regimen.
    3. The client will live as normal a life as possible.
    4. The client will verbalize understanding of treatments.

13. The client diagnosed with thalassemia, a hereditary anemia, is to receive a transfusion of packed RBCs. The cross-match reveals the presence of antibodies that cannot be cross-matched. Which precaution should the nurse implement when initiating the transfusion?
    1. Start the transfusion at 10–15 mL per hour for 15–30 minutes.
    2. Re–crossmatch the blood until the antibodies are identified.
    3. Have the client sign a permit to receive uncrossmatched blood.
    4. Have the unlicensed nursing assistant stay with the client.

14. The client is diagnosed with polycythemia vera. The nurse would prepare to perform which intervention?
    1. Type and cross-match for a transfusion.
    2. Assess for petechiae and purpura.
    3. Perform phlebotomy of 500 mL of blood.
    4. Monitor for low hemoglobin and hematocrit.

15. The client diagnosed with leukemia has had a bone marrow transplant. The nurse monitors the client's absolute neutrophil count (ANC). Which is the client's neutrophil count if the WBCs are 2.2 ($10^3$) mm, neutrophils are 25%, and bands are 5%._____

16. The client is diagnosed with leukemia and has leukocytosis. Which laboratory value would the nurse expect to assess?
    1. An elevated hemoglobin.
    2. A decreased sedimentation count.
    3. A decreased red cell distribution width.
    4. An elevated white blood cell count.

17. The client is placed on neutropenia precautions. Which information should the nurse teach the client?
    1. Shave with an electric razor and use a soft toothbrush.
    2. Eat plenty of fresh fruits and vegetables.
    3. Perform perineal care after every bowel movement
    4. Some blood in the urine is not unusual.

Hematological

18. The client is diagnosed with chronic myeloid leukemia and leukocytosis. Which signs/symptoms would the nurse expect to find when assessing this client?
    1. Frothy sputum and jugular vein distention.
    2. Dyspnea and slight confusion
    3. Right upper quadrant tenderness and nausea.
    4. Increased appetite and weight gain.

19. The client's CBC indicates an RBC 6.0 ($10^6$) mm, Hgb 14.2 g d/L, Hct 42%, and platelets 69 ($10^3$) mm. Which intervention should the nurse implement?
    1. Teach the client to use a soft-bristle toothbrush.
    2. Monitor the client for elevated temperature.
    3. Check the client's blood pressure.
    4. Hold venipuncture sites for one (1) minute.

20. The 24-year-old female client is diagnosed with idiopathic thrombocytopenia purpura (ITP). Which question would be important for the nurse to ask during the admission interview?
    1. "Do you become short of breath during activity?"
    2. "How heavy are your menstrual periods?"
    3. "Do you have a history of deep vein thrombosis?"
    4. "How often do you have migraine headaches?"

21. The client is diagnosed with hemophilia. Which safety precaution should the nurse encourage?
    1. Wear helmets and pads during contact sports.
    2. Take antibiotics prior to any dental work.
    3. Keep clotting factor VIII on hand at all times.
    4. Use ibuprofen, an NSAID, for mild pain.

22. The nurse writes a diagnosis of "potential for fluid volume deficit related to bleeding" for a client diagnosed with disseminated intravascular coagulation (DIC). Which would be an appropriate goal for this client?
    1. The client's clot formations will resolve in two (2) days.
    2. The saturation of the client's dressings will be documented.
    3. The client will use lemon-glycerin swabs for oral care.
    4. The client's urine output will be >30 mL per hour.

23. The client diagnosed with atrial fibrillation is admitted with warfarin (Coumadin) toxicity. Which HCP order would the nurse anticipate?
    1. Protamine sulfate, an anticoagulant antidote.
    2. Heparin sodium, an anticoagulant.
    3. Lovenox, a low molecular weight anticoagulant.
    4. Vitamin K, an anticoagulant agonist.

24. Fifteen minutes after the nurse has initiated a transfusion of packed red blood cells the client becomes restless and complains of itching on the trunk and arms. Which intervention should the nurse implement first?
    1. Collect urine for analysis.
    2. Notify the lab of the reaction.
    3. Administer diphenhydramine, an antihistamine.
    4. Stop the transfusion at the hub.

25. The HCP has ordered one (1) unit of packed RBCs for the client who is right-handed.
Which area would be the best place to insert the intravenous catheter?
1. A
2. B
3. C
4. D

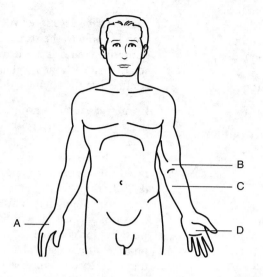

26. The nurse is administering a transfusion of packed red blood cells to a client. Which
interventions should the nurse implement? List in order of performance.
1. Start the transfusion slowly.
2. Have the client sign a permit.
3. Assess the IV site for size and patency.
4. Check the blood with another nurse at the bedside.
5. Obtain the blood from the laboratory.

1. 1. Iron supplements can be poorly tolerated. The supplements can cause nausea, abdominal discomfort, and constipation.
   2. There is benefit from oral preparations, but in severe cases of iron deficiency, the client may need parenteral replacement.
   3. Iron supplements cause constipation and should be taken one (1) hour before a meal or two (2) hours after a meal for the best absorption of the medication. As much as 50% of the iron is not absorbed when taken with food.
   4. At best only about 20%–35% of the medication is absorbed through the gastrointestinal tract (GI) tract.

2. 1. The normal RBC is 4.7–6.1 ($10^6$) for males and 4.2–5.4 ($10^6$) for females. The RBC is within normal limits.
   2. All the lab values are within normal limits. The nurse should continue to monitor the client.
   3. The normal WBC is 4.5–11 ($10^3$), so a biologic response modifier to increase the numbers of WBCs is not needed.
   4. The normal platelet count is 100–400 ($10^3$); there is no reason to institute bleeding precautions.

3. 1. The pulse of 116 and BP of 88/62 in addition to the other symptoms indicate the client is in shock. This is an emergency situation.
   2. The client is in shock; allergies to medications are not the most important thing.
   3. This may be the cause of the anemia and complications from the chemotherapy may be causing the shock, but the priority intervention is to treat the shock, regardless of the cause.
   4. These are normal blood gases so no immediate intervention regarding arterial blood gases is needed.

4. 1. A low hemoglobin level will not decrease pulmonary functioning. In fact, the lungs will try to compensate for the anemia by speeding up respirations to oxygenate the red blood cells and provide oxygen to the tissues.
   2. The client may have difficulty with activity intolerance, but this will be from lack of oxygen, not lack of ability of the muscles to function.
   3. General complications of severe anemia include heart failure, paresthesias, and confusion. The heart tries to compensate for the lack of oxygen in the tissues by becoming tachycardic. The heart will be able to maintain this compensatory mechanism for

only so long and then will show evidence of failure.
   4. The gastric secretions will not be altered. The blood supply to the stomach may be shunted to the more vital organs, leaving the acidic stomach to deal with the production of acid, and this could cause the client to develop a gastric ulcer.

5. 1. Isometric exercises are bodybuilding exercises; these types of exercises would deplete the client's energy stores.
   2. The client with activity intolerance will need assistance to perform activities of daily living.
   3. A high-protein diet may be needed, but this does not address activity intolerance.
   4. Activity intolerance is not a problem for a physical therapist. The client's blood counts must increase to increase the ability to perform activities.

6. 1. Red blood cell deficiency is anemia. The client should be taught to deal with the effects of anemia, not nausea.
   2. Anemia causes the client to experience dyspnea and fatigue. Teaching the client to pace activities and rest often, to eat a balanced diet, and to cope with changes in lifestyle is needed.
   3. Mucositis and diarrhea may occur with chemotherapy administration, but this client's problem is anemia.
   4. All clients with cancer should be assisted to discuss the impact of cancer on their lives, but this client's problem is anemia.

7. 1. After a bone marrow biopsy, it is important that the client form a clot to prevent bleeding. The nurse should hold direct pressure on the site for five (5) to ten (10) minutes.
   2. The nurse might premedicate for pain, but once the procedure is completed, a mild oral medication is usually sufficient to relieve any residual discomfort.
   3. The head of the bed can be in any position of comfort for the client.
   4. The procedure is performed on the iliac crest or the sternum and does not cause respiratory distress.

8. 1. The client is anemic, not neutropenic, so reverse isolation is not needed.
   2. This client will be receiving a form of dialysis to maintain life. Discontinuing treatments until the counts improve would be resigning the client to death.

Hematological

3. The red blood cell count would not appreciably improve from one day to the next unless a transfusion had been given.
4. **Erythropoietin is a biologic response modifier produced by the kidneys in response to a low red blood cell count in the body. It stimulates the body to produce more RBCs.**

9. 1. Alcohol consumption interferes with the absorption of nutrients.
2. The client will be short of breath with activity and therefore should pace activities.
3. Although all clients should be told to stop smoking, smoking will not directly affect the client's diagnosis.
4. **The client should eat a well-balanced diet to be able to manufacture blood cells.**
5. **The client should use an electric razor to diminish the risk of cuts and bleeding.**

10. 1. Aspirin is a an option for mild pain, but it would not be strong enough during a crisis.
2. NSAIDs are helpful because they relieve pain and decrease inflammation, but they are not used during a crisis because they are not strong enough.
3. Demerol breaks down in the body into normeperidine, which can cause seizures in large doses.
4. **Morphine is the drug of choice for a crisis; it does not have a ceiling effect and can be given in large amounts and frequent doses.**

11. 1. A bone marrow transplant is a treatment option for aplastic anemia and some clients with thalassemia, but not for spherocytosis.
2. **Hereditary spherocytosis is a relatively common hemolytic anemia (1:5000 people) characterized by an abnormal permeability of the red blood cell, which permits it to become spherical in shape. The spheres are then destroyed by the spleen. A splenectomy is the treatment of choice.**
3. The client may require blood transfusions, but preventing the destruction of RBCs by the spleen is the better option.
4. A liver biopsy will not affect the client's condition.

12. 1. All clients should know when to notify the HCP. This is not the primary goal of living with a chronic illness.
2. The client should be compliant with recommendations, but this is a lifestyle choice and not the primary goal.
3. **The primary goal for any client coping with a chronic illness is that the client will be able to maintain as normal a life as possible.**

4. This is a goal for a client with knowledge-deficit problems.

13. 1. **It can be difficult to cross-match blood when antibodies are present. If imperfectly cross-matched blood must be transfused, the nurse must start the blood very slowly and stay with the client, monitoring frequently for signs of a hemolytic reaction.**
2. The antibodies have been identified. The donor blood does not cross-match perfectly to the blood of the client.
3. The blood has been cross-matched. Client permits regarding uncross-matched blood are used for emergency transfusions when time does not allow an attempt to cross-match. In such a case, O− blood, the universal donor, will be used.
4. The nurse cannot delegate an unstable client to an unlicensed nursing assistant. The nurse must stay with the client.

14. 1. The client has too many red blood cells and does not need more.
2. Petechiae and purpura occur when a client does not have adequate platelets.
3. **The client has too many red blood cells, which can cause as much damage as too few. The treatment for this disease is to remove the excess blood; 500 mL at a time is removed.**
4. The client's hemoglobin and hematocrit are high, not low.

15. **660 ANC.** To determine the absolute neutrophils count, first the WBC count must be determined: 2.2 multiplied by 1000 ($10^3$) = 2,200. Multiply that by 30 (25% neutrophils + 5% bands) to obtain 6600 and divide that by 100 to determine the ANC of 660. The ANC is used to determine a client's risk of developing an infection.

16. 1. Clients with leukemia are usually anemic because of the bone marrow's inability to produce cells or, in this case, the bone marrow, stuck in high gear, producing immature white blood cells that are unable to function normally.
2. Sedimentation rates increase in some diseases, such as rheumatoid arthritis, but there will be no change in leukemia.
3. The red cell distribution width (RDW), shown in the CBC report, reports on the size of the red blood cell.
4. **An elevated white blood cell count is what is being described in the term "leukocytosis"—"leuko" means "white" and "cyto" refers to "cell." Leukocytosis is the opposite of leukopenia.**

17. 1. Shaving with an electric razor and using a soft toothbrush are interventions for thrombocytopenia.
2. Fresh fruits and vegetables are limited because they may harbor microbes.
3. **Perineal care after each bowel movement, preferably with an antimicrobial soap, is performed to reduce bacteria on the skin.**
4. Blood in the urine would indicate a complication and is not expected.

18. 1. Frothy sputum and jugular vein distention are symptoms of heart failure, which could occur as a complication of anemia.
2. **Clients with leukocytosis may be short of breath and somewhat confused as a result of decreased capillary perfusion to the lung and brain from excessive amounts of WBCs inhibiting blood flow through the capillaries.**
3. The client may have left upper quadrant pain and tenderness from WBC infiltration of the spleen, but the client will not have right upper quadrant tenderness.
4. The client may be anorectic and lose weight.

19. 1. **The client has a low platelet count (thrombocytopenia) and should be on bleeding precautions, such as using a soft bristle toothbrush**
2. Monitoring for a fever, a sign of infection, would be an intervention for low WBCs.
3. Assessing the blood pressure is not indicated for any of the blood cell count abnormalities.
4. Holding the venipuncture site would be done for a minimum of five (5) minutes.

20. 1. Thrombocytopenia is low platelets and would not cause shortness of breath.
2. **Because thrombocytopenia causes bleeding the nurse should assess for any type of bleeding that may be occurring. A young female client would present with excessive menstrual bleeding.**
3. The problems associated with ITP are bleeding, not clotting.
4. ITP does not cause migraine headaches.

21. 1. The client should not participate in contact sports because even minimal injury can cause massive bleeding.
2. The client should have factor VIII on hand for any dental procedure to make sure that he clots, but antibiotics are not needed.
3. **The client must have the clotting factor on hand in case of injury to prevent massive bleeding.**
4. NSAIDs prolong bleeding and should be avoided.

22. 1. The body dissolves clots over a period of several days to a week or more. The problem in DIC is that the body is bleeding and clotting simultaneously.
2. This is a nursing goal, not a client goal.
3. Lemon-glycerin swabs are drying to the mucosa and should be avoided because they will increase bleeding from the mucosa.
4. **The problem is addressing the potential for hemorrhage, and a urine output of greater than 30 mL per hour indicates the kidneys are being adequately perfused and the body is not in shock.**

23. 1. Protamine sulfate is the antidote for a heparin overdose, not for warfarin toxicity.
2. Administering heparin would increase the client's risk of bleeding.
3. Lovenox is a low molecular weight heparin and would increase the client's risk of bleeding.
4. **The antidote for warfarin (Coumadin) is vitamin K, vitamin K is an anticoagulant.**

24. 1. The question asks for a first action; urine will be collected for analysis, but this is not the first intervention.
2. The question asks for a first action. The lab should be notified, but this is not the first action to take.
3. Administering an antihistamine may be done, but it is more important to stop the transfusion that is causing the reaction.
4. **Any time the nurse suspects the client is having a reaction to blood or blood products, the nurse should stop the infusion at the spot closest to the client and not allow any more of the blood to enter the client's body.**

25. 1. The client is right-handed; therefore the nurse should attempt to place the IV catheter in the nondominant arm.
2. The antecubital area should not be used as an IV site because the movement of the elbow will crimp the cannula and it is uncomfortable for the client to keep the arm straight all the time.
3. **The left forearm is the best site to start the IV because it has larger veins that will accommodate an 18-gauge catheter, which should be used when administering blood. This area is less likely to have extravasation because there is no joint movement, and this site is on the client's nondominant side.**
4. The hand area usually has smaller veins that do not accommodate a larger gauge catheter, and hand movement can cause extravasation more readily than the forearm.

Hematological

26. In order of performance: 2, 3, 5, 4, 1
    2. The client must give consent prior to receiving blood; therefore this is the first intervention.
    3. Blood products should be administered within 30 minutes of obtaining the blood from the laboratory; therefore, the nurse should determine that the IV is patent and the catheter is large enough to administer blood, preferably an 18-gauge catheter, before obtaining the blood.
    5. The nurse must then obtain the blood from the laboratory.
    4. Blood must be checked by two registered nurses at the bedside to check the client's crossmatch bracelet with the unit of blood.
    1. After all of the previous steps are completed, then the nurse should start the infusion of the blood slowly for the first 15 minutes to determine if the client is going to have a reaction.

Hematological

*Any piece of knowledge I acquire today has a value at this moment exactly proportional to my skill to deal with it. Tomorrow when I know more, I recall that piece of knowledge and use it better.*—Mark Van Doren

# Respiratory Disorders

# 6

Respiratory disorders include some of the most common disorders that health-care providers and nurses encounter. They range from the simple cold to chronic conditions such as asthma to life-threatening diseases such as lung cancer. Whether it is teaching a client the correct way to blow the nose; administering oxygen, antibiotics, or pain-relieving medications; or checking ventilators, chest tubes, and other equipment used in the treatment of clients with respiratory disorders, the nurse must know the correct procedures, medications, and interventions to use. One of the most important interventions—and perhaps, the most important—is assessment and monitoring of the client's breathing status and oxygenation level. Oxygenation is the first priority in Maslow's hierarchy—and in terms of saving lives.

## KEYWORDS

adenoidectomy
ambu
antral
aphonia
bronchoscopy
Caldwell Luc
dorsiflexion
enteral
eupnea
exacerbation
extrinsic
hypoxemia
iatrogenic
intrinsic
laryngectomy
laryngoscopy
lobectomy
pleurodesis
pneumonectomy
polysomnography
rhinitis
rhinorrhea
rhonchi
thoracentesis
thoracotomy

## ABBREVIATIONS

Acute Respiratory Distress Syndrome (ARDS)
Arterial Blood Gases (ABG)
Blood Pressure (BP)
Capillary Refill Time (CRT)
Chronic Obstructive Pulmonary Disease (COPD)
Continuous Positive Airway Pressure (CPAP)
Directly Observed Treatment (DOT)
Electrocardiogram (ECG)
Endotracheal Tube (ET)
Exercise-Induced Asthma (EIA)
Health-Care Provider (HCP)
Hemoglobin and Hematocrit (Hgb & Hct)
International Normalized Ratio (INR)
Intravenous (IV)
Intravenous Push (IVP)
Licensed Practical Nurse (LPN)
Liters Per Minute (LPM)
Magnetic Resonance Imaging (MRI)
Nothing By Mouth (NPO)
Nursing Assistant (NA)
Partial Thromboplastin Time (PTT)
Percutaneous Gastrostomy (PEG) Tube
Prothrombin Time (PT)
Rule Out (R/O)
Severe Acute Respiratory Syndrome (SARS)
Shortness Of Breath (SOB)
Total Parenteral Nutrition (TPN)
Upper Respiratory Infection (URI)
When Required, As Needed (PRN)

## Upper Respiratory Infection (URI)

1. The home health-care nurse is talking on the telephone to a male client diagnosed with hypertension and hears the client sneezing. The client tells the nurse that he has been blowing his nose frequently. Which question should the nurse ask the client?
   1. "Have you had the flu shot in the last two (2) weeks?"
   2. "Are there any small children in the home?"
   3. "Are you taking over-the-counter-medicine for these symptoms?"
   4. "Do you have any cold sores associated with your sneezing?"

2. The school nurse is presenting a class to students at a primary school on how to prevent the transmission of the common cold virus. Which information should the nurse discuss?
   1. Instruct the children to always keep a tissue or handkerchief with them.
   2. Explain that children current with immunizations will not get a cold.
   3. Tell the children that they should go to the doctor if they get a cold.
   4. Include a demonstration of how to wash hands correctly.

3. Which information should the nurse teach the client diagnosed with acute sinusitis?
   1. Instruct the client to complete all the ordered antibiotics.
   2. Teach the client how to irrigate the nasal passages.
   3. Have the client demonstrate how to blow the nose.
   4. Give the client samples of a narcotic analgesic for the headache.

4. The client has been diagnosed with chronic sinusitis. Which signs and symptoms would alert the nurse to a potentially life-threatening complication?
   1. Muscle weakness.
   2. Purulent sputum.
   3. Nuchal rigidity.
   4. Intermittent loss of muscle control.

5. The client diagnosed with tonsillitis is scheduled to have surgery in the morning. Which assessment data should the nurse notify the health-care provider about prior to surgery?
   1. The client has a hemoglobin of 12.2 g/dL and hematocrit of 36.5%.
   2. The client has an oral temperature of 100.2°F and a dry cough.
   3. There are one (1) to two (2) white blood cells in the urinalysis.
   4. The client's current International Normalized Ratio (INR) is 1.0.

6. The influenza vaccine is in short supply. Which group of clients would the public health nurse consider priority when administering the vaccine?
   1. Elderly and chronically ill clients.
   2. Child-care workers and children younger than age four (4) years.
   3. Hospital chaplains and health-care workers.
   4. Schoolteachers and students living in a dormitory.

7. The client diagnosed with sinusitis who has undergone a Caldwell Luc procedure is complaining of pain. Which intervention should the nurse implement first?
   1. Administer the narcotic analgesic IVP.
   2. Perform gentle oral hygiene.
   3. Place the client in a semi-Fowler's position.
   4. Assess the client's pain.

8. The charge nurse on a surgical floor is making assignments. Which client should be assigned to the most experienced registered nurse (RN)?
   1. The 36-year-old client who has undergone an antral irrigation for sinusitis yesterday and has moderate pain.
   2. The six (6)-year-old client scheduled for a tonsillectomy and adenoidectomy this morning who will not swallow medication.
   3. The 18-year-old client who had a Caldwell Luc procedure three (3) days ago and has purulent drainage on the drip pad.
   4. The 45-year client diagnosed with a peritonsillar abscess who requires IVPB antibiotic therapy four (4) times a day.

9. The client diagnosed with influenza A is being discharged from the emergency department with a prescription for antibiotics. Which statement by the client indicates an understanding of this prescription?
   1. "These pills will make me feel better fast and I can return to work."
   2. "The antibiotics will help prevent me from developing a bacterial pneumonia."
   3. "If I had gotten this prescription sooner I could have prevented this illness."
   4. "I need to take these pills until I feel better; then I can stop taking the rest."

10. The nurse is developing a plan of care for a client diagnosed with laryngitis and identifies the client problem "altered communication." Which intervention should the nurse implement?
    1. Instruct the client to drink a mixture of brandy and honey several times a day.
    2. Encourage the client to whisper instead of trying to speak at a normal level.
    3. Provide the client with a blank note pad for writing any communication.
    4. Explain that the client's aphonia may become a permanent condition.

11. Which nursing task could be delegated to an unlicensed nursing assistant?
    1. Feed a client who is postoperative tonsillectomy the first meal of clear liquids.
    2. Encourage the client diagnosed with a cold to drink a glass of orange juice.
    3. Obtain a throat culture on a client diagnosed with bacterial pharyngitis.
    4. Escort the client diagnosed with laryngitis outside to smoke a cigarette.

12. The nurse is caring for a client diagnosed with a cold. Which is an example of an alternative therapy?
    1. Vitamin C, 2000 mg daily.
    2. Strict bed rest.
    3. Humidification of the air.
    4. Decongestant therapy.

## Lower Respiratory Infection

13. The nurse is assessing a 79-year-old client diagnosed with pneumonia. Which signs and symptoms would the nurse expect to find when assessing the client?
    1. Confusion and lethargy.
    2. High fever and chills.
    3. Frothy sputum and edema.
    4. Bradypnea and jugular vein distention.

14. The nurse is planning the care of a client diagnosed with pneumonia and writes a problem of "impaired gas exchange." Which would be an expected outcome for this problem?
    1. Performs chest physiotherapy three (3) times a day.
    2. Able to complete activities of daily living.
    3. Ambulates in the hall and back several times during each shift.
    4. Alert and oriented to person, place, time, and events.

15. The nurse in a long-term care facility is planning the care for a client with a percutaneous gastrostomy (PEG) feeding tube. Which interventions would the nurse include in the plan of care?
    1. Inspect the insertion line at the nare prior to instilling formula.
    2. Elevate the head of the bed after feeding the client.
    3. Place the client in the Sims position following each feeding.
    4. Change the dressing on the feeding tube every three (3) days.

16. The client diagnosed with a community-acquired pneumonia is being admitted to the medical unit. Which nursing intervention has the highest priority?
    1. Administer the oral antibiotic stat.
    2. Order the meal tray to be delivered as soon as possible.
    3. Obtain a sputum specimen for culture and sensitivity.
    4. Have the unlicensed nursing assistant weigh the client.

Respiratory

17. The 56-year-old client diagnosed with tuberculosis (TB) is being discharged. Which statement made by the client indicates an understanding of the discharge instructions?
    1. "I will take my medication for the full three (3) weeks prescribed."
    2. "I must stay on the medication for months if I am to get well."
    3. "I can be around my friends because I have started taking antibiotics."
    4. "I should get a TB skin test every three (3) months to determine if I am well."

18. The employee health nurse is administering tuberculin skin testing to employees who have possibly been exposed to a client with active tuberculosis. Which statement indicates the need for radiological evaluation instead of skin testing?
    1. The client's first skin test indicates a purple flat area at the site of injection.
    2. The client's second skin test indicates a red area measuring four (4) mm.
    3. The client's previous skin test was read as positive.
    4. The client has never shown a reaction to the tuberculin medication.

19. The nurse is caring for the client diagnosed with pneumonia. Which information should the nurse include in the teaching plan? Select all that apply.
    1. Place the client on oxygen by nasal cannula.
    2. Plan for periods of rest during activities of daily living.
    3. Place the client on a fluid restriction of 1000 mL per day.
    4. Restrict the client's smoking to two (2) to three (3) cigarettes per day.
    5. Monitor the client's pulse oximetry readings every four (4) hours.

20. While feeding the client diagnosed with aspiration pneumonia, the client becomes dyspneic, begins to cough, and is turning blue. Which nursing intervention would the nurse implement first?
    1. Suction the client's nares.
    2. Turn the client to the side.
    3. Place the client in the Trendelenburg position.
    4. Notify the health-care provider.

21. The day shift charge nurse on a medical unit is making rounds after report. Which client should be seen first?
    1. The 65-year-old client diagnosed with tuberculosis who has a sputum specimen to be sent to the lab.
    2. The 76-year-old client diagnosed with aspiration pneumonia who has a clogged feeding tube.
    3. The 45-year-old client diagnosed with pneumonia who has a pulse oximetry reading of 92%.
    4. The 39-year-old client diagnosed with bronchitis who has an arterial oxygenation level of 89%.

22. The client is admitted with a diagnosis of rule out tuberculosis. Which type of isolation procedures should the nurse implement?
    1. Standard Precautions.
    2. Contact Precautions.
    3. Droplet Precautions.
    4. Airborne Precautions.

23. The nurse observes the unlicensed nursing assistant (NA) entering an airborne isolation room and leaving the door open. Which action would be the nurse's best response?
    1. Close the door and discuss the NA's action when the NA comes out of the room.
    2. Make the NA come back outside the room and then reenter closing the door.
    3. Say nothing to the NA but report the incident to the nursing supervisor.
    4. Enter the client's room and discuss the matter with the NA immediately.

24. The client is admitted to a medical unit with a diagnosis of pneumonia. Which signs and symptoms would the nurse look for when assessing the client?
    1. Pleuritic chest discomfort and anxiety.
    2. Asymmetrical chest expansion and pallor.
    3. Leukopenia and CRT <3 seconds.
    4. Substernal chest pain and diaphoresis.

## Chronic Pulmonary Obstructive Disease (COPD)

25. When assessing the client with COPD, which health promotion information would be most important for the nurse to obtain?
    1. Number of years the client has smoked.
    2. Risk factors for complications.
    3. Ability to administer inhaled medication.
    4. Possibility for lifestyle changes.

26. The client diagnosed with an exacerbation of COPD is in respiratory distress. Which intervention should the nurse implement first?
    1. Assist the client into a sitting position at 90 degrees.
    2. Give oxygen at six (6) LPM via nasal cannula.
    3. Monitor vital signs with the client sitting upright.
    4. Notify the health-care provider about the client's status.

27. When assessing the client with the diagnosis of COPD, which data would require the nurse to take immediate action?
    1. Large amounts of thick white sputum.
    2. Oxygen flow meter set on eight (8) liters.
    3. Use of accessory muscles during inspiration.
    4. Presence of a barrel chest and dyspnea.

28. While the nurse is caring for the client diagnosed with COPD, which outcome would require a revision in the plan of care?
    1. The client has no signs of respiratory distress.
    2. The client shows an improved respiratory pattern.
    3. The client demonstrates intolerance to activity.
    4. The client participates in establishing goals.

29. The nurse is caring for the client diagnosed with end-stage COPD. Which data would warrant immediate intervention by the nurse?
    1. The client's pulse oximeter reading is 92%.
    2. The client's arterial blood gas level is 74.
    3. The client has SOB when walking to the bathroom.
    4. The client's sputum is rusty colored.

30. What statement made by the client diagnosed with chronic bronchitis indicates to the nurse that more teaching is needed?
    1. "I should contact my health-care provider if my sputum changes color or amount."
    2. "I will take my bronchodilator regularly to prevent having bronchospasms."
    3. "This metered dose inhaler gives a precise amount of medication with each dose."
    4. "I need to return to the HCP to have my blood drawn with my annual physical."

31. Which nursing diagnoses would be appropriate for the nurse to include in the plan of care for the client diagnosed with COPD? Select all that apply.
    1. Impaired gas exchange.
    2. Inability to tolerate temperature extremes.
    3. Activity intolerance.
    4. Inability to cope with changes in roles.
    5. Alteration in nutrition.

Respiratory

32. Which outcome would be appropriate for the client problem "ineffective gas exchange" for the client recently diagnosed with COPD?
    1. The client demonstrates the correct way to purse-lip breathe.
    2. The client lists three (3) signs/symptoms to report to the HCP.
    3. The client will drink at least 2500 mL of water daily.
    4. The client will be able to ambulate 100 feet with dyspnea.

33. The primary nurse observes the unlicensed nursing assistant removing the nasal cannula from the client diagnosed with COPD while ambulating the client to the bathroom. Which action should the primary nurse take?
    1. Praise the NA because this prevents the client from tripping on the oxygen tubing.
    2. Place the oxygen back on the client while sitting in the bathroom and say nothing.
    3. Explain to the NA in front of the client that the oxygen must be left in place at all times.
    4. Discuss the NA's action with the charge nurse so that appropriate action can be taken.

34. When assessing the client recently diagnosed with COPD, which sign and symptom should the nurse expect?
    1. Clubbing of the client's fingers.
    2. Infrequent respiratory infections.
    3. Chronic sputum production.
    4. Nonproductive hacking cough.

35. What statement made by the client would indicate that the nurse's discharge teaching was effective for the client diagnosed with COPD?
    1. "I need to get an influenza vaccine each year, even when there is a shortage."
    2. "I need to get a vaccine for pneumonia each year with my flu shot."
    3. "If I reduce my cigarette smoking to six (6) a day, I won't have difficulty breathing."
    4. "I need to restrict my drinking liquids to keep from having so much phlegm."

36. Which referral would be appropriate for a client diagnosed with COPD?
    1. The Asthma Foundation of America.
    2. The American Cancer Society.
    3. The American Lung Association.
    4. The American Heart Association.

## Reactive Airway Disease (Asthma)

37. The nurse is completing the admission assessment on a 13-year-old client diagnosed with asthma. Which signs and symptoms would the nurse expect to find?
    1. Fever and crepitus.
    2. Rales and hives.
    3. Dyspnea and wheezing.
    4. Normal chest shape and eupnea.

38. The nurse is planning the care of a client diagnosed with asthma and has written a problem of "anxiety." Which nursing intervention should be implemented?
    1. Stay with the client.
    2. Notify the health-care provider.
    3. Administer an anxiolytic medication.
    4. Encourage the client to drink fluids.

39. The case manager is arranging a care planning meeting regarding the care of a 65-year-old client diagnosed with adult-onset asthma. Which health-care disciplines should participate in the meeting? Select all that apply.
    1. Nursing.
    2. Pharmacy.
    3. Social Work.
    4. Occupational Therapy.
    5. Speech Therapy.

40. The client is diagnosed with mild intermittent asthma. Which medication should the nurse discuss with the client?
    1. Daily inhaled corticosteroids.
    2. Use of a "rescue inhaler."
    3. Use of systemic steroids.
    4. Leukotriene agonists.

41. The nurse knows the client understands teaching regarding mast cell stabilizer medications when the client makes which statement?
    1. "I should take two (2) puffs when I begin to have an asthma attack."
    2. "I must taper off the medications and not stop taking them abruptly."
    3. "These drugs will be most effective if taken at bedtime."
    4. "These drugs are not good at the time of an attack."

42. The client diagnosed with asthma is admitted to the emergency department with difficulty breathing and a blue color around the mouth. Which diagnostic test will be ordered to determine the status of the client?
    1. Complete blood count.
    2. Pulmonary function test.
    3. Allergy skin testing.
    4. Drug cortisol level.

43. The registered nurse and a licensed practical nurse are caring for five (5) clients on a medical unit. Which clients would the nurse assign to the licensed practical nurse? Select all that apply.
    1. The 32-year-old female diagnosed with exercise-induced asthma who has a forced vital capacity of 1000 mL.
    2. The 45-year-old male with adult-onset asthma who is complaining of difficulty completing all of the ADLs at one time.
    3. The 92-year-old client diagnosed with respiratory difficulty who is beginning to be confused and keeps climbing out of bed.
    4. The 6-year-old client diagnosed with intrinsic asthma who is scheduled for discharge and the mother needs teaching about the medications.
    5. The 20-year-old client diagnosed with asthma who has a pulse oximetry reading of 95% and wants to sleep all the time.

44. The charge nurse is making rounds. Which client should the nurse assess first?
    1. The 29-year-old client diagnosed with reactive airway disease who is complaining that the nurse caring for him was rude.
    2. The 76-year-old client diagnosed with heart failure who has 2+ edema of the lower extremities.
    3. The 15-year-old client diagnosed with diabetic ketoacidosis after a bout with the flu who has a blood glucose reading of 189 mg/dL.
    4. The 62-year-old client diagnosed with COPD and pneumonia who is receiving $O_2$ by nasal cannula at two (2) liters per minute.

45. The client diagnosed with exercise-induced asthma (EIA) is being discharged. Which information should the nurse include in the discharge teaching?
    1. Take two (2) puffs on the rescue inhaler and wait five (5) minutes before exercise.
    2. Warmup exercises will increase the potential for developing the asthma attacks.
    3. Use the bronchodilator inhaler immediately prior to beginning to exercise.
    4. Increase dietary intake of food high in monosodium glutamate (MSG).

46. The client diagnosed with restrictive airway disease, asthma, has been prescribed a glucocorticoid inhaled medication. Which information should the nurse teach regarding this medication?
    1. Do not abruptly stop taking this medication; it must be tapered off.
    2. Immediately rinse the mouth following administration of the drug.
    3. Hold the medication in the mouth for fifteen (15) seconds before swallowing.
    4. Take the medication immediately when an attack starts.

Respiratory

47. The nurse is discussing the care of a child diagnosed with asthma with the parent. Which referral would be important to include?
    1. Referral to a dietitian.
    2. Referral for allergy testing.
    3. Referral to the developmental psychologist.
    4. Referral to a home health nurse.

48. The nurse is discharging a client newly diagnosed with restrictive airway disease, asthma. Which statement indicates the client understands the discharge instructions?
    1. "I will call 911 if my medications don't control an attack."
    2. "I should wash my bedding in warm water."
    3. "I can still eat at the Chinese restaurant when I want."
    4. "If I get a headache I should take a nonsteroidal anti-inflammatory drug."

## Lung Cancer

49. The nurse is taking the social history from a client diagnosed with small cell carcinoma of the lung. Which information is significant for this disease?
    1. The client worked with asbestos for a short time many years ago.
    2. The client has no family history for this type of lung cancer.
    3. The client has numerous tattoos covering both upper and lower arms.
    4. The client has smoked two (2) packs of cigarettes a day for 20 years.

50. The nurse writes a problem of "impaired gas exchange" for a client diagnosed with cancer of the lung. Which interventions should be included in the plan of care? Select all that apply.
    1. Apply $O_2$ via nasal cannula.
    2. Have the dietitian plan for six (6) small meals per day.
    3. Place the client in respiratory isolation.
    4. Assess vital signs for fever.
    5. Listen to lung sounds every shift.

51. The nurse is discussing cancer statistics with a group from the community. Which information about death rates from lung cancer is accurate?
    1. Lung cancer is the number-two cause of cancer deaths in both men and women.
    2. Lung cancer is the number-one cause of cancer deaths in both men and women.
    3. Lung cancer deaths are not significant in relation to other cancers.
    4. Lung cancer deaths have continued to increase in the male population.

52. The nurse and an unlicensed nursing assistant are caring for a group of clients on a medical unit. Which information provided by the assistant warrants immediate intervention by the nurse?
    1. The client diagnosed with cancer of the lung has a small amount of blood in the sputum collection cup.
    2. The client diagnosed with chronic emphysema is sitting on the side of the bed and leaning over the bedside table.
    3. The client receiving Procrit, a biologic response modifier, has a T 99.2°, P 68, R 24, and BP of 198/102.
    4. The client receiving prednisone, a steroid, is complaining of an upset stomach after eating breakfast.

53. The client diagnosed with lung cancer has been told that the cancer has metastasized to the brain. Which intervention should the nurse implement?
    1. Discuss implementing an advance directive.
    2. Explain the use of chemotherapy for brain involvement.
    3. Teach the client to discontinue driving.
    4. Have the significant other make decisions for the client.

## Age-Adjusted Cancer Death Rates,* Males by Site, US, 1930–2001

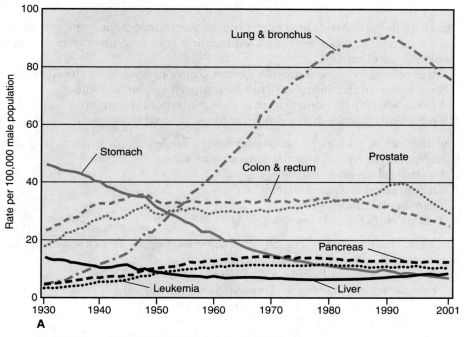

*Per 100,000 age-adjusted to the 2000 US standard population.

**Note:** Due to changes in the ICD coding numerator information has changed over time. Rates for cancers of the liver, lung & bronchus, and colon & rectum are affected by these coding changes.

**Source:** US Mortality Public Use Date Tapes 1960–2001, US Mortality Volumes 1930–1959, National Center for Health Statistics, Centers for Disease Control and Prevention, 2004.

American Cancer Society, Surveillance Research, 2005

## Age-Adjusted Cancer Death Rates,* Females by Site, US, 1930–2001

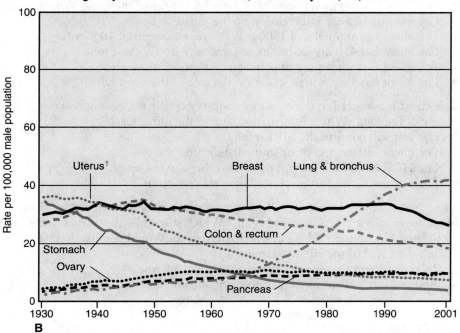

*Per 100,000 age-adjusted to the 2000 US standard population. †Uterus cancer death rates are for uterine cervix and uterine corpus combined.

**Note:** Due to changes in the ICD coding, numerator information has changed over time. Rates for cancers of the lung & bronchus, colon & rectum, and ovary are affected by these coding changes.

**Source:** US Mortality Public Use Date Tapes 1960–2001, US Mortality Volumes 1930–1959, National Center for Health Statistics, Centers for Disease Control and Prevention, 2004.

American Cancer Society, Surveillance Research, 2005

Respiratory

54. The client diagnosed with lung cancer is in an investigational program and receiving a vaccine to treat the cancer. Which information regarding investigational regimens should the nurse teach?
    1. Investigational regimens provide a better chance of survival for the client.
    2. Investigational treatments have not been proved helpful to clients.
    3. Clients will be paid to participate in an investigational program.
    4. Only clients that are dying qualify for investigational treatments.

55. The staff on an oncology unit is interviewing applicants for a position as the unit manager. Which type of organizational structure does this represent?
    1. Centralized decision-making.
    2. Decentralized decision-making.
    3. Shared governance.
    4. Pyramid with filtered-down decisions.

56. The client diagnosed with lung cancer is being discharged. Which statement made by the client indicates that more teaching is needed?
    1. "It doesn't matter if I smoke now. I already have cancer."
    2. "I should see the oncologist at my scheduled appointment."
    3. "If I begin to run a fever I should notify the HCP."
    4. "I should plan for periods of rest throughout the day."

57. The nurse working in an outpatient clinic is interviewing clients. Which information provided by the client warrants further investigation?
    1. The client uses Vicks VapoRub every night before bed.
    2. The client has had an appendectomy.
    3. The client takes a multiple vitamin pill every day.
    4. The client has been coughing up blood in the mornings.

58. The client is four (4) hours post-lobectomy for cancer of the lung. Which assessment data warrant immediate intervention by the nurse?
    1. The client has an intake of 1500 mL IV and an output of 1000 mL.
    2. The client has 450 mL of bright-red drainage in the chest tube.
    3. The client is complaining of pain at a "10" on a 1–10 scale.
    4. The client has absent lung sound on the side of the surgery.

59. The client is admitted to the outpatient surgery center for a bronchoscopy to rule out cancer of the lung. Which information should the nurse teach?
    1. The test will confirm the MRI results.
    2. The client can eat and drink immediately after the test.
    3. The HCP can do a biopsy of the tumor through the scope.
    4. There is no discomfort associated with this procedure.

60. The client diagnosed with oat cell carcinoma of the lung tells the nurse, "I am so tired of all this. I might as well just end it all." Which should be the nurse's first response?
    1. Respond by saying, "This must be hard for you. Would you like to talk?"
    2. Tell the HCP of the client's statement.
    3. Refer the client to a social worker or spiritual advisor.
    4. Find out if the client has a plan to carry out suicide.

## Cancer of the Larynx

61. The nurse is admitting a client with a diagnosis of rule out cancer of the larynx. Which information should the nurse teach?
    1. Demonstrate the proper method of gargling with normal saline.
    2. Perform voice exercises for 30 minutes three (3) times a day.
    3. Explain that a lighted instrument will be placed in the throat to biopsy the area.
    4. Teach the client to self-examine the larynx monthly.

62. The client is diagnosed with cancer of the larynx and is to have radiation therapy to the area. For which prophylactic procedure will the nurse prepare the client?
    1. Removal of the teeth.
    2. Taking anti-emetic medications every four (4) hours.
    3. Wearing sunscreen on the area at all times.
    4. Placement of a PEG tube.

63. The client is three (3) days post-partial laryngectomy. Which type of nutrition should the nurse offer the client?
    1. Total parenteral nutrition.
    2. Soft, regular diet.
    3. Partial parenteral nutrition.
    4. Clear liquid diet.

64. The nurse is preparing the client diagnosed with laryngeal cancer for a laryngectomy in the morning. Which intervention would have priority?
    1. Take the client to the intensive care unit for a visit.
    2. Explain that the client will need to ask for pain medication.
    3. Demonstrate the use of an anti-embolism hose.
    4. Find out if the client can read and write.

65. The client has had a total laryngectomy. Which referral is specific for this surgery?
    1. CanSurmount.
    2. Dialogue.
    3. Lost Chord Club.
    4. SmokEnders.

66. The nurse and unlicensed nursing assistant are caring for a group of clients on a surgical floor. Which information provided by the nursing assistant requires immediate intervention by the nurse?
    1. There is a small, continuous amount of bright-red drainage coming out from under the dressing of the client who had a radical neck dissection.
    2. The client who has had a right upper lobectomy is complaining that the patient controlled analgesia (PCA) pump is not giving any relief.
    3. The client diagnosed with cancer of the lung is complaining of being tired and short of breath.
    4. The client admitted with chronic obstructive pulmonary disease is making a whistling sound with every breath.

67. The charge nurse is assigning clients for the shift. Which client should be assigned to the new graduate nurse?
    1. The client diagnosed with cancer of the lung who has chest tubes.
    2. The client diagnosed with laryngeal spasms who has stridor.
    3. The client diagnosed with laryngeal cancer who has multiple fistulas.
    4. The client who is two (2) hours post-partial laryngectomy.

68. The nurse is writing a care plan for a client newly diagnosed with cancer of the larynx. Which problem would have the highest priority?
    1. Wound infection.
    2. Hemorrhage.
    3. Respiratory distress.
    4. Knowledge deficit.

69. The male client has had a radial neck dissection for cancer of the larynx. Which action by the client indicates a disturbance in body image?
    1. The client requests a consultation by the speech therapist.
    2. The client has a towel placed over the mirror.
    3. The client is attempting to shave himself.
    4. The client practices neck and shoulder exercises.

Respiratory

70. The HCP has recommended a total laryngectomy for a male client diagnosed with cancer of the larynx but the client refuses. Which intervention by the nurse illustrates the ethical principle of nonmalfeasance?
    1. The nurse listens to the client explain why he is refusing surgery.
    2. The nurse and significant other insist that the client have the surgery.
    3. The nurse refers the client to a counselor for help with the decision.
    4. The nurse asks a cancer survivor to come and discuss the surgery with the client.

71. The client diagnosed with cancer of the larynx has had four (4) weeks of radiation therapy to the neck. The client is complaining of severe pain when swallowing. Which scientific rationale explains the pain?
    1. The cancer has grown to obstruct the esophagus.
    2. The treatments are working on the cancer and the throat is edematous.
    3. Cancers are painful and this is expected.
    4. The treatments are also affecting the esophagus, causing ulcerations.

72. The client who has undergone a radical neck dissection and tracheostomy for cancer of the larynx is being discharged. Which discharge instructions should the nurse teach? Select all that apply.
    1. The client will be able to speak again after the surgery area has healed.
    2. The client should wear a protective covering over the stoma when showering.
    3. The client should clean the stoma and then apply a petroleum-based ointment.
    4. The client should use a humidifier in the room.
    5. The client can get a special telephone for communication.

## Pulmonary Embolus

73. The client is diagnosed with a pulmonary embolus and is receiving a heparin drip. The bag hanging is 20,000 units/500 mL of D5W infusing at 22 mL/hr. How many units of heparin is the client receiving each hour?_____

74. The client is suspected of having a pulmonary embolus. Which diagnostic test confirms the diagnosis?
    1. Plasma D-dimer test.
    2. Arterial blood gases.
    3. Chest x-ray.
    4. Magnetic resonance imaging (MRI).

75. Which assessment data would support that the client has experienced a pulmonary embolus?
    1. Calf pain with dorsiflexion of the foot.
    2. Sudden onset of chest pain and dyspnea.
    3. Left-sided chest pain and diaphoresis.
    4. Bilateral crackles and low-grade fever.

76. The client diagnosed with a pulmonary embolus is in the intensive care unit. Which assessment data would warrant immediate intervention from the nurse?
    1. The client's ABGs are pH 7.36, $PaO_2$ 95, $PaCO_2$ 38, $HCO_3$ 24.
    2. The client's telemetry exhibits occasional premature ventricular contractions.
    3. The client's pulse oximeter reading is 90%.
    4. The client's urinary output for the 12-hour shift is 800 mL.

77. The client has just been diagnosed with a pulmonary embolus. Which intervention should the nurse implement?
    1. Administer oral anticoagulants.
    2. Assess the client's bowel sounds.
    3. Prepare the client for a thoracentesis.
    4. Institute and maintain bed rest.

78. The nurse is preparing to administer the oral anticoagulant warfarin (Coumadin) to a client who has a PT/PTT of 22/39 and an INR 2.8. What action should the nurse implement?
    1. Assess the client for abnormal bleeding.
    2. Prepare to administer vitamin K (AquaMephyton).
    3. Administer the medication as ordered.
    4. Notify the HCP to obtain an order to increase the dose.

79. The nurse identified the client problem "decreased cardiac output" for the client diagnosed with a pulmonary embolus. Which intervention should be included in the plan of care?
    1. Monitor the client's arterial blood gases.
    2. Assess skin color and temperature.
    3. Check the client for signs of bleeding.
    4. Keep the client in the Trendelenburg position.

80. Which nursing interventions should the nurse implement for the client diagnosed with a pulmonary embolus who is undergoing thrombolytic therapy? Select all that apply.
    1. Keep protamine sulfate readily available.
    2. Avoid applying pressure to venipuncture sites.
    3. Assess for overt and covert signs of bleeding.
    4. Avoid invasive procedures and injections.
    5. Administer stool softeners as ordered.

81. Which statement by the client indicates the discharge teaching for the client diagnosed with a pulmonary embolus is effective?
    1. "I am going to use a regular-bristle toothbrush."
    2. "I will take antibiotics prior to having my teeth cleaned."
    3. "I can take enteric-coated aspirin for my headache."
    4. "I will wear a medic alert band at all times."

82. The client diagnosed with a pulmonary embolus is being discharged. Which intervention should the nurse discuss with the client?
    1. Increase fluid intake to two (2) to three (3) liters a day.
    2. Eat a low-cholesterol, low-fat diet.
    3. Avoid being around large crowds.
    4. Receive pneumonia and flu vaccines.

83. The nurse is preparing to administer medications to the following clients. Which medication would the nurse question administering?
    1. The oral coagulant warfarin (Coumadin) to the client with an INR of 1.9.
    2. Regular insulin to a client with a blood glucose level of 218 mg/dL.
    3. Hanging the heparin bag to a client with a PT/PTT of 12.9/98.
    4. A calcium channel blocker to the client with a BP of 112/82.

84. The client is getting out of bed and becomes very anxious and has a feeling of impending doom. The nurse thinks the client may be experiencing a pulmonary embolus. Which action should the nurse implement first?
    1. Administer oxygen ten (10) L via nasal cannula.
    2. Place the client in a high Fowler's position.
    3. Obtain a STAT pulse oximeter reading.
    4. Auscultate the client's lung sounds.

Respiratory

## Chest Trauma

85. The client is admitted to the emergency department with chest trauma. When assessing the client, which signs/symptoms would the nurse expect to find that support the diagnosis of pneumothorax?
    1. Bronchovesicular lung sounds and bradypnea.
    2. Unequal lung expansion and dyspnea.
    3. Frothy bloody sputum and consolidation.
    4. Barrel chest and polycythemia.

86. The client had a right-sided chest tube inserted two (2) hours ago for a pneumothorax. Which action should the nurse take if there is no fluctuation (tidaling) in the water-seal compartment?
    1. Obtain an order for a stat chest x-ray.
    2. Increase the amount of wall suction.
    3. Check the tubing for kinks or clots.
    4. Monitor the client's pulse oximeter reading.

87. Which intervention should the nurse implement for a male client who has had a left-sided chest tube for six (6) hours and refuses to take deep breaths because it hurts too much?
    1. Medicate the client and have the client take deep breaths.
    2. Encourage the client to take shallow breaths to help with the pain.
    3. Explain that deep breaths do not have to be taken at this time.
    4. Tell the client that if he doesn't take deep breaths, he could die.

88. The unlicensed nursing assistant is assisting the client with a chest tube to ambulate to the bathroom. Which situation warrants immediate intervention from the nurse?
    1. The client's chest tube is below the level of the chest.
    2. The nursing assistant has the chest tube attached to suction.
    3. The nursing assistant allowed the client out of the bed.
    4. The nursing assistant uses a bedside commode for the client.

89. The client has a right-sided chest tube. As the client is getting out of the bed it is accidentally pulled out of the pleural space. Which action should the nurse implement first?
    1. Notify the health-care provider to have chest tubes reinserted STAT.
    2. Instruct the client to take slow shallow breaths until the tube is reinserted.
    3. Take no action and assess the client's respiratory status every 15 minutes.
    4. Tape a petroleum jelly occlusive dressing on three (3) sides to the insertion site.

90. The nurse is presenting a class on chest tubes. Which statement describes a tension pneumothorax?
    1. A tension pneumothorax develops when an air-filled bleb on the surface of the lung ruptures.
    2. When a tension pneumothorax occurs, the air moves freely between the pleural space and the atmosphere.
    3. The injury allows air into the pleural space but prevents it from escaping from the pleural space.
    4. A tension pneumothorax results from a puncture of the pleura during a central line placement.

91. Which action should the nurse implement for the client with a hemothorax who has a right-sided chest tube and there is excessive bubbling in the water-seal compartment?
    1. Check the amount of wall suction being applied.
    2. Assess the tubing for any blood clots.
    3. Milk the tubing proximal to distal.
    4. Encourage the client to cough forcefully.

92. Which assessment data indicate that the chest tubes have been effective in treating the client with a hemothorax who has a right-sided chest tube?
    1. There is gentle bubbling in the suction compartment.
    2. There is no fluctuation (tidaling) in the water-seal compartment.
    3. There is 250 mL of blood in the drainage compartment
    4. The client is able to deep breathe without any pain.

93. The nurse is caring for a client with a right-sided chest tube secondary to a pneumothorax. Which interventions should the nurse implement when caring for this client? Select all that apply.
    1. Place the client in a low-Fowler's position.
    2. Assess chest tube drainage system frequently.
    3. Maintain strict bed rest for the client.
    4. Secure a loop of drainage tubing to the sheet.
    5. Observe the site for subcutaneous emphysema.

94. The charge nurse is making client assignments on a medical floor. Which client should the charge nurse assign to the LPN?
    1. The client with pneumonia who has a pulse oximeter reading of 91%.
    2. The client with a hemothorax who has Hgb of 9 mg/dL and Hct of 20%.
    3. The client with chest tubes who has jugular vein distention and BP of 96/60.
    4. The client who is two (2) hours post-bronchoscopy procedure.

95. The alert and oriented client is diagnosed with a spontaneous pneumothorax, and the physician is preparing to insert a left-sided chest tube. Which intervention should the nurse implement first?
    1. Gather the needed supplies for the procedure.
    2. Obtain a signed informed consent form.
    3. Assist the client into a side-lying position.
    4. Discuss the procedure with the client.

96. Which intervention should the nurse implement first for the client diagnosed with a hemothorax who has had a right-sided chest tube for three (3) days and has no fluctuation (tidaling) in the water compartment?
    1. Assess the client's bilateral lung sounds.
    2. Obtain an order for a STAT chest x-ray.
    3. Notify the health-care provider as soon as possible.
    4. Document the findings in the client's chart.

## Acute Respiratory Distress Syndrome

97. The unlicensed nursing assistant (NA) is bathing the client diagnosed with acute respiratory distress syndrome (ARDS). The bed is in a high position with the opposite side rail in the low position. Which action should the nurse implement?
    1. Demonstrate the correct technique for giving a bed bath.
    2. Encourage the NA to put the bed in the lowest position.
    3. Instruct the NA to get another person to help with the bath.
    4. Provide praise for performing the bath safely for the client and the NA.

98. The client diagnosed with ARDS is transferred to the intensive care department and placed on a ventilator. Which intervention should the nurse implement first?
    1. Confirm that the ventilator settings are correct.
    2. Verify that the ventilator alarms are functioning properly.
    3. Assess the respiratory status and pulse oximeter reading.
    4. Monitor the client's arterial blood gas results.

99. The nurse suspects the client may be developing ARDS. Which assessment data confirm the diagnosis of ARDS?
   1. Low arterial oxygen when administering high concentration of oxygen.
   2. The client has dyspnea and tachycardia and is feeling anxious.
   3. Bilateral breath sounds clear and pulse oximeter reading is 95%.
   4. The client has jugular vein distention and frothy sputum.

100. The client who smokes two (2) packs of cigarettes a day develops ARDS after a near drowning. The client asks the nurse, "What is happening to me? Why did I get this?" Which statement by the nurse is most appropriate?
   1. "Most people who drown end up developing ARDS."
   2. "Platelets and fluid enter the alveoli due to permeability instability."
   3. "Your lungs are filling up with fluid, causing breathing problems."
   4. "Smoking has caused your lungs to become weakened, so you got ARDS."

101. Which assessment data would indicate the client diagnosed with ARDS has experienced a complication secondary to the ventilator?
   1. The client's urine output is 100 mL in two (2) hours.
   2. The pulse oximeter reading is greater than 95%.
   3. The client has asymmetrical chest expansion.
   4. The telemetry reading shows sinus tachycardia.

102. The health-care provider ordered stat arterial blood gases (ABGs) for the client diagnosed with ARDS. The ABG results are pH 7.38, $PaO_2$ 92, $PaCO_2$ 38, $HCO_3$ 24. Which action should the nurse implement?
   1. Continue to monitor the client without taking any action.
   2. Encourage the client to take deep breaths and cough.
   3. Administer one (1) amp of sodium bicarbonate IVP.
   4. Notify the respiratory therapist of the ABG results.

103. The client with ARDS is on a mechanical ventilator. Which intervention should be included in the nursing care plan addressing the endotracheal tube care?
   1. Do not move or touch the ET tube.
   2. Obtain a chest x-ray daily.
   3. Determine if the ET cuff is deflated.
   4. Ensure that the ET tube is secure.

104. Which medication should the nurse anticipate the health-care provider ordering for the client diagnosed with ARDS?
   1. An aminoglycoside antibiotic.
   2. A synthetic surfactant.
   3. A potassium cation.
   4. A nonsteroidal anti-inflammatory drug.

105. The client diagnosed with ARDS is in respiratory distress and the ventilator is malfunctioning. Which intervention should the nurse implement first?
   1. Notify the respiratory therapist immediately.
   2. Ventilate with a manual resuscitation bag.
   3. Request STAT arterial blood gases.
   4. Auscultate the client's lung sounds.

106. The nurse is caring for the client diagnosed with ARDS. Which interventions should the nurse implement? Select all that apply.
   1. Assess the client's level of consciousness.
   2. Monitor urine output every shift.
   3. Turn the client every two (2) hours.
   4. Maintain intravenous fluids as ordered.
   5. Place the client in the Fowler's position.

107. Which instruction is most important for the nurse to discuss with the client diagnosed with ARDS who is being discharged from the hospital?
    1. Avoid smoking and exposure to smoke.
    2. Do not receive flu or pneumonia vaccines.
    3. Avoid any type of alcohol intake.
    4. It will take about one (1) month to recuperate.

108. The client diagnosed with ARDS is on a ventilator and the high alarm indicates that there is an increase in the peak airway pressure. Which intervention should the nurse implement first?
    1. Check the tubing for any kinks.
    2. Suction the airway for secretions.
    3. Assess the lip line of the ET tube.
    4. Sedate the client with a muscle relaxant.

# PRACTICE QUESTIONS ANSWERS AND RATIONALES

## Upper Respiratory Infection

1. 1. Influenza is a viral illness that might cause these symptoms; however, the immunization should not give the client the illness.
   2. Coming into contact with small children increases the risk of developing colds and the flu, but the client has a problem—not just a potential one.
   3. A client diagnosed with hypertension should not take many of the over-the-counter medications because they work by causing vasoconstriction, which will increase the hypertension.
   4. Cold sores are actually an infection by the herpes simplex virus. Colds and coldlike symptoms are caused by the rhinitis virus or influenza virus. The term "cold sore" is a common term that still persists in the populace.

   **TEST-TAKING HINT: The keys to answering this question are the words "hypertension" and "cold." Any time a client has a chronic illness, the client should discuss over-the-counter medications with the health-care provider or a pharmacist. Many of the routine medications for chronic illnesses interact with over-the-counter medications.**

2. 1. It is not feasible for a child to always have a tissue or handkerchief available.
   2. There is no immunization for the common cold. Colds are actually caused by at least 200 separate viruses and the viruses mutate frequently.
   3. Colds are caused by a virus and antibiotics do not treat a virus; therefore, there is no need to go to a health-care provider.
   4. Hand washing is the single most useful technique for prevention of disease.

   **TEST-TAKING HINT: Answer option "1" contains the word "always," an absolute term, and in most questions, absolute adjectives, such as "always," "never," and "only," make that answer option incorrect.**

3. 1. The client should be taught to take all antibiotics as ordered. Discontinuing antibiotics prior to the full dose results in the development of antibiotic-resistant bacteria. Sinus infections are difficult to treat and may become chronic and will then require several weeks of therapy or possibly surgery to control.
   2. If the sinuses are irrigated, it is done under anesthesia by a health-care provider.
   3. Blowing the nose will increase pressure in the sinus cavities and will cause the client increased pain.
   4. The nurse is not licensed to prescribe medications so this is not in the nurse's scope of practice. Also, narcotic analgesic medications are controlled substances and require written documentation of being prescribed by the health-care provider; samples are not generally available.

   **TEST-TAKING HINT: Note in this situation that an "all" is in the correct answer. There are very few cases in which absolute adjectives will describe the correct answer. The test taker must be aware that general rules will not always apply.**

4. 1. Muscle weakness is a sign/symptom of myalgia, but it is not a life-threatening complication of sinusitis.
   2. Purulent sputum would be a sign/symptom of a lung infection, but it is not a life-threatening complication of sinusitis.
   3. Nuchal rigidity is a sign/symptom of meningitis, which is a life-threatening potential complication of sinusitis resulting from the close proximity of the sinus cavities to the meninges.
   4. Intermittent loss of muscle control can be a symptom of multiple sclerosis, but it would not be a life-threatening complication of sinusitis.

   **TEST-TAKING HINT: A basic knowledge of anatomy and physiology would help to answer this question. The sinuses lie in the head and surround the orbital cavity. Options "1" and "4" refer to muscle problems, so both could be ruled out as a wrong.**

5. 1. The hemoglobin and hematocrit given are within normal range. This would not warrant notifying the health-care provider.
   2. A low-grade temperature and a cough could indicate the presence of an infection, in which case the health-care provider would not want to subject the client to anesthesia and the possibility of further complications. The surgery would be postponed.
   3. One (1) to two (2) WBCs in a urinalysis is not uncommon because of the normal flora in the bladder.
   4. The INR indicates that the client's bleeding time is within normal range.

   **TEST-TAKING HINT: In this question, all the answer options contain normal data except for one. The nurse would not call the health-care provider to notify him or her of normal values.**

Respiratory

**174**

6. 1. The elderly and chronically ill are at greatest risk for developing serious complications if they contract the influenza virus.
   2. It is recommended that people in contact with children receive the flu vaccine whenever possible, but these clients should be able to withstand a bout with the flu if their immune systems are functioning normally.
   3. It is probable that these clients will be exposed to the virus, but they are not as likely to develop severe complications with intact functioning immune systems.
   4. During flu season the more people that the individual comes into contact with, the greater the risk the client will be exposed to the influenza virus, but this group of people would not receive the vaccine before the elderly and chronically ill.

   **TEST-TAKING HINT: Sometimes the test taker may think the answer is too easy and obvious, but the test taker should not try to second guess the question. Item writers are not trying to trick the test taker; they are trying to evaluate knowledge.**

7. 1. The client has complained of pain, and the nurse, after determining the severity of the pain and barring any complications in the client, will administer pain medication after completion of the assessment.
   2. Oral hygiene helps to prevent the development of infections and promotes comfort, but it will not relieve the pain.
   3. Placing the client in a semi-Fowler's position will reduce edema of inflamed sinus tissue, but it will not immediately affect the client's perception of pain.
   4. Prior to intervening the nurse must assess to determine the amount of pain and possible complications occurring that could be masked if narcotic medication is administered.

   **TEST-TAKING HINT: Whenever there is an assessment answer among the answer options, the test taker should look carefully at what is being assessed. If the option says to assess the problem identified in the question, it will usually be the correct answer. Remember, the first step in the nursing process is assessment.**

8. 1. This client is one (1)-day postoperative and has moderate pain, which is to be expected after surgery. A less experienced nurse can care for this client.
   2. A child about to go to surgery involving the throat area can be expected to have painful swallowing. This does not require the most experienced nurse.
   3. The postoperative client with purulent drainage could be developing an infection. The experienced nurse would be needed to assess and monitor the client's condition.
   4. Any nurse that is capable of administering IVPB medications can care for this client.

   **TEST-TAKING HINT: In this type of question the test taker must determine if the situation described is expected or within normal limits. The one (1) answer option that gives data that are not expected or within normal limits is the one (1) that will require a nurse with the greatest amount of knowledge and experience.**

9. 1. A person with a viral infection should not return to work until the virus has run its course because the antibiotics help prevent complications of the virus, but they do not make the client get better faster.
   2. **Secondary bacterial infections often accompany influenza, and antibiotics are often prescribed to help prevent the development of a bacterial infection.**
   3. Antibiotics will not prevent the flu. Only the flu vaccine will prevent the flu.
   4. When people take portions of the antibiotic prescription and stop taking the remainder, an antibiotic-resistant strain of bacteria may develop, and the client may experience a return of symptoms—but this time, the antibiotics will not be effective.

   **TEST-TAKING HINT: Knowing drug classifications and how the drugs within that classification work would assist the test taker to determine the correct answer. Antibiotics work to destroy bacterial invasions of the body.**

10. 1. The client with laryngitis is instructed to avoid all alcohol. Alcohol causes increased irritation of the throat.
    2. Whispering places added strain on the larynx.
    3. **Voice rest is encouraged for the client experiencing laryngitis.**
    4. Aphonia, or inability to speak, is a temporary condition associated with laryngitis.

    **TEST-TAKING HINT: Encouraging the use of alcohol, with the exception of a glass of red wine, is not accepted medical practice; therefore, this option "1" could be eliminated. Option "4" has an absolute—"permanent"—in it and therefore could be eliminated from consideration.**

Respiratory

11. 1. Tonsillectomies cause throat edema and difficulty swallowing; the nurse must observe the client's ability to swallow before this task can be delegated.
    2. Clients with colds are encouraged to drink 2000 mL of liquids a day. The unlicensed nursing assistant could do this.
    3. Throat swabs for culture must be done correctly or false-negative results can occur. The nurse should obtain the swab.
    4. Clients with laryngitis are instructed not to smoke. Smoking is discouraged in all health-care facilities. Sending nursing personnel outside to encourage an unhealthy practice is not the best use of the personnel.

    **TEST-TAKING HINT: Interventions that could require assessing, teaching, and evaluating should not be delegated. Levels of activities being delegated should be appropriate for the level of training of the staff member carrying out the task. Tasks delegated should conform to safe health-care practice.**

12. 1. Alternative therapies are therapies that are not accepted medical practice. These may be encouraged as long as they do not interfere with the medical regimen. Vitamin C in large doses is thought to improve the immune system's functions.
    2. Bed rest is accepted standard advice for a client with a cold.
    3. Humidifying the air helps to relieve congestion and is a standard practice.
    4. Decongestant therapy is standard therapy for a cold.

    **TEST-TAKING HINT: Only one of the answer options is not common advice for a client with a cold. When all options but one (1) match, then the one (1) odd one should be selected as the correct answer.**

## Lower Respiratory Infection

13. 1. The elderly client diagnosed with pneumonia may present with weakness, fatigue, lethargy, confusion, and poor appetite but not have any of the classic signs and symptoms of pneumonia.
    2. Fever and chills are classic symptoms of pneumonia, but they are usually absent in the elderly client.
    3. Frothy sputum and edema are signs and symptoms of heart failure, not pneumonia.
    4. The client has tachypnea (fast respirations), not bradypnea (slow respirations), and jugular vein distention accompanies heart failure.

**TEST-TAKING HINT: The question gives an age range—"elderly"—so age can be expected to affect the disease process—in this case, causing atypical symptoms. The prefix "brady" means "slow" when attached to a word. Knowing the definition of medical prefixes can assist the test taker in determining the correct answer.**

14. 1. Clients do not perform chest physiotherapy; this is normally done by the respiratory therapist. This is a staff goal, not a client goal.
    2. This would be a goal for self-care deficit but not for impaired gas exchange.
    3. This would be a goal for the problem of activity intolerance.
    4. Impaired gas exchange results in hypoxia, the earliest sign and symptom of which is a change in the level of consciousness.

**TEST-TAKING HINT: The test taker should match the answer option to the listed nursing problem. Option "1" is a staff goal to accomplish. When writing goals for the client, it is important to remember they are written in terms of what is expected of the client. Options "2" and "3" are appropriately written client goals, but they do not evaluate gas exchange.**

15. 1. A gastrostomy tube is placed directly into the stomach through the abdominal wall; the nare is the opening of the nostril.
    2. Elevating the head of the bed uses gravity to keep the formula in the gastric cavity and help prevent it from refluxing into the esophagus, which predisposes the client to aspiration.
    3. The Sims position is the left lateral side-lying flat position. This position is used for administering enemas and can be used to prevent aspiration in clients sedated by anesthesia. The sedated client would not have a full stomach.
    4. Dressings on PEG tubes should be changed at least daily. If there is no dressing, the insertion site is still assessed daily.

**TEST-TAKING HINT: The test taker should try to picture the positioning of the client to determine the correct answer. In "4" the test taker should question if the time given, three (3) days, is the correct time interval for performing this intervention.**

16. 1. Broad-spectrum IV antibiotics are priority, but before antibiotics are administered, it is important to obtain culture specimens to determine the correct antibiotic for the client's infection. Clients are placed on oral medications only after several days of IVPB therapy.
    2. Meal trays are not priority over cultures.

3. To determine the antibiotic that will effectively treat an infection, specimens for culture are taken prior to beginning the medication. Administering antibiotics prior to cultures may make it impossible to determine the actual agent causing the pneumonia.

4. Admission weights are important to determine appropriate dosing of medication, but they are not priority over sputum collection.

**TEST-TAKING HINT: Answer option "1" has a medication classification and a route, and the test taker should question if the route is appropriate for the client being admitted. Clients will not die from a delayed meal, but a client could die from delayed IV antibiotic therapy.**

17. 1. Clients diagnosed with TB will need to take the medications for six (6) months to a year.

2. Compliance with treatment plans for TB includes multi-drug therapy for six (6) months to one (1) year for the client to be free of the TB bacteria.

3. Clients are no longer contagious when three (3) morning sputum specimens are cultured negative, but this will not occur until after several weeks of therapy.

4. The TB skin test only determines possible exposure to the bacteria, not active disease.

**TEST-TAKING HINT: The test taker should determine if the time of three (3) weeks in "1," months in "2," or immediately in "3" is the correct time interval.**

18. 1. A purple flat area indicates that the client became bruised when the intradermal injection was given, but it has no bearing on whether the test is positive.

2. A positive skin test is 10 mm or greater with induration, not redness.

3. If the client has ever reacted positively, then the client should have a chest x-ray to look for causation and inflammation.

4. These are negative findings and do not indicate the need to have x-ray determination of disease.

**TEST-TAKING HINT: The test taker should note descriptive adjectives such as "purple," "flat," or "4 mm" before determining the correct answer. Option "4" has the absolute word "never" and absolutes usually indicate incorrect answers.**

19. 1. The client diagnosed with pneumonia will have some degree of gas-exchange deficit. Administering oxygen would help the client.

2. Activities of daily living require energy and therefore oxygen consumption. Spacing the activities allows the client to rebuild oxygen reserves between activities.

3. Clients are encouraged to drink at least 2000 mL daily to thin secretions.

4. Cigarette smoking depresses the action of the cilia in the lungs. Any smoking should be prohibited.

5. Pulse oximetry readings provide the nurse with an estimate of oxygenation in the periphery.

**TEST-TAKING HINT: Maslow's Hierarchy of Needs lists oxygenation as the top priority. Therefore the test taker should select interventions addressing oxygenation.**

20. 1. The nares are the opening of the nostrils. Suctioning, if done, would be of the posterior pharynx.

2. Turning the client to the side allows for the food to be coughed up and come out of the mouth, rather than be aspirated into the lungs.

3. Placing the client in the Trendelenburg position would increase the risk of aspiration.

4. An immediate action is needed to protect the client.

**TEST-TAKING HINT: In a question that asks the test taker to determine the first action, all the answer options may be correct for the situation. The test taker must determine which has the greatest potential for improving the client's condition.**

21. 1. The specimen needs to be taken to the lab within a reasonable time frame, but an unlicensed nursing assistant can take specimens to the lab.

2. Clogged feeding tubes occur with some regularity. Delay in feeding a client will not result in permanent damage.

3. A pulse oximetry reading of 92% means that the arterial blood oxygen saturation is somewhere around 60%–70%.

4. Arterial oxygenation normal values are 80%–100%.

**TEST-TAKING HINT: Be sure to read all the answer options. Pulse oximetry readings do not give the same information as arterial blood gas readings.**

22. 1. Standard precautions are used to prevent exposure to blood and body secretions on all clients. TB is caused by airborne bacteria.

2. Contact precautions are used for wounds.

3. Droplet precautions are used for infections

that are spread by sneezing or coughing but are not transmitted over distances of more than three (3) to four (4) feet.

4. Tuberculosis bacteria are capable of disseminating over distances on air currents. Clients with tuberculosis are placed in negative air pressure rooms where the air in the room is not allowed to cross-contaminate the air in the hallway.

**TEST-TAKING HINT: Standard precautions and contact precautions can be ruled out as the correct answer if the test taker is aware that TB is usually a respiratory illness. This at least gives the reader a 1:2 chance of selecting the correct answer if the answer is not known.**

23. 1. Closing the door reestablishes the negative air pressure, which prevents the air from entering the hall and contaminating the hospital environment. When correcting an individual, it is always best to do so in a private manner.
    2. The employee is an adult and as such should be treated with respect and corrected accordingly.
    3. Problems should be taken care of at the lowest level possible. The nurse is responsible for any task delegated, including the appropriate handling of isolation.
    4. Correcting staff should never be done in the presence of the client. This undermines the nursing assistant and creates doubt of the staff's competency in the client's mind.

**TEST-TAKING HINT: An action must be taken; the test taker must determine which action would have the desired results with the least amount of disruption to client care. Correcting the nursing assistant in this manner has the greatest chance of creating a win–win situation.**

24. 1. Pleuritic chest pain and anxiety from diminished oxygenation occur along with fever, chills, dyspnea, and cough.
    2. Asymmetrical chest expansion occurs if the client has a collapsed lung from a pneumothorax or hemothorax, and the client would be cyanotic from decreased oxygenation.
    3. The client would have leukocytosis, not leukopenia, and a capillary refill time (CRT) of <3 seconds is normal.
    4. Substernal chest pain and diaphoresis are symptoms of MI.

**TEST-TAKING HINT: Options "1" and "4" have chest pain as part of the answer. The adjectives describing the chest pain determine the correct answer.**

## Chronic Pulmonary Obstructive Disease

25. 1. This would be information needed to treat the cause but not the most important in health promotion.
    2. The risk factors for complications would be important in planning care.
    3. Assessing the ability to deliver medications would be important when teaching the client.
    4. The possibility of lifestyle changes is most important in health promotion. The most important is smoking cessation. The nurse needs to assess if the client has the willingness to consider cessation of smoking and carry out the plan. If the client refuses to stop, treatment will need to be altered.

**TEST-TAKING HINT: The test taker needs to read the question for words such as "health promotion." These words make all the other answer options wrong because they do not promote health.**

26. 1. The client should be assisted into a sitting position either on the side of the bed or in the bed. This position decreases the work of breathing. Some clients find it easier sitting on the side of the bed leaning over the bed table. The nurse needs to maintain the client's safety.
    2. Oxygen will be applied as soon as possible, but the least amount possible. If levels of oxygen are too high, the client may stop breathing.
    3. Vital signs need to be monitored, but this is not the first priority. If the equipment is not in the room, another member of the health-care team should bring it to the nurse. The nurse should stay with the client.
    4. The health-care provider will need to be notified, but the client needs to be treated first. The nurse should get assistance if possible so that the nurse can treat this client quickly.

**TEST-TAKING HINT: When a question asks for the test taker to choose the intervention to implement first, the test taker should treat life-threatening events first. In this situation the client is in respiratory distress so the nurse must act quickly to prevent the progression to respiratory failure. "Notify the health-care provider" is usually not the first intervention. There are usually assessment data to obtain before calling.**

27. 1. A large amount of thick sputum is a common symptom of COPD. There is no cause for immediate intervention.

2. The nurse should decrease the oxygen rate. Hypoxemia is the stimulus for breathing in the client with COPD. If the hypoxemia improves and the oxygen level increases, the drive to breathe may be eliminated. Careful monitoring is important to prevent complications.
3. It is common for clients with COPD to use accessory muscles when inhaling. These clients tend to lean forward.
4. In clients with COPD, there is a characteristic barrel chest from chronic hyperinflation, and dyspnea is common.

**TEST-TAKING HINT:** This question requires interpreting the data to determine which is abnormal or unexpected and thus is the one that needs intervention before the client is harmed. At first the test taker may be tempted to choose "4" because of the word "dyspnea" or "3" because of the use of accessory muscles, but these are common occurrences for that client or, in other words, normal for the client. If the data describes a normal scenario for that client, the test taker should look for the option that is different or describes an occurrence that is not expected or that is incorrect—in this case, the oxygen being given too rapidly.

28. 1. The expected outcome of showing no signs of respiratory distress would indicate that the plan of care is effective and should be continued.
2. An improved respiratory pattern indicates that the plan should be continued because the client is improving.
3. The expected outcome should be that the client is showing an improved activity tolerance; because the client is not meeting the expected outcome, the plan of care needs revision. The nurse needs to collaborate with the health-care team and with the client to establish interventions that will assist in improving the client's outcome.
4. The client needs to participate in planning the course of care. The client is meeting the expected outcome.

**TEST-TAKING HINT:** This question is similar to an "except" question. The test taker should look at each answer option for a positive outcome. Nurses want their clients to improve so the expected outcomes should be an improvement of some problem. The test taker should decide which outcome is not desired.

29. 1. The client with end-stage COPD would have decreased peripheral oxygen levels; therefore, this would not warrant immediate intervention.

2. The client's ABGs would normally have a low oxygen level; therefore, this would not warrant immediate intervention.
3. The client would have shortness of breath (SOB) when ambulating to the bathroom.
4. Rusty-colored sputum may indicate blood in the sputum and would require further assessment by the nurse.

**TEST-TAKING HINT:** The test taker could rule out options "1" and "2" as correct answers because both describe the same data of decreased oxygen, which is characteristic of COPD.

30. 1. When sputum changes in color, amount, or both, this indicates infection and the client should report this information to the health-care provider.
2. Bronchodilators should be taken routinely to prevent bronchospasms.
3. Clients use the metered dose inhalers because they deliver a precise amount of medication with correct use.
4. Clients need to have blood levels drawn every six (6) months when taking bronchodilators.

**TEST-TAKING HINT:** When evaluating whether the client has learned the information presented, the test taker is observing for incorrect information. The test taker should pay close attention to numbers such as "every 12 months." Is that adequate for the stable client?

31. 1. The client diagnosed with COPD has difficulty exchanging oxygen with carbon dioxide, which is manifested by physical signs such as fingernail clubbing and metabolic acidosis as seen on arterial blood gases.
2. Clients need to avoid extremes in temperatures. Warm temperatures cause an increase in the metabolism and increase the need for oxygen. Cold temperatures cause bronchospasms.
3. When a client has difficulty breathing the client can become fatigued so that the client can stop breathing. Activities should be timed so rest periods are available to prevent fatigue.
4. Many clients have difficulty adapting to the role changes brought about because of the disease process. Many cannot maintain the activities involved in meeting responsibilities at home and at work. Clients should be assessed for these issues.
5. Clients often lose weight because so much effort is expended to breathe.

**TEST-TAKING HINT: This is an example of an alternate question. There may be more than one (1) answer. The test taker should consider all options independently and understand that the question is not a trick.**

32. 1. Pursed-lip breathing helps keep the alveoli open to allow for better oxygen and carbon dioxide exchange.
    2. This would be an appropriate outcome for a knowledge-deficit problem.
    3. This outcome does not ensure the client has an effective airway; increasing fluid does not ensure an effective airway.
    4. This would be an outcome for the client problem of activity intolerance.

**TEST-TAKING HINT: The test taker needs to identify the outcome for the client problem cited—namely, "ineffective gas exchange." The only answer option dealing with the airway is "1," pursed-lip breathing.**

33. 1. The client diagnosed with COPD needs oxygen at all times, especially when exerting energy such as when ambulating to the bathroom.
    2. The client needs the oxygen, and the nurse should not correct the NA in front of the client; it is embarrassing for the NA, and the client loses confidence in the staff.
    3. The nurse should not verbally correct an NA in front of the client; the nurse should correct the behavior and then talk to the NA in private.
    4. The primary nurse should confront the NA and take care of the situation. Continued unsafe client care would warrant notifying the charge nurse.

**TEST-TAKING HINT: The test taker must know management concepts and the nurse should first address the behavior with the person directly then follow the chain of command. Remember, the nurse should treat a subordinate the way they would want to be treated and not embarrass the NA in front of the client.**

34. 1. Clubbing fingers is the result of chronic hypoxemia, which would be expected with chronic COPD but not with recently diagnosed COPD.
    2. These clients have frequent respiratory infections.
    3. Sputum production, along with cough and dyspnea on exertion, are the early signs/symptoms of COPD.
    4. These clients have a productive cough, not a nonproductive cough.

**TEST-TAKING HINT: The test taker must be observant of adjectives such as "recently diagnosed," which helps to rule out incorrect answers such as "1." Option "2" has the word "infrequent." The test taker must notice these words.**

35. 1. Clients diagnosed with COPD should receive the influenza vaccine each year. If there is a shortage, these clients have top priority.
    2. The pneumococcal vaccine should be given every five (5) to seven (7) years. It is important to prevent respiratory illnesses when possible with these clients.
    3. Reducing the number of cigarettes smoked does not stop the progression of COPD, and the client will continue to experience signs and symptoms such as shortness of breath or dyspnea on exertion.
    4. Clients diagnosed with COPD should increase their fluid intake unless contraindicated for another health condition. The increased fluid assists the client in expectorating the thick sputum.

**TEST-TAKING HINT: Nurses are expected to serve as community resources. The nurse should be knowledgeable about health promotion activities such as immunizations. One (1) option describes a desired goal, but the other three (3) do not.**

36. 1. The asthma foundation would not be appropriate for a client diagnosed with chronic lung disease.
    2. The American Cancer Society is helpful for a client with lung cancer but not for a client with COPD.
    3. The American Lung Association has information that is helpful for a client with COPD.
    4. Many clients with COPD end up with heart problems, but the American Heart Association does not have information for clients with COPD.

**TEST-TAKING HINT: The test taker should be familiar with organizations, but if the test taker had no idea what the answer was, the only option containing a word referring to respiration—"lung"—is option "3."**

## Reactive Airway Disease (Asthma)

37. 1. Fever is a sign of infection and crepitus is air trapped in the layers of the skin.

2. Rales indicate fluid in the lung, and hives are a skin reaction to a stimulus such as occurs with an allergy to a specific substance.

3. During an asthma attack the muscles surrounding the bronchioles constrict, causing a narrowing of the bronchioles. The lungs then respond with the production of secretions that further narrow the lumen. The resulting symptoms include wheezing from air passing through the narrow, clogged spaces, and dyspnea.

4. During an attack, the chest will be expanded from air being trapped and not being exhaled. A chest x-ray will reveal a lowered diaphragm and hyperinflated lungs.

**TEST-TAKING HINTS: The test taker must have a basic knowledge of common medical terms to answer this question. Dyspnea, wheezing, and rales are common terms used when describing respiratory function and lung sounds. Crepitus and eupnea are not as commonly used, but they are also terms that describe respiratory processes and problems.**

38. 1. Anxiety is an expected sequela of being unable to meet the oxygen needs of the body. Staying with the client lets the client know the nurse will intervene and that the client is not alone.

2. Because anxiety is an expected occurrence with asthma, it is not necessary to notify the health-care provider.

3. An anxiolytic medication could decrease respiratory drive and increase the respiratory distress. Also, the medication will require a delayed time period to begin to work.

4. Drinking fluids will not treat an asthma attack or anxiety.

**TEST-TAKING HINTS: Before choosing an answer option that directs the test taker to notify a health-care provider, the test taker should determine if the option is describing an expected event or data for the disease process being discussed. If it is expected, then notifying the health-care provider would not be the correct answer.**

39. 1. Nursing is the one discipline that is with the client around the clock. Therefore nurses have knowledge of the client that the other disciplines might not know.

2. The pharmacist will be able to discuss the medication regimen that the client is receiving and make suggestions regarding other medications or medication interactions.

3. The social worker may be able to assist with financial information or home care arrangements.

4. Occupational therapists help clients with activities of daily living and modifications to home environments; nothing in the stem indicates a need for these services.

5. Speech therapists assist clients with speech and swallowing problems; nothing in the stem indicates a need for these services

**TEST-TAKING HINTS: Cost containment issues are always a concern the nurse must address. The use of limited resources (health-care personnel) should be on an as-needed basis only. Cost containment must be considered when using people or supplies.**

40. 1. Daily inhaled steroids are used for mild, moderate, or severe persistent asthma, not for intermittent asthma.

2. Clients with intermittent asthma will have exacerbations that are treated with rescue inhalers. Therefore, the nurse should teach the client about rescue inhalers.

3. Systemic steroids are used frequently by clients with severe persistent asthma, not with mild intermittent asthma.

4. Leukotriene agonists are prescribed for clients diagnosed with mild persistent asthma.

**TEST-TAKING HINTS: In the stem there are two (2) words that give the test taker a clue about which answer is correct. "Mild" and "intermittent" are words that tell the test taker that the client is not experiencing frequent or escalating symptoms. Steroid medications can have multiple side effects.**

41. 1. Mast cell stabilizers require ten (10) to 14 days to begin to be effective. Some clients diagnosed with exercise-induced asthma derive benefit from taking the drugs immediately before exercising, but these drugs must be in the system for a period of time before effectiveness can be achieved.

2. Tapering of medications is done for systemic steroids because of adrenal functioning.

3. The drugs are taken daily, before exercise, or both.

4. Mast cell drugs are routine maintenance medications and do not treat an attack.

**TEST-TAKING HINTS: The test taker must be knowledgeable about medications. There are not many test-taking hints. If the test taker knows that a specific option applies to a medication other than the one (1) mentioned in the stem, the test taker can eliminate that option.**

Respiratory

42. 1. A complete blood count determines the oxygen-carrying capacity of the hemoglobin in the body, but it will not identify the immediate problem.
  2. Pulmonary functions tests are completed to determine the forced vital capacity (FVC), the forced expiratory vital capacity in the first second (FEV1), and the peak expiratory flow (PEF). A decline in the FVC, FEV1, and PEF indicate respiratory compromise.
  3. Allergy skin testing will be done to determine triggers for allergic asthma, but it is not done during an attack.
  4. Drug cortisol levels do not relate to asthma.

  **TEST-TAKING HINTS: If the test taker is unsure about the correct response, it is a helpful to choose the option that directly relates to the topic. Asthma is a pulmonary problem and only one (1) distracter has the word "pulmonary" in it.**

43. 1. A forced vital capacity of 1000 mL is considered normal for most females.
  2. The client should be encouraged to pace the activities of daily living; this is expected for a client diagnosed with asthma.
  3. Confusion could be a sign of decreased oxygen to the brain and requires the RN's expertise.
  4. The client's mother requires teaching, which is the registered nurse's responsibility.
  5. A pulse oximetry level of 95% is normal.

  **TEST-TAKING HINTS: The licensed practical nurse should be assigned clients who are stable and do not require teaching.**

44. 1. The charge nurse is responsible for all clients. At times it is necessary to see clients with a psychosocial need before other clients who have situations that are expected and are not life threatening.
  2. Two (2) + edema of the lower extremities is expected in a client diagnosed with heart failure.
  3. A blood glucose reading of 189 mg/dL is not within normal range, but it is not in a range that indicates the client is catabolizing the fats and proteins in the body. No ketones will be produced at this blood glucose level, so the ketoacidosis has resolved itself.
  4. Most clients diagnosed with COPD are receiving oxygen at a low level.

  **TEST-TAKING HINT: All of the answer options except one (1) have expected data listed.**

45. 1. Rescue inhalers are used to treat attacks, not prevent them.

  2. Warmup exercises decrease the risk of developing an asthma attack.
  3. Using a bronchodilator immediately prior to exercising will reduce bronchospasms.
  4. Monosodium glutamate, a food preservative, has been shown to initiate asthma attacks.

  **TEST-TAKING HINTS: Answer option "1" has two words that are opposed—"rescue" and "wait"—which might lead the test taker to eliminate this option. Remember basic concepts, which are contradicted in option "2." There are a few disease processes that encourage intake of sodium, but asthma is not one of them, which would cause "4" to be eliminated.**

46. 1. This applies to systemically administered steroids, not to inhaled steroids.
  2. The steroids must pass through the oral cavity before reaching the lungs. Allowing the medication to stay within the oral cavity will suppress the normal flora found there, and the client could develop a yeast infection of the mouth, oral candidiasis.
  3. Holding the medication in the mouth increases the risk of an oral yeast infection, and the medication is inhaled, not swallowed.
  4. Inhaled steroids are not used first, the beta andrenergic inhalers are used for acute attack.

  **TEST-TAKING HINTS: Answer option "3" suggests that an inhaled medication is swallowed; the two (2) terms do not match.**

47. 1. Children with asthma can eat a regular diet if the child is not allergic to the components of the diet.
  2. Because asthma can be a reaction to an allergen, it is important to determine which substances may trigger an attack.
  3. The stem did not indicate the child is developmentally delayed.
  4. The child does not require a home health nurse only on the basis of asthma; the school nurse or any child-care provider should be informed of the child's diagnosis, and the parents must know that the individual caring for the child is prepared to intervene during an attack.

  **TEST-TAKING HINTS: The test taker must be aware of the disease process, determine causes, and then make a decision based on interventions required.**

48. 1. The client must be able to recognize a life-threatening situation and initiate the correct procedure.
  2. Bedding is washed in hot water to kill dust mites.
  3. Many Chinese dishes are prepared with mono-

sodium glutamate, an ingredient that can initiate an asthma attack.

4. Nonsteroidal anti-inflammatory medications, aspirin, and beta blockers have been known to initiate asthma attacks.

**TEST-TAKING HINTS: Dietary questions or answer options should be analyzed for the content. The test taker should decide, "What about Chinese foods could be a problem for a client diagnosed with asthma?" or "What might be good for the client about this diet?"**

## Lung Cancer

49. 1. Working with asbestos is significant for mesothelioma of the lung, a cancer with a very poor prognosis, but not for small cell carcinoma.
   2. Family history is not the significant risk factor for small cell carcinoma. Smoking is the number-one risk factor.
   3. Tattoos may be implicated in the development of blood-borne pathogen disease (if sterile needles were not used), but they do not have any association with cancer.
   4. Smoking is the number-one risk factor for developing cancer of the lung. More than 85% of lung cancers are attributable to inhalation of chemicals. There are more than 400 chemicals in each puff of cigarette smoke, 17 of which are known to cause cancer.

**TEST-TAKING HINT: If the test taker did not know this information, option "3" has no anatomical connection to the lungs and could be eliminated. This information has been widely disseminated in the media for more than 40 years since the Surgeon General's office first warned about the dangers of smoking in the early 1960s.**

50. 1. Respiratory distress is a common finding in clients diagnosed with lung cancer. As the tumor grows and takes up more space or blocks air movement, the client may need to be taught positioning for lung expansion. The administration of oxygen will help the client to use the lung capacity that is available to get oxygen to the tissues.
   2. Clients with lung cancer frequently become fatigued trying to eat. Providing six (6) small meals spaces the amount of food the client eats throughout the day.
   3. Cancer is not communicable, so the client does not need to be in isolation.
   4. Clients with cancer of the lung are at risk

for developing an infection from lowered resistance as a result of treatments or from the tumor blocking secretions in the lung. Therefore, monitoring for the presence of fever, a possible indication of infection, is important.

5. Assessment of the lungs should be completed on a routine and PRN basis.

**TEST-TAKING HINT: This alternative type question is an all-or-nothing situation. The RN-NCLEX examination requires the test taker to get each answer option correct to receive credit for the question. Each option has the potential to be right or wrong.**

51. 1. Lung cancer is the number-one cause of cancer deaths in the United States.
   2. **Lung cancers are responsible for almost twice as many deaths among males as any other cancer and more deaths than breast cancer in females.**
   3. Lung cancers are the most deadly cancers among the United States population.
   4. Lung cancer deaths have remained relatively stable among the male population but have continued to steadily increase among females.

**TEST-TAKING HINT: The nurse must be able to interpret data to the public. The nurse will be asked about incidence of diseases and severity.**

52. 1. This is expected from this client and does not warrant immediate attention.
   2. This is called a three (3)-point stance. It is a position many clients with lung disease will assume because it assists in the expansion of the lung.
   3. Biologic response modifiers that stimulate the bone marrow can increase the client's blood pressure to dangerous levels. This BP is very high and warrants immediate attention.
   4. This client can be seen after taking care of the client in "3." The nurse should intervene, but it is not a life-threatening situation.

**TEST-TAKING HINT: Even if the test taker did not know the side effect of Procrit, a BP of 198/102 warrants immediate attention.**

53. 1. This situation indicates a terminal process, and the client should make decisions for the end of life.
   2. Radiation therapy is used for tumors in the brain. Chemotherapy as a whole will not cross the blood–brain barrier.
   3. There is no indication the client cannot drive at this point. Clients may develop seizures from the tumors at some point.

Respiratory

4. The client should make decisions for himself or herself as long as possible. However, the client should discuss personal wishes with the person named in an advance directive to make decisions.

**TEST-TAKING HINT:** The ethical principle of autonomy could help the test taker to discard "4" as an answer.

54. 1. If the investigational regimen proves to be effective, then this statement is true. However, many investigational treatments have not proved to be efficacious.
2. Investigational treatments are just that—treatments being investigated to see if they are effective in the care of clients diagnosed with cancer. There is no guarantee the treatments will help the client.
3. Clients receive medical care and associated treatments and laboratory tests at no cost, but they are not paid. This is against the ethical principles.
4. Frequently clients who have failed standard treatments and have no other hope of a treatment are the clients involved in investigational protocols, but the protocols can be used for any client who volunteers for investigational treatment.

**TEST-TAKING HINT:** The test taker should think about the word "investigational" and understand its meaning. Investigational means looking into something. This should lead the test taker to choose "2."

55. 1. A centralized system of organization means decisions are made at the top and given to the staff underneath to accept and implement.
2. A decentralized decision-making pattern means that there is a fairly flat accountability chart. The unit manager has more autonomy in managing the unit, but that does not mean the staff has input into decisions.
3. Shared governance is a system where the staff is empowered to make decisions such as scheduling and hiring of certain staff. Staff members are encouraged to participate in developing policies and procedures to reach set goals.
4. A pyramid decision-making tree is an example of a centralized system.

**TEST-TAKING HINT:** Answer options "1" and "4" basically say the same thing and could be eliminated for this reason.

56. 1. Research indicates that smoking will still interfere with the client's response to treatment.

2. It is expected for the client to follow up with a specialist regarding subsequent treatment.
3. Clients diagnosed with cancer and undergoing treatment are at risk for developing infections.
4. Lung cancers produce fatigue as a result of physiologic drains on the body in the areas of lack of adequate oxygen to the tissues, the tumor burden on the body, and the toll taken by the effects of the treatments. Cancer-related fatigue syndrome is a very real occurrence.

**TEST-TAKING HINT:** Two (2) options—"2" and "3"—are instructions given to all clients regardless of disease process.

57. 1. This is an individual cultural/familial situation and should be encouraged unless it interferes with the medical treatment plan. The nurse should be nonjudgmental when clients discuss their cultural practices if the nurse expects the clients to be honest about health practices.
2. An appendectomy in the past should be documented, but no further information is required.
3. Many clients take a multi-vitamin.
4. Coughing up blood could indicate a lung cancer and should be investigated.

**TEST-TAKING HINT:** The test taker should read all distracters carefully. "Further investigation" means something abnormal is occurring. Coughing up blood is always abnormal.

58. 1. This is an adequate output. After a major surgery, clients will frequently have an intake greater than the output because of the fluid shift occurring as a result of trauma to the body.
2. This is about a pint of blood loss and could indicate the client is hemorrhaging.
3. The nurse should intervene and medicate the client, but pain, although a client comfort issue, is not life threatening.
4. The client will have a chest tube to assist in reinflation of the lung, and absent lung sounds are expected at this point in the client's recovery.

**TEST-TAKING HINT:** Blood is always a priority.

59. 1. Bronchoscopies are not performed to confirm another test; they are performed to confirm diagnoses, such as cancer, pneumocystis pneumonia, tuberculosis, fungal infections, and other lung diseases.
2. The client's throat will be numbed with a local anesthetic to prevent gagging during the procedure. The client will not be able to eat or drink until this medication has worn off.
3. The HCP can take biopsies and wash of the lung tissue for pathological diagnosis during the procedure.

4. Most HCPs use an anesthetic procedure called twilight sleep to perform endoscopies, but there is no guarantee the client will not experience some discomfort.

**TEST-TAKING HINT: The test taker must read each stem and answer option carefully. When in medicine does one (1) test confirm another? Tests are done to confirm diagnoses. Option "4" has a false promise.**

60. 1. The nurse might enter into a therapeutic conversation, but client safety is the priority.
    2. The nurse must first assess the seriousness of the client's statement and whether he or she has a plan to carry out suicide. Depending on the client's responses, the nurse will notify the HCP.
    3. The client can be referred for assistance in dealing with the disease and its ramifications, but this is not the priority.
    4. The priority action any time a client makes a statement regarding taking his or her own life is to determine if the client has thought it through enough to have a plan. A plan indicates an emergency situation.

**TEST-TAKING HINT: In a question that asks for a first response, all answer options may be actions the nurse would take. Ranking the options in order of action—"4," "1," "2," "3"—may help the test taker to make a decision. Applying Maslow's Hierarchy of Needs, safety comes first.**

## Cancer of the Larynx

61. 1. Gargling with salt water is good for sore throats, but it does not diagnose cancer of the larynx.
    2. Clients thought to have a vocal cord problem are encouraged to practice voice rest. Vocal cord exercises would not assist in the diagnosis of cancer.
    3. A laryngoscopy will be done to allow for visualization of the vocal cords and to obtain a biopsy for pathological diagnosis.
    4. There is no monthly self-examination of the larynx. To visualize the vocal cords the HCP must numb the throat and pass a fiberoptic instrument through the throat and into the trachea.

**TEST-TAKING HINT: The test taker must understand that if the question states the client is admitted to "rule out" a disease, then diagnostic tests and procedures will be done to determine if, in fact, the client has the diagnosis that the HCP suspects.**

62. 1. The teeth will be in the area of radiation and the roots of teeth are highly sensitive to radiation, which results in root abscesses. The teeth are removed and the client is fitted for dentures prior to radiation.
    2. An anti-emetic on a routine scheduled basis is prophylactic for nausea, and the schedule is 30 minutes before a meal. Radiation to the throat does not encompass nausea-producing areas.
    3. Sunscreen is used to prevent the penetration of ultraviolet (UV) rays from entering the dermis. Radiation is gamma rays.
    4. Placement of a PEG tube is a treatment for a client who has developed severe esophagitis from irradiation of the esophagus, but the tube does not prevent the esophagitis from occurring.

**TEST-TAKING HINT: The test taker could eliminate "4" as a form of nutritional treatment, not prophylaxis. The test taker must recognize which anatomical structures would lay within the radiation beam. The teeth of the lower jaw definitely are within the port, and the upper teeth possibly would be in range.**

63. 1. The client is three (3) days post a partial removal of the larynx and should be eating by this time.
    2. The client should be eating normal foods by this time. The consistency should be soft to allow for less chewing of the food and easier swallowing because a portion of the throat musculature has been removed. The client should be taught to turn the head toward the affected side when swallowing to help prevent aspiration.
    3. The client should be capable of enteral nutrition at this time.
    4. The client should have progressed to a diet with a more normal consistency and amount.

**TEST-TAKING HINT: The keys to this question are "three (3) days" and "partial." Clients are progressed rapidly after surgery to as normal a life as possible.**

64. 1. This is a good preoperative intervention, but it is not priority.
    2. The client should be taught about how the pain medication will be given, but this is not the highest priority.
    3. The client should be told about an anti-embolism hose, but it is not necessary to demonstrate the hose because the nurse will apply and remove the hose initially.
    4. The client is having the vocal cords removed and will be unable to speak. Communication is a high priority for this

client. If the client is able to read and write, a Magic Slate or pad of paper should be provided. If the client is illiterate, the nurse and the client should develop a method of communication using pictures.

**TEST-TAKING HINT: If the question asks for the test taker to choose the highest priority, the test taker could ask, "If this is not done, what will be the outcome for the client?" In "1" the client will not be prepared for the intensive care environment, but in "4" the client will be in strange place and may not be able to communicate with health-care providers.**

65. 1. CanSurmount is a program of cancer survivors who volunteer to talk to clients about having cancer or what the treatments are like. This group is based on the success of Reach to Recovery for breast cancer, but it is not specific to a particular cancer.
  2. Dialogue is a cancer support group that brings together clients diagnosed with cancer to discuss the feelings that are associated with having cancer.
  3. **The Lost Chord Club is an American Cancer Society–sponsored group of survivors of larynx cancer. These clients are able to discuss the feelings and needs of clients that have had laryngectomies because they have all had this particular surgery.**
  4. SmokEnders is a group of clients working together to stop smoking. It is a group that anyone that smokes could be referred to.

**TEST-TAKING HINT: The larynx is commonly referred to as the "vocal chords." If the test taker were not aware of the various support groups, option "3" has "lost" and "chords" in it and would be the best choice.**

66. 1. **The most serious complication resulting from a radical neck dissection is rupture of the carotid artery. A continuous bright-red drainage indicates bleeding, and this client should be assessed immediately.**
  2. Pain is a priority but not over hemorrhaging.
  3. Clients with cancer of the lung have fatigue and are short of breath; these are expected findings.
  4. Clients with chronic lung problems are taught pursed-lip breathing to assist in expelling air. This type of breathing often produces a whistling sound.

**TEST-TAKING HINT: If the test taker is not sure of the answer and airway compromise is not one of the answer options, then an option dealing with bleeding would be a good choice.**

67. 1. Chest tubes are part of the nursing education curriculum. The new graduate should

be capable of caring for this client or at least knowing when to get assistance.
  2. This client is in respiratory compromise and an experienced nurse should care for the client.
  3. A client with multiple fistulas in the neck area is at high risk for airway compromise and should be assigned to a more experienced nurse.
  4. This client is at risk for developing edema of the neck area and should be cared for by a more experienced nurse.

**TEST-TAKING HINT: The question is asking for the least compromised client. The client in option "1" already has chest tubes in place and is presumably stable.**

68. 1. Wound infection is a concern, but in the list of the answer options it is not the highest priority. A wound infection can be treated, but a client who is not breathing is in a life-threatening situation and the problem must be addressed immediately.
  2. Hemorrhage is normally a priority, but bleeding is not priority over not breathing.
  3. **Respiratory distress is the highest priority. There is a chance to stop the bleeding or treat an infection, but a client who is not breathing dies very quickly.**
  4. Knowledge deficit is the lowest on this priority list. It is a psychosocial problem and these problems rank lower in priority than physiological ones.

**TEST-TAKING HINT: In cardiopulmonary resuscitation the steps are airway, breathing, and then circulation. This concurs with Maslow's Hierarchy of Needs, which places oxygenation at the top of the hierarchy.**

69. 1. This request indicates the client is accepting the situation and trying to deal with it.
  2. **Placing a towel over the mirror indicates the client is having difficulty looking at his reflection, a body-image problem.**
  3. In attempting to shave himself the client is participating in self-care activities and also must look at his neck in the mirror, both good steps toward adjustment.
  4. Neck and shoulder exercises are done to strengthen the remaining musculature, but they have nothing to do with body image.

**TEST-TAKING HINT: The test taker must try to match the problem with the answer choices. This would eliminate "1" and "4." Shaving himself is a positive action, and the question asks for an action that indicates a disturbance in body image.**

70. 1. This is an example of nonmalfeasance where the nurse "does no harm." In

attempting to discuss the client's refusal, the nurse is not trying to influence the client; the nurse is merely attempting to listen therapeutically.

2. This is an example of paternalism, telling the client what he should do, and it is also coercion, an unethical action.

3. This is an example of beneficence, "to do good"; it is a positive action and a step up from nonmalfeasance.

4. This is an example of beneficence.

**TEST-TAKING HINT: If the test taker was not aware of the terms of ethical principles, then dissecting the word "nonmalfeasance" into its portions might help. "Non" means "nothing" or "none," and "mal" means "bad," so "no bad action" could be inferred. This would eliminate "2."**

71. 1. The cancer may have grown, but this would not be indicated by the type of pain described.
2. Painful swallowing is caused by esophageal irritation.
3. Most cancers are not painful unless obstructing an organ or pressing on a nerve. This is not what is being described.
4. The esophagus is extremely radiosensitive, and esophageal ulcerations are common. The pain can become so severe that the client cannot swallow saliva. This is a situation in which the client will be admitted to the hospital for IV narcotic pain medication and possibly total parenteral nutrition.

**TEST-TAKING HINT: The test taker must remember not to jump to conclusions and to remember what a word is actually saying. Swallowing is an action involving the esophagus so the best choice would be either "2" or "4," which have the word "esophagus" in them.**

72. 1. This surgery removed the vocal cords. The client will not be able to speak again unless the client learns esophageal speech, uses an electric larynx, or a transesophageal puncture that has been surgically created.
2. The client breathes through a stoma in the neck. Care should be taken not to allow water to enter the stoma.
3. The stoma should be cleaned, but petroleum-based products should not be allowed near the stoma. Petroleum-based products are contraindicated because they are not water-soluble and could contribute to an occlusion. They should also not be used around oxygen because they are flammable.
4. The client has lost the use of the nasal passages to humidify the inhaled air, and

artificial humidification is useful until the client's body adapts to the change.
5. There is special equipment available for clients who cannot hear or speak.

**TEST-TAKING HINT: Answer option "1" can be eliminated as a false promise and would undermine the nurse–client relationship.**

## Pulmonary Embolus

73. 880 units. If there are 20,000 units of heparin in 500 mL of D5W, then there are 40 units in each mL.

20,000 ÷ 500 = 40 units
If 22 mL are infused per hour, then 880 units of heparin are infused each hour.
40 × 22 = 880

**TEST-TAKING HINT: The test taker must know how to calculate heparin drips from two aspects: the question may give the mL/hr and the test taker has to determine units/hr or the question may give units/hr and the test taker has to determine mL/hr. Remember to learn how to use the drop-down calculator on the computer. During RN-NCLEX the test taker can request an erase slate.**

74. 1. The plasma D-dimer test is highly specific for the presence of a thrombus; an elevated D-dimer indicates a thrombus formation and lysis.
2. ABGs evaluate oxygenation level, but they do not diagnose a pulmonary embolism.
3. A CXR shows pulmonary infiltration and pleural effusions, but it does not diagnose a PE.
4. MRI is a noninvasive test that detects a deep vein thrombosis, but it does not diagnose a pulmonary embolus.

**TEST-TAKING HINT: The keys to answering this question are the words "confirms diagnosis." The test taker should eliminate "2" and "3" based on the fact that these are diagnostic tests used for many disease processes and conditions.**

75. 1. This is a sign of a deep vein thrombosis, which is a precursor to a PE, but it is not a sign of a pulmonary embolism.
2. The most common signs of a PE are sudden onset of chest pain when taking a deep breath and shortness of breath.
3. These are signs of a myocardial infarction.
4. These could be signs of pneumonia or other pulmonary complications, but not specifically a PE.

**TEST-TAKING HINT: The key to selecting "2" as the correct answer is sudden onset. The test**

Respiratory

taker would need to note "left-sided" in "3" to eliminate this as a possible correct answer, and "4" is nonspecific for a PE.

76. 1. These ABGs are within normal limits and would not warrant immediate intervention.
    2. Occasional premature ventricular contractions are not unusual for any client and would not warrant immediate intervention.
    3. The normal pulse oximeter reading is 93%–100%. A reading of 90% indicates the client has an arterial oxygen level of around 60.
    4. A urinary output of 800 mL over 12 hours indicates an output of greater than 30 mL/hour, and this would not warrant immediate intervention by the nurse.

    **TEST-TAKING HINT:** This question is asking the test taker to select assessment data that are abnormal, unexpected, or life threatening in relationship to the client's disease process. A pulse oximeter reading of less than 93% indicates severe hypoxia and requires immediate intervention.

77. 1. The intravenous anticoagulant heparin will be administered immediately after diagnosis of a PE, not oral anticoagulants.
    2. The client's respiratory system will be assessed, not the gastrointestinal system.
    3. A thoracentesis is used to aspirate fluid from the pleural space; it is not a treatment for a PE.
    4. Bed rest reduces metabolic demands and tissue needs for oxygen.

    **TEST-TAKING HINT:** The test taker must be aware of adjectives such as "oral" in option "1," which make this option incorrect. The test taker should apply the body system of the disease process to eliminate "2" as a correct answer.

78. 1. The client would not be experiencing abnormal bleeding with this INR.
    2. This is the antidote for an overdose of anticoagulant and the INR does not indicate this.
    3. A therapeutic INR is 2–3; therefore, the nurse should administer the medication.
    4. There is no need to increase the dose; this result is within the therapeutic range.

    **TEST-TAKING HINT:** The test taker must know normal laboratory values; this is the only way the test taker will be able to answer this question. The test taker should make a list of laboratory values that must be memorized for successful test taking.

79. 1. Arterial blood gases would be included in the client problem "impaired gas exchange."

    2. These assessment data monitor tissue perfusion, which evaluates for decreased cardiac output.
    3. This would be appropriate for the client problem "high risk for bleeding."
    4. The client should not be put in a position with the head lower than the legs because this would increase difficulty breathing.

    **TEST-TAKING HINT:** The test taker must think about which answer option addresses the problem of not getting enough blood out of the heart. Decreased blood to the extremities results in cyanosis and cold extremities.

80. 1. Heparin is administered during thrombolytic therapy, and the antidote is protamine sulfate and should be available to reverse the effects of the anticoagulant.
    2. Firm pressure reduces the risk for bleeding into the tissues.
    3. Obvious (overt) as well as hidden (covert) signs of bleeding should be assessed for.
    4. Invasive procedures increase the risk of tissue trauma and bleeding.
    5. Stool softeners help prevent constipation and straining, which may precipitate bleeding from hemorrhoids.

    **TEST-TAKING HINT:** Thrombolytic therapy is ordered to help dissolve the clot that resulted in the PE. Therefore, all nursing interventions should address bleeding tendencies. The test taker must select all interventions that are applicable in these alternative questions.

81. 1. The client should use a soft-bristle toothbrush to reduce the risk of bleeding.
    2. This is appropriate for a client with a mechanical valve replacement, not a client receiving anticoagulant therapy.
    3. Aspirin, enteric-coated or not, is an antiplatelet, which may increase bleeding tendencies and should be avoided.
    4. The client should wear a medic alert band at all times so that if any accident or situation occurs, the health-care providers will know the client is receiving anticoagulant therapy.

    **TEST-TAKING HINT:** This is a higher-level question in which the test taker must know that a client with a pulmonary embolus would be prescribed anticoagulant therapy on discharge from the hospital. If the test taker had no idea of the answer, however, the option stating "wear a medic alert band" would be a good choice because many disease processes require the client to take long-term medication and a health-care provider should be aware of this.

82. 1. Increasing fluids will help increase fluid volume, which will, in turn, help prevent the development of deep vein thrombosis, the most common cause of PE.
    2. Pulmonary emboli are not caused by atherosclerosis; therefore, this is not an appropriate discharge instruction for a client with pulmonary embolism.
    3. Infection does not cause a PE; therefore, this is not an appropriate teaching instruction.
    4. Pneumonia and flu do not cause pulmonary embolism.

    **TEST-TAKING HINT: The test taker must know that deep vein thrombosis is the most common cause of pulmonary embolus and preventing dehydration is an important intervention. The test taker can attempt to eliminate answers by trying to figure out which disease process is appropriate for the intervention.**

83. 1. An INR of 2–3 is therapeutic; therefore, the nurse would administer this medication.
    2. This is an elevated blood glucose level; therefore, the nurse should administer the insulin.
    3. A normal PTT is 39 seconds; therefore, 58–78 is 1.5 to 2 times the normal value and is within the therapeutic range. A PTT of 98 means the client is not clotting and the medication should be held.
    4. This is a normal blood pressure and the nurse should administer the medication.

    **TEST-TAKING HINT: This question is asking the test taker to select a distracter that has assessment data that are unsafe for administering the medication. The test taker must know normal laboratory values to administer medication safely.**

84. 1. The client needs oxygen, but the nurse can do something that will help the client before applying oxygen.
    2. Placing the client in this position facilitates maximal lung expansion and reduces venous return to the right side of the heart, thus lowering pressures in the pulmonary vascular system.
    3. This is needed, but it is not the first intervention.
    4. Assessing the client is indicated, but it is not the first intervention in this situation.

    **TEST-TAKING HINT: The test taker must select the option that will directly help the client breathe easier. Therefore, assessment is not the first intervention and option "4" can be eliminated as the correct answer. Oxygenation is important but positioning the client is the easiest and first intervention. The test taker**

should not immediately jump to conclusions. Always read the stem and think about what will help the client.

## Chest Trauma

85. 1. The client with pneumothorax would have absent breath sounds and tachypnea.
    2. Unequal lung expansion and dyspnea would indicate a pneumothorax.
    3. Consolidation occurs when there is no air moving through the alveoli as in pneumonia; frothy sputum occurs with congestive heart failure.
    4. Barrel chest and polycythemia are signs of chronic obstructive pulmonary disease.

    **TEST-TAKING HINT: The test taker can use "chest trauma" or "pneumothorax" to help select the correct answer. Both of these words should cause the test taker to select "2" because unequal chest expansion would result from trauma.**

86. 1. A STAT chest x-ray would not be needed to determine why there is no fluctuation in the water-seal compartment.
    2. Increasing the amount of wall suction does not address why there is no fluctuation in the water-seal compartment.
    3. The key to the answer is "2 hours." The air from the pleural space is not able to get to the water-seal compartment, and the nurse should try to determine why. Usually the client is lying on the tube, it is kinked, or there is a dependent loop.
    4. The stem does not state that the client is in respiratory distress, and a pulse oximeter reading detects hypoxemia but does not address any fluctuation in the water-seal compartment.

    **TEST-TAKING HINT: The test taker should apply the nursing process to answer the question correctly. The first step in the nursing process is assessment and "check" (option "3") is a word that can be used synonymously for assess. Monitoring (option "4") is also assessing, but the test taker should not check a diagnostic test result before caring for the client.**

87. 1. The client must take deep breaths to help push the air out of the pleural space into the water-seal drainage, and deep breaths will help prevent the client from developing pneumonia or atelectasis.
    2. The client must take deep breaths; shallow breaths could lead to complications.
    3. Deep breaths must be taken to prevent complications.

4. This is a cruel intervention; the nurse can medicate the client and then encourage deep breathing.

**TEST-TAKING HINT: If the test taker reads options "2" and "3" and notices that both reflect the same idea—namely, that deep breaths are not necessary—then both can either be eliminated as incorrect answers or kept as possible correct answers. Option "4" should be eliminated based on being a very rude and threatening comment.**

88. 1. Keeping the drainage system lower than the chest promotes drainage and prevents reflux.
    2. The chest tube system can function as a result of gravity and does not have to be attached to suction. Keeping it attached to suction could cause the client to trip and fall. Therefore, this is a safety issue and the nurse should intervene and explain this to the nursing assistant.
    3. Ambulation facilitates lung ventilation and expansion; drainage systems are portable to allow ambulation while chest tubes are in place.
    4. The client should ambulate, but getting up and using the bedside commode is better than staying in the bed, so no action would be needed.

**TEST-TAKING HINT: "Warrants immediate intervention" means the test taker must identify the situation in which the nurse should intervene and correct the action, demonstrate a skill, or somehow intervene with the unlicensed assistant's behavior.**

89. 1. The health-care provider will have to be notified, but this is not the first intervention. Air must be prevented from entering the pleural space from the outside atmosphere.
    2. The client should breathe regularly or take deep breaths until the tubes are reinserted.
    3. The nurse must take action and prevent air from entering the pleural space.
    4. Taping on three sides prevents the development of a tension pneumothorax by inhibiting air from entering the wound during inhalation but allowing it to escape during exhalation.

**TEST-TAKING HINT: The word "first intervention" in the stem of the question indicates to the test taker that possibly more than one (1) intervention could be indicated in the situation but only one (1) is implemented first. Remember, do not select assessment first without reading the question. If the client is in any type of crisis, then the nurse should first do something to help the client's situation.**

90. 1. This is incorrect information. It is the description of a spontaneous pneumothorax.
    2. This is the description of an open pneumothorax.
    3. **This describes a tension pneumothorax. It is a medical emergency requiring immediate intervention to preserve life.**
    4. This is called an iatrogenic pneumothorax, which also may be caused by thoracentesis or lung biopsy. A tension pneumothorax could occur from this procedure, but it does not describe a tension pneumothorax.

**TEST-TAKING HINT: The test taker must always be clear about what the question is asking before answering the question. If the test taker can eliminate options "1" and "2" and can't decide between "3" and "4," the test taker must go back to the stem and clarify what the question is asking.**

91. 1. **Checking to see if someone has increased the suction rate is the simplest action for the nurse to implement; if it is not on high, then the nurse must check to see if the problem is with the client or the system.**
    2. No fluctuation (tidaling) would cause the nurse to assess the tubing for a blood clot.
    3. The tube is milked to help dislodge a blood clot that may be blocking the chest tube causing no fluctuation (tidaling) in the water-seal compartment. The chest tube is never stripped, which creates a negative air pressure and would suck lung tissue into the chest tube.
    4. Encouraging the client to cough forcefully will help dislodge a blood clot that may be blocking the chest tube, causing no fluctuation (tidaling) in the water-seal compartment.

**TEST-TAKING HINT: The test taker should always think about assessing the client if there is a problem and the client is not in immediate danger. This would cause the test taker to eliminate options "3" and "4." If the test taker thinks about bubbling, he or she should know it has to do with suctioning.**

92. 1. This is an expected finding in the suction compartment of the drainage system that indicates adequate suctioning is being applied.
    2. **At three (3) days post-insertion, no fluctuation (tidaling) indicates the lung has reexpanded, which indicates the treatment has been effective.**
    3. Blood in the drainage bottle is expected for a hemothorax but does not indicate the chest tubes have reexpanded the lung.

4. Taking a deep breath without pain is good, but it does not mean the lungs have reexpanded.

**TEST-TAKING HINT: The test taker must be knowledgeable about chest tubes to be able to answer this question. The test taker must know the normal time frame and what is expected for each compartment of the chest tube drainage system.**

93. 1. The client should be in a high-Fowler's position to facilitate lung expansion.
2. The system must be patent and intact to function properly.
3. The client can have bathroom privileges, and ambulation facilitates lung ventilation and expansion.
4. Looping the tubing prevents direct pressure on the chest tube itself and keeps tubing off the floor, addressing both a safety and an infection control issue.
5. Subcutaneous emphysema is air under the skin, which is a common occurrence at the chest tube insertion site.

**TEST-TAKING HINT: The test taker should be careful with adjectives. In option "1" the word "low" makes it incorrect; in option "3," the word "strict" makes this option incorrect.**

94. 1. This pulse oximeter reading indicates the client is hypoxic and therefore is not stable and should be assigned to an RN.
2. This H&H are very low; therefore the client is not stable and should be assigned to an RN.
3. Jugular vein distention and hypotension are signs of a tension pneumothorax, which is a medical emergency, and the client should be assigned to an RN.
4. A client that is two (2) hours post-bronchoscopy procedure could safely be assigned to an LPN.

**TEST-TAKING HINT: The test taker must understand that the LPN should be assigned the least critical client or the client that is stable and not exhibiting any complications secondary to the admitting disease or condition.**

95. 1. The nurse should gather a thoracotomy tray and the chest tube drainage system and take it to the client's bedside, but it is not the first intervention.
2. The insertion of a chest tube is an invasive procedure and so requires informed consent. Without a consent form, this procedure cannot be done on an alert and oriented client.
3. This is a correct position to place the client for

a chest tube insertion, but it is not the first intervention.
4. The physician will discuss the procedure with the client, then informed consent must be obtained, and then the nurse can do further teaching.

**TEST-TAKING HINT: The test taker must know that invasive procedures require informed consent and legally it must be obtained first before anyone can touch the client.**

96. 1. Assessment of the lung sounds could indicate that the client's lung has reexpanded because it has been three (3) days since the chest tube has been inserted.
2. This should be done to ensure that the lung has reexpanded, but it is not the first intervention.
3. The HCP will need to be notified so that the chest tube can be removed, but it is not the first intervention.
4. This situation needs to be documented, but it is not the first intervention.

**TEST-TAKING HINT: When the stem asks the test taker to identify the first intervention, all four (4) answer options could be interventions that are appropriate for the situation, but only one (1) is the first intervention. Remember to apply the nursing process: the first step is assessment.**

## Acute Respiratory Distress Syndrome (ARDS)

97. 1. The opposite side rail should be elevated so the client will not fall out of the bed. Safety is priority, so the nurse should demonstrate the proper way to bathe a client in the bed.
2. The bed should be at a comfortable height for the NA to bathe the client, not in the lowest position.
3. The NA can bathe a client without assistance if the client's safety can be ensured.
4. The NA is not ensuring the client's safety because the opposite side rail is not elevated to prevent the client from falling out of the bed.

**TEST-TAKING HINT: Although the test taker should not always be concerned with the disease process of the client, many times the answer may be selected based on basic nursing skills that do not require an understanding of the client's disease process.**

98. 1. Maintaining ventilator settings and checking to ensure they are specifically set as prescribed is appropriate, but it is not the first intervention.

2. Making sure alarms are functioning properly is appropriate, but checking a machine is not priority.

3. Assessment is the first part of the nursing process and is the first intervention the nurse should implement when caring for a client on a ventilator.

4. Monitoring lab results is an appropriate intervention for the client on a ventilator, but monitoring laboratory data is not the priority intervention.

**TEST-TAKING HINT:** The test taker should apply the nursing process, which identifies assessment as the first step. Therefore, if the test taker is not sure of the answer, the best educated selection is to select an option that addresses assessment data.

99. 1. The classic sign of ARDS is decreased arterial oxygen level ($PaO_2$) while administering high levels of oxygen; the oxygen is unable to cross the alveolar membrane.

2. These are early signs of ARDS, but they could also indicate pneumonia, atelectasis, and other pulmonary complications and so they do not confirm the diagnosis of ARDS.

3. Clear breath sounds and the oxygen saturation indicate the client is not experiencing any respiratory difficulty or compromise.

4. These are signs of congestive heart failure; ARDS is noncardiogenic (without signs of cardiac involvement) pulmonary edema.

**TEST-TAKING HINT:** If the test taker does not know the signs/symptoms of ARDS, the test taker should eliminate distracter "2" because this could be any respiratory disorder and would not confirm any specific disorder. Option "3" are normal data so that would not support the diagnosis of a specific respiratory disorder. JVD (option "4") usually occurs with heart problems and this should cause the test taker to eliminate it.

100. 1. This is an incorrect statement. ARDS has multiple etiologies, such has hemorrhagic shock, septic shock, drug overdose, burns, and near drowning; but many people with near drowning do not develop ARDS.

2. The layperson may not know what the term "alveoli" means and the near drowning is the initial insult that caused the ARDS.

3. This is a very basic explanation of ARDS and explains why the client is having trouble breathing.

4. ARDS does not occur more in clients who smoke; the etiology is unknown, but an initial insult occurs 24 to 48 hours before the development of ARDS.

**TEST-TAKING HINT:** The test taker should select the distracter that presents facts and is easiest for the client to understand. The test taker should not select the distracter that has medical jargon that the client may not understand. The test taker as a rule can eliminate any distracter that has medical jargon in the answer.

101. 1. A urine output of 30 mL/hr indicates the kidneys are functioning properly.

2. This indicates that the client is being adequately oxygenated.

3. Asymmetrical chest expansion indicates the client has had a pneumothorax, which is a complication of mechanical ventilation.

4. An increased heart rate does not indicate a complication; this could result from numerous reasons that are not specifically because of the ventilator.

**TEST-TAKING HINT:** The test taker should be looking for an answer option that describes something that is abnormal, unexpected, or life threatening because of the word "complication" in the stem. Understanding medical suffixes and prefixes could help the test taker select the correct answer. Any time there is an "a" before the word, it means "without," as in "asymmetrical" means "without symmetry."

102. 1. These arterial blood gases are within normal limits and therefore the nurse should not take any action except to continue to monitor the client.

2. The nurse would recommend deep breaths and coughing if the client's ABGs revealed respiratory acidosis.

3. Sodium bicarbonate is administered when the client is in metabolic acidosis.

4. This is a normal ABG and therefore the respiratory therapist does not need to be notified.

**TEST-TAKING HINT:** This question requires the test taker to know what normal arterial blood gas results are pH 7.35–7.45, $PaO_2$ 80–100, $PaCO_2$ 35–45, $HCO_3$ 22–26. The test taker must know how to evaluate the results.

103. 1. Alternating the ET tube will help prevent a pressure ulcer on the client's tongue and mouth.

2. A CXR is done immediately after insertion of the ET tube, but not daily.

3. The cuff should be inflated but to no more than 25 cm $H_2O$ to ensure there is no air leakage, and it must be checked every 4–8 hours, not daily.

4. The ET tube should be secure to ensure that it does not enter the right main bronchus. The ET tube should be one (1) inch above the bifurcation of the bronchi.

**TEST-TAKING HINT: The test taker must be knowledgeable about ventilator care. Radiation is dangerous; therefore a daily CXR (option "2") may be eliminated as the correct answer.**

104. 1. Unless the initial insult is an infection, an aminoglycoside antibiotic would not be a medication the nurse would anticipate being ordered.
2. Surfactant therapy may be prescribed to reduce the surface tension in the alveoli. The surfactant helps maintain open alveoli, decreases the work of breathing, improves compliance, and helps prevent atelectasis.
3. A potassium cation, such as Kayexalate, helps remove potassium from the bloodstream in the gastrointestinal tract and would not be prescribed for a client with ARDS.
4. NSAIDs are under investigation for treating ARDS because they block the inflammatory response, but the nurse should not anticipate this being prescribed by the health-care provider.

**TEST-TAKING HINT: Acute respiratory distress syndrome (ARDS) would indicate a problem with the lungs; if the test taker knew that surfactant is needed by the lungs to expand, this would be an appropriate selection as the correct answer.**

105. 1. The nurse must first address the client's acute respiratory distress and then notify other members of the multidisciplinary team.
2. If the ventilator system malfunctions, the nurse must ventilate the client with a manual resuscitation bag (ambu) until the problem is resolved.
3. The nurse must first address the client's respiratory distress before requesting any laboratory data.
4. Assessment is not always priority. In this situation, the client is in "obvious acute respiratory distress"; therefore the nurse needs to intervene to help the client breathe.

**TEST-TAKING HINT: When the question asks the test taker to select the first intervention and the client is in a life-threatening situation, the nurse should select an intervention that directly helps the client. In this situation, assessment does not help the client breathe better. Ventilating the client is the**

only option that has the nurse doing something directly to help the client breathe.

106. 1. Altered level of consciousness is the earliest sign of hypoxemia.
2. Urine output of less than 30 mL/hr indicates decreased cardiac output, which requires immediate intervention; it should be assessed every one (1) or two (2) hours, not once during a shift.
3. The client is at risk for complications of immobility; therefore the nurse should turn the client at least every two (2) hours to prevent pressure ulcers.
4. The client is at risk for fluid volume overload. Therefore the nurse should monitor and maintain the fluid intake.
5. Fowler's position facilitates lung expansion and reduces the workload of breathing.

**TEST-TAKING HINT: The client with ARDS is critically ill, and interventions should address complications of immobility, decreased cardiac output, and respiratory distress. Remember that how often an intervention is implemented is important when selecting the correct answer for the question. More than one (1) answer is possible in these alternate type questions.**

107. 1. Not smoking is vital to prevent further lung damage.
2. The client should get vaccines to help prevent further episodes of serious respiratory distress.
3. Avoiding alcohol intake is appropriate for many serious illnesses, but it is not the most important when discussing ARDS.
4. It usually takes about six (6) months to recover maximal respiratory function after ARDS.

**TEST-TAKING HINT: ARDS means something is wrong with the respiratory system. Therefore the test taker should select an answer option that has something to do with the lungs and possible lung damage.**

108. 1. When peak airway pressure is increased, the nurse should implement the intervention that is less invasive for the client. This alarm goes off with a plugged airway, "bucking" in the ventilator, decreasing lung compliance, kinked tubing, or pneumothorax.
2. The alarm may indicate that the client needs suctioning, but the nurse should always do the least invasive procedure when troubleshooting a ventilator alarm.

Respiratory

3. The lip line on the ET tube determines how far the ET tube is in the trachea. It should always stay the same number, but it would not have anything to do with the ventilator alarms.

4. This may be needed, but the nurse should not sedate the client unless absolutely necessary.

**TEST-TAKING HINT:** If the test taker has no idea what peak airway pressure is, the test taker should not give up on being able to figure out the correct answer. When something is going wrong with a machine, the nurse should either assess or do something for the client. Always select the easiest and least invasive intervention to help the client.

1. Which diagnostic test should the nurse anticipate the health-care provider ordering to rule out the diagnosis of asthma?
   1. A bronchoscopy.
   2. An immunoglobulin E.
   3. An arterial blood gas.
   4. A bronchodilator reversibility test.

2. Which statement indicates the client diagnosed with asthma needs more teaching concerning the medication regimen?
   1. "I will take Singulair, a leukotriene, every day to prevent allergic asthma attacks."
   2. "I need to use my Intal, Cromolyn inhaler 15 minutes before I begin my exercise."
   3. "I need to take oral glucocorticoids every day to prevent my asthma attacks."
   4. "If I have an asthma attack, I need to use my Albuterol, a beta$_2$ agonist, inhaler."

3. Which intervention should the emergency department nurse implement first for the client admitted for an acute asthma attack?
   1. Administer glucocorticoids intravenously.
   2. Encourage the client to cough forcefully.
   3. Establish and maintain a 20-gauge saline lock.
   4. Assess breath sounds every 15 minutes.

4. Which isolation procedure should be instituted for the client admitted to rule out severe acute respiratory syndrome (SARS)?
   1. Airborne isolation.
   2. Droplet isolation.
   3. Reverse isolation.
   4. Strict isolation.

5. The client is admitted with a diagnosis of rule out severe acute respiratory syndrome (SARS). Which information is most important for the nurse to ask related to this diagnosis?
   1. Current prescription and over-the-counter medication use.
   2. Dates of and any complications associated with recent immunizations.
   3. Any problems with recent or past use of blood or blood products.
   4. Recent travel to mainland China, Hong Kong, or Taiwan.

6. The nurse suspects the client admitted with a near drowning is developing acute respiratory distress syndrome (ARDS). Which data would support the nurse's suspicion?
   1. The client's arterial blood gases are within normal limits.
   2. The client appears anxious, has dyspnea, and is tachypneic.
   3. The client has intercostal retractions and is using accessory muscles.
   4. The client's bilateral lung sounds have crackles and rhonchi.

7. Which arterial blood gases (ABGs) would the nurse expect in the client diagnosed with acute respiratory distress syndrome (ARDS) after receiving oxygen at ten (10) LPM via nasal cannula?
   1. pH 7.38, PaO$_2$ 94, PaCO$_2$ 44, HCO$_3$ 24.
   2. pH 7.46, PaO$_2$ 82, PaCO$_2$ 34, HCO$_3$ 22.
   3. pH 7.48, PaO$_2$ 59, PaCO$_2$ 30, HCO$_3$ 26.
   4. pH 7.33, PaO$_2$ 94, PaCO$_2$ 44, HCO$_3$ 20.

8. The nurse is planning the activities for the client diagnosed with asbestosis. What activity should the nurse schedule at 0900 if breakfast is served at 0800?
   1. Assist with the client's bath and linen change.
   2. Administer an inhalation bronchodilator treatment.
   3. Provide the client with a one (1)-hour rest period.
   4. Have respiratory therapy perform chest physiotherapy.

9. When assessing the client diagnosed with asbestosis, which data would require immediate intervention by the nurse?
   1. The client develops an S3 heart sound.
   2. The client has clubbing of the fingers.
   3. The client is fatigued in the afternoon.
   4. The client has basilar crackles in all lobes.

10. Which clinical manifestation would the nurse expect to find in the client newly diagnosed with intrinsic lung cancer?
    1. Dysphagia.
    2. Foul-smelling breath.
    3. Hoarseness.
    4. Weight loss.

11. Which priority intervention should the nurse implement for the client diagnosed with coal workers' pneumoconiosis?
    1. Monitor client's intake and output.
    2. Assess for black-streaked sputum.
    3. Monitor the white blood cell count daily.
    4. Assess the client's activity level every shift.

12. Which statement indicates the client with a total laryngectomy needs more teaching concerning the care of the tracheostomy?
    1. "I must avoid hair spray and powders."
    2. "I should take a shower instead of a tub bath."
    3. "I will need to cleanse around the stoma daily."
    4. "I can use an electric larynx to speak."

13. The occupational nurse for a mining company is planning a class on the risks of working with toxic substances to comply with the "Right to Know Law." Which information should the nurse include in the presentation? Select all that apply.
    1. A client who smokes cigarettes has a drastically increased risk for lung cancer.
    2. Floors need to be clean and dust needs to be wet to prevent transfer of dust.
    3. The air needs to be monitored at specific times to evaluate for exposure.
    4. All surface areas need to be painted every year to prevent the accumulation of dust.
    5. Employees should wear the appropriate personal protective equipment.

14. Which data would be significant when assessing a client diagnosed with rule out Legionnaires' disease?
    1. The amount of cigarettes smoked a day and the age when started.
    2. Symptoms of aching muscles, high fever, malaise, and coughing.
    3. Exposure to a saprophytic water bacterium transmitted into the air.
    4. Decreased bilateral lung sounds in the lower lobes.

15. Which assessment data indicate the client diagnosed with Legionnaires' disease is experiencing a complication?
    1. The client has an elevated body temperature.
    2. The client has <30 mL urine output an hour.
    3. The client has a decrease in body aches.
    4. The client has an elevated white blood cell count.

16. Which statement indicates the need for further teaching for the client diagnosed with sleep apnea?
    1. "If I lose weight and stop smoking cigarettes I may not need treatment for sleep apnea."
    2. "The continuous positive airway pressure (CPAP) holds my airway open with pressure."
    3. "The CPAP will help me stay awake during the day while I am at work."
    4. "It is all right to have a couple of beers at night because I have this CPAP machine."

Respiratory

17. The nurse is preparing to administer influenza vaccines to a group of elderly clients in a long-term care facility. Which client should the nurse question receiving the vaccine?
    1. The client diagnosed with congestive heart failure.
    2. The client with a documented allergy to eggs.
    3. The client who has had an anaphylactic reaction to penicillin.
    4. The client who has an elevated blood pressure and pulse.

18. The nurse is preparing the client for a polysomnography to confirm sleep apnea. Which preprocedure instruction should the nurse include?
    1. The client should not eat or drink past midnight.
    2. The client will receive a sedative for relaxation.
    3. The client will sleep in a laboratory for evaluation.
    4. The client will wear a monitor at home for this test.

19. The client in the intensive care unit diagnosed with end-stage chronic obstructive pulmonary disease has a Swan-Ganz mean pulmonary artery pressure of 35 mm Hg. Which order would the nurse question?
    1. Administer intravenous fluids of normal saline at 125 mL/hr.
    2. Provide supplemental oxygen per nasal cannula at 2 liters/min.
    3. Continuous telemetry monitoring with strips every four (4) hours.
    4. Administer a loop diuretic intravenously every six (6) hours.

20. The nurse and an unlicensed nursing assistant (NA) are caring for an elderly client diagnosed with emphysema. Which nursing tasks could be delegated to the NA to improve gas exchange? Select all that apply.
    1. Keep the head of the bed elevated.
    2. Encourage deep breathing exercises.
    3. Record pulse oximeter reading.
    4. Assess level of conscious.
    5. Auscultate breath sounds.

21. When preparing the plan of care for the client's post-pleurodesis procedure, which collaborative intervention should the nurse include?
    1. Monitor the amount and color of drainage from the chest tube.
    2. Perform a complete respiratory assessment every two (2) hours.
    3. Administer morphine sulfate, an opioid analgesic, intravenously.
    4. Keep a sterile dressing and bottle of sterile normal saline at the bedside.

22. Which nursing diagnosis would be appropriate for the client that is one (1) day post-operative for a thoracotomy?
    1. Alteration in comfort.
    2. Altered level of conscious.
    3. Alteration in elimination pattern.
    4. Knowledge deficit.

23. The nurse is caring for the client diagnosed with bacterial pneumonia. Which priority intervention should the nurse implement?
    1. Assess respiratory rate and depth.
    2. Provide for adequate rest period.
    3. Administer oxygen as prescribed.
    4. Teach slow abdominal breathing.

24. The nurse is caring for a client diagnosed with pneumonia who is having shortness of breath and difficulty breathing. Which intervention should the nurse implement first?
    1. Take the client's vital signs.
    2. Check the client's pulse oximeter reading.
    3. Elevate the client's head of the bed.
    4. Notify the respiratory therapist STAT.

Respiratory

25. The post-anesthesia care nurse is caring for the client diagnosed with lung cancer who had a thoracotomy and is experiencing frequent premature ventricular contractions (PVC). Which intervention should the nurse implement first?
    1. Request STAT arterial blood gases.
    2. Administer lidocaine intravenous push.
    3. Assess for possible causes.
    4. Request a STAT electrocardiogram (ECG).

26. The nurse is caring for the postoperative client diagnosed with lung cancer recovering from a thoracotomy. Which data would require immediate intervention by the nurse?
    1. The client refuses to perform shoulder exercises.
    2. The client complains of a sore throat and is hoarse.
    3. The client has crackles that clear with cough.
    4. The client is coughing up pink frothy sputum.

27. What information should be included in the teaching plan for the mother of a client diagnosed with cystic fibrosis? Select all that apply.
    1. Perform postural drainage and percussion every four (4) hours.
    2. Modify activities to accommodate daily physiotherapy.
    3. Increase fluid intake to one (1) liter daily to thin secretions.
    4. Recognize and report signs and symptoms of respiratory infections.
    5. Avoid anyone suspected of having an upper respiratory infection.

28. Which symptom would the nurse expect for the client to report to support the diagnosis of cystic fibrosis?
    1. Wheezing with a productive cough.
    2. Excessive salty sweat secretions.
    3. Multiple vitamin deficiencies.
    4. Clubbing of all fingers.

29. The client is diagnosed with bronchiolitis obliterans. Which data indicate the glucocorticoid therapy is effective?
    1. The client has an elevation in the blood glucose.
    2. The client has a decrease in sputum production.
    3. The client has an increase in the temperature.
    4. The client appears restless and is irritable.

30. The nurse is discharging the client diagnosed with bronchiolitis obliterans for discharge. Which priority intervention should the nurse include?
    1. Refer the client to the American Lung Association.
    2. Notify the physical therapy department to arrange for activity training.
    3. Arrange for oxygen therapy to be used at home.
    4. Discuss advance directives with the client.

31. The client admitted for recurrent aspiration pneumonia is at risk for bronchiectasis. Which intervention should the nurse anticipate the health-care provider to order?
    1. Administer intravenous antibiotics for seven (7) days.
    2. Insert a subclavian line and initiate total parenteral nutrition.
    3. Provide a low-calorie and low-sodium restricted diet.
    4. Encourage the client to turn, cough, and deep breathe frequently.

32. Which collaborative intervention should the nurse implement when caring for the client diagnosed with bronchiectasis?
    1. Prepare the client for an emergency tracheostomy.
    2. Discuss postoperative teaching for a lobectomy.
    3. Administer bronchodilators with postural drainage.
    4. Obtain informed consent form for chest tube insertion.

33. The nurse is discussing the results of a tuberculosis skin test. Which explanation should the nurse give the client?
    1. A red area is a positive reading that means the client has tuberculosis.
    2. The skin test is the only procedure needed to diagnose tuberculosis.
    3. A positive reading means exposure to the tuberculosis bacilli.
    4. Do not get another skin test for one (1) year if the skin test is positive.

34. The client diagnosed with tuberculosis has been treated with antitubercular medications for six (6) weeks. Which data would indicate the medication has been effective?
    1. A decrease in the white blood cells in the sputum.
    2. The client's symptoms are improving.
    3. No change in the chest x-ray.
    4. The skin test is now negative.

35. The nurse is caring for a client on a mechanical ventilator and the alarm goes off. The nurse is unable to determine what is wrong with the ventilator and the client is in respiratory distress. Which action should the nurse implement first?
    1. Notify the respiratory therapist immediately.
    2. Use the ambu bag to ventilate the client.
    3. Elevate the head of the client's bed.
    4. Assess the client's oxygen saturation.

36. The client diagnosed with deep vein thrombosis (DVT) suddenly complains of severe chest pain and a feeling of impending doom. Which complication would the nurse suspect the client has experienced?
    1. Myocardial infarction.
    2. Pneumonia.
    3. Pulmonary embolus.
    4. Pneumothorax.

37. The nurse is preparing to administer warfarin (Coumadin), an oral anticoagulant, to a client diagnosed with a pulmonary embolus. Which data would cause the nurse to question administering the medication?
    1. The client's partial thromboplastin time (PTT) is 38.
    2. The client's International Normalized Ratio (INR) is 5.
    3. The client's prothrombin time (PT) is 22.
    4. The client's erythrocyte sedimentation rate (ESR) is 10.

38. The nurse is caring for a client diagnosed with a pneumothorax who had chest tubes inserted four (4) hours ago. There is no fluctuating (tidaling) in the water-seal compartment of the closed chest drainage system. Which action should the nurse take first?
    1. Milk the chest tube.
    2. Check the tubing for kinks.
    3. Instruct the client to cough.
    4. Assess the insertion site.

39. The health-care provider has ordered a continuous intravenous infusion of aminophylline. The client weighs 165 pounds. The infusion order is 0.3 mg/kg/hr. The bag is mixed with 500 mg of aminophylline in 250 mL of D5W. What rate should the nurse set the pump? _____

40. The client diagnosed with a viral upper respiratory infection, the common cold, is taking an antihistamine. Which statement indicates the client needs more teaching concerning the medication?
    1. "If my mouth gets dry I will suck on hard candy."
    2. "I will not drink beer or any type of alcohol."
    3. "I need to be careful when I drive my car."
    4. "This medication will make me sleepy."

Respiratory

41. The client with a viral upper respiratory infection, the common cold, asks the nurse, "Is it all right to take echinacea for my cold?" Which statement is the best response?
    1. "You should discuss that with your health-care provider."
    2. "No, you should not take any type of herbal medicine."
    3. "Yes, but do not take it for more than 3 days."
    4. "Echinacea may help with the symptoms of your cold."

42. Which intervention should the nurse implement for the client experiencing bronchospasms?
    1. Administer intravenous epinephrine, a bronchodilator.
    2. Administer albuterol, a bronchodilator, via nebulizer.
    3. Request a STAT portable chest x-ray at the bedside.
    4. Insert a small nasal trumpet in the right nostril.

43. The nurse is caring for a female client that is very anxious, has a respiratory rate of 40, and is complaining of her fingers tingling and her lips feeling numb. Which intervention should the nurse implement?
    1. Have the client take slow, deep breaths.
    2. Instruct her to put her head between her legs.
    3. Determine why she is feeling so anxious.
    4. Administer Xanax, an antianxiety agent.

44. The client with pneumonia that has the following arterial blood gases: pH 7.33, $PaO_2$ 94, $PaCO_2$ 47, $HCO_3$ 25. Which intervention should the nurse implement?
    1. Administer sodium bicarbonate.
    2. Administer oxygen via nasal cannula.
    3. Have the client cough and deep breathe.
    4. Instruct the client to breathe in a paper bag.

45. When assessing the client diagnosed with a lung abscess, which information would the nurse expect to find to support the diagnosis?
    1. Tympanic sounds elicited by percussion over the site.
    2. Inspiratory and expiratory wheezes heard over the upper lobes.
    3. Decreased breath sounds with a pleural friction rub.
    4. Asymmetric movement of the chest wall with inspiration.

46. The public health department nurse is caring for the client diagnosed with active tuberculosis who has been placed on directly observed therapy (DOT). Which statement best describes this therapy?
    1. The nurse accounts for all medications administered to the client.
    2. The nurse must complete federal, state, and local forms for this client.
    3. The nurse must report the client to the Centers for Disease Control.
    4. The nurse must watch the client take the medication daily.

47. When caring for the client with a respiratory disorder, which intervention should the nurse implement first?
    1. Administer a respiratory treatment.
    2. Assess the client's radial pulses daily.
    3. Monitor the client's vital signs daily.
    4. Assess the client's capillary refill time.

48. The nurse is preparing to hang the next bag of aminophylline, a bronchodilator, for the client diagnosed with asthma. The current theophylline level is 18 mcg/mL. Which intervention should the nurse implement?
    1. Hang the next bag and continue the infusion.
    2. Do not hang the next bag and decrease the rate.
    3. Notify the health-care provider of the level.
    4. Confirm the current serum theophylline level.

49. Which intervention should the nurse implement first when administering the first dose of intravenous antibiotic to the client diagnosed with a respiratory infection?
    1. Monitor the client's current temperature.
    2. Monitor the client's white blood cells.
    3. Determine if a culture has been collected.
    4. Determine the compatibility of fluids.

50. Which nursing interventions should the nurse implement for the client who has a respiratory disorder? Select all that apply.
    1. Administer oxygen via a nasal cannula.
    2. Assess the client's lung sounds.
    3. Encourage the client to cough and deep breathe.
    4. Monitor the client's pulse oximeter reading.
    5. Increase the client's fluid intake.

51. The client in the intensive care unit on a mechanical ventilator is bucking the ventilator, causing the alarms to sound. Which assessment data should the nurse obtain? List in the order of priority.
    1. Assess the ventilator alarms.
    2. Assess the client's pulse oximetry reading.
    3. Assess the client's lung sounds.
    4. Assess for symmetry of the client's chest expansion.
    5. Assess the client's endotracheal tube for secretions.

1. 1. A bronchoscope visualizes the bronchial tree under sedation, but it does not confirm the diagnosis of asthma.
   2. An immunoglobulin E is a blood test for the presence of an antibody protein indicating allergic reactions.
   3. Arterial blood gases analyze levels that provide information about the exchange of oxygen and carbon dioxide, but they are not diagnostic of asthma.
   4. **During a bronchodilator reversibility test, the client's positive response to a bronchodilator confirms the diagnosis of asthma.**

2. 1. Leukotrienes, such as Singulair, should be taken daily to prevent an asthma attack that is triggered by the allergen response.
   2. Cromolyn inhalers, such as Intal, are used to prevent exercise-induced asthma attacks.
   3. **Glucocorticoids are given orally or intravenously during acute exacerbations of asthma, not on a daily basis because of the long-term complications of steroid therapy.**
   4. Albuterol, a beta$_2$ agonist, is used during attacks because of the fast action.

3. 1. Glucocorticoids are a treatment of choice, but they are not the first intervention.
   2. Encouraging the client to cough will help the client expectorate sputum if needed.
   3. A saline lock is needed for intravenous fluids, but it is not the first intervention.
   4. **Assessment is the first step of the nursing process and should be implemented first.**

4. 1. Airborne isolation is used when the infectious agent can remain in the air and be transported greater than three (3) feet and includes wearing specially fitted masks to prevent transmission.
   2. **SARS is an influenza-type virus that is transmitted by particle droplets. Therefore, the client should be placed in droplet isolation.**
   3. Reverse isolation is a term for using equipment to prevent the client from being exposed to organisms from other people.
   4. Strict isolation is an old term used to describe isolation to prevent transmission of organisms to other people.

5. 1. This information is important during an admission interview but is not specific to SARS.
   2. The information would not be specific to the diagnosis of SARS.
   3. This would be important to ask prior to the administration of any blood products, but it is not specific for SARS.
   4. **Recent travel to mainland China, Taiwan, and Hong Kong is a risk factor for SARS.**

6. 1. The client would have low arterial oxygen when developing ARDS.
   2. **Initial manifestations of ARDS usually develop 24 to 48 hours after the initial insult leading to hypoxia and include anxiety, dyspnea, and tachypnea.**
   3. As ARDS progresses, the client has more difficulty breathing, resulting in intercostal retractions and use of accessory muscles.
   4. Lungs are initially clear; crackles and rhonchi develop in later stages of ARDS.

7. 1. This ABG is within normal limits and would not be expected in a client with ARDS.
   2. These ABG levels indicate respiratory alkalosis, but the oxygen level is within normal limits and would not be expected in a client with ARDS.
   3. **ABGs initially show hypoxemia with a Pao$_2$ of less than 60 mm/Hg and respiratory alkalosis resulting from tachypnea.**
   4. This ABG is metabolic acidosis and would not be expected in a client with ARDS.

8. 1. Bathing is too strenuous an activity immediately after eating.
   2. Inhalation bronchodilators should be given one (1) hour after meals. The nurse should realize that the client will require 20–30 minutes to eat, and scheduling these activities at 0900 would not give the client sufficient time to digest the food or rest before the activity.
   3. **Periods of rest should be alternated with periods of activity.**
   4. Chest physiotherapy should be given at least one (1) hour after meals. The nurse should realize that the client will require 20–30 minutes to eat, and scheduling these activities at 0900 would not give the client sufficient time to digest the food or rest before the activity.

9. 1. **The appearance of S3 heart sounds indicates that the client is developing heart failure, which is a medical emergency.**
   2. Clubbing of the fingers indicates that the client has a chronic respiratory condition, but this would not require immediate intervention.
   3. Fatigue is a common occurrence in clients with respiratory conditions, such as asbestosis, as a result of the effort required to breathe.
   4. Bibasilar crackles are common symptoms experienced by clients with asbestosis and do not require immediate intervention.

10. 1. Dysphagia is a late sign of intrinsic lung cancer.
    2. Foul-smelling breath is a late sign of intrinsic lung cancer.

3. Hoarseness is an early clinical manifestation of intrinsic lung cancer.

4. Weight loss is a late sign of most types of cancers, not just intrinsic lung cancer.

11. 1. Fluids should be encouraged to help to liquefy sputum; therefore, intake and output should be monitored, but this is not the priority intervention.

2. **Black-streaked sputum is a classic sign of coal workers' pneumoconiosis (black lung), and the sputum should be assessed for color and amount. Remember Maslow's Hierarchy of Needs when answering priority questions.**

3. The client's white blood cells should be monitored to assess for infection, but it is not priority and is not done daily.

4. Activity tolerance is important to assess for clients with all respiratory diseases, but it is not the priority intervention.

12. 1. The client should not let any spray or powder enter the stoma because it goes directly into the lung.

2. **The client should not allow water to enter the stoma; therefore, the client should take a tub bath, not a shower.**

3. The stoma site should be cleansed to help prevent infection.

4. The client's vocal cords were removed; therefore, the client must use an alternate form of communication.

13. 1. **Clients who smoke cigarettes and work with toxic substances have increased risk of lung cancer because many of the substances are carcinogenic.**

2. **When floors and surfaces are kept clean, toxic dust particles, such as asbestos and silica, are controlled and this decreases exposure. Covering areas with water controls dust.**

3. The quality of air is monitored to determine what toxic substances are present and in what amount. The information is then used in efforts to minimize the amount of exposure.

4. Applying paint to a surface does not eliminate or minimize exposure.

5. **Employees must wear protective coverings, goggles, and other equipment needed to eliminate exposure to the toxic substances.**

14. 1. Smoking cigarettes is important to assess in any respiratory disease, but it is not specific to Legionnaires' disease.

2. Aching muscles, high fever, malaise, and coughing are symptoms of most respiratory

illnesses, including influenza and pneumonia, but these symptoms are not specific to Legionnaires' disease.

3. **Legionnaires' disease is caused by a saprophytic water bacterium that is transmitted through the air from places where the bacteria are found: rivers, lakes, evaporative condensers, respiratory apparatuses, or water distribution centers.**

4. Abnormal breath sounds can be heard in many respiratory illnesses.

15. 1. The temperature is elevated and does not indicate a complication.

2. **Multiple organ failure is a common complication of Legionnaires' disease, and if the client does not have a urine output of 30 mL an hour, it indicates the complication of renal failure.**

3. A decrease in body aches does not indicate a complication.

4. An elevation of white blood cells is expected in a client with Legionnaires' disease and is not a complication.

16. 1. The contributing factors of sleep apnea are obesity, smoking, drinking alcohol, and a short neck. In some situations modifying lifestyle will improve sleep apnea.

2. Many clients need a continuous positive airway pressure (CPAP) machine that continuously administers positive pressure to assist sleep during the night.

3. When clients have sleep apnea, the buildup of carbon dioxide causes the client to arouse constantly from sleep to breathe. This, in turn, causes the client to be sleepy during the day.

4. **Drinking alcohol before sleep sedates the client, causing the muscles to relax, which, in turn, causes an obstruction of the client's airway. Thus, drinking alcohol should be avoided even if the client uses a CPAP machine.**

17. 1. There would be no reason to question administering a vaccine to a client with heart failure.

2. **In clients who are allergic to egg protein, a significant hypersensitivity response may occur when they are receiving the influenza vaccine.**

3. There would be no reason to question administering a vaccine to a client who has had a reaction to penicillin.

4. There would be no reason to question administering a vaccine to a client who has elevated blood pressure and pulse.

18. 1. Preparation for the polysomnography does not require being NPO after midnight.

2. The examination is a recording of the natural sleep of the client so no sedative would be administered.

3. The polysomnography is completed in a sleep laboratory to observe all the stages of sleep. Equipment is attached to the client to monitor depth, stage, movement, respiratory effort, and oxygen saturation level during sleep.

4. The client could perform this test at home, but the evaluation is not as reliable and the visual observation is not included; therefore, this is not recommended.

19. 1. Normal mean pulmonary artery pressure is about 15 mm Hg and an elevation indicates right ventricular heart failure or cor pulmonale, which occurs in chronic obstructive pulmonary disease. The nurse should question this order because this rate is too high and sodium should be restricted.

2. Supplemental oxygen should be administered at the lowest amount; therefore this order should not be questioned.

3. Clients with hypoxia and cor pulmonale are at risk for dysrhythmias so monitoring the ECG is an appropriate intervention.

4. Loop diuretics are administered to decrease the fluid and decrease the circulatory load on the right side of the heart; therefore, this order would not be questioned.

20. 1. Keeping the head of the bed elevated maximizes lung excursion and improves gas exchange and can be delegated.

2. Encouraging breathing exercises can be delegated.

3. Recording pulse oximeter readings can be delegated.

4. Assessment cannot be delegated. Confusion is one of the first symptoms of hypoxia in the elderly.

5. Auscultation is a technique of assessment that cannot be delegated.

21. 1. Monitoring the amount and color of drainage from the chest tube is an independent nursing intervention.

2. Respiratory assessment is an independent intervention.

3. Administering medication is a collaborative intervention because it requires a health-care provider's order.

4. Keeping supplies at the bedside is an independent intervention that the nurse may take in case the chest tube becomes dislodged.

22. 1. Pain and discomfort are major problems for clients who have had a thoracotomy be-

cause the chest wall has been opened and closed.

2. The client would be on a mechanical ventilator and have an adequate airway; therefore, altered consciousness would not be an appropriate diagnosis.

3. Clients are out of bed the first day after surgery; therefore, elimination is not an appropriate nursing diagnosis.

4. The client should have received instructions prior to surgery.

23. 1. Because tachypnea and dyspnea may be early indicators of respiratory compromise, the assessment of respiratory rate and depth is the priority intervention.

2. Rest reduces metabolic demands, fatigue, and the work of breathing, which promotes a more effective breathing pattern, but it is not priority over assessment.

3. Oxygen therapy increases the alveolar oxygen concentration reducing hypoxia and anxiety, but it is not priority over assessment.

4. This breathing pattern promotes lung expansion, but it is not priority over assessment.

24. 1. Taking the client's vital signs will not help the client's shortness of breath and difficulty in breathing.

2. Checking the pulse oximeter reading will not help the client's shortness of breath and difficulty breathing.

3. Elevating the head of the bed promotes lung expansion and will directly help the client's breathing.

4. Notifying the respiratory therapist will not help the client's shortness of breath and difficulty breathing.

25. 1. ABGs may show hypoxia, which is a cause of PVCs, but it is not the first intervention the nurse should implement.

2. Lidocaine is the treatment of choice for PVCs, but it is not the first intervention.

3. The nurse should assess for possible causes of the PVCs; these causes may include hypoxia or hypokalemia.

4. An ECG further evaluates the heart function, but it is not the first intervention.

26. 1. The client refusing to perform shoulder exercises is pertinent, but it does not require immediate intervention.

2. Sore throats and hoarseness are common post-intubation and would not require immediate intervention.

3. Crackles that clear with coughing would not require immediate intervention.

4. Pink frothy sputum indicates pulmonary

edema and would require immediate intervention.

27. 1. Clients and family members should be taught chest physiotherapy including postural drainage, chest percussion, and vibration and breathing techniques to keep the lungs clear of the copious secretions.
    2. Daily activities should be modified to accommodate the client's treatments.
    3. Clients should increase fluids up to 3000 mL each day to thin secretions and ease expectoration.
    4. Clients should be taught the signs and symptoms of infections to report to the health-care provider.
    5. Clients with CF are susceptible to respiratory infections and should avoid anyone who is suspected of having an infection.

28. 1. Wheezing and productive coughs are symptoms experienced by clients with respiratory diseases, but they are not specific to cystic fibrosis.
    2. The excessive excretion of salt from the sweat glands is specific to cystic fibrosis. Repeated values greater than 60 mEq/L of sweat chloride is diagnostic for CF.
    3. Multiple vitamin deficiencies are experienced with some pulmonary diseases, but they are not specific to cystic fibrosis.
    4. Clubbing of the fingers is an indicator of chronic hypoxia, but it is not specific to the diagnosis of cystic fibrosis.

29. 1. An elevation in the blood glucose level is a common side effect of corticosteroids and does not indicate effectiveness of the treatment for bronchiolitis obliterans.
    2. A decrease in sputum production indicates that the client is improving and the medication is effective; long-term use of corticosteroids is indicated for a client with bronchiolitis obliterans.
    3. An elevated temperature indicates that the client is becoming worse; therefore, the medication is not effective.
    4. Restlessness and irritability can be side effects of treatment with corticosteroids or they could be signs of hypoxemia, which would indicate the medication is not effective.

30. 1. The American Lung Association is an excellent resource for educational material, but it is not the priority intervention for the client.
    2. Physical therapy is an appropriate intervention, but it is not the priority intervention.
    3. The client with bronchiolitis obliterans will need long-term use of oxygen.

4. Advance directives are an important intervention, but are not the priority interventions.

31. 1. Antibiotics should be administered intravenously for seven (7) to ten (10) days. Bronchiectasis is an irreversible condition caused by repeated damage to the bronchial walls secondary to repeated aspiration of gastric contents.
    2. Total parental nutrition is not an expected treatment for a client with bronchiectasis.
    3. Clients should have a high-calorie and high-protein diet as a result of high expenditure of energy used to breathe and tissue healing.
    4. Turning, coughing, and deep breathing are appropriate independent nursing interventions that do not require a health-care provider's order.

32. 1. Medical treatment for bronchiectasis does not include a tracheostomy.
    2. Removing a lobe of the lung is not the expected medical treatment for a client with bronchiectasis.
    3. Administering bronchodilators is a collaborative intervention (requiring an order from a health-care provider) appropriate for this client.
    4. Insertion of chest tubes is not an expected treatment for bronchiectasis.

33. 1. A red and raised area at the injection site indicates that the client has been exposed to tuberculosis bacilli, but it does not indicate active disease.
    2. The skin test indicates that the client has been exposed to the tuberculosis bacilli, but further tests must be performed to confirm the diagnosis of tuberculosis.
    3. A positive reading indicates that the client has been exposed to the bacilli.
    4. Once a positive reading occurs, then the client should never take the skin test again.

34. 1. Antitubercular medications target the tubercular bacilli, not white blood cells.
    2. As the bacilli are being destroyed, the client should begin to feel better and have fewer symptoms.
    3. At six (6) weeks, the chest x-ray may not have changes.
    4. The skin test will always be positive.

35. 1. The nurse needs to notify the respiratory therapist to fix the ventilator, but it is not the first intervention.
    2. The nurse must first disconnect the client from the ventilator and bag the client until the ventilator can be fixed.

Respiratory

3. Elevating the head of the bed will help lung expansion, but it is not the first intervention.
4. When the client is in a life-threatening situation, the nurse should not assess the client's oxygen saturation first; the nurse first should attempt to do something to correct the life-threatening situation.

36. 1. The most common complication of a DVT is a pulmonary embolus, although chest pain is a sign of a myocardial infarction.
2. These signs and symptoms should not make the nurse think the client has pneumonia.
3. **Part of the clot in the deep veins of the legs dislodges and travels up the inferior vena cava, lodges in the pulmonary artery, and causes the chest pain; the client often feels as if they are going to die.**
4. Chest pain is a sign of pneumothorax, but it is not a complication of deep vein thrombosis.

37. 1. The PTT is not monitored to determine a serum therapeutic level for warfarin; normal is 30 to 45.
2. **The INR therapeutic range is 2–3 for a client receiving warfarin. The INR may be allowed to go to 3.5 if the client has a mechanical cardiac valve, but nothing in the stem of the question indicates this.**
3. The PT is monitored for oral anticoagulant therapy and should be 1.5 to 2 times the normal of 12; therefore, 22 is within therapeutic range and would not warrant the nurse questioning administering this medication.
4. The ESR is not monitored for oral anticoagulant therapy.

38. 1. No fluctuation in the water-seal chamber four (4) hours post-insertion indicates the tubing is blocked; the nurse can milk the chest tube, but it is not the first action.
2. **The nurse should implement the easiest intervention first. The nurse should check to see if the tubing is kinked, causing a blockage between the pleural space and the water-seal bottle.**
3. Coughing may help push the clot in the tubing into the drainage bottle, but the first intervention is to check and see if the client is lying on the tubing or the tube is kinked somewhere.
4. The insertion site can be assessed, but it will not help determine why there is no fluctuation in the water-seal drainage compartment.

39. 11 mL/hr First, convert pounds to kilograms
$$165 \text{ pounds} \div 2.2 = 75 \text{ kg}$$
Then, determine how many milligrams of aminophylline per hour should be administered:
$$0.3 \text{ mg} \times 75 \text{ kg} = 22.5 \text{ mg/hour}$$

Then, determine how much aminophylline is delivered per liter:
$$500 \text{ mg} \div 250 \text{ mL} = 2 \text{ mg/1 mL}$$
If 2 mg/1 mL is delivered, then to deliver the prescribed 22.5 mg/hour, the rate must be set at
$$22.5 \div 2 = 11.25 \text{ mL/hr}$$

40. 1. Antihistamines dry respiratory secretions through an anticholinergic effect; therefore, the client will have a dry mouth.
2. Antihistamines cause drowsiness; therefore the client should not drink any type of alcohol.
3. Antihistamines cause drowsiness so the client should not drive or operate any type of machinery.
4. Antihistamines cause drowsiness; therefore, the client understands the teaching.

41. 1. The nurse can answer client's questions concerning herbal medication. Passing the buck should be eliminated as a possible correct answer.
2. The nurse should not be judgmental. If the client does not have comorbid conditions, is not taking other medications, or is not pregnant, herbal medications may be helpful in treating the common cold.
3. Echinacea should not be taken for more than two (2) weeks, not three (3) days. Nothing cures the common cold; the cold must run its course.
4. **Echinacea is an herb that may reduce the duration and symptoms of the common cold, but nothing cures the common cold. If the client does not have comorbid conditions, is not taking other medications, and is not pregnant, herbal medications may be helpful in treating the common cold.**

42. 1. Epinephrine is administered intravenously during an arrest in a code situation, but it is not a treatment of choice for bronchospasms.
2. **Albuterol given via nebulizer is administered to stop the bronchospasms. If the client continues to have the bronchospasms, intubation may be needed.**
3. A STAT portable x-ray will be ordered, but the goal is to prevent respiratory arrest.
4. Nasal trumpet airways would not be helpful in stopping the bronchospasm and respiratory arrest.

43. 1. **The client is hyperventilating and blowing off too much $CO_2$, which is why her fingers are tingling and her mouth is numb; she needs to retain $CO_2$ by taking slow deep breaths.**
2. Putting the head between the legs sometimes helps a client who is going to faint.

3. The client is hyperventilating; determining why is not appropriate at this time.

4. Medications take up to 30 minutes to one (1) hour to work and are not an appropriate intervention for the client who is hyperventilating.

44. 1. Sodium bicarbonate is administered for metabolic acidosis.

2. The arterial oxygen level is within normal limits—80–100; therefore, the client does not need oxygen.

3. **The client is retaining $CO_2$, which causes respiratory acidosis, and the nurse should help the client remove the $CO_2$ by instructing them to cough and deep breathe.**

4. Breathing in a paper bag is not recommended for clients in respiratory acidosis.

45. 1. Dull sounds would be heard over the site of a lung abscess as a result of the solid mass.

2. Crackles may be heard but wheezes would indicate a narrowing of airways, not exudate-filled airways.

3. **Diminished or absent sounds are heard with intermittent pleural friction rubs. A lung abscess is the accumulation of pus in an area where pneumonia was present that becomes encapsulated and can extend to the bronchus or pleural space.**

4. Even with a lung abscess, the chest should move with symmetry.

46. 1. Nurses are responsible for accounting for medications, but that is not the rationale for DOT.

2. Nurses complete forms as required by all governmental agencies, but this is not the rationale for DOT.

3. Documentation of events concerning the client's treatment is completed, but this is not the rationale for DOT.

4. **To ensure the compliance with all medications regimens, the health department has adapted a directly observed therapy (DOT) where the nurse actually observes the client taking the medication every day.**

47. 1. The nurse should gather data before implementing an intervention.

2. The radial pulse would indicate the cardiovascular status of the client, not the respiratory status, and the nurse should assess the apical pulse.

3. Daily vital signs would not indicate the respiratory status of the client.

4. **Assessing the client's capillary time has the highest priority for the nurse because it indicates the oxygenation of the client.**

48. 1. The therapeutic level is 10 to 20 mcg/mL; therefore, the nurse should hang the bag and continue the infusion to maintain the level.

2. There is no reason not to hang the next bag of aminophylline.

3. There is no need to notify the health-care provider for a level of 18 mcg/mL.

4. There is no need for the nurse to confirm the laboratory results.

49. 1. The client's current temperature would not affect the administration of the antibiotic.

2. The client's white blood cells may be elevated because of the infection, but that would not affect administering the medication.

3. **A culture needs to be collected prior to the first dose of antibiotic, or the culture and sensitivity will be skewed and the appropriate antibiotic needed to treat the respiratory infection may not be identified.**

4. Compatibility of fluids should be assessed prior to administering each intravenous antibiotic, but when administering the first dose of an antibiotic the nurse must check to make sure the sputum culture was obtained.

50. 1. A client with a respiratory disorder may have decreased oxygen saturation; therefore, administering oxygen via a nasal cannula is appropriate.

2. The client's lungs sounds should be assessed to determine how much air is being exchanged in the lungs.

3. Coughing and deep breathing will help the client expectorate sputum, thus clearing the bronchial tree.

4. The pulse oximeter evaluates how much oxygen is reaching the periphery.

5. Increasing fluids will help thin secretions, making them easier to expectorate.

51. In order of priority: 5, 2, 3, 4, 1

5. The most common cause of bucking the ventilator is obstructed airway, which could be secondary to secretions in the airway.

2. Clients in the ICU are constantly monitored by pulse oximetry; therefore, the nurse should determine if the client has decreased oxygenation saturation and if so the nurse should start to "bag" the client.

3. The nurse should assess the client's lung fields to determine if air movement is occurring.

4. A complication of mechanical ventilation is a pneumothorax, and the nurse should assess for this.

1. The machine is alerting the nurse that a problem with the client is occurring; the nurse should assess the client, not the machine.

Respiratory

*Science is knowledge; wisdom is organized life.*—Immanuel Kant

# 7

# Gastrointestinal Disorders

The many organs that make up the gastrointestinal system—the mouth, esophagus, stomach, upper and lower intestine, and related organs—are subject to many disorders/diseases. Some are relatively minor, such as temporary constipation or a short bout of diarrhea and gastroenteritis. Others, such as diverticulosis and inflammatory bowel disease, may be chronic, requiring the client to follow specific diet and other lifestyle modifications. Some chronic diseases, including gastroesophageal reflux, may eventually lead to life-threatening problems such as esophageal cancer. Still other diseases affect the gastrointestinal tract. One—colon cancer—is one of the most common cancers in the United States. In addition, eating disorders rooted in psychological problems can be serious if not addressed promptly and effectively. Because gastrointestinal diseases/disorders are so common, the nurse must be aware of the sign/symptoms of each, what is considered normal or abnormal for the disease process, and how the specific problem is treated.

## KEYWORDS

ascites
asterixis
borborygmus
caput medusae
cathartic
cruciferous
dyspepsia
dysphagia
eructation
esophagogastroduodenoscopy
evisceration
exacerbation
feces
hematemesis
hypoalbuminemia
jaundice
lower esophageal sphincter
melena
nosocomial
odynophagia
oligomenorrhea
peritonitis
pruritus
pyrosis
sedentary
steatorrhea
tenesmus
water brash

## ABBREVIATIONS

Acquired Immunodeficiency Syndrome (AIDS)
Blood Pressure (BP)
Body Mass Index (BMI)
Esophagogastroduodenoscopy (EGD)
Gastroesophageal Reflux Disease (GERD)
Gastrointestinal (GI)
Head Of Bed (HOB)
Health-Care Provider (HCP)
Inflammatory Bowel Disease (IBD)
Intake and Output (I & O)
International Normalized Ratio (INR)
Intravenous (IV)
Nasogastric (N/G) tube
Nonsteroidal Anti-Inflammatory Drugs (NSAIDs)
Nothing by Mouth (NPO)
Partial Thromboplastin Time (PTT)
Patient Controlled Analgesic (PCA)
Percutaneous Gastronomy (PEG)
Prothrombin Time (PT)
Pulse (P)
Red Blood Cells (RBC)
Three Times a Day (t.i.d.)
Total Parenteral Nutrition (TPN)
Unlicensed Nursing Personnel (UAP)
When Required, As Needed (PRN)
White Blood Cells (WBC)
Within Normal Limits (WNL)

## Gastroesophageal Reflux

1. The male client in a health-care provider's office tells the nurse that he has been experiencing "heartburn" at night that awakens him. Which assessment question should the nurse ask?
   1. "How much weight have you gained recently?"
   2. "What have you done to alleviate the heartburn?"
   3. "Do you consume many milk and dairy products?"
   4. "Have you been around anyone with a stomach virus?"

2. The nurse caring for a client diagnosed with gastroesophageal reflux disease (GERD) writes the nursing problem of "behavior modification." Which intervention should be included for this problem?
   1. Teach the client to sleep with a foam wedge under the head.
   2. Encourage the client to decrease the amount of smoking.
   3. Instruct the client to take over-the-counter medication for relief of pain.
   4. Discuss the need to attend Alcoholics Anonymous to quit drinking.

3. The nurse is preparing a client diagnosed with GERD for discharge following an esophagogastroduodenoscopy. Which statement indicates the client understands the discharge instructions?
   1. "I should not eat for twenty-four (24) hours following this procedure."
   2. "I can lie down whenever I want after a meal. It won't make a difference."
   3. "The stomach contents won't bother my esophagus but will make me nauseous."
   4. "I should avoid drinking orange juice and eating tomatoes until my esophagus heals."

4. The nurse is planning the care of a client diagnosed with lower esophageal sphincter dysfunction. Which dietary modifications should be included in the plan of care?
   1. Allow any of the client's favorite foods as long as the amount of the food is limited.
   2. Have the client perform eructation exercises several times a day.
   3. Eat four (4) to six (6) small meals a day and limit fluids during mealtimes.
   4. Encourage the client to consume a glass of red wine with one (1) meal a day.

5. The nurse is caring for a client diagnosed with gastroesophageal reflux disease (GERD). Which nursing interventions should be implemented?
   1. Place the client prone in bed and administer nonsteroidal anti-inflammatory medications.
   2. Have the client remain upright at all times and walk for 30 minutes three (3) times a week.
   3. Instruct the client to maintain a right lateral side-lying position and take antacids before meals.
   4. Elevate the head of the bed 30 degrees and discuss lifestyle modifications with the client.

6. The nurse is caring for an adult client diagnosed with gastroesophageal reflux disease (GERD). Which condition is the most common comorbid disease associated with GERD?
   1. Adult-onset asthma.
   2. Pancreatitis.
   3. Peptic ulcer disease.
   4. Increased gastric emptying.

7. The nurse is administering morning medications at 0730. Which medication would have priority?
   1. A proton pump inhibitor.
   2. A nonnarcotic analgesic.
   3. A histamine receptor antagonist.
   4. A mucosal barrier agent.

8. The nurse is preparing a client diagnosed with gastroesophageal reflux disease (GERD) for surgery. Which information should be brought to the attention of the health-care provider?
   1. The client's Bernstein esophageal test was positive.
   2. The client's abdominal x-ray shows a hiatal hernia.
   3. The client's WBC count is 14,000 mg/dL.
   4. The client's hemoglobin is 13.8 mg/dL.

9. The charge nurse is making assignments. Staffing includes a registered nurse with five (5) years of medical-surgical experience, a newly graduated registered nurse, and two (2) unlicensed nursing assistants. Which client should be assigned to the most experienced nurse?
   1. The 39-year-old client diagnosed with lower esophageal dysfunction who is complaining of pyrosis.
   2. The 54-year-old client diagnosed with Barrett's esophagitis who is scheduled to have an endoscopy this morning.
   3. The 46-year-old client diagnosed with gastroesophageal reflux disease who has wheezes in all five (5) lobes.
   4. The 68-year-old client who is three (3) days post-op hiatal hernia and needs to be ambulated four (4) times today.

10. Which statement made by the client would alert the nurse that the client may be experiencing GERD?
    1. "My chest hurts when I walk up the stairs in my home."
    2. "I take antacid tablets with me wherever I go."
    3. "My spouse tells me I snore very loudly at night."
    4. "I drink six (6) to seven (7) soft drinks every day."

11. The nurse is performing an admission assessment on a client diagnosed with gastroesophageal reflux disease (GERD). Which signs and symptoms would indicate GERD?
    1. Pyrosis, water brash, and flatulence.
    2. Weight loss, dysarthria, and diarrhea.
    3. Decreased abdominal fat, proteinuria, and constipation.
    4. Mid-epigastric pain, positive *H. pylori* test, and melena.

12. The client diagnosed with gastroesophageal reflux disease (GERD) is at greater risk for which disease?
    1. Hiatal hernia.
    2. Gastroenteritis.
    3. Esophageal cancer.
    4. Gastric cancer.

## Inflammatory Bowel Disease

13. The client is diagnosed with ulcerative colitis. When assessing this client, which sign/symptom would the nurse expect to find?
    1. Twenty bloody stools a day.
    2. Oral temperature of 102°F.
    3. Hard, rigid abdomen.
    4. Urinary stress incontinence.

14. The client is prescribed prednisone, a steroid, for an acute episode of inflammatory bowel disease. Which intervention should the nurse discuss with the client?
    1. Take this medication on an empty stomach.
    2. Notify the HCP if you experience a moon face.
    3. Be sure to take this medication as prescribed.
    4. Take the medication in the morning only.

15. The client diagnosed with inflammatory bowel disease has a serum potassium level of 3.4 mEq/L. Which action should the nurse implement first?
    1. Notify the health-care provider.
    2. Assess the client for leg cramps.
    3. Request telemetry for the client.
    4. Prepare to administer potassium IV.

16. The client is diagnosed with an acute exacerbation of ulcerative colitis. Which intervention should the nurse implement?
    1. Provide a low-residue diet.
    2. Monitor intravenous fluids.
    3. Assess vital signs daily.
    4. Administer antacids orally.

17. The client diagnosed with IBD is prescribed total parental nutrition (TPN). Which intervention should the nurse implement?
    1. Check the client's glucose level.
    2. Administer an oral hypoglycemic.
    3. Assess the peripheral intravenous site.
    4. Monitor the client's oral food intake.

18. The client is diagnosed with an acute exacerbation of IBD. Which priority intervention should the nurse implement first?
    1. Weigh the client daily and document it in the client's chart.
    2. Teach coping strategies such as dietary modifications.
    3. Record the frequency, amount, and color of stools.
    4. Monitor the client's oral fluid intake every shift.

19. The client diagnosed with Crohn's disease is crying and tells the nurse, "I can't take it anymore. I never know when I will get sick and end up here in the hospital." Which statement would be the nurse's best response?
    1. "I understand how frustrating this must be for you."
    2. "You must keep thinking about the good things in your life."
    3. "I can see you are very upset. I'll sit down and we can talk."
    4. "Are you thinking about doing anything like committing suicide?"

20. The client diagnosed with ulcerative colitis has had an ileostomy. Which statement indicates the client needs more teaching concerning the ileostomy?
    1. "My stoma should be pink and moist."
    2. "I will irrigate my ileostomy every morning."
    3. "If I get a red, bumpy, itchy rash I will call my HCP."
    4. "I will change my pouch if it starts leaking."

21. The client diagnosed with IBD is prescribed sulfasalazine (Asulfidine), a sulfonamide antibiotic. Which statement best describes the rationale for administering this medication?
    1. It is administered rectally to help decrease colon inflammation.
    2. This medication slows gastrointestinal motility and reduces diarrhea.
    3. This medication kills the bacteria that cause the exacerbation.
    4. It acts topically on the colon mucosa to decreases inflammation.

22. The client is diagnosed with Crohn's disease, also known as regional enteritis. Which statement by the client would support this diagnosis?
    1. "My pain goes away when I have a bowel movement."
    2. "I have bright red blood in my stool all the time."
    3. "I have episodes of diarrhea and constipation."
    4. "My abdomen is hard and rigid and I have a fever."

23. The client diagnosed with ulcerative colitis is prescribed a low-residue diet. Which meal selection indicates the client understands the diet teaching?
    1. Grilled hamburger on a wheat bun and fried potatoes.
    2. A chicken salad sandwich and lettuce and tomato salad.
    3. Roast pork, white rice, and plain custard.
    4. Fried fish, whole grain pasta, and fruit salad.

24. The client with ulcerative colitis is scheduled for an ileostomy. The nurse is aware that the client's stoma will be located in which area of the abdomen?

    1. A
    2. B
    3. C
    4. D

## Peptic Ulcer Disease

25. Which assessment data support the client's diagnosis of gastric ulcer?
    1. Presence of blood in the client's stool for the past month.
    2. Complaints of a burning sensation that moves like a wave.
    3. Sharp pain in the upper abdomen after eating a heavy meal.
    4. Comparison of complaints of pain with ingestion of food and sleep.

26. The client has been seen by the health-care provider and the suspected diagnosis is peptic ulcer disease. Which diagnostic test would confirm this diagnosis?
    1. Esophagogastroduodenoscopy (EGD).
    2. Magnetic resonance imaging (MRI).
    3. Occult blood test.
    4. Gastric acid stimulation.

27. When the nurse is conducting the initial interview, which specific data should the nurse obtain from the client who is suspected of having peptic ulcer disease?
    1. History of side effects experienced from all medication.
    2. Use of nonsteroidal anti-inflammatory drugs (NSAIDs).
    3. Any known allergies to drugs and environmental factors.
    4. Medical histories of at least three (3) generations.

28. When assessing the client with the diagnosis of peptic ulcer disease, which physical examination should the nurse implement first?
    1. Auscultate the client's bowel sounds in all four quadrants.
    2. Palpate the abdominal area for tenderness.
    3. Percuss the abdominal borders to identify organs.
    4. Assess the tender area progressing to nontender.

29. The client diagnosed with peptic ulcer disease is admitted into the hospital. Which nursing diagnosis should the nurse include in the plan of care to observe for physiological complications?
    1. Alteration in bowel elimination patterns.
    2. Knowledge deficit in the causes of ulcers.
    3. Inability to cope with changing family roles.
    4. Potential for alteration in gastric emptying.

30. The client has been admitted to the hospital with hemorrhaging from a duodenal ulcer. Which collaborative interventions should the nurse implement? Select all that apply.
    1. Perform a complete pain assessment.
    2. Evaluate BP lying, sitting, and standing
    3. Administer antibiotics intravenously.
    4. Administer blood products.
    5. Monitor intake of a soft, bland diet.

31. When planning the care for a client diagnosed with peptic ulcer disease, which expected outcome should the nurse include?
    1. The client's pain is controlled with the use of NSAIDs.
    2. The client maintains lifestyle modifications.
    3. The client has no signs and symptoms of hemoptysis.
    4. The client takes antacids with each meal.

32. The nurse has been assigned to care for a client diagnosed with peptic ulcer disease. When the nurse is evaluating care, which assessment data require further intervention?
    1. Bowel sounds auscultated fifteen (15) times in one (1) minute.
    2. Belching after eating a heavy and fatty meal late at night.
    3. A decrease in systolic BP of 20 mm Hg from lying to sitting.
    4. A decreased frequency of distress located in the epigastric region.

33. Which medication should the nurse question before administering to the client with peptic ulcer disease?
    1. E-mycin, an antibiotic.
    2. Prilosec, a proton pump inhibitor.
    3. Flagyl, an antimicrobial agent.
    4. Tylenol, a nonnarcotic analgesic.

34. The nurse has administered an antibiotic, a proton pump inhibitor, and Pepto-Bismol for peptic ulcer disease secondary to *H. pylori*. Which data would indicate to the nurse that the medications are effective?
    1. A decrease in alcohol intake.
    2. Maintaining a bland diet.
    3. A return to previous activities.
    4. A decrease in gastric distress.

35. Which assessment data would indicate to the nurse that the client's gastric ulcer has perforated?
    1. Complaints of sudden, sharp, substernal pain.
    2. Rigid, boardlike abdomen with rebound tenderness.
    3. Frequent, clay-colored, liquid stool.
    4. Complaints of vague abdominal pain in the right upper quadrant.

36. The client with a history of peptic ulcer disease has been admitted into the hospital intensive care unit with frank gastric bleeding. Which priority intervention should the nurse implement?
    1. Maintain a strict record of intake and output.
    2. Insert a nasogastric tube and begin saline lavage.
    3. Assist the client with keeping a detailed calorie count.
    4. Provide a quite environment to promote rest.

## Colorectal Disease

37. The occupational health nurse is preparing a presentation to a group of factory workers about preventing colon cancer. Which information should be included in the presentation?
    1. Wear a high filtration mask when around chemicals.
    2. Eat several servings of cruciferous vegetables daily.
    3. Take a multiple vitamin every day.
    4. Do not engage in high-risk sexual behaviors.

38. The nurse is admitting a male client to a medical floor with a diagnosis of adenocarcinoma of the rectosigmoid colon. Which assessment data support this diagnosis?
    1. The client reports up to 20 bloody stools per day.
    2. The client states that he has a feeling of fullness after a heavy meal.
    3. The client has diarrhea alternating with constipation.
    4. The client complains of right lower quadrant pain with rebound tenderness.

39. The 85-year-old male client diagnosed with cancer of the colon asks the nurse, "Why did I get this cancer?" Which statement is the nurse's best response?
    1. Cancer of the colon is associated with a lack of fiber in the diet.
    2. Cancer of the colon has a greater incidence among those younger than age 50 years.
    3. Cancer of the colon has no known risk factors.
    4. Cancer of the colon is rare among male clients.

40. The nurse is planning the care of a client who has had an abdominal perineal resection for cancer of the colon. Which interventions should the nurse implement? Select all that apply.
    1. Provide meticulous skin care to stoma.
    2. Assess the flank incision.
    3. Maintain the indwelling catheter.
    4. Irrigate the J-P drains every shift.
    5. Position the client semi-recumbent.

41. The client who has had an abdominal perineal resection is being discharged. Which discharge information should the nurse teach?
    1. The stoma should be a white, blue, or purple color.
    2. Limit ambulation to prevent the pouch from coming off.
    3. Take pain medication when the pain level is at an "8."
    4. Empty the pouch when it is one-third to one-half full.

42. The nurse caring for a client one (1) day postoperative sigmoid resection notes a moderate amount of dark reddish brown drainage on the midline abdominal incision. Which intervention should the nurse implement first?
    1. Mark the drainage on the dressing with the time and date.
    2. Change the dressing immediately using sterile technique.
    3. Notify the health-care provider immediately.
    4. Reinforce the dressing with a sterile gauze pad.

43. The client complains to the nurse of unhappiness with the health-care provider. Which intervention should the nurse implement next?
    1. Call the HCP and suggest he or she talk with the client.
    2. Determine what about the HCP is bothering the client.
    3. Notify the nursing supervisor to arrange a new HCP to take over.
    4. Explain to the client that until discharge, the client will have to keep the HCP.

44. The client with a new colostomy is being discharged. Which statement made by the client indicates the need for further teaching?
    1. "If I notice any skin breakdown I will call the HCP."
    2. "I should drink only liquids until the colostomy starts to work."
    3. "I should not take a tub bath until the HCP okays it."
    4. "I should not drive or lift more than five (5) pounds."

45. The nurse is preparing to hang a new bag of total parental nutrition on a client that has had an abdominal perineal resection. The bag has 1500 mL of 50% dextrose, 10 mL of trace elements, 20 mL of multivitamins, 20 mL of potassium chloride, and 500 mL of lipids. The bag is to infuse over the next 24 hours. At what rate should the nurse set the pump? _____

46. The nurse is caring for clients in an outpatient clinic. Which information should the nurse teach regarding the American Cancer Society's recommendations for the early detection of colon cancer?
    1. Beginning at age 60, a digital rectal exam should be done yearly.
    2. After the client reaches middle age, a yearly fecal occult test should be done.
    3. At age 50, a colonoscopy and then once every five (5) to ten (10) years.
    4. A flexible sigmoidoscopy should be done yearly after age 40.

Gastrointestinal

47. The nurse writes a psychosocial problem of "risk for altered sexual functioning related to new colostomy." Which intervention should the nurse implement?
    1. Tell the client that there should be no intimacy for at least three (3) months.
    2. Ensure that the client and significant other are able to change the ostomy pouch.
    3. Demonstrate with charts possible sexual positions for the client to assume.
    4. Teach the client to protect the pouch from becoming dislodged during sex.

48. The client presents with a complete blockage of the large intestine from a large tumor. Which health-care provider's order would the nurse question?
    1. Obtain consent for a colonoscopy and biopsy.
    2. Start an IV of 0.9% saline at 125 mL/hour.
    3. Administer 3 liters of Go-LYTELY.
    4. Give tap water enemas until it is clear.

## Diverticulosis/Diverticulitis

49. The client admitted to the medical unit with diverticulitis is complaining of severe pain in the left lower quadrant and has an oral temperature of 100.6°F. Which action should the nurse implement first?
    1. Notify the health-care provider.
    2. Document the findings in the chart.
    3. Administer an oral antipyretic.
    4. Assess the client's abdomen.

50. The nurse is teaching the client diagnosed with diverticulosis. Which instruction should the nurse include in the teaching session?
    1. Discuss the importance of drinking 1000 mL of water daily.
    2. Instruct the client to exercise at least three (3) times a week.
    3. Teach the client about a eating a low-residue diet.
    4. Explain the need to have daily bowel movements.

51. The client is admitted to the medical unit with a diagnosis of acute diverticulitis. Which health-care provider's order should the nurse question?
    1. Insert a nasogastric tube.
    2. Start IV D5W at 125 mL/hr.
    3. Put client on a clear liquid diet.
    4. Place client on bed rest with bathroom privileges.

52. The nurse is discussing the therapeutic diet for the client diagnosed with diverticulosis. Which meal indicates the client understands the discharge teaching?
    1. Fried fish, mashed potatoes, and iced tea.
    2. Ham sandwich, applesauce, and whole milk.
    3. Chicken salad on whole-wheat bread and water.
    4. Lettuce, tomato, and cucumber salad and coffee.

53. The client is two (2) hours post-colonoscopy. Which assessment data would warrant intermediate intervention by the nurse?
    1. The client has a soft, nontender abdomen.
    2. The client has a loose, watery stool.
    3. The client has hyperactive bowel sounds.
    4. The client's pulse is 104 and BP is 98/60.

54. The nurse is preparing to administer an aminoglycoside antibiotic to the client just admitted with a diagnosis of acute diverticulitis. Which intervention should the nurse implement?
    1. Obtain a serum trough level.
    2. Ask about drug allergies.
    3. Monitor the peak level.
    4. Assess the vital signs.

55. The client diagnosed with acute diverticulitis is complaining of severe abdominal pain. On assessment, the nurse finds a hard, rigid abdomen and T 102°F. Which intervention should the nurse implement?
    1. Notify the health-care provider.
    2. Prepare to administer a Fleet's enema.
    3. Administer an antipyretic suppository.
    4. Continue to monitor the client closely.

56. The nurse is preparing to administer a 250-mL intravenous antibiotic to the client. The medication must infuse in one (1) hour. An intravenous pump is not available and the nurse must administer the medication via gravity with IV tubing 10 gtts/min. At what rate should the nurse infuse the medication?_____

57. The client with acute diverticulitis has a nasogastric tube draining green liquid bile. Which action should the nurse implement?
    1. Document the findings as normal.
    2. Assess the client's bowel sounds.
    3. Determine the client's last bowel movement.
    4. Insert the N/G tube at least 2 more inches.

58. The nurse is teaching a class on diverticulosis. Which interventions should the nurse discuss when teaching ways to prevent an acute exacerbation of diverticulosis? Select all that apply.
    1. Eat a high-fiber diet.
    2. Increase fluid intake.
    3. Elevate the HOB after eating.
    4. Walk 30 minutes a day.
    5. Take an antacid every two (2) hours.

59. Which client would be most likely to have the diagnosis of diverticulosis?
    1. A 60-year-old male with a sedentary lifestyle.
    2. A 72-year-old female with multiple childbirths.
    3. A 63-year-old female with hemorrhoids.
    4. A 40-year-old male with a family history of diverticulosis.

60. The client is admitted to the medical floor with acute diverticulitis. Which collaborative intervention would the nurse anticipate the health-care provider ordering?
    1. Administer total parenteral nutrition.
    2. Maintain NPO and nasogastric tube.
    3. Maintain on a high-fiber diet and increase fluids.
    4. Obtain consent for abdominal surgery.

## Gallbladder Disorders

61. The client is four (4) hours postoperative open cholecystectomy. Which data would warrant immediate intervention by the nurse?
    1. Absent bowel sounds in all four (4) quadrants.
    2. The T-tube with 60 mL of green drainage.
    3. Urine output of 100 mL in the past three (3) hours.
    4. Refusal to turn, deep breathe, and cough.

62. The client two (2) hours postoperative laparoscopic cholecystectomy is complaining of severe pain in the right shoulder. Which nursing intervention should the nurse implement?
    1. Apply a heating pad to the abdomen for 15 to 20 minutes.
    2. Administer morphine sulfate intravenously after diluting with saline.
    3. Contact the surgeon for an order to x-ray the right shoulder.
    4. Apply a sling to the right arm that was injured in surgery.

63. The nurse is teaching a client recovering from a laparoscopic cholecystectomy. Which statement indicates the discharge teaching was effective?
    1. "I will take my lipid-lowering medicine at the same time each night."
    2. "I may experience some discomfort when I eat a high-fat meal."
    3. "I need someone to stay with me for about a week after surgery."
    4. "I should not splint my incision when I deep breathe and cough."

64. When assessing the client recovering from an open cholecystectomy, which signs and symptoms should the nurse report to the health-care provider? Select all that apply.
    1. Clay-colored stools.
    2. Yellow-tinted sclera.
    3. Dark yellow urine.
    4. Feverish chills.
    5. Abdominal pain.

65. The nurse is caring for the immediate postoperative client who had a laparoscopic cholecystectomy. Which task could the nurse delegate to the unlicensed nursing assistant?
    1. Check the abdominal dressings for bleeding.
    2. Increase the IV fluid if the blood pressure is low.
    3. Document the amount of output on the I & O sheet.
    4. Listen to the breath sounds in all lobes.

66. Which assessment data should the nurse expect to find for the client who had an upper gastrointestinal (UGI) series?
    1. Chalky white stools.
    2. Increased heart rate.
    3. A firm hard abdomen.
    4. Hyperactive bowel sounds.

67. The client is one (1) hour post-endoscopic retrograde cholangiopancreatogram (ERCP). Which intervention should the nurse include in the plan of care?
    1. Instruct the client to cough forcefully.
    2. Encourage early ambulation.
    3. Assess for return of a gag reflex.
    4. Administer held medications.

68. Which expected outcome would be appropriate for the client scheduled to have a cholecystectomy?
    1. Decreased pain management.
    2. Ambulate first day postoperative.
    3. No break in skin integrity.
    4. Knowledge of postoperative care.

69. Which assessment data indicate that the client recovering from an open cholecystectomy requires pain medication?
    1. The client's pulse is 65 beats per minute.
    2. The client has shallow respirations.
    3. The client's bowel sounds are 20 per minute.
    4. The client uses a pillow to splint when coughing.

70. Which laboratory value would the nurse expect to find indicating a chronic inflammation in the client with cholecystitis?
    1. An elevated white blood cell (WBC) count.
    2. A decreased lactate dehydrogenase (LDH)
    3. An elevated alkaline phosphatase.
    4. A decreased direct bilirubin level.

71. Which nursing diagnosis would be highest priority for the client who had an open cholecystectomy surgery?
    1. Alteration in nutrition.
    2. Alteration in skin integrity.
    3. Alteration in urinary pattern.
    4. Alteration in comfort.

72. The client is six (6) hours postoperative open cholecystectomy and the nurse finds a large amount of red drainage on the dressing. Which intervention should the nurse implement?
    1. Measure the abdominal girth.
    2. Palpate the lower abdomen for a mass.
    3. Turn client onto side to assess for further drainage.
    4. Remove the dressing to determine the source.

## Liver Failure

73. The client diagnosed with end-stage liver failure is admitted to the medical unit diagnosed with esophageal bleeding. The HCP inserts and inflates a triple-lumen nasogastric tube (Sengstaken-Blakemore). Which nursing action should the nurse implement for this treatment?
    1. Assess the gag reflex every shift.
    2. Stay with the client at all times.
    3. Administer the laxative lactulose (Chronulac).
    4. Monitor the client's ammonia level.

74. The client has had a liver biopsy. Which post-procedure intervention should the nurse implement?
    1. Instruct the client to void immediately.
    2. Keep the client NPO for eight (8) hours.
    3. Place the client on the right side.
    4. Monitor blood urea nitrogen (BUN) and creatinine level.

75. The client diagnosed with end-stage liver failure is admitted with hepatic encephalopathy. Which dietary restriction should be implemented by the nurse to address this complication?
    1. Restrict sodium intake to 2 g/day.
    2. Limit oral fluids to 1500 mL/day.
    3. Decrease the daily fat intake.
    4. Reduce protein intake to 60 to 80 g/day.

76. The client diagnosed with end-stage renal failure with ascites is scheduled for a paracentesis. Which client teaching should the nurse discuss with the client?
    1. Explain that the procedure will be done in the operating room.
    2. Instruct the client that a Foley catheter will have to be inserted.
    3. Tell the client that vital signs will be taken frequently after the procedure.
    4. Provide instructions on holding the breath when the HCP inserts the catheter.

77. The client diagnosed with liver failure is experiencing pruritus secondary to severe jaundice. Which action by the unlicensed assistant warrants intervention by the primary nurse?
    1. Assisting the client to take a hot soapy shower.
    2. Applying an emollient to the client's legs and back.
    3. Putting mittens on both hands of the client.
    4. Patting the client's skin dry with a clean towel.

78. The nurse identifies the client problem as "excess fluid volume" for the client in liver failure. Which short-term goal would be most appropriate for this problem?
    1. The client will not gain more that two (2) kg a day.
    2. The client will have no increase in abdominal girth.
    3. The client's vital signs will remain within normal limits (WNL).
    4. The client will receive a low-sodium diet.

79. The client is in end-stage liver failure and has vitamin K deficiency. Which interventions should the nurse implement? Select all that apply.
    1. Avoid rectal temperatures.
    2. Use only a soft toothbrush.
    3. Monitor the platelet count.
    4. Use small-gauge needles.
    5. Assess for asterixis.

80. The client is in end-stage liver failure. Which gastrointestinal assessment data would the nurse expect to find when assessing the client?
    1. Hypoalbuminemia and muscle wasting.
    2. Oligomenorrhea and decreased body hair.
    3. Clay-colored stools and hemorrhoids.
    4. Dyspnea and caput medusae.

81. Which assessment question would be priority for the nurse to ask the client diagnosed with end-stage liver failure secondary to alcoholic cirrhosis?
    1. How many years have you been drinking alcohol?
    2. Have you completed an advanced directive?
    3. When did you have your last alcoholic drink?
    4. What foods did you eat at your last meal?

82. The client has end-stage liver failure secondary to alcoholic cirrhosis. Which complication indicates the client is at risk for developing hepatic encephalopathy?
    1. Gastrointestinal bleeding.
    2. Hypoalbuminemia.
    3. Splenomegaly.
    4. Hyperaldosteronism.

83. The client is diagnosed with end-stage liver failure. The client asks the nurse, "Why is my doctor decreasing the doses of my medications?" Which statement is the nurse's best response?
    1. "You are worried that your doctor has decreased the dosage."
    2. "You really should ask your doctor. I am sure there is a good reason."
    3. "You may have an overdose of the medication because your liver is damaged."
    4. "The half-life is altered because the liver is damaged."

84. The client is admitted with end-stage liver failure and is prescribed the laxative lactulose (Chronulac). Which statement indicates the client needs more teaching concerning this medication?
    1. "I should have two to three soft stools a day."
    2. "I must check my ammonia level daily."
    3. "If I have diarrhea, I will call my doctor."
    4. "I should check my stool for any blood."

## Hepatitis

85. The client is in the preicteric phase of hepatitis. Which signs/symptoms would the nurse expect the client to exhibit during this phase?
    1. Clay-colored stools and jaundice.
    2. Normal appetite and pruritus.
    3. Being afebrile and left upper quadrant pain.
    4. Complaints of fatigue and diarrhea.

86. Which type of hepatitis is transmitted by the fecal–oral route via contaminated food, water, or direct contact with an infected person?
    1. Hepatitis A.
    2. Hepatitis B.
    3. Hepatitis C.
    4. Hepatitis D.

87. Which type of precaution should the nurse implement to protect from being exposed to any of the hepatitis viruses?
    1. Airborne precautions.
    2. Standard precautions.
    3. Droplet precautions.
    4. Exposure precautions.

88. The school nurse is discussing ways to prevent an outbreak of hepatitis A with a group of high school teachers. Which action is the most important intervention that the school nurse must explain to the school teachers?
    1. Do not allow students to eat or drink after each other.
    2. Drink bottled water as much as possible.
    3. Encourage protected sexual activity.
    4. Thoroughly wash hands.

89. Which instruction should the nurse discuss with the client who is in the icteric phase of hepatitis C?
    1. Decrease alcohol intake.
    2. Encourage rest periods.
    3. Eat a large evening meal.
    4. Drink diet drinks and juices.

90. The public health nurse is discussing hepatitis B with a group in the community. Which health promotion activities should the nurse discuss with the group? Select all that apply.
    1. Do not share needles or equipment.
    2. Use barrier protection during sex.
    3. Get the hepatitis B vaccines.
    4. Obtain immune globulin injections.
    5. Avoid any type of hepatotoxic medications.

91. The client with hepatitis asks the nurse, "I went to an herbalist, who recommended I take milk thistle. What do you think about that?" Which statement is the nurse's best response?
    1. "You are concerned about taking an herb."
    2. "The herb has been used to treat liver disease."
    3. "I would not take anything that is not prescribed."
    4. "Why would you want to take any herbs?"

92. The nurse writes the client problem "imbalanced nutrition: less than body requirements" for the client diagnosed with hepatitis. Which intervention should the nurse include in the plan of care?
    1. Provide a high-calorie intake diet.
    2. Discuss total parenteral nutrition (TPN).
    3. Instruct the client to decrease salt intake.
    4. Encourage the client to increase water intake.

93. The female nurse sticks herself with a dirty needle. Which action should the nurse implement first?
    1. Notify the infection control nurse.
    2. Cleanse the area with soap and water.
    3. Request post-exposure prophylaxis.
    4. Check the hepatitis status of the client.

94. The client diagnosed with liver problems asks the nurse, "Why are my stools clay-colored?" On which scientific rationale should the nurse base the response?
    1. There is an increase in serum ammonia level.
    2. The liver is unable to excrete bilirubin.
    3. The liver is unable to metabolize fatty foods.
    4. A damaged liver cannot detoxify vitamins.

95. Which statement by the client diagnosed with hepatitis would warrant immediate intervention by the clinic nurse?
    1. "I will not drink any type of beer or mixed drink."
    2. "I will get adequate rest so that I don't get exhausted."
    3. "I had a big hearty breakfast this morning."
    4. "I took some cough syrup for this nasty head cold."

96. Which task would be most appropriate for the nurse to delegate to the unlicensed nursing assistant?
    1. Draw the serum liver function test.
    2. Evaluate the client's intake and output.
    3. Assist the client to the bedside commode.
    4. Help the ward clerk transcribe orders.

## Gastroenteritis

97. The female client came to the clinic complaining of abdominal cramping and has had at least 10 episodes of diarrhea every day for the last 2 days. The client reported that she had been in Mexico on a mission trip and just returned yesterday. Which intervention should the nurse implement?
    1. Instruct the client to take a cathartic laxative daily.
    2. Encourage the client to drink lots of Gatorade.
    3. Discuss the need to increase protein in the diet.
    4. Explain that the client should weigh herself daily.

98. Which intervention should the nurse include when discussing ways to help prevent potential episodes of gastroenteritis from *Clostridium* botulism?
    1. Make sure that all hamburger meat is well cooked.
    2. Ensure that all dairy products are refrigerated.
    3. Discuss that campers should drink only bottled water.
    4. Discard all canned goods that are damaged.

99. The client is diagnosed with salmonellosis secondary to eating some slightly cooked hamburger meat. Which clinical manifestations would the nurse expect the client to report?
    1. Abdominal cramping, nausea, and vomiting.
    2. Neuromuscular paralysis and dysphagia.
    3. Gross amounts of explosive bloody diarrhea.
    4. Frequent "rice water stool" with no fecal odor.

100. The client is diagnosed with gastroenteritis. Which laboratory data would warrant immediate intervention by the nurse?
    1. A serum sodium level of 137 mEq/L.
    2. An arterial blood gas of pH 7.37, $PaO_2$ 95, $PaCO_2$ 43, $HCO_3$ 24.
    3. A serum potassium level of 3.3 mEq/L.
    4. A stool sample that is positive for fecal leukocytes.

101. The client diagnosed with gastroenteritis is being discharged from the emergency department. Which intervention should the nurse include in the discharge teaching?
    1. If diarrhea persists for more than 96 hours, contact the physician.
    2. Instruct the client to wash hands thoroughly before handling any type of food.
    3. Explain the importance of decreasing steroids gradually as instructed.
    4. Discuss how to collect all stool samples for the next 24 hours.

102. Which medication would the nurse expect the health-care provider to order to treat the client diagnosed with botulism secondary to eating contaminated canned goods?
    1. An antidiarrheal medication.
    2. An aminoglycoside antibiotic.
    3. An antitoxin medication.
    4. An ACE inhibitor medication.

103. Which nursing problem is priority for the 76-year-old client diagnosed with gastroenteritis from staphylococcal food poisoning?
    1. Fluid volume deficit.
    2. Nausea.
    3. Risk for aspiration.
    4. Impaired urinary elimination.

104. Which assessment data would the nurse expect to find in the client diagnosed with acute gastroenteritis?
    1. Decreased gurgling sounds on auscultation of the abdominal wall.
    2. A hard, firm edematous abdomen on palpation.
    3. Frequent, small melena-type liquid bowel movements.
    4. Bowel assessment reveals loud, rushing bowel sounds.

105. The 79-year-old client diagnosed with acute gastroenteritis is admitted to the medical unit. Which nursing task would be most appropriate for the nurse to delegate to the unlicensed nursing assistant?
    1. Evaluate the client's intake and output.
    2. Take the client's vital signs.
    3. Change the client's intravenous solution.
    4. Assess the client's perianal area.

106. The emergency department nurse knows the client diagnosed with acute gastroenteritis understands the discharge teaching when the client makes which statement?
    1. "I will probably have some leg cramps while I have gastroenteritis."
    2. "I should decrease my fluid intake until the diarrhea subsides."
    3. "I should reintroduce solid foods very slowly into my diet."
    4. "I should only drink bottled water until the abdominal cramping stops."

107. Which nursing interventions should be included in the care plan for the 84-year-old client diagnosed with acute gastroenteritis? Select all that apply.
    1. Assess the skin turgor on the back of the client's hands.
    2. Monitor the client for orthostatic hypotension.
    3. Record the frequency and characteristics of sputum.
    4. Use standard precautions when caring for the client.
    5. Institute safety precautions when ambulating the client.

108. The nurse has received the A.M. shift report. Which client should the nurse assess first?
    1. The 44-year-old client diagnosed with peptic ulcer disease who is complaining of acute epigastric pain.
    2. The 74-year-old client diagnosed with acute gastroenteritis who has had four (4) diarrhea stools during the night.
    3. The 65-year-old client diagnosed with inflammatory bowel disease who has a hard, rigid abdomen and elevated temperature.
    4. The 15-year-old client diagnosed with food poisoning who has vomited several times during the night shift.

## Abdominal Surgery

109. The male client has had abdominal surgery and is now diagnosed with peritonitis. Which assessment data support the client's diagnosis of peritonitis?
    1. Absent bowel sounds and potassium level of 3.9 mEq/L.
    2. Abdominal cramping and hemoglobin of 14 gm/dL.
    3. Profuse diarrhea and stool specimen shows *Campylobacter*.
    4. Hard, rigid abdomen and white blood cell count 22,000 mm.

110. The client has had abdominal surgery and tells the nurse, "I felt as something just gave way in my stomach." Which action should the nurse implement first?
    1. Notify the surgeon immediately.
    2. Instruct the client to splint the incision.
    3. Assess for serosanguineous wound drainage.
    4. Administer pain medication intravenously.

111. The client is one (1) day postoperative major abdominal surgery. Which client problem is priority?
    1. Impaired skin integrity.
    2. Fluid and electrolyte imbalance.
    3. Altered bowel elimination.
    4. Altered body image.

112. The client has a large abdominal wound that has eviscerated. Which intervention should the nurse implement?
    1. Apply sterile normal saline dressing.
    2. Use sterile gloves to replace protruding parts.
    3. Place the client in the reverse Trendelenburg position.
    4. Administer intravenous antibiotic stat.

113. The client is diagnosed with peritonitis. Which assessment data indicate the client's condition is improving?
    1. The client is using more pain medication on a daily basis.
    2. The client's nasogastric tube is draining coffee-ground material.
    3. The client has a decrease in temperature and a soft abdomen.
    4. The client has had two (2) soft, formed bowel movements.

114. The client has developed a paralytic ileus after abdominal surgery. Which intervention should the nurse include in the plan of care?
    1. Administer a laxative of choice.
    2. Encourage client to increase oral fluids.
    3. Encourage the client to take deep breaths.
    4. Maintain a patent nasogastric tube.

115. The client who has had an abdominal surgery has a Jackson Pratt (JP) drainage tube. Which assessment data would warrant immediate intervention by the nurse?
    1. The bulb is round and has 40 mL of fluid.
    2. The drainage tube is pinned to the dressing.
    3. The JP insertion site is pink and has no drainage.
    4. The JP bulb has suction and is sunken in.

116. The post-anesthesia care nurse is caring for a client who has had abdominal surgery. The client is complaining of nausea. Which intervention should the nurse implement first?
    1. Medicate the client with a narcotic analgesic IVP.
    2. Assess the nasogastric tube for patency.
    3. Check the temperature for elevation.
    4. Hyperextend the neck to prevent stridor.

117. The nurse is completing the shift assessment on the client recovering from abdominal surgery who has a PCA pump. The client has shallow respirations and refuses to deep breathe. Which intervention should the nurse implement?
    1. Insist that the client take deep breaths.
    2. Notify the surgeon to request a chest x-ray.
    3. Determine the last time the client used the PCA pump.
    4. Administer oxygen 2 L/min via nasal cannula.

118. The client has a nasogastric tube. The health-care provider orders IV fluid replacement based on the previous hour's output plus the baseline IV fluid ordered of 125 mL/hr. From 0800 to 0900 the client's N/G tube drained 45 mL. At 0900, what rate should the nurse set the IV pump?_____

119. The nurse is caring for the following clients on a surgical unit. Which client would the nurse assess first?
    1. The client who had an inguinal hernia repair and has not voided in four (4) hours.
    2. The client who was admitted with abdominal pain who suddenly has no pain.
    3. The client four (4) hours postoperative abdominal surgery with no bowel sounds.
    4. The client who is one (1) day postoperative appendectomy who is being discharged.

120. The 84-year-old client comes to the clinic complaining of right lower abdominal pain. Which question would be most appropriate for the nurse to ask the client?
    1. "When was your last bowel movement?"
    2. "Did you have a high-fat meal last night?"
    3. "How long have you had this pain?"
    4. "Have you been experiencing any gas?"

## Eating Disorders

121. The female client presents to the clinic for an examination because she has not had a menstrual cycle for several months and wonders if she could be pregnant. The client is 5'10" tall and weighs 45 kg. Which assessment data should the nurse obtain first?
    1. Ask the client to recall what she ate for the last 24 hours.
    2. Determine what type of birth control the client has been using.
    3. Reweigh the client to confirm the data.
    4. Take the client's pulse and blood pressure.

122. The occupational health nurse observes the chief financial officer eat large lunch meals. The client disappears into the restroom after a meal for about 20 minutes. Which observation by the nurse would indicate the client has bulimia?
    1. The client jogs two (2) miles a day.
    2. The client has not gained weight.
    3. The client's teeth are a green color.
    4. The client has smooth knuckles.

123. The nurse is caring for a client diagnosed with bulimia nervosa. Which nursing intervention should the nurse implement after the client's evening meal?
    1. Praise the client for eating all the food on the tray.
    2. Stay with the client for 45 minutes to an hour.
    3. Allow the client to work out on the treadmill.
    4. Place the client on bed rest until morning.

124. The nurse writes a nursing diagnosis of "altered nutrition: less than body requirements related to low self-esteem" for a client diagnosed with anorexia. Which client goal should be included in the plan of care?
    1. The nurse will prevent the client from doing excessive exercise.
    2. The client eats 50% of the meals provided.
    3. Dietary will provide high-protein milk shakes t.i.d.
    4. The client will verbalize one positive attribute.

125. The client diagnosed with anorexia nervosa is admitted to the hospital. The client is 67 inches tall and weighs 40 kg. Which client problem has the highest priority?
   1. Altered nutrition.
   2. Low self-esteem.
   3. Disturbed body image.
   4. Altered sexuality.

126. Which diagnostic tests should be monitored for the client diagnosed with severe anorexia nervosa?
   1. Liver function tests.
   2. Kidney function tests.
   3. Cardiac function tests.
   4. Bone density scan.

127. The female client is more than 10% over ideal body weight. Which nursing intervention should the nurse implement first?
   1. Ask the client why she is eating too much.
   2. Refer the client to a gymnasium for exercise.
   3. Have the client set a realistic weight loss goal.
   4. Determine the client's eating patterns.

128. The client who is morbidly obese has undergone gastric bypass surgery. Which immediate postoperative intervention has the greatest priority?
   1. Monitor respiratory status.
   2. Weigh the client daily.
   3. Teach a healthy diet.
   4. Assist the client in behavior modification.

129. The client who is obese presents to the clinic before beginning a weight loss program. Which interventions should the nurse teach? Select all that apply.
   1. Walk for 30 minutes three (3) times a day.
   2. Determine situations that initiate eating behavior.
   3. Weigh at the same time every day.
   4. Limit sodium in the diet.
   5. Refer to a weight support group.

130. The 22-year-old female who is obese is discussing weight loss programs with the nurse. Which information should the nurse teach?
   1. Jog for two (2) to three (3) hours every day.
   2. Lifestyle behaviors must be modified.
   3. Eat one large meal every day in the evening.
   4. Eat 1000 calories a day and don't take vitamins.

131. The 36-year-old female client diagnosed with anorexia nervosa tells the nurse "I am so fat. I won't be able to eat today." Which response by the nurse is most appropriate?
   1. "Can you tell me why you think you are fat?"
   2. "You are skinny. Many women wish they had your problem."
   3. "If you don't eat, we will have to restrain you and feed you."
   4. "Not eating might cause physical problems."

132. The client is being admitted to the outpatient psychiatric clinic diagnosed with bulimia. While assessing the client, which question should the nurse ask to identify behaviors that suggest bulimia?
   1. "When was the last time you exercised?"
   2. "What over-the-counter medications do you take?"
   3. "How long have you had a positive self-image?"
   4. "Do you eat a lot of high-fiber foods for bowel movements?"

## Constipation/Diarrhea Disorders

133. The client being admitted from the emergency department is diagnosed with a fecal impaction. Which nursing intervention should be implemented?
    1. Administer an antidiarrheal medication, every day and PRN.
    2. Perform bowel training every two (2) hours.
    3. Administer oil retention enemas.
    4. Prepare for an upper gastrointestinal (UGI) series x-ray.

134. Which statement made by the client admitted with electrolyte imbalance from frequent cathartic use demonstrates an understanding of the discharge teaching?
    1. "In the future I will eat a banana every time I take the medication."
    2. "I don't have to have a bowel movement every day."
    3. "I should limit the fluids I drink with my meals."
    4. "If I feel sluggish, I will eat a lot of cheese and dairy products."

135. The client has been experiencing difficulty and straining when expelling feces. Which intervention should be taught to the client?
    1. Explain that some blood in the stool will be normal for the client.
    2. Instruct the client in manual removal of feces.
    3. Encourage the client to use a cathartic laxative on a daily basis.
    4. Place the client on a high-residue diet.

136. The client has had a stool that is dark, watery, and shiny in appearance. Which intervention should be the nurse's first action?
    1. Check for a fecal impaction.
    2. Encourage the client to drink fluids.
    3. Check the chart for sodium and potassium levels.
    4. Apply a protective barrier cream to the perianal area.

137. The charge nurse has completed report. Which client should be seen first?
    1. The client diagnosed with Crohn's disease who had two (2) semi-formed stools on the previous shift.
    2. The elderly client admitted from another facility who is complaining of constipation.
    3. The client diagnosed with AIDS who had a 200-mL diarrhea stool and has elastic skin tissue turgor.
    4. The client diagnosed with hemorrhoids who had some spotting of bright red blood on the toilet tissue.

138. The dietician and nurse in a long-term care facility are planning the menu for the day. Which foods would be recommended for the immobile clients for whom swallowing is not an issue?
    1. Cheeseburger and milk shake.
    2. Canned peaches and a sandwich on whole-wheat bread.
    3. Mashed potatoes and mechanically ground red meat.
    4. Biscuits and gravy with bacon.

139. The client diagnosed with AIDS is experiencing voluminous diarrhea. Which interventions should the nurse implement? Select all that apply.
    1. Monitor diarrhea, charting amount, character, and consistency.
    2. Assess the client's tissue turgor every day.
    3. Encourage the client to drink carbonated soft drinks.
    4. Weigh the client daily in the same clothes and at the same time.
    5. Assist the client with a warm sitz bath PRN.

140. The nurse, a licensed practical nurse, and an unlicensed nursing assistant are caring for clients on a medical floor. Which nursing task would be most appropriate to assign to the licensed practical nurse?
    1. Assist the unlicensed nursing assistant to learn to perform blood glucose checks.
    2. Monitor the potassium levels of a client with diarrhea.
    3. Administer a bulk laxative to a client diagnosed with constipation.
    4. Assess the abdomen of a client who has had complaints of pain.

141. The client is placed on percutaneous gastrostomy (PEG) tube feedings. Which occurrence would warrant immediate intervention by the nurse?
    1. The client tolerates the feedings being infused at 50 mL/hour.
    2. The client pulls the nasogastric feeding tube out.
    3. The client complains of being thirsty.
    4. The client has green, watery stool.

142. The client presents to the emergency department experiencing frequent watery, bloody stools after eating some undercooked meat at a fast food restaurant. Which intervention should be implemented first?
    1. Provide the client with a specimen collection hat to collect a stool sample.
    2. Initiate antibiotic therapy intravenously.
    3. Have the laboratory draw a complete blood count.
    4. Administer the antidiarrheal medication Lomotil.

143. The nurse is planning the care of a client diagnosed with infectious diarrhea. Which independent problem should be included in the plan of care?
    1. Risk for hypovolemic shock.
    2. Bacteremia.
    3. Fluid volume deficit.
    4. Increased knowledge of transmission.

144. The nurse is caring for clients on a medical unit. Which client information should be brought to the attention of the HCP immediately?
    1. A serum sodium of 139 mEq/L in a client diagnosed with obstipation.
    2. The client diagnosed with fecal impaction who had two (2) hard formed stools.
    3. A serum potassium level of 3.0 mEq/L in a client diagnosed with diarrhea.
    4. The client with diarrhea who had two (2) semi-liquid stools totaling 300 mL.

## Gastroesophageal Reflux

1. 1. Clients with heartburn are frequently diagnosed as having gastroesophageal reflux disease (GERD). GERD can occasionally cause weight loss, but not weight gain.
   2. Most clients with GERD have been self-medicating with over-the-counter medications prior to seeking advice from a health-care provider. It is important to know what the client has been using to treat the problem.
   3. Milk and dairy products contain lactose, which would be important if considering lactose intolerance, but it is not important for "heartburn."
   4. Heartburn is not a symptom of a viral illness.

   TEST-TAKING HINT: **Clients will use common terms such as "heartburn" to describe symptoms. The nurse must be able to interpret or clarify the meaning of terms used with the client. Part of the assessment of a symptom requires determining what aggravates and alleviates the symptom.**

2. 1. The client should elevate the head of the bed on blocks or use a foam wedge to use gravity to help keep the gastric acid in the stomach and prevent reflux into the esophagus. Behavior modification is changing one's behavior.
   2. The client should be encouraged to quit smoking altogether. Referral to support groups for smoking cessation should be made.
   3. The nurse would be prescribing medication; this is not in the nurse's scope of practice.
   4. The client should be instructed to discontinue using alcohol, but the stem does not indicate the client is an alcoholic.

   TEST-TAKING HINT: **Clients are not encouraged to decrease smoking. Current research indicates that smoking is damaging to many body systems, including the gastrointestinal system. The nurse must always practice in the scope of practice for which the nurse is licensed. Do not assume anything not in the stem of a question.**

3. 1. The client is allowed to eat as soon as the gag reflex has returned.
   2. An esophagogastroduodenoscopy is a diagnostic procedure, not a cure. Therefore the client still has GERD and should be instructed to stay in an upright position for two (2) to three (3) hours after eating.
   3. Stomach contents are acidic and will erode the esophageal lining.
   4. Orange and tomato juices are acidic, and the client diagnosed with GERD should avoid acidic foods until the esophagus has had a chance to heal.

   TEST-TAKING HINT: **This question assumes the test taker has knowledge of diagnostic procedures for specific disease processes.**

4. 1. The client is instructed to avoid spicy and acidic foods and any food that produces symptoms.
   2. Eructation means belching, which is a symptom of GERD.
   3. Clients should eat small, frequent meals and limit fluids with the meals to prevent reflux into the esophagus from a distended stomach.
   4. Clients are encouraged to forgo all alcoholic beverages because alcohol relaxes the lower esophageal sphincter and increases the risk of reflux.

   TEST-TAKING HINT: **The word "any" in answer option "1" should give the test taker a clue that unless there are absolutely no dietary restrictions, this is an incorrect answer. Option "2" requires knowledge of medical terminology.**

5. 1. The client is encouraged to lie with the head of the bed elevated, but this is difficult to achieve when on the stomach. NSAIDs inhibit prostaglandin synthesis in the stomach, which places the client at risk for developing gastric ulcers. The client is already experiencing gastric acid difficulty.
   2. The client will need to lie down at some time, and walking will not help with GERD.
   3. If lying on the side, the left side-lying position, not the right side, will allow less chance of reflux into the esophagus. Antacids are taken one (1) and three (3) hours after a meal.
   4. The head of the bed should be elevated to allow gravity to help in preventing reflux. Lifestyle modifications of losing weight, making dietary modifications, attempting smoking cessation, discontinuing the use of alcohol, and not stooping or bending at the waist all help to decrease reflux.

   TEST-TAKING HINT: **Answer option "2" has an "all," which should alert the test taker that this is an incorrect response. If the test taker has no idea of the answer, lifestyle modifications are an educated guess for most chronic problems.**

6. 1. Of adult-onset asthma cases, 80%–90% are caused by gastroesophageal reflux disease (GERD).
   2. Pancreatitis is not related to GERD.

3. Peptic ulcer disease is related to *H. pylori* bacterial infections and can lead to increased levels of gastric acid, but it is not related to reflux.

4. GERD is not related to increased gastric emptying. Increased gastric emptying would be a benefit to a client with decreased functioning of the lower esophageal sphincter.

**TEST-TAKING HINT: Adjectives such as "increased" should always be examined to determine how to interpret the answer option.**

7. 1. Proton pump inhibitors can be administered at routine dosing times, usually 0900 or after breakfast.

2. Pain medication is important, but a nonnarcotic medication, such as Tylenol, can be administered after a medication that must be timed.

3. A histamine receptor antagonist can be administered at routine dosing times.

4. A mucosal barrier agent must be administered on an empty stomach for the medication to coat the stomach.

**TEST-TAKING HINT: Basic knowledge of how medications work is required to administer medications for peak effectiveness.**

8. 1. In a Bernstein's test, acid is instilled into the distal esophagus; this causes immediate heartburn for a client diagnosed with GERD. This would not warrant notifying the HCP.

2. Hiatal hernias are frequently the cause of GERD; therefore, this finding would not warrant notifying the HCP.

3. The client's WBC is elevated, indicating a possible infection, which warrants notifying the HCP.

4. This is a normal hemoglobin result and would not warrant notifying the HCP.

**TEST-TAKING HINT: When the test taker is deciding when to notify a health-care provider, the answer should be data that are not normal for the disease process or that signal a potential or life-threatening complication.**

9. 1. Pyrosis is heartburn and is expected in a client diagnosed with GERD. The new graduate can care for this client.

2. Barrett's esophagitis is a complication of GERD; new graduates can prepare a client for a diagnostic procedure.

3. This client is exhibiting symptoms of asthma, a complication of GERD; therefore, the client should be assigned to the most experienced nurse.

4. This client can be cared for by the new graduate, and ambulating can be delegated to the unlicensed nursing assistant.

**TEST-TAKING HINT: The most experienced nurse should be assigned to the client whose assessment and care require more experience and knowledge about the disease process, potential complications, and medications. The adjective in the stem "most experienced" is the key to answering this question.**

10. 1. Pain in the chest when walking up stairs would indicate angina.

2. Frequent use of antacids indicates an acid-reflux problem.

3. Snoring loudly could indicate sleep apnea, but not GERD.

4. Carbonated beverages increase stomach pressure. Six (6) to seven (7) soft drinks a day would not be tolerated by a client with GERD.

**TEST-TAKING HINT: The stem of the question indicates an acid problem. The drug classification of antacid or "against acid" gives the test taker a hint as to the correct answer.**

11. 1. Pyrosis is heartburn, water brash is the feeling of saliva secretion as a result of reflux, and flatulence is gas—all symptoms of GERD.

2. Gastroesophageal reflux disease does not cause weight loss.

3. There is no change in abdominal fat, no proteinuria (the result of a filtration problem in the kidney), and no alteration in bowel elimination for the client diagnosed with GERD.

4. Mid-epigastric pain, a positive *H. pylori* test, and melena are associated with gastric ulcer disease.

**TEST-TAKING HINT: Frequently, incorrect answer options will contain the symptoms of a disease of the same organ system.**

12. 1. A hiatal hernia places the client at risk for GERD; GERD does not predispose the client for developing a hiatal hernia.

2. Gastroenteritis is an inflammation of the stomach and intestine, usually caused by a virus.

3. Barrett's esophagitis results from long-term erosion of the esophagus as a result of reflux of stomach contents secondary to GERD. This is a precursor to esophageal cancer.

4. The problems associated with GERD result from the reflux of acidic stomach contents into the esophagus, which is not a precursor to gastric cancer.

**TEST-TAKING HINT: The test taker may associate hiatal hernia with GERD. One (1) can be a result of the other, and this can confuse the test taker If the test taker did not have any idea of the correct answer, "3" has the word**

"esophageal" in it, as does the stem of the question, and therefore the test taker should select this as the correct answer.

## Inflammatory Bowel Disease

13. 1. The colon is ulcerated and unable to absorb water, resulting in bloody diarrhea. Ten (10) to twenty bloody diarrhea stools is the most common symptom of ulcerative colitis.
    2. Although there is an inflammation of the colon, there is usually not an elevated temperature, and if it is elevated, it is a low-grade fever.
    3. A hard, rigid abdomen indicates peritonitis, which is a complication of ulcerative colitis but not an expected symptom.
    4. Stress incontinence is not a symptom of colitis.

    **TEST-TAKING HINT: If the test taker is not sure of the answer, the test taker should use knowledge of anatomy and physiology to help identify the correct answer. The colon is responsible for absorbing water, and if the colon can't do its job, then water will not be absorbed, causing diarrhea, answer option "3." Colitis is inflammation of the colon; therefore, option "4" referring to the urinary system can be eliminated.**

14. 1. This medication can cause erosion of the stomach and should be taken with food.
    2. A moon face is an expected side effect of prednisone.
    3. This medication must be tapered off to prevent adrenal insufficiency; therefore, the client must take this medication as prescribed.
    4. There is no need to take this medication only in the morning. It is usually taken three (3) to four (4) times a day.

    **TEST-TAKING HINT: The test taker should know that very few medications must be taken on an empty stomach, which would cause "1" to be eliminated. All medications should be taken as prescribed—don't think that the answer is too easy.**

15. 1. The HCP needs to be notified so that potassium supplements can be ordered, but this is not the first intervention.
    2. **Leg cramps are a sign of hypokalemia; hypokalemia can lead to cardiac dysrhythmias and can be life threatening. Assessment is priority for a potassium level that is just below normal level, which is 3.5 to 5.5 mEq/L.**
    3. Hypokalemia can lead to cardiac dysrhythmias;

therefore, requesting telemetry is appropriate, but it is not the first intervention.
    4. The client will need potassium to correct the hypokalemia, but it is not the first intervention.

    **TEST-TAKING HINT: When the question asks which action should be implemented first, remember that assessment is the first step in the nursing process. If the answer option that addresses assessment is appropriate for the situation in the question, then the test taker should select it as the correct answer.**

16. 1. The client's bowel should be placed on rest and no foods or fluids should be introduced into the bowel.
    2. **The client requires fluids to help prevent dehydration from diarrhea and to replace the fluid lost through normal body functioning.**
    3. The vital signs must be taken more often than daily in a client who is having an acute exacerbation of ulcerative colitis.
    4. The client will receive anti-inflammatory and antidiarrheal medications, not antacids, which are used for gastroenteritis.

    **TEST-TAKING HINT: "Acute exacerbation" is the key phrase in the stem of the question. The test taker should remember the concept that any lower gastrointestinal disorder should require NPO. The word "acute" should cause the test taker to eliminate any intervention that is "daily."**

17. 1. **TPN is high in dextrose, which is glucose; therefore the client's blood glucose level must be monitored closely.**
    2. The client may be on sliding-scale regular insulin coverage for the high glucose level.
    3. The TPN must be administered via a subclavian line because of the high glucose level.
    4. The client would be NPO to put the bowel at rest, which is the rationale for administering the TPN.

    **TEST-TAKING HINT: The test taker may want to select "3" because it has the word "assess," but remember to note the adjective "peripheral," which makes this option incorrect. Remember the words "check" and "monitor" are words that mean assess.**

18. 1. Weighing the client daily will help identify if the client is experiencing malnutrition, but it is not the priority intervention during an acute exacerbation.
    2. Coping strategies help develop healthy ways to deal with this chronic disease that has remissions and exacerbations, but it is not the priority intervention.

3. The severity of the diarrhea helps determine the need for fluid replacement. The liquid stool should be measured as part of the total output.
4. The client will be NPO when there is an acute exacerbation of IBD to allow the bowel to rest.

**TEST-TAKING HINT:** The test taker can apply Maslow's Hierarchy of Needs and select the option that is the intervention addressing a physiological need.

19. 1. The nurse should never tell a client that they understand what they are going through.
2. This is not addressing the client's feelings.
3. The client is crying and is expressing feelings of powerlessness; therefore the nurse should allow the client to talk.
4. The client is crying and states "I can't take it anymore," but this is not a suicidal comment or situation.

**TEST-TAKING HINT:** There are rules that can be applied to therapeutic responses. Do not say "understand" and do not ask "why." Select an option that has some type of feeling that is being reflected in the statement.

20. 1. A pink and moist stoma indicates viable tissue and adequate circulation. A purple stoma indicates necrosis.
2. An ileostomy will drain liquid all the time and should not routinely be irrigated; only specially trained nurses are allowed to irrigate an ileostomy. A sigmoid colostomy may need daily irrigation to evacuate feces.
3. A red, bumpy, itchy rash indicates infection with the yeast *Candida albicans*, which should be treated with medication.
4. The ileostomy drainage has enzymes and bile salts that are irritating and harsh to the skin; therefore, the pouch should be changed if any leakage occurs.

**TEST-TAKING HINT:** This is an "except" question and the test taker must identify which option is not a correct action for the nurse to implement. Sometimes flipping the question— "Which interventions indicate the client understands the teaching?"—can assist in identifying the correct answer.

21. 1. Asulfidine cannot be administered rectally. Corticosteroids may be administered by enema for the local effect of decreasing inflammation but minimizing the systemic effects.
2. Antidiarrheal agents slow the gastrointestinal motility and reduce diarrhea.
3. IBD is not caused by bacteria.
4. This antibiotic is poorly absorbed from the gastrointestinal tract and acts topically on the colonic mucosa to inhibit the inflammatory process.

**TEST-TAKING HINT:** If the test taker doesn't know the answer, then the test taker could eliminate "2" and "4" because they do not contain the word inflammation; IBD is inflammatory bowel disease.

22. 1. The terminal ileum is the most common site for regional enteritis and causes right lower quadrant pain that is relieved by defecation.
2. Stools are liquid or semi-formed and usually do not contain blood.
3. Episodes of diarrhea and constipation may be a sign/symptom of colon cancer, not Crohn's disease.
4. A fever and hard rigid abdomen are signs/symptoms of peritonitis, a complication of Crohn's disease.

**TEST-TAKING HINT:** The test taker should eliminate option "2" because of the word "all," which is an absolute. There are very few absolutes in the health-care arena.

23. 1. Fried potatoes, along with pastries and pies, should be avoided.
2. Raw vegetables should be avoided because this is roughage.
3. A low-residue diet is a low-fiber diet. Products made of refined flour or finely milled grains, along with roasted, baked, or broiled meats, are recommended.
4. Fried foods should be avoided, and whole grain is high in fiber. Nuts and fruits with peels should be avoided.

**TEST-TAKING HINT:** The test taker must know about therapeutic diets prescribed by health-care providers. Remember low-residue is the same as low-fiber.

24. 1. The cure for ulcerative colitis is a total colectomy, which is removing the entire large colon and bringing the terminal end of the ileum up to the abdomen in the right lower quadrant. This is an ileostomy.
2. This is the left-lower quadrant
3. This is the transcending colon.
4. This is the right upper quadrant.

## Peptic Ulcer Disease

25. 1. The presence of blood does not specifically indicate diagnosis of an ulcer. The client could have hemorrhoids or cancer that would result in the presence of blood.

2. A wavelike burning sensation is a symptom of gastroesophageal reflux.
3. Sharp pain in the upper abdomen after eating a heavy meal is a symptom of gallbladder disease.
4. In a client diagnosed with a gastric ulcer, pain usually occurs 30–60 minutes after eating, but not at night. In contrast, a client with a duodenal ulcer has pain during the night that is often relieved by eating food. Pain occurs 1–3 hours after meals.

**TEST-TAKING HINT: This question asks the test taker to identify assessment data that are specific to the disease process. Many diseases have similar symptoms, but the timing of symptoms or their location may help rule out some diseases and provide the health-care provider with a key to diagnose a specific disease— in this case, peptic ulcer disease. Nurses are usually the major source for information to the health-care team.**

26. 1. **The EGD is an invasive diagnostic test that visualizes the esophagus and stomach to accurately diagnose an ulcer and evaluate the effectiveness of the client's treatment.**
2. MRIs show cross-sectional images of tissue or blood flow.
3. An occult blood test shows the presence of blood, but not the source.
4. A gastric acid stimulation test is used to understand the pathophysiology of ulcer disease, but it has limited usefulness.

**TEST-TAKING HINT: If the test taker has no idea what the correct answer is, knowledge of anatomy can help identify the answer. A peptic ulcer is an ulcer n the stomach, and the word "esophagogastroduodenoscopy" has "gastro," which refers to the stomach. Therefore this would be best option to select as the correct answer.**

27. 1. A history of problems the client has experienced with medications is taken during the admission interview. This information does not specifically address peptic ulcer disease.
2. **Use of NSAIDs places the client at risk for peptic ulcer disease and hemorrhage. Any client suspected of having peptic ulcer disease should be questioned specifically about the use of NSAIDs.**
3. In taking the history of clients, allergies are included for safety, but this is not specific for peptic ulcer disease.
4. Information needs to be collected about past generations so that the nurse can analyze any potential health problems, but this is not specific for peptic ulcer disease.

**TEST-TAKING HINT: The words "specific to peptic ulcer disease" indicate that there will be appropriate data in one (1) or more of the answer options but only one (1) is specific to peptic ulcer disease. The test taker needs to read the question carefully to select the correct answer.**

28. 1. **Auscultation should be used prior to palpation or percussion when assessing the abdomen. If the nurse manipulates the abdomen, the bowel sounds can be altered and give false information.**
2. Palpation gives appropriate information that the nurse needs to collect, but if done prior to auscultation, the sounds will be altered.
3. Percussion of the abdomen would not give specific information about peptic ulcer disease.
4. Tender areas should be assessed last to prevent guarding and altering the assessment. This would include palpation, which should be done after auscultation.

**TEST-TAKING HINT: The word "first" requires the test taker to rank in order the interventions needed to be performed. The test taker should visualize caring for the client. This will assist the test taker in making the correct choice.**

29. 1. There is no indication from the question that there is a problem or potential problem with bowel elimination.
2. Knowledge deficit does not address physiological complications.
3. This client may have problems from changing roles within the family, but the question asks for potential physiological complications, not psychosocial problems.
4. **Potential for alteration in gastric emptying is caused by edema or scarring associated with peptic ulcer disease, which may cause a feeling of "fullness," vomiting of undigested food, or abdominal distention.**

**TEST-TAKING HINT: This question asks the test taker to identify a physiological problem that identifies a complication of the disease process. Therefore, options "2" and "3" that do not address physiological problems could be eliminated.**

30. 1. A pain assessment is an independent intervention that the nurse should implement frequently.
2. Evaluating blood pressure is an independent intervention that the nurse should implement. If the client is able, B/Ps should be taken lying, sitting, and standing to assess for orthostatic hypotension.

3. This is a collaborative intervention that the nurse should implement. It requires an order from the HCP.

4. Administering blood products is collaborative, requiring an order from the HCP.

5. The diet needs an order by the health-care provider, but it would not be given to a client with a bleeding ulcer. These clients are allowed nothing by mouth until the bleeding stops.

**TEST-TAKING HINT:** Descriptive words such as "collaborative" or "independent" can be the deciding factor when determining if an answer option is correct or incorrect. These are key words that the test taker should identify. Collaborative interventions require an HCP's order or an intervention from another health-care discipline.

31. 1. Use of NSAIDs increases and causes problems associated with peptic ulcer disease.

2. **Maintaining lifestyle changes such as following an appropriate diet and reducing stress indicates that the client is complying with the medical teachings. Such compliance is the goal of treatment to prevent complications.**

3. Hemoptysis is coughing up blood, which is not a sign or symptom of peptic ulcer disease, so not coughing up blood would not be an expected outcome for a client with peptic ulcer disease.

4. Antacids should be taken one (1) to three (3) hours after meals, not with each meal.

**TEST-TAKING HINT:** Expected outcomes are positive completion of goals, and maintaining lifestyle modifications would be an appropriate goal for any client with any chronic illness.

32. 1. The range for normoactive bowel sounds is from five (5) to thirty-five (35) times per minute. This would require no intervention.

2. Belching after a heavy, fatty meal is a symptom of gallbladder disease. Eating late at night may cause symptoms of esophageal disorders.

3. **A decrease of 20 mm Hg in blood pressure after changing position from lying, to sitting, to standing is orthostatic hypotension. This could indicate that the client is bleeding.**

4. A decrease in the quality and quantity of discomfort shows an improvement in the client's condition. This would not require further intervention.

**TEST-TAKING HINT:** When the questions ask about further intervention, the test taker should examine the answer options for an outcome that would not be expected and would require further assessment.

33. 1. E-mycin is irritating to stomach, and its use in a client with peptic ulcer disease should be questioned.

2. Prilosec, a proton pump inhibitor, decreases gastric acid production and its use should not be questioned by the nurse.

3. Flagyl, an antimicrobial, is given to treat peptic ulcer disease secondary to *H. pylori* bacteria.

4. Tylenol can be safely administered to a client with peptic ulcer disease.

**TEST-TAKING HINT:** The test taker needs to understand how medications work, adverse effects of medications, when to question the safety of giving a specific medication, and how to administer the medication safely. By learning classifications, the test taker should be able to make a knowledgeable selection in most cases.

34. 1. Decreasing the alcohol intake indicates that the client is making some lifestyle changes.

2. Maintaining a bland diet would indicate that dietary restrictions are being followed.

3. The return to previous activities would indicate that the client has not adapted to the lifestyle changes and has returned to the previous behaviors that precipitated the peptic ulcer disease.

4. **Antibiotics, proton pump inhibitors, and Pepto-Bismol are administered to decrease the irritation of the ulcerative area and cure the ulcer. A decrease in gastric distress indicates the medication is effective.**

**TEST-TAKING HINT:** To determine the effectiveness of a medication, the test taker must know why the medication is being administered. Peptic ulcer disease causes gastric distress. If gastric distress is relieved, then the medication is effective.

35. 1. Sudden sharp pain felt in the substernal area is indicative of angina or myocardial infarction.

2. **A rigid boardlike abdomen with rebound tenderness is the classic sign and symptom of peritonitis, which is a complication of a perforated gastric ulcer.**

3. Clay-colored stools indicate liver disorders, such as hepatitis.

4. Clients with gallbladder disease report vague to sharp abdominal pain in the right upper quadrant.

**TEST-TAKING HINT:** The only two (2) answer options that have the word "abdomen" are "2" or "4." Therefore, the test taker should select one (1) of these two (2) because a gastric ulcer involves the stomach.

36. 1. Maintaining a strict record of intake and output is important to evaluate the progression of

the client's condition, but it is not the most important intervention.

2. Inserting a nasogastric tube and lavaging the stomach with saline is the most important intervention because this directly stops the bleeding.

3. A calorie count is important information that can assist in the prevention and treatment of a nutritional deficit, but this intervention does not address the client's immediate and life-threatening problem.

4. Promoting a quiet environment aids in the reduction of stress, which can cause further bleeding, but this will not stop the bleeding.

**TEST-TAKING HINT:** The test taker is required to rank the importance of interventions in the question. Using Maslow's Hierarchy of Needs to rank real physiologic needs first, the test taker should realize that inserting a nasogastric tube and beginning lavage is solving a circulation or fluid deficit problem.

## Colorectal Disease

37. 1. Some cancers have a higher risk of development when the client is exposed to occupationally exposed chemicals, but cancer of the colon is not one of them.

2. Cruciferous vegetables, such as broccoli, cauliflower, and cabbage, are high in fiber. One of the risks for cancer of the colon is a high-fat, low-fiber, and high-protein diet. The longer the transit time (the time from ingestion of the food to the elimination of the waste products) the greater the chance of developing cancer of the colon.

3. A multiple vitamin may improve immune system function, but it does not prevent colon cancer.

4. High-risk sexual behavior places the client at risk for sexually transmitted diseases. A history of multiple sexual partners and initial sexual experience at an early age does increase the risk for the development of cancer of the cervix in females.

**TEST-TAKING HINT:** The colon processes waste products from eating foods, and option "2" is the only option to mention food. Therefore, "2" would be the best option to select if the test taker did not know the correct answer.

38. 1. Frequent bloody stools are a symptom of inflammatory bowel disease (IBD). IBD is a risk factor for cancer of the colon, but the symptoms are different when the colon becomes cancerous.

2. Most people have a feeling of fullness after a heavy meal; this does not indicate cancer.

3. The most common symptom of colon cancer is a change in bowel habits, specifically diarrhea alternating with constipation.

4. Lower right quadrant pain with rebound tenderness would indicate appendicitis.

**TEST-TAKING HINT:** The test taker could eliminate "4" based on anatomical position. The rectosigmoid area is in the left lower quadrant.

39. 1. A long history of low-fiber, high-fat, high-protein diets results in a prolonged transit time. This allows the carcinogenic agents in the waste products to have a greater exposure to the lumen of the colon.

2. The older the client, the greater the risk of developing cancer of the colon.

3. Risk factors for cancer of the colon include increasing age; family history of colon cancer or polyps; history of IBD; genital or breast cancer; and eating a high-fat, high-protein, low-fiber diet.

4. Males have a slightly higher incidence of colon cancers than do females.

**TEST-TAKING HINT:** The test taker should realize that cancers in general have an increasing incidence with age. Cancer etiologies are not an exact science, but most cancers have some risk factor, if only advancing age.

40. 1. Colostomy stomas are portions of the large intestines pulled through the abdominal wall through which feces exits the body. Feces can be irritating to the abdominal skin, so careful and thorough skin care is needed.

2. There are midline and perineal incisions, not flank incisions.

3. Because of the perineal wound, the client will have an indwelling catheter to keep urine out of the incision.

4. Jackson Pratt drains are emptied every shift, but they are not irrigated.

5. The client should not sit upright because this would cause pressure on the perineum.

**TEST-TAKING HINT:** The test taker could eliminate "2" because flank and abdominal/perineal are not in the same areas. This is an alternative question requiring the test taker to choose more than one (1) option.

41. 1. The stoma should be light to a medium pink, the color of the intestines. A blue or purple color would indicate a lack of circulation to the stoma and is a medical emergency.

2. The stoma should be pouched securely for the client to be able to participate in normal daily

activities. The client should be encouraged to ambulate to aid in recovery.

3. Pain medication should be taken before the pain level reaches a five (5). Delaying taking medication will delay the onset of pain relief and the client will not get a full benefit from the medication.

4. **The pouch should be emptied when it is one-third to one-half full to prevent the contents from becoming too heavy for the seal to hold and to prevent leakage from occurring.**

**TEST-TAKING HINT: Normal mucosa is pink, not white, and clients are always encouraged to ambulate after surgery to prevent the complications related to immobility. Remember basic concepts when answering questions, especially postoperative nursing care.**

42. 1. **The nurse should mark the drainage on the dressing to determine if active bleeding is occurring because dark reddish-brown drainage indicates old blood. This allows the nurse to assess what is actually happening.**

2. Surgical dressings are initially changed by the surgeon; the nurse should not remove the dressing until the surgeon orders the dressing change to be done by the nurse.

3. The nurse should assess the situation before notifying the HCP.

4. The nurse may need to reinforce the dressing if the dressing becomes too saturated, but this would be after a thorough assessment is completed.

**TEST-TAKING HINT: The question is asking the test taker to determine which intervention must be implemented first, and assessment is the first step of the nursing process. Options "2," "3," and "4" would not be implemented prior to assessing. Marking the dressing allows the nurse to assess the dressing and determine whether active bleeding is occurring.**

43. 1. The nurse should first inform the HCP of the client's concerns and then allow the HCP and client to discuss the situation.

2. **The nurse should determine what is concerning the client. It could be a misunderstanding or a real situation where the client's care is unsafe or inadequate.**

3. If a new HCP is to be arranged, it is the HCP's responsibility to arrange for another HCP to take over the care of the client.

4. The choice of HCP is ultimately the client's. If the HCP cannot arrange for another HCP, the client may have to be discharged and obtain a new health-care provider.

**TEST-TAKING HINT: The nurse should assess the situation; the first step in the nursing process is assessment.**

44. 1. If the tissue around the stoma becomes excoriated, the client will be unable to pouch the stoma adequately, resulting in discomfort and leakage. The client understands the teaching.

2. **The client should be on a regular diet, and the colostomy will have been working for several days prior to discharge. The client's statement indicates the need for further teaching.**

3. Until the incision is completely healed the client should not sit in bath water because of the potential contamination of the wound by the bath water. The client understands the teaching.

4. The client has had major surgery and should limit lifting to minimal weight. The client understands the teaching.

**TEST-TAKING HINT: This is an abdominal surgery and all instructions for major surgery apply. This is an "except" question; therefore three (3) options would indicate the client understands the teaching.**

45. **85 mL/hours.** First determine the total amount to be infused over 24 hours.

1500 + 500 + 20 + 20 = 2040 mL over 24 hours.

Then, determine the rate per hour.

2040 ÷ 24 = 85 mL/hour

**TEST-TAKING HINT: Check and recheck calculations. Division should be carried out to the second or third decimal place before rounding.**

46. 1. A digital rectal exam is done to detect rectal cancer and should be started at age 40 years.

2. "Middle age" is a relative term; specific ages are used for recommendation.

3. **The American Cancer Society recommends a colonoscopy at age 50 and every five (5) to ten (10) years thereafter and a flexible sigmoidoscopy and barium enema every five (5) years.**

4. A flexible sigmoidoscopy should be done at five (5)-year intervals between the colonoscopy.

**TEST-TAKING HINT: A digital examination is an examination that is performed by the examiner's finger and does not examine the entire colon.**

47. 1. Intimacy involves more than sexual intercourse. The client can be sexually active whenever the wounds are healed sufficiently to not cause pain.

2. This is an appropriate nursing intervention for home care, but it has nothing to do with sexual activity.

3. The nurse is not a sexual counselor who would have these types of charts. The nurse should address sexuality with the client but would not be considered an expert capable of explaining the advantages and disadvantages of sexual positioning.

4. A pouch that becomes dislodged during the sexual act would cause embarrassment for the client whose body image has already been dealt a blow.

**TEST-TAKING HINT:** Answer option "2" does not address the issue and "3" is outside of the nurse's professional expertise. Option "1" could be eliminated because of the word "no," which is an absolute word.

48. 1. The client will need to have diagnostic tests so this is an appropriate intervention.

2. The client who has an intestinal blockage will need to be hydrated.

3. This client has an intestinal blockage from a solid tumor blocking the colon. Although the client needs to be cleaned out for the colonoscopy, this would cause severe cramping without a reasonable benefit to the client and could cause a medical emergency.

4. Tap water enemas until it is clear would be instilling water from below the tumor to try and rid the colon of any feces in that portion of the colon and the client can expel this water.

**TEST-TAKING HINT:** The stem states a "complete blockage," which indicates the client would need surgery. Therefore, options "1" and "2" would be appropriate for surgery. The stem asks the test taker which order would be questioned so this is an "except" question.

## Diverticulosis/Diverticulitis

49. 1. These are classic signs/symptoms of diverticulitis; therefore the HCP would not need to be notified.

2. These are normal findings for a client diagnosed with diverticulitis, but on admission the nurse should assess the client and document the findings in the client's chart.

3. The nurse should not administer any food or medications.

4. The nurse should assess the client to determine if the abdomen is soft and nontender. A rigid tender abdomen may indicate peritonitis.

**TEST-TAKING HINT:** The test taker must remember to apply the nursing process when answering test questions. Assessment is the first step in the nursing process. Although the signs/symptoms are normal and could be documented, the nurse should always assess.

50. 1. The client should drink at least 3000 mL of water daily to help prevent constipation.

2. The client should exercise daily to help prevent constipation.

3. The client should eat a high-fiber diet to help prevent constipation.

4. The client should have regular bowel movements, preferably daily. Constipation may cause diverticulitis, which is a potentially life-threatening complication of diverticulosis.

**TEST-TAKING HINT:** The test taker must be sure to distinguish between "osis" and "itis." diverticulosis is the condition of having small pouches in the colon, and preventing constipation is the most important action the client can take to prevent diverticulitis, inflammation of the diverticulum.

51. 1. The client will have a nasogastric tube because the client will be NPO, which will decompress the bowel and help remove hydrochloric acid.

2. Preventing dehydration is a priority with the client who is NPO.

3. The nurse should question a clear liquid diet because the bowel must be put on total rest, which means NPO.

4. The client is in severe pain and should be on bed rest, which will help rest the bowel.

**TEST-TAKING HINT:** This is an "except" question. Therefore the test taker must identify which answer option is incorrect for the stem. Sometimes flipping the question helps in selecting the correct answer. In this question, the test taker could ask, "Which HCP order would be expected for a client diagnosed with diverticulitis?" The option that is not expected would be the correct answer.

52. 1. Fried foods increase cholesterol. Mashed potatoes do not have the peel, which is needed for increased fiber.

2. Applesauce does not have the peel, which is needed for increased fiber, and the option does not identify which type of bread; whole milk is high in fat.

3. Chicken and whole-wheat bread are high in fiber, which is the therapeutic diet prescribed for clients with diverticulosis. An adequate intake of water helps prevent constipation.

4. Tomatoes and cucumbers both have seeds, and many health-care providers recommend that people with diverticulosis avoid seeds because of the possibility of the seeds entering the diverticulum and becoming trapped, leading to peritonitis.

**TEST-TAKING HINT: The test taker must know that a high-fiber diet is prescribed for diverticulosis and at least five (5) to six (6) foods that are encouraged or discouraged for the different types of diets. High-fiber foods are foods with peels (potato, apple) and whole-wheat products.**

53. 1. The client's abdomen should be soft and nontender; therefore, this finding would not require immediate intervention.
    2. The client had to clean the bowel prior to the colonoscopy; therefore, watery stool would be expected.
    3. The client was NPO and received bowel preparation prior to the colonoscopy; therefore, hyperactive bowel sounds might occur and would not warrant immediate intervention.
    4. **Bowel perforation is a potential complication of a colonoscopy. Therefore signs of hypotension—decreased BP and increased pulse—would warrant immediate intervention from the nurse.**

**TEST-TAKING HINT: This is an "except" question. The test taker is being asked to select which data are abnormal for a procedure. The test taker should remember that any invasive procedure could possibly lead to hemorrhaging, and signs of shock should always be considered a possible correct answer.**

54. 1. A peak and trough is drawn after the client has received at least three (3) to four (4) doses of medication, not on the initial dose because the client has just been admitted.
    2. **The nurse should always ask about allergies to medication when administering medications, but especially when administering antibiotics, which are notorious for allergic reactions.**
    3. The peak and trough would not be drawn prior to the first dose; it is ordered after multiple doses.
    4. The nurse should question when to administer the medication, but there is no vital sign that would prevent the nurse from administering this medication.

**TEST-TAKING HINT: The test taker must read the stem closely to realize the client was just admitted and that therefore this would be the first dose of medication to be given. This**

would cause the test taker to eliminate "1" and "3" as possible correct answers. Both "2" and "4" are assessment data, but the test taker should ask which one will directly affect the administration of the medication.

55. 1. **These are signs of peritonitis, which is life threatening. The health-care provider should be notified immediately.**
    2. A Fleet's enema will not help a life-threatening complication of diverticulitis.
    3. A medication administered to help decrease the client's temperature will not help a life-threatening complication.
    4. **These are signs/symptoms that indicate a possible life-threatening situation and require immediate intervention.**

**TEST-TAKING HINT: In most instances, the test taker should not select the option that says to notify the HCP immediately, but in some situations, it is the correct answer. The test taker should look at all the other options and determine if the option is information the HCP would require or if it is an independent intervention that will help the client.**

56. **42 gtts per minute.** The nurse must use the formula:

$$\frac{\text{amount to be infused} \times \text{drops per minute}}{\div \text{minutes for infusion}}$$

$$\frac{250 \text{ mL} \times 10 \text{ gtts} = 2500}{60 \text{ minutes}} = 41.8 \text{ gtts per minute}$$

**TEST-TAKING HINT: The test taker must know how to calculate dosage and calculation questions. Remember to use the drop-down calculator if needed; the test taker can also ask for an erase slate during state board examinations.**

57. 1. **Green bile contains hydrochloric acid and should be draining from the N/G tube; therefore the nurse should take no action and should document the findings.**
    2. There is no reason for the nurse to take further action because this is normal.
    3. The client's last bowel movement would not affect the N/G drainage.
    4. Bile draining from the N/G tube indicates that the tube is in the stomach and there is no need to advance the tube further.

**TEST-TAKING HINT: The test taker must know what drainage is normal for tubes inserted into the body. Any type of blood or coffee-ground drainage would be abnormal and require intervention by the nurse.**

58. 1. A high-fiber diet will help to prevent constipation, which is the primary reason for diverticulitis.

2. Increased fluids will help keep the stool soft and prevent constipation.
3. This will not do anything to help prevent diverticulitis.
4. Exercise will help prevent constipation.
5. There are no medications used to help prevent an acute exacerbation of diverticulitis. Antacids are used to neutralize hydrochloric acid in the stomach.

**TEST-TAKING HINT: This is an alternate-type question where the test taker must select all answer options that apply. To prevent diverticulitis, the nurse must discuss interventions that will prevent constipation. To identify the correct answers, the test taker should think about what part of the GI system is affected. Knowing that diverticulosis occurs in the sigmoid colon would help eliminate "3" and "5" because these would be secondary to stomach disorders.**

59. 1. A sedentary lifestyle may lead to obesity and contribute to hypertension or heart disease but usually not to diverticulosis.
2. Multiple childbirths are not a risk factor for developing diverticulosis.
3. **Hemorrhoids would indicate the client has chronic constipation, which is a strong risk factor for diverticulosis. Constipation increases the intraluminal pressure in the sigmoid colon, leading to weakness in the intestinal lining, which, in turn, causes outpouchings, or diverticula.**
4. A family history is not a risk factor. Having daily bowel movements and preventing constipation will decrease the chance of developing diverticulosis.

**TEST-TAKING HINT: The test taker must know that constipation is the leading risk factor for diverticulosis, and if the test taker knows that hemorrhoids are caused by constipation it would lead the test taker to select "3" as the correct answer.**

60. 1. Total parenteral nutrition is not an expected order for this client.
2. **The bowel must be put at rest. Therefore, the nurse should anticipate orders for maintaining NPO and a nasogastric tube.**
3. These orders would be instituted when the client is getting better and the bowel is not inflamed.
4. Surgery is not the first consideration when the client is admitted into the hospital.

**TEST-TAKING HINT: Collaborative means the nurse must care for the client with another discipline and the health-care provider would have to order all of the distracters. The test**

taker should remember the concept that with lower gastrointestinal problems, food and fluid probably should be stopped.

## Gallbladder Disorders

61. 1. After abdominal surgery, it is not uncommon for bowel sounds to be absent.
2. This is a normal amount and color of drainage.
3. The minimum urine output is 30 mL/hr.
4. Refusing to turn, deep breathe, and cough puts the client at risk for pneumonia. This client needs immediate intervention to prevent complications.

**TEST-TAKING HINT: The test taker should recognize normal data such as the normal urine output and normal data for postoperative clients. The test taker should apply basic concepts when answering questions. Normal or expected outcomes do not require action.**

62. 1. **A heating pad should be applied for 15 to 20 minutes to assist the migration of the $CO_2$ used to insufflate the abdomen.**
2. Morphine sulfate would not affect the etiology of the pain.
3. The surgeon would not order an x-ray for this condition.
4. There is no indication that an injury occurred during surgery. A sling would not benefit the migration of the $CO_2$.

**TEST-TAKING HINT: The test taker must understand laparoscopic surgery to be able to answer this question. Option "4" could be eliminated because of the "injured during surgery" phrase that is making an assumption.**

63. 1. This surgery does not require lipid-lowering medications, but eating high-fat meals may cause discomfort.
2. **After removal of the gallbladder, some clients experience abdominal discomfort when eating fatty foods.**
3. Laparoscopic cholecystectomy surgeries are performed in day surgery, and clients usually do not need assistance for a week.
4. Using a pillow to splint the abdomen provides support for the incision and should be continued after discharge.

**TEST-TAKING HINT: When answering questions that state "teaching is effective," the test taker should look for the correct information. Basic concepts should help the test taker answer questions and, because pain often occurs after surgeries, answer option "2" would probably be a correct answer if the test taker had no idea which option is correct.**

64. 1. Clay-colored stools are caused by recurring stricture of the common bile duct, which is a sign of post-cholecystectomy syndrome.
2. Yellow-tinted sclera and skin indicate residual effects of stricture of the common bile duct, which is a sign of post-cholecystectomy syndrome.
3. Dark yellow urine indicates a residual effect of a stricture of the common bile duct, which is a sign of post-cholecystectomy syndrome.
4. Fever and chills indicate residual or recurring calculi, inflammation, or stricture of common bile duct, which is a sign of post-cholecystectomy syndrome.
5. Abdominal pain indicates a residual effect of a stricture of common bile duct, inflammation, or calculi, which is a sign of post-cholecystectomy syndrome.

**TEST-TAKING HINT:** The test taker must use knowledge of anatomy to answer this question. All answer options have something to do with the abdominal area, and the common bile duct is anatomically near the hepatic duct, which causes the liver signs/symptoms.

65. 1. This is assessment and cannot be delegated.
2. This intervention would require analysis.
3. This intervention would be appropriate for the nursing assistant to implement.
4. This would require assessment and cannot be delegated.

**TEST-TAKING HINT:** The nurse cannot delegate teaching, assessing, and evaluating to a nursing assistant. The nurse cannot delegate any nursing task unless the client is stable and the task does not require judgment.

66. 1. A UGI requires the client to swallow barium, which passes through the intestines, making the stools a chalky white color.
2. This would be abnormal data and would be cause for further assessment.
3. This would not be expected from the test.
4. This is a serious finding and should be treated.

**TEST-TAKING HINTS:** Answer option "2" could be eliminated because it does not have anything to do with the gastrointestinal system. A firm hard abdomen is very seldom ever expected, so "3" could be eliminated.

67. 1. This intervention may irritate the client's throat.
2. This would not enhance safety.
3. The endoscopic retrograde cholangiopancreatogram (ERCP) requires that an anesthetic spray be used prior to insertion of the endoscope. If medications, food, or fluid is given orally prior to the return of the gag reflex, the client may aspirate, causing pneumonia that could be fatal.
4. Medications would not be given until the gag reflex has returned.

**TEST-TAKING HINTS:** The test taker must notice adjectives such as "endoscopic," which means the procedure includes going down the mouth; "3" is the only option that has anything to do with the mouth. If the test taker had no idea of the correct answer, selecting a distracter addressing assessment would be appropriate because assessment is the first step of the nursing process.

68. 1. The expected outcome would be increased pain management for both preoperative and postoperative care.
2. Postoperative care would include ambulation.
3. Prevention of an additional break in skin integrity would be a desired postoperative outcome. The incision would be a break in skin integrity.
4. This would be an expected outcome for the client scheduled for surgery. This indicates that preoperative teaching has been effective.

**TEST-TAKING HINT:** The time element is important in this question. The "expected outcome" that is required is for before the client's surgery. Option "1" is wrong because of the adjective "decreased." Adjectives commonly determine the accuracy of answer options.

69. 1. The nurse would expect an increased pulse in the client who is in acute pain.
2. Clients having abdominal pain frequently have shallow respirations. When assessing clients for pain, the nurse should discuss pain medication with any client who has shallow respirations.
3. These are normal data and would not require further action.
4. Splinting the abdomen allows the client to increase the strength of the cough by increasing comfort and would not indicate a need for pain medication.

**TEST-TAKING HINT:** The stem asks which data would warrant pain medication. Therefore the test taker should select an answer that is not expected or is not normal for clients who are postoperative abdominal surgery.

70. 1. This value would be elevated in clients with chronic inflammation.
2. This value would indicate liver abnormalities.

3. This value would indicate liver abnormalities.

4. This value would indicate an obstructive process.

**TEST-TAKING HINT: If the test taker does not know what the values mean, the test taker should look to the disease process. The "itis" means inflammation, and an educated guess would be that WBCs are elevated in inflammatory processes.**

71. 1. This may be an appropriate client problem, but it is not priority.
2. This may be an appropriate client problem, but is not priority.
3. This may be an appropriate client problem, but is not priority.
4. Acute pain management is the highest priority client problem after surgery because pain may indicate a life-threatening problem.

**TEST-TAKING HINT: When a question asks for the highest priority, the test taker should look for life-threatening problems that would be the highest priority for intervention. Pain may be expected, but it may indicate a complication.**

72. 1. This intervention would help further assess internal bleeding, not external bleeding.
2. This would assess the bladder, not bleeding.
3. Turning the client to the side to assess the amount of drainage and possible bleeding is important prior to contacting the surgeon.
4. The first dressing change is usually done by the surgeon; the nurse would reinforce the dressing.

**TEST-TAKING HINT: The adjectives "large" and "red" indicate that the client is bleeding, and assessment is always priority when the client is having a possible complication of a surgery. Remember assessment is the first step in the nursing process.**

## Liver Failure

73. 1. The client's throat is not anesthetized during the insertion of a nasogastric tube, so the gag reflex does not need to be assessed.
2. While the balloons are inflated, the client must not be left unattended in case they become dislodged and occlude the airway. This is a safety issue.
3. This laxative is administered to decrease the ammonia level, but the question does not say that the client's ammonia level is elevated.

4. Esophageal bleeding does not cause the ammonia level to be elevated.

**TEST-TAKING HINT: In most cases, the test taker should not select an option that contains the word "all," but in some instances, it may be the correct answer. Although the ammonia level is elevated in liver failure, the test taker must be clear as to what the question is asking. "Inflate" is the key to answering the question correctly.**

74. 1. The client should empty the bladder immediately prior to the liver biopsy, not after the procedure.
2. Foods and fluids are usually withheld two (2) hours after the biopsy, after which the client can resume the usual diet.
3. Direct pressure is applied to the site, and then the client is placed on the right side to maintain site pressure.
4. BUN and creatinine levels are monitored for kidney function, not liver function, and the renal system is not affected with the liver biopsy.

**TEST-TAKING HINT: The adjective "post-procedure" should help the test taker rule out option "1." Knowing the anatomical position of the liver should help the test taker select "3" as the correct answer. The test taker must know laboratory data for each organ, which would help rule out "4" as a possible correct answer.**

75. 1. Sodium is restricted to reduce ascites and generalized edema, not for hepatic encephalopathy.
2. Fluids are calculated based on diuretic therapy, urine output, and serum electrolyte values; fluids do not affect hepatic encephalopathy.
3. A diet high in calories and moderate in fat intake is recommended to promote healing.
4. Ammonia is a byproduct of protein metabolism and contributes to hepatic encephalopathy. Reducing protein intake should decrease ammonia levels.

**TEST-TAKING HINT: The test taker could eliminate options "1" and "2" based on the knowledge that sodium and water work together and address edema, not encephalopathy. The test taker's knowledge of biochemistry—protein breaks down to ammonia, carbohydrates break down to glucose, and fat breaks down to ketones—may be helpful in selecting the correct answer.**

76. 1. The procedure is done in the client's room, with the client either seated on the side of the bed or in a chair.

2. The client should empty the bladder prior to the procedure to avoid bladder puncture, but there is no need for a Foley catheter to be inserted.

3. The client is at risk for hypovolemia; therefore, vital signs will be assessed frequently to monitor for signs of hemorrhaging.

4. The client does not have to hold the breath when the catheter is inserted into the peritoneum; this is done when obtaining a liver biopsy.

**TEST-TAKING HINT: If the test taker had no idea what the answer is, knowing that vital signs are assessed after all procedures should make the test taker select this option.**

77. 1. Hot water increases pruritus, and soap will cause dry skin, which increases pruritus; therefore, the nurse should discuss this with the assistant.

2. This will help prevent dry skin, which will help decrease pruritus; therefore this would not require any intervention by the primary nurse.

3. Mittens will help prevent the client from scratching the skin and causing skin breakdown.

4. The skin should be patted dry, not rubbed, because rubbing the skin will cause increased irritation.

**TEST-TAKING HINT: A concept that is accepted for most clients during A.M. care is not to use hot water because it causes dilatation of vessels, which may cause orthostatic hypotension. This is not the rationale for not using hot water with a client who has pruritus, but sometimes the test taker can apply broad concepts when answering questions.**

78. 1. Two (2) kg is more than four (4) pounds, which indicates severe fluid retention and is not an appropriate goal.

2. Excess fluid volume could be secondary to portal hypertension. Therefore, no increase in abdominal girth would be an appropriate short-term goal, indicating no excess of fluid volume.

3. Vital signs are appropriate to monitor, but they do not yield specific information about fluid volume status.

4. Having the client receive a low-sodium diet does not ensure that the client will comply with the diet. The short-term goal must evaluate if the fluid volume is within normal limits.

**TEST-TAKING HINT: Remember that goals evaluate the interventions; therefore option "4" could be eliminated as the correct answer because it is an intervention, not a goal. Short-**

term weight fluctuations tend to reflect fluid balance, and any weight gain in 24 hours indicates retention of fluid, which is not an appropriate goal.

79. 1. Vitamin K deficiency causes impaired coagulation; therefore rectal thermometers should be avoided to prevent bleeding.

2. Soft toothbrushes will help prevent bleeding of the gums.

3. Platelet count, PTT/PT, and INR should be monitored to assess coagulation status.

4. Injections should be avoided, if at all possible, because the client is unable to clot, but if they are absolutely necessarily, the nurse should use small-gauge needles.

5. Asterixis is a flapping tremor of the hands when the arms are extended and indicates an elevated ammonia level, but it is not associated with vitamin K deficiency.

**TEST-TAKING HINT: The test taker must know the function of specific vitamins. Vitamin K is responsible for blood clotting. This is an alternate-type question, which requires the test taker to select all interventions that apply; the test taker should select interventions that address bleeding.**

80. 1. Hypoalbuminemia, decreased albumin, and muscle wasting are metabolic effects, not gastrointestinal effects.

2. Oligomenorrhea is no menses, which is a reproductive effect, and decreased body hair is an integumentary effect.

3. Clay-colored stools and hemorrhoids are gastrointestinal effects of liver failure.

4. Dyspnea is a respiratory effect, and caput medusae (dilated veins around the umbilicus) is an integumentary effect, although it is on the abdomen.

**TEST-TAKING HINT: The adjective "gastrointestinal" is the key word that guides the test taker to select the correct answer. The test taker must rule out options that do not involve gastrointestinal symptoms. Although liver failure affects every body system, the question asks for a gastrointestinal effect.**

81. 1. It really doesn't matter how long the client has been drinking alcohol. The diagnosis of alcoholic cirrhosis indicates the client has probably been drinking for many years.

2. An advance directive is important for the client who is terminally ill, but it is not the priority question.

3. The nurse must know when the client had the last alcoholic drink to be able to determine when and if the client will experience

delirium tremens, the physical withdrawal from alcohol.

4. This is not a typical question asked by the nurse unless the client is malnourished, which is not information given in the stem.

**TEST-TAKING HINT: Because the word "alcohol" is in the stem of the question, and if the test taker had no idea what the correct answer is, the test taker should select options that have the word "alcohol" in them and look closely at options "1" and "3."**

82. 1. Blood in the intestinal tract is digested as a protein, which increases serum ammonia levels and increases the risk of developing hepatic encephalopathy.
2. Decreased albumin would cause the client to develop ascites.
3. An enlarged spleen increases the rate at which RBCs, WBCs, and platelets are destroyed, which causes the client to develop anemia, leukopenia, and thrombocytopenia, but not hepatic encephalopathy.
4. An increase in aldosterone causes sodium and water retention that, in turn, causes the development of ascites and generalized edema.

**TEST-TAKING HINT: Some questions require the test taker to have specific knowledge to be able to identify the correct answer. This is one (1) of these questions.**

83. 1. This is a therapeutic response and used to encourage the client to verbalize feelings, but it does not provide factual information.
2. This is passing the buck; the nurse should be able to answer this question.
3. **This is the main reason the HCP decreases the client's medication dose, and it is an explanation appropriate for the client.**
4. This is the medical explanation as to why the medication dose is decreased, but it should not be used to explain to a layperson.

**TEST-TAKING HINT: The test taker should provide factual information when the client asks "why." Therefore, "1" and "2" could be eliminated as possible correct answers. Both "3" and "4" explain the rationale for decreasing the medication dose, but the nurse should answer in terms the client can understand. Would a layperson know what half-life means?**

84. 1. Two to soft three stools a day indicates the medication is effective.
2. There is no instrument that can be used at home to test daily ammonia levels. The ammonia level is a serum level that requires venipuncture and laboratory diagnostic equipment.

3. Diarrhea indicates an overdosage, possibly requiring that the dosage be decreased. The HCP would need to make this change in dosage, so the client is correct.
4. The client should check the stool for bright-red blood as well as dark, tarry stool.

**TEST-TAKING HINT: This is an "except" question. The test taker must realize that three (3) options indicate an understanding of the teaching. If the test taker does not know the answer, notice that all the options except "2" have something to do with stool, and laxative affects the stool.**

## Hepatitis

85. 1. Clay-colored stools and jaundice occur in the icteric phase of hepatitis.
2. These signs/symptoms occur in the icteric phase of hepatitis.
3. Fever subsides in the icteric phase, and the pain is in the right upper quadrant.
4. **"Flu-like" symptoms are the first complaints of the client in the preicteric phase of hepatitis, which is the initial phase and may begin abruptly or insidiously.**

**TEST-TAKING HINT: The test taker must use anatomy knowledge in ruling out incorrect answers; "3" could be ruled out because the liver is in the right upper quadrant.**

86. 1. **The hepatitis A virus is in the stool of infected people up to two (2) weeks before symptoms develop.**
2. Hepatitis B virus is spread through contact with infected blood and body fluids.
3. Hepatitis C virus is transmitted through infected blood and body fluids.
4. Hepatitis D virus only causes infection in people who are also infected with hepatitis B or C.

**TEST-TAKING HINT: This is a knowledge question; the nurse must be aware of how the various types of hepatitis virus are transmitted.**

87. 1. Airborne precautions are required for transmission that occurs by dissemination of either airborne droplet nuclei or dust particles containing the infectious agent.
2. **Standard Precautions apply to blood, all body fluids, secretions, and excretions, except sweat, regardless of whether they contain visible blood.**
3. Droplet transmission involves contact of the conjunctivae of the eyes or mucous membranes of the nose or mouth with large-particle

droplets generated during coughing, sneezing, talking, or suctioning.

4. There is no such precaution known as exposure precautions.

**TEST-TAKING HINT: The test taker must know that standard precautions are used by all health-care workers who have direct contact with clients or with their body fluids or have indirect contact with objects used by the clients who are infected, such as would be involved in emptying trash, changing linens, or cleaning the room.**

88. 1. Eating after each other should be discouraged, but it is not the most important intervention.
2. Only bottled water should be consumed in Third World countries, but that precaution is not necessary in American high schools.
3. Hepatitis B and C, not hepatitis A, are transmitted by sexual activity.
4. Hepatitis A is transmitted via the fecal–oral route. Good hand washing helps to prevent its spread.

**TEST-TAKING HINTS: The test taker must realize that good hand washing is the most important action in preventing transmission of any of the hepatitis viruses. Often, the test taker will not select the answer option that seems too easy—but remember, do not overlook the obvious.**

89. 1. The client must avoid alcohol altogether, not decrease intake, to prevent further liver damage and promote healing.
2. Adequate rest is needed for maintaining optimal immune function.
3. Clients are more often anorexic and nauseated in the afternoon and evening; therefore the main meal should be in the morning.
4. Diet drinks and juices provide few calories, and the client needs an increased caloric diet for healing.

**TEST-TAKING HINT: The test taker must be aware of key words in both the stem and answer options. The "icteric" phase means the acute phase. The word "decrease" should cause the test taker to eliminate "1" as a possible correct answer, and "large" should cause the test taker to eliminate "3" as a possible correct answer.**

90. 1. Hepatitis B can be transmitted by sharing any type of needles, especially those used by drug abusers.
2. Hepatitis B can be transmitted through sexual activity; therefore the nurse should recommend abstinence, mutual monogamy, or barrier protection.

3. Three doses of hepatitis B vaccine provide immunity in 90% of healthy adults.
4. Immune globulin injections are administered as post-exposure prophylaxis (after being exposed to hepatitis B), but encouraging these injections is not a health promotion activity.
5. Hepatotoxic medications should be avoided in clients who have hepatitis or who have had hepatitis. The health-care provider prescribes medications, and the person in the community does not know which medications are hepatotoxic.

**TEST-TAKING HINT: In this select-all-that apply type question, there may be only one (1) correct answer, there may be several, or all five options may be correct answers.**

91. 1. This is a therapeutic response and the nurse should provide factual information.
2. Milk thistle has an active ingredient, silymarin, which has been used to treat liver disease for more than 2000 years. It is a powerful oxidant and promotes liver cell growth.
3. The nurse should not discourage complementary therapies.
4. This is a judgmental statement and the nurse should encourage the client to ask questions.

**TEST-TAKING HINT: The test taker may not have any idea what milk thistle is but should apply test-taking strategies that include not selecting options with "why" ("4") unless interviewing the client. Only use therapeutic responses when unable to provide factual information. At times, the test taker may not like any answer option but should always apply the rules to help determine the correct answer.**

92. 1. Sufficient energy is required for healing. Adequate carbohydrate intake can spare protein. The client should eat approximately 16 carbohydrate kilocalories for each kilogram of ideal body weight daily.
2. TPN is not routinely prescribed for the client with hepatitis; the client would have to have lost a large of amount of weight and be unable to eat anything for TPN to be ordered.
3. Salt intake does not affect the healing of the liver.
4. Water intake does not affect healing of the liver, and the client should not drink so much water as to decrease caloric food intake.

**TEST-TAKING HINT: The test taker should key in on "less than body requirement" in the stem and select the answer that addresses increasing calories, which eliminates options "3" and "4."**

**93.** 1. The nurse must notify the infection control nurse as soon as possible so that treatment can start if needed, but this is not the first intervention.
2. **The nurse should first clean the needle stick with soap and water to help remove any virus that is on the skin.**
3. Post-exposure prophylaxis may be needed, but this is not the first action.
4. The infection control nurse will check the status of the client that the needle was used on before the nurse stuck herself.

**TEST-TAKING HINT: The question requires the test taker to identify the first intervention. The test taker should think about which intervention will directly help the nurse—and that is to clean the area.**

**94.** 1. The serum ammonia level is increased in liver failure, but it is not the cause of clay-colored stools.
2. **Bilirubin, the byproduct of red blood cell destruction, is metabolized in the liver and excreted via the feces, which is what gives the feces the dark color. If the liver is damaged, the bilirubin is excreted via the urine and skin.**
3. The liver excretes bile into the gallbladder and the body uses the bile to digest fat, but it does not affect the feces.
4. Vitamin deficiency, resulting from the liver's inability to detoxify vitamins, may cause steatorrhea, but it does not cause clay-colored stool.

**TEST-TAKING HINT: The test taker should have a grasp of physiology to help answer this question. Clay-colored stool indicates no color in the feces. Because color in the feces is caused by bilirubin, lack of color would be the result of the liver's inability to excrete bilirubin.**

**95.** 1. The client should avoid alcohol to prevent further liver damage and promote healing.
2. Rest is needed for healing of the liver and to promote optimum immune function.
3. Clients with hepatitis need increased caloric intake, so this is a good statement.
4. **The client needs to understand that some types of cough syrup have alcohol and all alcohol must be avoided to prevent further injury to the liver; therefore this statement requires intervention.**

**TEST-TAKING HINT: If the test taker did not know the answer, the test taker could apply the rule that any over-the-counter (OTC) medications should be avoided unless approved by a health-care provider.**

**96.** 1. The laboratory technician draws serum blood studies, not the nursing assistant.
2. The nursing assistant can obtain the intake and output, but the nurse must evaluate the data to determine if the results are normal for the client's disease process or condition.
3. **The nursing assistant can assist a client to the bedside commode.**
4. The ward clerk has specific training that allows the transcribing of health-care provider orders.

**TEST-TAKING HINT: The test taker must be knowledgeable of delegation rules; the nurse cannot delegate assessing, teaching, medication administration, evaluating, and any task for an unstable client.**

## Gastroenteritis

**97.** 1. The client would be taking antidiarrheal medication, not medications to stimulate bowel movements.
2. **The client probably has traveler's diarrhea, and oral rehydration is the preferred choice for replacing fluids lost as a result of diarrhea. An oral glucose electrolyte solution, such as Gatorade, All-Sport, or Pedialyte, is recommended.**
3. The client should be encouraged to stay on liquids and eat bland foods of all three (3) food groups—carbohydrates, proteins, and fats.
4. There is no need for the client to weigh herself daily. Symptoms usually resolve within two (2) to three (3) days without complications.

**TEST-TAKING HINT: Be sure to note the adjectives and adverbs in the stem and the answer options, such as "cathartic" laxative and weight "daily." These words are very often important in ruling out answers and identifying the correct answer.**

**98.** 1. This will help prevent gastroenteritis secondary to staphylococcal food poisoning.
2. This will help prevent gastroenteritis secondary to foods kept at room temperature, causing staphylococcal food poisoning.
3. This will help prevent gastroenteritis secondary to *Escherichia coli* and contaminated water.
4. **Any food that is discolored or comes from a can or jar that has been damaged or does not have a tight seal should be destroyed without tasting or touching it.**

**TEST-TAKING HINT: The test taker should be careful with words such as "all," "only," and "never"; there are very few absolutes in the health-care field. However, when all options**

**have these words, the test taker must find another way to choose the correct answer.**

99. 1. Symptoms develop 8–48 hours after ingesting the *Salmonella* bacteria and include diarrhea, abdominal cramping, nausea, and vomiting, along with low-grade fever, chills, and weakness.
   2. This occurs with botulism, a severe life-threatening form of food poisoning caused by *Clostridium botulinum.*
   3. This is a clinical manifestation of hemorrhagic colitis caused by *Escherichia coli.*
   4. This gray-cloudy diarrhea that has no fecal odor, blood, or pus is caused by cholera, which is endemic in parts of Asia, the Middle East, and Africa.

   **TEST-TAKING HINT: Often when two (2) answer options have the same clinical manifestation, such as diarrhea and stool, this should make the test taker realize that these two (2) options are either a right or wrong answer so the other two (2) options can be eliminated.**

100. 1. The normal serum sodium level is 135–145 mEq/L; therefore an intervention by the nurse is not needed.
   2. These are normal arterial blood gas results; therefore, the nurse would not need to intervene.
   3. In gastroenteritis, diarrhea often results in metabolic acidosis and loss of potassium. The normal serum potassium level is 3.5–5.5 mEq/L; therefore a 3.3 mEq/L would require immediate intervention. Hypokalemia (a low potassium level) can lead to life-threatening cardiac dysrhythmias.
   4. A stool specimen showing fecal leukocytes would support the diagnosis of gastroenteritis and not warrant immediate intervention by the nurse.

   **TEST-TAKING HINT: Read the stem and make sure the test taker understands what the question is asking—in this case, "which requires immediate intervention?" Therefore the test taker is identifying an answer that is not normal for the disease process.**

101. 1. If the diarrhea persists more than 48 hours, notify the physician. Diarrhea for more than 96 hours could lead to metabolic acidosis, hypokalemia, and possible death.
   2. This should be done by the client at all times, but especially when the client has gastroenteritis. The bacteria in feces may be transferred to other people via food if hands are not washed properly.

3. Steroids are not used in the treatment of gastroenteritis; antidiarrheal medication is usually prescribed.
4. The client may be asked to provide a stool specimen for culture, ova, parasites, and fecal leukocytes, but the client would not be asked for a 24-hour stool collection.

**TEST-TAKING HINT: If the test taker did not know the answer to this question, hand washing should be selected because it is the number one (1) intervention for preventing any type of contamination or nosocomial infection.**

102. 1. Antidiarrheal medications are contraindicated with botulism because the toxin needs to be expelled from the body. A laxative may be ordered to promote removal of the toxin from the bowel.
   2. Aminoglycoside antibiotics will not be ordered because there is no bacterium with botulism; it is a toxin.
   3. **A botulism antitoxin neutralizes the circulating toxin and is prescribed for a client with botulism.**
   4. An ACE inhibitor is prescribed for a client diagnosed with cardiovascular disease.

   **TEST-TAKING HINT: The key word in this question is "treat." Because botulism does not end in "itis, and thus is not an infection, the use of an antibiotic (option "2") can be eliminated. Antidiarrheal medication treats the diarrhea, which is a symptom of a disease, not a disease itself.**

103. 1. Fluid volume deficit secondary to diarrhea is the priority because of the potential for metabolic acidosis and hypokalemia, which are both life threatening, especially in the elderly.
   2. Nausea may occur, but it is not priority. However, excessive vomiting could lead to potential complications.
   3. Risk for aspiration could result from vomiting; however, vomiting does not usually occur in food poisoning, but it may be secondary to botulism.
   4. Impaired urinary elimination is not a priority. The client has diarrhea, not urine output problems.

   **TEST-TAKING HINT: Always notice the client's age because it is usually a significant clue as to what the correct answer will be. Prioritizing questions may have more than one (1) potential appropriate nursing problem but only one (1) has priority. Remember Maslow's Hierarchy of Needs.**

**104.** 1. The client would have increased gurgling sounds revealing hyperactive bowel movements.
2. A hard, firm, edematous abdomen would not be expected in a client with gastroenteritis; this would indicate a possible complication and require further assessment.
3. The client would have increased liquid bowel movements, diarrhea, but would not have blood in the stool, which is the definition of melena.
4. Borborygmi, or loud, rushing bowel sounds, indicates increased peristalsis, which occurs in clients with diarrhea and is the primary clinical manifestation in a client diagnosed with acute gastroenteritis.

**TEST-TAKING HINT: The test taker should realize that in an acute condition, the assessment data would be abnormal, which may help select the correct answer for some questions, However, in this question, all of the answer options are abnormal data so this will not help in this situation.**

**105.** 1. The assistant can calculate the client's intake and output, but the nurse must evaluate the data to determine if it is normal for the elderly client diagnosed with acute gastroenteritis.
2. The assistant can take the vital signs for a client who is stable; the nurse must interpret and evaluate the vital signs.
3. The assistant cannot administer medications, and IV solutions are considered to be medications.
4. The nurse cannot delegate assessment. The client may have an excoriated perianal area secondary to diarrhea; therefore, the nurse should assess the client.

**TEST-TAKING HINT: The nurse should not delegate any nursing task that requires judgment or assessment and cannot delegate the administration of medications. Words like "evaluate" mean the same thing as assess; therefore option "1," "3," and "4" can be eliminated.**

**106.** 1. Leg cramps could indicate hypokalemia, which is a potential complication of excessive diarrhea and should be reported to the health-care provider.
2. The client should increase the fluid intake because oral rehydration is the primary treatment for gastroenteritis to replace lost fluid as a result of diarrhea and to prevent dehydration.

3. Reintroducing solid foods slowly, in small amounts, will allow the bowel to rest and the mucosa to return to health after acute gastroenteritis states.
4. Bottled water should be consumed when contaminated water is suspected, and an oral glucose–electrolyte solution, such as Gatorade or Pedialyte, should be recommended.

**TEST-TAKING HINT: Both answer options "2" and "4" refer to fluids, which should make the test taker either eliminate both of these or select from one (1) of these two (2) as the right answer.**

**107.** 1. The nurse should assess the elderly skin turgor over the sternum because loss of subcutaneous fat associated with aging makes skin turgor assessment on the arms less reliable.
2. Orthostatic hypotension indicates fluid volume deficit, which can occur in an elderly client who is having many episodes of diarrhea, which occurs with acute gastroenteritis.
3. The nurse should record frequency and characteristics of stool, not sputum, in the client diagnosed with gastroenteritis.
4. Standard precautions, including wearing gloves and hand washing, help prevent the spread of the infection to others.
5. The elderly client is at risk for orthostatic hypotension; therefore safety precautions should be instituted to ensure the client doesn't fall as a result of a decrease in blood pressure.

**TEST-TAKING HINT: This is an alternate-type question that requires the test taker to choose all interventions that apply. The test taker should look at each option and consider if this is an intervention for an "elderly" client. The elderly are a special population that usually have specific interventions that address the aging process no matter what the disease process.**

**108.** 1. Epigastric pain is expected in a client diagnosed with peptic ulcer disease.
2. Four (4) diarrheal stools would not be unusual in a client diagnosed with gastroenteritis.
3. A hard, rigid abdomen and an elevated temperature are abnormal in any circumstance and the nurse should assess this client first. These are clinical manifestations of peritonitis, a potentially life-threatening condition.

4. Vomiting is expected in a client diagnosed with food poisoning.

**TEST-TAKING HINT: When managing clients the nurse must be able to prioritize care. Therefore, the test taker must be able to determine which client's complaints, signs, or symptoms are not expected of the disease process. Always look at the client's age because it may help the test taker determine the best answer.**

## Abdominal Surgery

109. 1. Absent bowel sounds would indicate a paralytic ileus, not peritonitis, and this is a normal potassium level (3.5 to 5.5 mEq/L).
    2. Abdominal cramping would not make the nurse suspect peritonitis, and the hemoglobin is normal (13–17 g/dL)
    3. *Campylobacter* is a cause of profuse diarrhea, but it does not support a diagnosis of peritonitis.
    4. A hard, rigid abdomen indicates an inflamed peritoneum (abdominal wall cavity) resulting from an infection, which results in an elevated WBC level.

**TEST-TAKING HINT: The "itis" of peritonitis means inflammation, and if the test taker has no idea what the answer is, an elevated WBC count should provide a key to selecting "4" as the correct answer.**

110. 1. The nurse may notify the surgeon if warranted, but that is not the first intervention.
    2. The nurse should instruct the client to splint the incision when coughing but then take further action.
    3. Assessing the surgical incision is the first intervention because this may indicate the client has wound dehiscence.
    4. The nurse should never administer pain medication without assessing for potential complications.

**TEST-TAKING HINT: The stem is asking which intervention is first. This means that all four (4) answer options could be possible actions but only one (1) is first. The test taker should use the nursing process and select the option that addresses assessment because it is the first step in the nursing process.**

111. 1. The client has a surgical incision, which impairs the skin integrity, but it is not the priority because it is sutured under sterile conditions.
    2. After abdominal surgery, the body distrib-

utes fluids to the affected area as part of the healing process. These fluids are shifted from the intravascular compartment to the interstitial space, which causes potential fluid and electrolyte imbalance.

3. Bowel elimination is a problem, but after general anesthesia wears off, the bowel sounds will return and this is not a life-threatening problem.
4. Psychosocial problems are not priority over actual physiological problems.

**TEST-TAKING HINT: When identifying priority problems the test taker can eliminate any psychosocial problem as a potential correct answer if there are applicable physiological problems.**

112. 1. Evisceration is a life-threatening condition in which the abdominal contents have protruded through the ruptured incision. The nurse must protect the bowel from the environment by placing a sterile normal saline dressing on it. The saline prevents the intestines from drying out and necrosing.
    2. The nurse should not attempt to replace the protruding bowel.
    3. This position places the client with the head of the bed elevated, which will make the situation worse.
    4. Antibiotics will not protect the protruding bowels, which must be priority. Antibiotics will be administered at a later time to prevent infection, but this is not urgent.

**TEST-TAKING HINT: The test taker must understand the term "evisceration" to answer this question.**

113. 1. The client needing more pain medication indicates the client's condition is getting worse.
    2. Coffee-ground material indicates old blood.
    3. Because the signs of peritonitis are elevated temperature and rigid abdomen, a reversal of these signs would indicate the client is getting better.
    4. Two soft-formed bowel movements are good, but this does not have anything to do with peritonitis.

**TEST-TAKING HINT: The "itis" of peritonitis means inflammation. Peritonitis is inflammation of the peritoneum, or abdominal wall, caused by an infection. An infection is usually associated with an elevated temperature, so a decrease in temperature would be a sign that the client is improving. A soft abdomen is also**

a good sign. Knowing that the word "peritoneum" means "abdominal wall" could help the test taker choose option "3," which is the only option that contains the word abdomen.

114. 1. The client would be NPO; therefore no medication would be administered.
2. The client would be NPO; therefore no food or fluids would be administered.
3. Deep breathing will help prevent pulmonary complications, but it will not address the client's paralytic ileus.
4. A paralytic ileus is the absence of peristalsis; therefore the bowel will be unable to process any oral intake. A nasogastric tube is inserted to decompress the bowel until there is surgical intervention or bowel sounds return spontaneously.

**TEST-TAKING HINT: If the test taker realizes that the stem of the question says that the part of the gastrointestinal system, the ileus, is paralyzed, the test taker should know that allowing the client to take anything by mouth would be an inappropriate action, so options "1" and "2" could be eliminated. Deep breathing addresses the respiratory system, not the gastrointestinal system, so "3" could also be eliminated.**

115. 1. The JP bulb should be depressed, which indicates suction is being applied. A round bulb indicates that the bulb is full and needs to be emptied and suction reapplied.
2. The tube should be pinned to the dressing to prevent accidentally pulling the drain out of the insertion site.
3. The insertion site should be pink and without any signs of infection, which include drainage, warmth, and redness.
4. The JP bulb should be sunken in or depressed, indicating that suction is being applied.

**TEST-TAKING HINT: The stem is asking which data need intervention by the nurse. Option "2" can be ruled out because all tubes and drains should be secured. A pink insertion site with no drainage is expected, which would cause the test taker to eliminate this option as a possible correct answer.**

116. 1. Medicating the client with an analgesic could increase the client's nausea unless the nausea is caused by pain. The nurse should assess the etiology to determine the interventions.
2. A client who has had abdominal surgery usually has a nasogastric tube (NGT) in place. If the NGT is not patent, this will

cause nausea. Irrigating the NGT may relieve nausea.
3. Checking the temperature will not treat the nausea.
4. Hyperextending the neck will assist the client to breathe but will not treat nausea.

**TEST-TAKING HINT: Assessment is the first step in the nursing process. Checking the NGT for patency and taking the temperature are the only assessment activities. Temperature does not correlate with nausea. Medication may be administered but it would be an antiemetic, not a narcotic analgesic.**

117. 1. The nurse cannot force the client to do anything; this would be considered assault.
2. There are no data that support the need for a chest x-ray.
3. Shallow respirations and refusal to deep breathe could be the result of abdominal pain. The nurse should assess the client for pain and determine the last time the PCA pump was used.
4. Based on the information given, the client does not need oxygen.

**TEST-TAKING HINT: If the test taker has no idea of what the answer is, identify key words in the stem "abdominal surgery" and "PCA" and select an answer option that is related to one (1) of these key words. "Determine" can be substituted for the word "assess," which is the first step of the nursing process.**

118. 170 mL/hr. The N/G drainage of 45 mL must be added to the 125 mL/hr IV rate, which equals 170 (125 + 45=170). The nurse should infuse 170 mL in the next hour.

**TEST-TAKING HINT: The stem states the previous hour's N/G output plus the baseline IV rate. The test taker must observe the key words in the stem. Don't forget to use the pull-down calculator when taking RN-NCLEX.**

119. 1. A client who has not voided within four (4) hours after any surgery would not be priority. This is an acceptable occurrence, but if the client hasn't voided for eight (8) hours, then the nurse would assess further.
2. This could indicate a ruptured appendix, which could lead to peritonitis, a life-threatening complication; therefore, the nurse should assess this client first.
3. Bowel sounds should return within 24 hours after abdominal surgery. Absent bowel sounds at four (4) hours postoperative would not be of great concern to the nurse.

4. The client being discharged would be stable and not a priority for the nurse.

**TEST-TAKING HINT: The stem is asking which client the nurse should see first. Therefore, the test taker should look for life-threatening or serious complications or abnormal assessment data for the disease process.**

120. 1. The last bowel movement would not help identify the cause of the client's right lower abdominal pain. This might be appropriate for a client with left lower abdominal pain.
2. Information about a high-fat meal would be asked if the nurse suspected the client had a gallbladder problem.
3. **Elderly clients usually display a high tolerance to pain and frequently may have a ruptured appendix with minimal pain, therefore the nurse should assess the characteristic and etiology of the pain.**
4. The passage of flatus (gas) does not help determine the cause of right lower abdominal pain.

**TEST-TAKING HINT: The test taker should go back to basics and assess the client.**

## Eating Disorders

121. 1. **This client is 5'10" tall and weighs 99 pounds (45 kg × 2.2 = 99). Menses will cease if the client is severely emaciated. This occurs in clients diagnosed with anorexia nervosa; the nurse should attempt to determine how much the client eats. A 24-hour dietary recall is a step toward assessing the client's eating patterns.**
2. This could be asked, but the client is asking about missing menstrual periods. Birth control does not interfere with having a period; if anything, some forms of birth control will make the cycles more regular.
3. The nurse can look at the client and see a very thin young woman, which should confirm that more assessment is needed, not reweighing.
4. The pulse and blood pressure will not give the nurse any information as to why the client's menstrual cycles have ceased.

**TEST-TAKING HINT: The stem of the question gives information about the client's height and weight, and the test taker must determine if this is important information. Information in the stem must be eliminated**

as not pertinent to the question or closely regarded to let the test taker know what the real problem is.

122. 1. Many clients jog one (1) to two (2) miles per day as part of their exercise program. This does not indicate bulimia.
2. This may be an end result of bulimia, but it does not identify bulimia.
3. **Bulimia is characterized by bingeing and purging by inducing vomiting after a meal. Stomach contents are acidic and the acid wears away the enamel on the teeth, leaving the teeth a green color.**
4. The client would have calluses on the knuckles from pushing them into the throat to induce vomiting.

**TEST-TAKING HINT: The stem requires the test taker to integrate two (2) pieces of information: large lunch meals and spending a relatively long time in the restroom after the meal. The test taker must determine what the client might be achieving by the behavior and then what result would show up that the nurse might observe—in this case, greenish teeth.**

123. 1. Clients diagnosed with bulimia will eat the entire meal and more food if available. This is not unusual behavior for a client diagnosed with bulimia.
2. **By having someone stay with the client for 45 minutes to one (1) hour after a meal, the client will be prevented from inducing vomiting and ridding the body of the meal before it can be metabolized.**
3. Clients diagnosed with anorexia nervosa tend to overexercise to prevent weight gain and to lose imagined excess weight.
4. Bed rest is not needed for this client.

**TEST-TAKING HINT: The test taker must be able to differentiate between bulimia and anorexia. It can be difficult to keep these processes separate, especially because some clients have both anorexia and bulimia.**

124. 1. The goal is written in terms of client behavior; this option is a nursing intervention, not a client goal.
2. This is written in terms of client behavior and is measurable—eats 50% of meals provided. However, goals should address the etiology of the problem, and this does not. This would be an appropriate goal for a diagnosis of body weight less than needed related to inadequate nutritional intake.
3. This is a dietary intervention.

4. The etiology of the diagnosis of anorexia is "low self-esteem." Therefore the goal must address the client's low self-esteem.

**TEST-TAKING HINT: The test taker could eliminate distracters "1" and "3" as health-care discipline interventions and then choose between the two (2) client goals. The test taker must know the rules about goals and interventions and the nursing diagnosis.**

125. 1. The client is 67 inches tall (5′7″) and weighs 88 pounds (40 kg × 2.2 = 88). This client is severely underweight and nutrition is the priority.
2. Clients with anorexia have a chronic low self-esteem problem, but this is a psychosocial problem and actual physical problems are priority.
3. Disturbed body image is a psychosocial problem that has now manifested itself in a physical one. The physical problem is priority; this would be an appropriate long-term goal.
4. This client thinks that her body is not appealing and this could be a problem, but it is a psychosocial issue and not priority.

**TEST-TAKING HINT: The test taker must decide which problem is priority when all the problems could apply to the client. Unless the client is considering suicide and has a plan to carry it out, physical problems are priority.**

126. 1. The client diagnosed with anorexia will have muscle tissue wasting; liver function tests will not monitor for this.
2. Kidney functions will not monitor nutrition or muscle wasting.
3. The heart is a muscle; in severe anorexia (more than 60% under ideal body weight) muscle tissue is catabolized to provide energy to the body. The client is at risk for death from cardiac complications.
4. The client's entire body will be involved in the process as a result of malnutrition, but bone density tests are not done.

**TEST-TAKING HINT: The test taker needs to be aware of the complications associated with specific disease processes.**

127. 1. The client does not owe the nurse an explanation.
2. If the HCP determines that it is safe for the client to exercise, a gymnasium might be recommended, but walking is the best exercise and this can be done in the neighborhood or at an enclosed shopping mall.
3. The client should set realistic weight loss goals. A realistic weight loss goal is one (1) to

one and one half (1 1/2) pounds per week, but this should be done after assessing the client.
4. Determining the client's eating patterns and what triggers the client to eat—stress or boredom, for example—and where and when the client consumes most of the calories—snacking in front of the TV at night, for example—are needed to assist the client to change eating behaviors.

**TEST-TAKING HINT: This question is an example of using the nursing process to arrive at the correct answer. Assessing the client has priority.**

128. 1. The client that is morbidly obese will have a large abdomen that prevents the lungs from expanding and predisposes the client to respiratory complications.
2. The client may be weighed daily, but this is not priority.
3. The client should be taught proper nutrition for weight loss, but this is not the priority in the immediate postoperative period.
4. This is very important for the long term but respiratory status is priority.

**TEST-TAKING HINT: Regardless of the procedure or the size of the client, respiratory status is priority in the immediate postoperative period. The test taker should apply Maslow's Hierarchy of Needs.**

129. 1. Exercise recommendations for weight loss are to exercise for 30 minutes at least 3 times per week.
2. The client should be aware of situations that trigger the consumption of food when the client is not hungry, such as anger, boredom, and stress. Food-seeking behaviors are usually not associated only with hunger in the client who is obese.
3. The client should weigh herself or himself about once a week. If weight is not observed to be going down every day, the client gets discouraged and feels powerless to control the weight, and this can lead to diet failure.
4. Sodium is limited in clients with hypertension, not obesity.
5. Weight loss support groups such as Weight Watchers or TOPS (Take Off Pounds Sensibly) are helpful to keep the client participating in a weight loss program.

**TEST-TAKING HINT: This is an alternate-type question. The test taker must judge each answer option for itself; one (1) option does not eliminate another. RN-NCLEX gives**

Gastrointestinal

credit for the entire question. The test taker must get all the answers right or the answer will be counted as incorrect.

130. 1. Jogging is not an appropriate exercise for a client who is obese: there is too much stress on the heart and joints.
2. If lifestyle behaviors, patterns of eating, and daily exercise are not modified, the client who loses weight will regain the weight and usually more.
3. The client should eat frequent small meals during the day to keep from being hungry. Breakfast should not be skipped.
4. Diets containing fewer than 1200 calories per day need to be supplemented with a multivitamin to provide the body with the nutrients needed to stay healthy.

TEST-TAKING HINT: The test taker could eliminate "4" on the basis that health-care professionals should not tell clients not to take a multivitamin.

131. 1. The client does not have to explain actions to the nurse; the nurse should not ask "why."
2. This is belittling the client.
3. The client is 36 years old and has the right to refuse to eat, even to the detriment of her body. Restraining the client could be considered assault.
4. This is a factual statement to the client about the possible results if the client refuses nourishment.

TEST-TAKING HINT: The test taker could eliminate "1" on the basis of "why." Option "2" is not therapeutic or factual information.

132. 1. Clients diagnosed with anorexia exercise excessively; clients diagnosed with bulimia do not.
2. Clients diagnosed with bulimia frequently take cathartic laxatives to prevent absorption of calories from the food consumed.
3. Clients diagnosed with bulimia and anorexia have low self-esteem. They feel ugly or unlovable if they are overweight (by their perception).
4. High-fiber foods do help the body to produce larger stools, but this client would use a cathartic laxative.

TEST-TAKING HINT: The test taker must distinguish between bulimia and anorexia to answer this question. Clients with anorexia are usually underweight, whereas clients with bulimia may be of a normal or slightly larger size.

## Constipation/Diarrhea Disorders

133. 1. An antidiarrheal medication would slow down the peristalsis in the colon, worsening the problem.
2. The client has an immediate need to evacuate the bowel, not bowel training.
3. Oil retention enemas will help to soften the feces and evacuate the stool.
4. A UGI series would add barium to the already hardened stool in the colon. Barium enemas x-ray the colon; a UGI x-rays the stomach and jejunum.

TEST-TAKING HINT: If the test taker understands that fecal impaction is the opposite of diarrhea, then option "1" can be eliminated. Knowledge of anatomy and physiology eliminates "4" because stool is formed in the colon and transported to the anus, part of the lower gastrointestinal tract.

134. 1. Bananas are encouraged for clients with potassium loss from diuretics; a banana is not needed for harsh laxative (cathartic) use. Harsh laxatives should be discouraged because they cause laxative dependence and a narrowing of the colon with long-term use.
2. It is not necessary to have a bowel movement every day to have normal bowel functioning.
3. Limiting fluids will increase the problem; the client should be encouraged to increase the fluids in the diet.
4. If the client were feeling "sluggish" from not being able to have a bowel movement, these foods would increase constipation because they are low in residue (fiber).

TEST-TAKING HINT: The test taker must understand terms such as "cathartic." Limiting fluids is used for clients in renal failure or congestive heart failure, but increasing fluids is recommended for most other conditions.

135. 1. Blood may indicate a hemorrhoid, but it is not normal to expel blood when having a bowel movement.
2. Nurses manually remove feces; it is not a self-care activity.
3. Cathartic use on a daily basis creates dependence and a narrowing of the lumen of the colon, creating a much more serious problem.
4. A high-residue diet provides bulk for the colon to use in removing the waste prod-

ucts of metabolism. Bulk laxatives and fiber from vegetables and bran assist the colon to work more effectively.

**TEST-TAKING HINT: Blood is not normal in any circumstance. It may be expected but is not "normal" unless inside a vessel.**

136. 1. This is a symptom of diarrhea moving around an impaction higher up in the colon. The nurse should assess for an impaction when observing this finding.
2. Encouraging the client to drink fluids should be done, but this is not the first intervention.
3. The sodium level is usually not a problem for clients experiencing diarrhea, but the potassium level may be checked. However, again, this is not the first intervention.
4. A protective cream can be applied to an excoriated perineum, but first the nurse should assess the situation.

**TEST-TAKING HINT: The first step of the nursing process is assessment, after which a nursing diagnosis and interventions follow. The nurse should assess first.**

137. 1. This client is improving; semi-formed stools are better than diarrhea.
2. This client has just arrived so the nurse does not know if the complaint is valid and needs intervention unless this client is seen and assessed. The elderly have difficulty with constipation as a result of decreased gastric motility, medications, poor diet, and immobility.
3. The client has diarrhea, but only 200 mL, and has elastic tissue turgor that lets the nurse know the client is not dehydrated.
4. This is not normal, but it is expected for a client with hemorrhoids.

**TEST-TAKING HINT: The test taker should notice descriptive words such as "elderly," which should alert the test taker that the age range has an implication in answering the question. Answer options "3" and "4" are expected for the disease processes.**

138. 1. Cheeseburgers and milk shakes are low-residue foods that can make constipation worse.
2. Canned peaches are soft and can be chewed and swallowed easily while providing some fiber, and whole-wheat bread is higher in fiber than white bread. These foods will be helpful for clients whose gastric motility is slowed as a result of lack of exercise or immobility.

3. These foods do not provide the needed fiber.
4. These are refined flour foods or processed meat (fat). These will not help clients to prevent constipation.

**TEST-TAKING HINT: The test taker must realize that the consequences of immobility include constipation. Then the test taker should try to eliminate processed foods from the choices.**

139. 1. It is important to keep track of the amounts, color, and other characteristics of all body fluids lost.
2. Skin turgor should be assessed at least every six (6) to eight (8) hours, not daily.
3. Carbonated soft drinks increase flatus in the GI tract, and the increased sugar will act as an osmotic laxative and increase the diarrhea.
4. Daily weights are the best method of determining fluid loss and gain.
5. Sitz baths will assist in keeping the client's perianal area clean without having to rub. The warm water is soothing, providing comfort.

**TEST-TAKING HINT: The test taker should note the time frame for any answer option. Every day is not often enough to assess for dehydration in a client who is experiencing massive (voluminous) fluid loss. If the test taker were not aware of the definition, then an associated word "volume" would be a hint.**

140. 1. The nurse will be responsible for signing off on the unlicensed nursing assistant as to being competent to perform the blood glucose. The nurse should do this to determine the competency of the assistant.
2. The lab values may require the nurse to interpret and act on the results. The nurse cannot delegate anything that requires professional judgment.
3. The licensed practical nurse could administer a laxative.
4. The nurse cannot delegate assessment.

**TEST-TAKING HINT: State boards of nursing have agreed that nurses cannot delegate any activity that requires professional judgment, assessment, teaching, or evaluation.**

141. 1. The client is tolerating the feeding change so there is no need for an immediate action.
2. The client has a PEG tube; therefore, the nasogastric feeding tube can be removed.
3. This should be addressed; the client may require some ice chips in the mouth or some oral care, but this must wait until an assess-

ment of the client's ability to swallow has been completed.

4. This client needs to be cleaned immediately; the abdomen must be assessed; and a determination must be made regarding the type of feeding and the additives and medications being administered and skin damage occurring. This client is priority.

**TEST-TAKING HINT: The test taker must identify assessment data that indicate a complication secondary to the disease process when the stem asks which warrants immediate intervention.**

142. 1. This client may have developed an infection from the undercooked meat. The nurse should try to get a specimen for the laboratory to analyze and for the nurse to be able to assess. The client's complaint of "bloody diarrhea" needs to be investigated by the nurse, who should observe the amount, color, and characteristics of the stool.
   2. Antibiotic therapy is initiated in only the most serious cases of infectious diarrhea; the diarrhea must be assessed first. A specimen for culture should be obtained, if possible, before beginning medication.
   3. A complete blood count will provide an estimate of blood loss, but it is not the first intervention.
   4. An antidiarrheal medication would be administered after the specimen collection.

**TEST-TAKING HINT: All answer options in a priority-setting question may be actions the nurse would take, but the right answer will be the one (1) that should be taken before the others. Collecting a stool sample is assessment, which is the first step in the nursing process.**

143. 1. The risk for hypovolemic shock would require that the HCP be informed and that there be an order for treatment. It is a collaborative problem.
   2. Bacteremia is a bacterial infection in the circulatory system. This is a collaborative problem.
   3. The treatment of a fluid volume deficit is an independent nursing problem; the nurse can assess and intervene with oral fluids.
   4. The client might have a decreased knowledge of transmission. Increase in knowledge is not a problem.

**TEST-TAKING HINT: The question is asking for an independent nursing problem; only one (1) problem appears in any text as a nursing problem/diagnosis. Knowledge problems are always written as knowledge deficit.**

144. 1. Normal serum sodium levels are 135–152 mEq/L, so this falls within the normal range.
   2. The client diagnosed with a fecal impaction is beginning to move the stool; this indicates an improvement.
   3. Normal potassium levels are 3.5–5.5 mEq/L. The level stated in this option is below normal. Imbalances in potassium levels can be caused by diarrhea and can cause cardiac dysrhythmias.
   4. This client has been having diarrhea and now is having semi-liquid stools, so this client is getting better.

**TEST-TAKING HINT: The test taker must determine if the client is experiencing a potentially life-threatening complication, such as potential for cardiac dysrhythmias. Answer options "1," "2," and "4" are expected for the disease process and are normal or show improvement.**

1. The nurse is caring for the client with active herpes simplex 1 lesions. Which intervention should the nurse implement to prevent the spread of the virus?
   1. Wash hands completely only before providing care.
   2. Wear clean gloves to prevent transfer of the virus.
   3. Scrub the lesions with soap and water twice daily.
   4. Apply 1% Lidocaine (hydrocortisone) cream to the lesions.

2. The client receiving antibiotic therapy complains of white, cheesy plaques in the mouth that bleed when removed. Which action should the nurse implement?
   1. Notify the health-care provider to obtain an antifungal medication.
   2. Explain that the patches will go away naturally in about two (2) weeks.
   3. Instruct the client to rinse the mouth with diluted hydrogen peroxide and water daily.
   4. Allow the client to verbalize feelings about having the plaques.

3. Which instruction should be discussed with the client diagnosed with gastroesophageal reflux disease (GERD)?
   1. Eat a low-carbohydrate, low-sodium diet.
   2. Lie down for 30 minutes after eating.
   3. Do not eat spicy foods or acidic foods.
   4. Drink two (2) glasses of water before bedtime.

4. When assessing the oral cavity of an elderly client, which data should the nurse report to the health-care provider?
   1. The client's tongue is rough and beefy red.
   2. The client's tonsils are at a +1 on a grading scale.
   3. The client's mucosa is pink and moist.
   4. The client's uvula rises with the mouth open.

5. Which complaint would be significant for the nurse to assess in the adolescent male client who uses oral tobacco?
   1. The client complains of clear to white sputum.
   2. The client has an episodic blister on the upper lip.
   3. The client complains of a nonhealing sore in the mouth.
   4. The client has bilateral ducts at the second molars.

6. The female client is diagnosed with ulcerative colitis. Which sign/symptom would warrant immediate intervention by the nurse?
   1. The client has 20 bloody stools a day.
   2. The client's oral temperature is 99.8°F.
   3. The client's abdomen is hard and rigid.
   4. The client complains of urinating when she coughs.

7. Which expected outcome would be appropriate for the client diagnosed with aphthous stomatitis?
   1. The client will be able to cope with perceived stress.
   2. The client will consume a balanced diet.
   3. The client will deny any difficulty swallowing.
   4. The client will take antacids as prescribed.

8. The nurse is administering a proton pump inhibitor to the client diagnosed with peptic ulcer disease. Which statement supports the rationale for administering this medication?
   1. It prevents the final transport of hydrogen ions into the gastric lumen.
   2. It blocks receptors that control hydrochloric acid secretion by the parietal cells.
   3. It protects the ulcer from the destructive action of the digestive enzyme pepsin.
   4. It neutralizes the hydrochloric acid secreted by the stomach.

9. Which task can the nurse delegate to the unlicensed nursing assistant to improve the desire to eat in a client diagnosed with anorexia?
   1. Administer an antiemetic 30 minutes before the meal.
   2. Provide mouth care with lemon glycerin swabs prior to the meal.
   3. Create a social atmosphere by interacting with the client.
   4. Encourage the client's parents to sit with the client during meals.

10. The male client with rule out colon cancer is two (2) hours post-sigmoidoscopy procedure. Which intervention would warrant immediate intervention by the nurse?
    1. The client has hyperactive bowel sounds.
    2. The client is eating a hamburger that his family brought.
    3. The client is sleepy and wants to sleep.
    4. The client's BP is 96/60 and apical pulse is 108.

11. The nurse identifies the client problem "alteration in gastrointestinal system" for the elderly client. Which statement reflects the most appropriate rationale for this diagnosis?
    1. Elderly clients have a better mechanical handling of food with dentures.
    2. Elderly clients have an increase in digestive enzymes, which helps with digestion.
    3. Elderly clients have an increased need for laxatives because of a decrease in bile.
    4. Elderly clients have an increase in bacteria in the GI system, resulting in diarrhea.

12. The nurse is teaching a class on diverticulosis. Which interventions should the nurse discuss when teaching ways to prevent an acute exacerbation of diverticulitis? Select all that apply.
    1. Eat a low-fiber diet.
    2. Drink 2500 mL of water daily.
    3. Avoid eating foods with seeds.
    4. Walk 30 minutes a day.
    5. Take an antacid every two (2) hours.

13. The nurse in an outpatient clinic is caring for a client who is 67 inches tall and weighs 100 kg. The client complains of occasional pyrosis that resolves with standing or with taking antacids. What treatment should the nurse expect the HCP to order?
    1. Place the client on a weight loss program.
    2. Instruct the client to eat three (3) balanced meals.
    3. Tell the client to take an antiemetic before each meal.
    4. Discuss the importance of decreasing alcohol intake.

14. The client is one (1) hour postoperative laparoscopic cholecystectomy. Which intervention should the nurse implement?
    1. Assess the client's abdominal dressing for bleeding.
    2. Monitor the client's T-tube output every one (1) hour.
    3. Discuss discharge teaching with the significant other.
    4. Check the client's upper right quadrant stoma site.

15. Which information should the nurse teach the client post–barium enema procedure?
    1. The client should not eat or drink anything for four (4) hours.
    2. The client should remain on bed rest until the sedative wears off.
    3. The client should take a mild laxative to help expel the barium.
    4. The client will have normal elimination color and pattern immediately.

16. The client diagnosed with a hiatal hernia has been scheduled for a laparoscopic Nissen fundoplication. Which statement indicates that the nurse's teaching has been effective?
    1. "I will have three (3) or four (4) small incisions."
    2. "I will be able to go home the same day of surgery."
    3. "I will not have any pain because this is laparoscopic surgery."
    4. "I will be returning to work the day after my surgery."

17. The client has been diagnosed with esophageal diverticula. Which lifestyle modification should be taught by the nurse?
    1. Raise the foot of the bed to 45 degrees to increase peristalsis.
    2. Eat the evening meal at least two (2) hours prior to bed.
    3. Eat a low-fat, low-cholesterol, high-fiber diet.
    4. Wear an abdominal binder to strengthen the abdominal muscles.

18. The client weighs 160 pounds and is 5'1" tall. Calculate the body mass index (BMI) using the following formula:

$$BMI = \frac{703 \times \text{weight in pounds}}{(\text{height in inches})^2}$$

19. Based on the client's body mass index (BMI) from Question 18, which category should the nurse document in the client's medical records?
    1. Underweight.
    2. Overweight.
    3. Ideal weight.
    4. Obese.

### Body Mass Index

| Category | BMI Lower Range | BMI Upper Range |
| --- | --- | --- |
| Underweight | >19 | — |
| Ideal weight | 19 | 24.9 |
| Overweight | 25 | 30 |
| Obese | 30.1 | — |

20. Which intervention should the nurse implement specifically for the client in end-stage liver failure who is experiencing hepatic encephalopathy?
    1. Assess the client's neurological status.
    2. Prepare to administer a loop diuretic.
    3. Check the client's stool for bleeding.
    4. Assess the abdominal fluid wave.

21. Which priority teaching information should the nurse discuss with the client to help prevent contracting hepatitis B?
    1. Explain the importance of good hand washing.
    2. Tell the client to take the hepatitis B vaccine in three (3) doses.
    3. Tell the client not to ingest unsanitary food or water.
    4. Discuss how to implement standard precautions.

22. The nurse is working in an emergency department of a community hospital. During the past 2 hours, 15 clients have been diagnosed with *Salmonella* food poisoning. Which information should the nurse discuss with clients?
    1. Explain that the incubation period is 48 to 72 hours.
    2. Explain that the source of this poisoning is contaminated water.
    3. Explain that one (1) source of potential contamination is eggs.
    4. Explain that the bacterial contaminant is from canned foods.

23. Which intervention should the nurse include when discussing ways to prevent food poisoning?
    1. Wash hands for ten (10) seconds after handling raw meat.
    2. Clean all cutting boards between meats and fruits.
    3. Maintain food temperatures at 140°F during extended servings.
    4. Explain that fruits do not require washing prior to eating or preparing.

24. Which nursing diagnosis would be appropriate for the nurse to identify for the client with diarrhea?
    1. Alteration in skin integrity.
    2. Chronic pain perception.
    3. Fluid volume excess.
    4. Ineffective coping.

25. The nurse is assessing a client complaining of abdominal pain. Which data would support the diagnosis of a bowel obstruction?
    1. Steady, aching pain in one specific area.
    2. Sharp back pain radiating to the flank.
    3. Sharp pain that increases with deep breaths.
    4. Intermittent colicky pain near the umbilicus.

26. The nurse is caring for the client scheduled for an abdominal perineal resection for Stage IV colon cancer. When preparing the plan of care during surgery, which client problem should the nurse include in the plan?
    1. Fluid volume deficit.
    2. Impaired tissue perfusion.
    3. Infection of surgical site.
    4. Immunosuppression.

27. The nurse is assessing the client in end-stage liver failure who has been diagnosed with portal hypertension. Which intervention should the nurse include in the plan of care?
    1. Assess the abdomen for a tympanic wave.
    2. Monitor the client's blood pressure.
    3. Percuss the liver for size and location.
    4. Weigh the client twice each week.

28. The nurse is caring for the client diagnosed with ascites from hepatic cirrhosis. What information should the nurse report to the health-care provider?
    1. A decrease in the client's daily weight of one (1) pound.
    2. An increase in urine output after administration of a diuretic.
    3. An increase in abdominal girth of two (2) inches.
    4. A decrease in the serum direct bilirubin to 0.6 mg/dL.

29. The nurse is caring for the client diagnosed with hepatic encephalopathy. Which sign and symptom would indicate that the disease is progressing?
    1. The client has a decrease in serum ammonia level.
    2. The client is not able to circle choices on the menu.
    3. The client is able to take deep breaths as directed.
    4. The client is now able to eat previously restricted food items.

30. The client is scheduled for a colostomy as a result of colon cancer, and the surgeon tells the client the stool will be a formed consistency. Where would the nurse teach the client the stoma will be located?

    1. A
    2. B
    3. C
    4. D

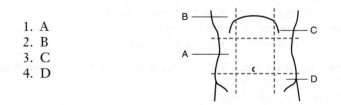

31. The nurse is speaking to a support group for clients diagnosed with Crohn's disease. Which information would be most important for the nurse to discuss with the clients?
    1. Discuss coping skills that assist with adaptation to lifestyle modifications.
    2. Teach about drug administration, dosages, and scheduled times.
    3. Teach dietary changes necessary to control symptoms.
    4. Explain the care of the colostomy and necessary equipment.

32. The nurse is caring for a client diagnosed with ulcerative colitis. Which symptom(s) supports this diagnosis?
    1. Increased appetite and thirst.
    2. Elevated hemoglobin.
    3. Multiple bloody, liquid stools.
    4. Exacerbations unrelated to stress.

33. The nurse is teaching the client diagnosed with inflammatory bowel disease (IBD) about the therapeutic diet. Which food selection would be the best choice for a meal?
    1. Roast beef on wheat bread and a milk shake.
    2. Hamburger, French fries, and a Coke.
    3. Pepper steak, brown rice, and iced tea.
    4. Roasted turkey, asparagus, and water.

34. The elderly client has been diagnosed with acute gastritis. Which client problem would be priority for this client?
    1. Fluid volume deficit.
    2. Altered nutrition: less than body requirements.
    3. Impaired tissue perfusion.
    4. Alteration in comfort.

35. The nurse is caring for the client diagnosed with chronic gastritis. Which symptom(s) would support this diagnosis?
    1. Rapid onset of mid-sternal discomfort.
    2. Epigastric pain relieved by eating food.
    3. Dyspepsia and hematemesis.
    4. Nausea and projectile vomiting.

36. The nurse identifies the client problem of "fluid volume deficit" for a client diagnosed with gastritis. Which intervention should be included in the plan of care?
    1. Obtain permission for a blood transfusion.
    2. Prepare the client for total parenteral nutrition.
    3. Monitor the client's lung sounds every shift.
    4. Assess the client's intravenous site.

37. The nurse working in a skilled nursing facility is collaborating with the dietician concerning the meals of a client who is immobile. Which foods would be most appropriate for this client?
    1. Oatmeal and wheat toast.
    2. Cream of wheat and biscuits.
    3. Cottage cheese and canned peaches.
    4. Tuna on croissant and applesauce.

38. Which intervention should the nurse implement when administering a potassium supplement?
    1. Determine the client's allergies.
    2. Assess the client's apical heart rate.
    3. Monitor the client's blood pressure.
    4. Monitor the client's complete blood count.

39. The nurse is preparing the client for a fiberoptic colonoscopy for colon polyps. Which task can be delegated to the unlicensed nursing assistant?
    1. Administer the polyethylene glycol electrolyte lavage solution.
    2. Explain to the client why that morning's breakfast is withheld.
    3. Start an intravenous site with 0.9% normal saline fluid.
    4. Administer a cleansing enema until the return is clear.

40. The nurse is caring for the client that is one (1)-day post-upper gastrointestinal series (UGI). Which assessment data warrant immediate intervention?
    1. No bowel movement.
    2. Oxygen saturation 96%.
    3. Vital signs within normal baseline.
    4. Intact gag reflex.

41. The client is complaining of painful swallowing secondary to mouth ulcers. Which statement indicates the nurse's teaching has been effective?
    1. "I will brush my teeth with a soft-bristle toothbrush."
    2. "I will rinse my mouth with Listerine mouth wash."
    3. "I will swish with antifungal solution and then swallow."
    4. "I will avoid spicy foods, tobacco, and alcohol."

42. When assessing the integumentary system of the client with anorexia nervosa, which finding would support the diagnosis?
    1. Preoccupation with calories.
    2. Thick body hair.
    3. Sore tongue.
    4. Dry, brittle hair.

43. The nurse is teaching the client diagnosed with colon cancer who is scheduled for a colostomy the next day. Which behavior indicates the best method of applying adult teaching principles?
    1. The nurse repeats the information as indicated by the client's questions.
    2. The nurse teaches in one session all the information that the client needs.
    3. The nurse uses a video so that the client can hear the medical terms.
    4. The nurse waits until the client asks questions about the surgery.

44. The nurse is caring for the client one (1) day postoperative sigmoid colostomy operation. Which independent nursing intervention should the nurse implement?
    1. Change the infusion rate of the intravenous fluid.
    2. Encourage the client to discuss his or her feelings.
    3. Administer opioid narcotic medications for pain management.
    4. Assist the client out of bed to sit in the chair twice daily.

45. The nurse is caring for the client recovering from intestinal surgery. Which assessment finding would require immediate intervention?
    1. Presence of thin pink drainage in the Jackson Pratt.
    2. Guarding when the nurse touches the abdomen.
    3. Tenderness around the surgical site during palpation.
    4. Complaints of chills and feeling feverish.

46. The client has been diagnosed with hemorrhoids. Which statement from the client indicates that further teaching is needed?
    1. "I should increase fruits, bran, and fluids in my diet."
    2. "I will use warm compresses and take sitz baths daily."
    3. "I must take a laxative every night and have a stool daily."
    4. "I can use an analgesic ointment or suppository for pain."

47. The nurse is preparing the postoperative nursing care plan for the client recovering from a hemorrhoidectomy. Which intervention should the nurse implement?
    1. Establish a rapport with the client to decrease embarrassment of assessing site.
    2. Encourage the client to lie in the lithotomy position twice a day.
    3. Milk the tube inserted during surgery to allow the passage of flatus.
    4. Digitally dilate the rectal sphincter to express old blood.

48. The client has recently been diagnosed with irritable bowel syndrome (IBS). Which intervention should the nurse teach the client to reduce symptoms?
    1. Instruct the client to avoid drinking fluids with meals.
    2. Explain the need to decrease intake of flatus-forming foods.
    3. Teach the client how to perform gentle perianal care.
    4. Encourage the client to see a psychologist.

49. The nurse at the scene of a knife fight is caring for a young man who has a knife stuck in his abdomen. Which action should the nurse implement?
    1. Stabilize the knife.
    2. Remove the knife gently.
    3. Turn the client on the side.
    4. Apply pressure to the insertion site.

50. The nurse writes the problem "risk for impaired skin integrity" for a client with a sigmoid colostomy. Which expected outcome would be appropriate for this client?
    1. The client will have intact skin around the stoma.
    2. The client will be able to change the ostomy bag.
    3. The client will express anxiety about the body changes.
    4. The client will maintain fluid balance.

51. The client is admitted into the emergency department complaining of acute epigastric pain and reports vomiting a large amount of bright-red blood at home. Which interventions should the nurse implement? List in order of priority.
    1. Assess the client's vital signs.
    2. Insert a nasogastric tube.
    3. Begin iced saline lavage.
    4. Start an IV with an 18-gauge needle.
    5. Type and crossmatch for a blood transfusion.

1. 1. Hand washing before and after care is a minimum measure to prevent transfer of the virus; it is a basic standard precaution.
   2. **Clean gloves should be worn when providing care to prevent the transfer of the herpes simplex 1 virus.**
   3. Scrubbing the lesions would transfer the virus along the nerves and spread the disease process.
   4. Herpes simplex is treated with acyclovir (Zovirax), an antiviral medication; it is not treated with Lidocaine cream.

2. 1. **Candidiasis, or thrush, presents as white, cheesy plaques that bleed if rubbed and is a side effect of antibiotic therapy. Candidiasis is treated with antifungal solution, which is swished around the mouth, held for at least one (1) minute, and then swallowed. Candidiasis can be prevented if acidophilus is administered concurrently with antibiotic therapy.**
   2. White painless patches that disappear in approximately two (2) weeks are leukoplakia, caused by tobacco use, which may be cancerous and should be evaluated by an HCP.
   3. A solution of hydrogen peroxide is not recommended to treat candidiasis.
   4. The nurse needs to treat the client's mouth, not listen to feelings.

3. 1. The client should eat a low-fat, high-fiber diet.
   2. The client should not lie down for at least two (2) hours after each meal to prevent gastric reflux.
   3. **The client should avoid irritants, such as spicy foods or acidic foods, as well as alcohol, caffeine, and tobacco, because they increase gastric secretions.**
   4. The client should avoid food or drink two (2) hours before bedtime or lying down after eating.

4. 1. **A rough, beefy-red tongue may indicate that the client has pernicious anemia and should be evaluated by the health-care provider.**
   2. A score of +1 on the tonsil grading scale shows that the tonsils are extending to the pharyngopalatine arch, which is normal.
   3. Mucosa should be pink and moist; therefore the nurse would not need to notify the health-care provider.
   4. Symmetrical movement of the uvula is normal and should not be reported to the health-care provider.

5. 1. Clear to white sputum would not be significant in the client using oral tobacco.
   2. Episodic blisters on the lips are herpes simplex 1 and would not be specific to this client.
   3. **Presence of any nonhealing sore on the lips or mouth may be oral cancer, the risk for which is increased by using oral tobacco.**
   4. Bilateral Stensen's ducts visible at the site of the second molars are normal assessment data.

6. 1. The colon is ulcerated and unable to absorb water, so 10 to 20 bloody diarrhea stools is the most common symptom of ulcerative colitis and would not warrant immediate intervention.
   2. This is not an elevated temperature and would not warrant immediate intervention by the nurse.
   3. **A hard, rigid abdomen indicates peritonitis, which is a complication of ulcerative colitis and warrants immediate intervention.**
   4. Stress incontinence is not a symptom of colitis and would not warrant immediate intervention.

7. 1. **The cause of canker sores, aphthous stomatitis, is unknown. The small ulcerations of the soft oral tissue are linked to stress, trauma, allergies, viral infections, and metabolic disorders. Therefore, being able to cope with stress would be a desired outcome.**
   2. The client with recurrent erythematous macule cankers will not have malnutrition; therefore a balanced diet would not be applicable to this client.
   3. The client with cankers should not have difficulty swallowing.
   4. Antacids are not a treatment for canker sores.

8. 1. **This is the rationale for proton pump inhibitors.**
   2. This is the rationale for histamine receptor antagonists.
   3. This is the rationale for mucosal protective agents.
   4. This is the rationale for antacids.

9. 1. Unlicensed nursing assistants cannot administer medications, and this would not be appropriate for a client with anorexia.
   2. Mouth care should be provided before and after meals, but not with alcohol mouth wash and lemon glycerin swabs, which decrease the appetite.
   3. **The NA assisting the client with meals needs to increase interaction to improve the client's appetite and make it an enjoyable occasion.**

4. Often the parents are the cause of the client's stress and anxiety, which may have led to the client's anorexia; therefore, the parents should not be asked to stay with the client.

10. 1. The client has been NPO and had laxatives; therefore, hyperactive bowel sounds would not warrant immediate intervention.
    2. The client is able to eat after the procedure, so this would not warrant immediate intervention.
    3. The client received sedation during the procedure. That, plus being up all the night before having bowel movements, may have made the client exhausted and sleepy.
    4. **These are signs/symptoms of hypovolemic shock that require immediate intervention by the nurse.**

11. 1. The elderly client does not have a better way of breaking down food with dentures.
    2. The secretion of digestive enzymes and bile is decreased in the elderly, and this results in an alteration in nutrition and elimination.
    3. Bile does not affect motility of the intestines. The need for laxatives is caused by client misunderstanding about the frequency of bowel movements and to decreased fluid and fiber intake.
    4. **When the motility of the gastrointestinal tract decreases, bacteria remain in the gut longer and multiply, which results in diarrhea.**

12. 1. A high-fiber diet will prevent constipation, the primary reason for diverticulitis. A low-fiber (residue) diet would be prescribed for acute diverticulitis.
    2. **Increased fluids will help keep the stool soft and prevent constipation.**
    3. **It is controversial if seeds cause an exacerbation of diverticulosis, but this is an appropriate intervention to teach until proved otherwise.**
    4. **Exercise will help prevent constipation, which causes an exacerbation of diverticulitis.**
    5. There are no medications used to help prevent an acute exacerbation of diverticulitis. Antacids are used to neutralize hydrochloric acid in the stomach.

13. 1. **Obesity increases the risk of pyrosis (heartburn); therefore losing weight could help decrease the incidents.**
    2. Eating small, frequent meals along with decreased intake of spicy foods have been linked to the prevention of heartburn (pyrosis).
    3. Antiemetics decrease nausea, which is not a problem with heartburn. Antacids neutralize the acid of the stomach and are used to treat heartburn.
    4. Drinking alcoholic beverages increases heartburn and should be avoided, not decreased.

14. 1. The client has three (3) to four (4) band-aid incisions in the upper quadrant, not an abdominal dressing.
    2. The client will not have a T-tube with a laparoscopic cholecystectomy.
    3. **A laparoscopic cholecystectomy is done in day surgery. The nurse must make sure the significant others taking care of the client are knowledgeable of postoperative care.**
    4. The client does not have a stoma.

15. 1. The client may resume the regular diet.
    2. The client will not be sedated for this procedure; therefore the client does not need to be on bed rest.
    3. **The nurse needs to teach the client to take a mild laxative to help evacuate the barium and return to the client's normal bowel routine. Failure to pass the barium could cause constipation when the barium hardens.**
    4. The client can expect to pass white- or light-colored stools until the barium has completely been evacuated.

16. 1. **In a laparoscopic Nissen fundoplication, there are four (4) to five (5) incisions approximately one (1) inch apart that allow for the passage of equipment to visualize the abdominal organs and perform the operation.**
    2. Many clients come through the day surgery department, but some must remain in the hospital for more than one (1) day, so this may be a false statement.
    3. There is no surgery that does not cause pain.
    4. This is still surgery and the client should not return to work the next day; the client should wait at least one (1) week before returning to work.

17. 1. The client needs to elevate the head, not the foot, of the bed to prevent the reflux of stomach contents.
    2. **The evening meal should be eaten at least two (2) hours prior to retiring. Small, frequent meals and semi-soft foods ease the passage of food, which can decrease signs and symptoms of the disease process.**
    3. This diet is recommended for a client with coronary artery disease, not for esophageal diverticula.

4. Restrictive clothing should be avoided, and abdominal binders do not strengthen muscles and would not benefit this client.

18. BMI of 30.2

$$BMI = \frac{703 \times weight\ in\ pounds}{(height\ in\ inches)^2}$$

$$\frac{112480}{3721} = 30.22\ BMI$$

19. 1. This client is not underweight. Less than 19 would be underweight.
2. This client is not overweight. Between 25 and 30 is overweight.
3. This client is not ideal weight. The BMI would be 19–24.9.
4. **This client is obese, with a BMI greater than 30.**

20. 1. **The increased serum ammonia level associated with liver failure causes the hepatic encephalopathy, which, in turn, leads to neurological deficit.**
2. Administering a loop diuretic would be appropriate for ascites and portal hypertension.
3. Checking the stool for bleeding would be appropriate for esophageal varices and decreased vitamin K.
4. Assessing the abdominal fluid wave would be appropriate for ascites and portal hypertension.

21. 1. This would be appropriate for prevention of hepatitis A.
2. **The hepatitis B vaccine will prevent the client from contracting this disease.**
3. This would be appropriate for prevention of hepatitis A.
4. The nurse uses standard precautions, not the client.

22. 1. The incubation period for *Salmonella* food poisoning is 8 to 48 hours.
2. *Salmonellae* bacteria are not transmitted to humans via water.
3. **Eggs, poultry, pet turtles, and chickens are sources of the *Salmonellae* bacteria, which cause food poisoning.**
4. *Clostridium botulinum* is transmitted via improperly canned food.

23. 1. Hand washing for ten (10) seconds is not long enough to remove any bacteria. Hands should be washed for at least 30 seconds before handling food or eating.
2. Cutting surfaces used for meats should be different from those used for fruits and vegetables to prevent contamination.

3. Foods that are being served for an extended time should be kept at 140°F.
4. All fruits and vegetables should be washed before eating or preparing.

24. 1. **When clients have multiple liquid stools, the rectal area can become irritated. The integrity of the skin can be impaired.**
2. Pain experienced by this client would be acute, rather than chronic.
3. Fluid volume deficit would be appropriate, rather than fluid volume excess.
4. Ineffective coping is a psychosocial problem and is not appropriate for a client with diarrhea.

25. 1. Steady, aching pain is associated with a peritoneal inflammation, which may be secondary to a ruptured spleen or perforated ulcer or other abdominal organ.
2. Sharp pain in the back and flank indicates kidney involvement.
3. Sharp pain that increases with deep breaths indicates muscular involvement.
4. **Intermittent and colicky pain located near the umbilicus is indicative of a small bowel obstruction; lumbar pain is indicative of colon involvement.**

26. 1. Fluid deficit would be a potential problem, not an actual problem. The client's fluid balance should be managed by intravenous fluids. Assessment should support the balance.
2. **The perfusion of the surgical site is compromised as a result of the surgical incision, especially when a graft is used.**
3. Infection would be a potential problem, but not at the time of surgery.
4. After surgery, not during surgery, the client may require chemotherapy, which would cause immunosuppression.

27. 1. **A client who has been diagnosed with portal hypertension should be assessed for a fluid wave to check for ascites.**
2. High blood pressure is not the etiology of portal hypertension.
3. In portal hypertension, the liver usually cannot be percussed.
4. Weighing the client should be done daily, not twice each week.

28. 1. A decrease in weight would indicate a loss in fluid and would not be reported to the healthcare provider.
2. An increase in urine output would indicate that the diuretic was effective.
3. **An increase in abdominal girth would indicate that the ascites is increasing, meaning**

that the client's condition is becoming more serious and should be reported to the health-care provider.

4. The normal direct bilirubin value is 0.1 to 0.4 mg/dL; therefore, a decrease in the value although it is still elevated would not be reported.

29. 1. An increase in serum ammonia levels is seen in clients that have hepatic encephalopathy and coma.
    2. **The inability to circle food items on the menu indicates deterioration in the client's cognitive status.**
    3. Being able to follow commands indicates that the client's neurological status is intact.
    4. Consuming foods that provide adequate nutrition indicates the client is getting better and able to follow client teaching.

30. 1. Stools would be liquid in the ascending colon.
    2. Stools would be mushy in the right transverse colon.
    3. The left transverse colostomy would have semi-mushy stool.
    4. **Sigmoid colon is located in the left lower quadrant, and the client would expel solid feces.**

31. 1. **The objectives for support groups are to help members cope with chronic diseases and help manage symptom control.**
    2. Drug administration, dosage, and scheduled times should be discussed in the hospital prior to discharge or in the health-care provider's office; therefore, it is not a priority at the group support meeting.
    3. Dietary changes should be taught at the time the disease is diagnosed, but it is not a priority at the group support meeting.
    4. Colostomy may be the surgical option for clients who do not respond to medical treatment, but other nonsurgical treatments would be topics of discussions during support group meetings.

32. 1. Clients suffering from ulcerative colitis have anorexia, not an increased appetite.
    2. The hemoglobin and hematocrit would be decreased, not elevated, as a result of blood loss.
    3. **Clients report as many as 10 to 20 liquid bloody stools in a day.**
    4. Stressful events have been linked to an increase in symptoms. The nurse needs to assess for perceived stress in the client's life that produces symptoms.

33. 1. Wheat bread and all whole grains should be avoided, and most clients cannot tolerate milk products.
    2. Fried foods such as hamburger and French fries should be avoided. Raw fruits and vegetables such as lettuce and tomatoes are usually not tolerated.
    3. Whole grains such as brown rice should be avoided. White rice can be eaten. Spicy meats and foods should be avoided.
    4. **Meats can be eaten if prepared by roasting, baking, or broiling. Vegetables should be cooked, not raw, and skins should be removed. A low-residue diet should be eaten.**

34. 1. **Pediatric and geriatric clients are the most at risk for fluid volume and electrolyte imbalances, and the nurse should always be alert to this possible complication.**
    2. Altered nutrition may be appropriate, depending on how long the client has been unable to eat, but it would not be priority over fluid volume deficit.
    3. Impaired tissue perfusion may be appropriate if the mucosal lining of the stomach is unable to heal, but it is not priority over fluid volume deficit.
    4. Alteration in comfort may be appropriate, but is not priority over fluid volume deficit.

35. 1. Acute gastritis is characterized by sudden epigastric pain or discomfort, not mid-sternal chest pain.
    2. **Chronic pain in the epigastric area that is relieved by ingesting food is a sign of chronic gastritis.**
    3. Dyspepsia (heartburn) and hematemesis (vomiting blood) are frequent symptoms of acute gastritis.
    4. Projective vomiting is not a sign of chronic gastritis.

36. 1. There are no data that suggest the client needs a blood transfusion.
    2. TPN is not a treatment for a client with fluid volume deficit. TPN provides calories for nutritional deficits, not fluid deficits.
    3. If the client's problem was fluid volume excess, assessing lung sounds would be appropriate.
    4. **This would be the most appropriate intervention to implement because fluid infusion is the treatment of choice for this problem. The effectiveness of the client's treatment would be altered if the intravenous site becomes infected or infiltrated.**

37. 1. **Oatmeal and wheat toast are high-fiber foods that are recommended for clients**

Gastrointestinal

who are immobile to help prevent constipation.

2. Cream of wheat and biscuits are low-fiber foods.

3. Cottage cheese and canned peaches are low-fiber foods.

4. Tuna is a good source of protein for the client, but croissants have a high fat content and would be a factor in weight gain if consistently eaten. Applesauce is low in fiber.

38. 1. The nurse should inquire about drug allergies before administering all medications, not just potassium.

2. **Cardiac dysrhythmias occur when serum potassium levels are too low or too high. Many dysrhythmias can be detected by assessing the regularity of the heart rate.**

3. The blood pressure does not evaluate for dysrhythmias, a possible result of abnormal potassium levels.

4. The complete blood count does not include the potassium level; a chemistry panel would be needed.

39. 1. The polyethylene glycol electrolyte lavage solution is a medication and therefore cannot be delegated.

2. Teaching is the responsibility of the nurse and cannot be delegated.

3. Starting an intravenous site and managing the delivery of the fluid is the responsibility of the nurse and cannot be delegated.

4. **The administration of enemas can be delegated to the unlicensed nursing assistant.**

40. 1. **The nurse should monitor the client for the first bowel movement to document elimination of barium that should be eliminated within two (2) days. If the client does not have a bowel movement, a laxative may be needed to help the client to eliminate the barium before it becomes too hard to pass.**

2. An oxygen saturation of 96% is acceptable and does not require intervention.

3. Vital signs should be monitored to recognize and treat complications before the client is in danger. Baseline is a desired outcome.

4. The client's throat is not anesthetized for this procedure, so the gag reflex is not pertinent information in this procedure.

41. 1. A soft-bristle toothbrush will not affect painful swallowing.

2. An alcohol mouthwash would be irritating to the oral cavity and increase pain.

3. An antifungal medication should be used with candidiasis and would not be an effective treatment for plain mouth ulcers.

4. **Substances that are irritating should be avoided during the outbreaks of ulcers in the mouth. Spicy foods, alcohol, and tobacco are common irritants that the client should avoid.**

42. 1. The preoccupation with food, calories, and preparing meals are psychosocial behaviors that suggest the client has an eating disorder.

2. Clients who have anorexia nervosa have thin, fine body hair.

3. Iron deficiency anemia causes clients to experience a sore tongue.

4. **Thin, brittle hair occurs in clients with anorexia.**

43. 1. **The nurse should realize the client is anxious about the diagnosis of cancer and the impending surgery. Therefore the nurse should be prepared to repeat information as necessary. The teaching principle that the nurse needs to consider is that anxiety decreases learning.**

2. Small manageable sessions increase learning, especially when the client is anxious.

3. Videos are not the best teaching tool for adults. Short videos are useful for children.

4. The nurse should assess the client's readiness and willingness to learn and not wait until the client asks questions about the surgery.

44. 1. The rate of the intravenous fluid is a collaborative nursing intervention because it requires an order from the health-care provider.

2. **Encouraging the client to verbalize feelings about body changes assists the client to accept these changes.**

3. Medication administration is a collaborative intervention because it requires an order by the health-care provider.

4. Activity level immediately postoperative requires an order by the health-care provider.

45. 1. Thin pink drainage would be expected in the Jackson Pratt (JP) bulb.

2. Guarding would be a normal occurrence when touching a tender area on the abdomen and would not require immediate intervention.

3. Tenderness around the surgical site would be a normal finding and would not require intervention.

4. **Complaints of chills, sudden onset of fever, tachycardia, nausea, and hiccups are symptoms of peritonitis, which is a life-threatening complication.**

46. 1. Clients with hemorrhoids need to eat high-fiber diets and increase fluid intake to keep the stools soft and prevent constipation; therefore, the teaching is effective.

2. Warm compresses or sitz baths decrease pain; therefore, the teaching is effective.

3. Laxatives can be harsh to the bowel and are habit-forming, so they should not be taken daily. Stool softeners that soften stool can be taken daily.

4. Analgesic ointments, suppositories, and astringents can be used to decrease pain and decrease edema; therefore, the teaching has been effective.

47. 1. The site of the surgery can cause embarrassment when the nurse assesses the site; therefore, the nurse should establish a positive relationship.

2. The lithotomy position is with the client's legs in stirrups for procedures such as Pap smears and some surgeries such as transurethral resection of the prostate, not for the client who is postoperative hemorrhoidectomy.

3. A tube is not placed in the client's rectum after this surgery.

4. The rectal sphincter does not need to be digitally dilated.

48. 1. This will help prevent abdominal distention, which causes symptoms of IBS. Do not confuse inflammatory bowel disease (IBD) and irritable bowel syndrome (IBS).

2. Flatus (gas) forming foods will help prevent symptoms of IBD, not IBS.

3. Clients with IBS do have altered bowel habits such as diarrhea and constipation, but perianal care will not prevent IBS.

4. IBS does have a psychological component, but a client recently diagnosed should be taught other interventions before a psychologist is recommended.

49. 1. Do not remove any penetrating object in the abdomen; removal could cause further internal damage.

2. Removal of the knife could cause further internal damage.

3. The client should be kept on the back and the knife should be stabilized.

4. The nurse should stabilize the knife and get the client to the emergency department; pressure could increase abdominal damage.

50. 1. Intact skin around the stoma is the most appropriate outcome for the problem of "impaired skin integrity."

2. Being able to change the ostomy bag is a goal for a knowledge-deficit problem.

3. Expressing anxiety about the body changes would be a goal for an alteration in body image.

4. Maintaining a balance in fluid would be a goal for a nursing diagnosis of risk for fluid deficit.

51. In order of priority: 1, 4, 5, 2, and 3

1. The nurse should assess the vital signs to determine if the client is in hypovolemic shock.

4. The nurse should start the IV line to replace fluid volume.

5. While the nurse is starting the IV, a blood sample for typing and cross-matching should be obtained and sent to the laboratory.

2. An N/G tube should be inserted so that direct iced saline can be instilled to cause constriction, which will decrease the bleeding.

3. The iced saline lavage will help decrease bleeding.

*A little knowledge that acts is worth infinitely more than much knowledge that is idle.—*
Kahlil Gibran

# Endocrine Disorders

**8**

The endocrine system, along with the nervous system, controls or influences the activities of other body systems. The major glands of the endocrine system—the pituitary, thyroid, parathyroid, adrenals, pancreas, and ovaries (in females) and testes (in men)—play a major role in regulating activities of the body, including metabolism, fluid balance, reaction to stress, and sexual function. As with organs in other systems, these glands are subject to many disorders, some relatively minor and easily treated and others life threatening. This chapter focuses on diabetes mellitus, one of the most common and major endocrine system disorders; on other pancreatic disorders; and on adrenal, pituitary, and thyroid disorders. Disorders affecting the glands that are involved in reproduction and sexual functioning are discussed in Chapter 10.

## KEYWORDS

Addisonian crisis
aldosteronism
androgen
antidiuretic
endogenous
euthyroid
exogenous
fluid deprivation test
glucocorticoid
hyperparathyroidism
hyperthyroidism
hypoparathyroidism
hypothyroidism
iatrogenic
ketone
Kussmaul breathing
mineralocorticoid
pruritus
tenesmus
turgor
vasopressin
water challenge test

## ABBREVIATIONS

Adrenocorticotropic Hormone (ACTH)
Antidiuretic Hormone (ADH)
Arterial Blood Gas (ABG)
At Bedtime (hs)
Beats Per Minute (bpm)
Before Meals (bc)
Blood Pressure (BP)
Blood Urea Nitrogen (BUN)
Computed Tomography (CT)
Diabetes Insipidus (DI)
Diabetes Mellitus (DM)
Diabetic Ketoacidosis (DKA)
Endoscopic Retrograde Cholangiopancreatogram (ERCP)
Health-Care Provider (HCP)
Hyperosmolar Hyperglycemic State (HHS)
Intake & Output (I & O)
Intensive Care Department (ICD)
Intravenous (IV)
Intravenous Push (IVP)
Nasogastric (N/G)
Nothing by Mouth (NPO)
Percutaneous Endoscopic Gastrostomy (PEG)
Premature Ventricular Contraction (PVC)
Prothrombin Time (PT)
Rule Out (R/O)
Syndrome of Inappropriate Antidiuretic Hormone (SIADH)
Within Normal Limits (WNL)

## Diabetes Mellitus

1. The client, an 18-year-old female, 5′4″ tall, weighing 113 kg, comes to the clinic for a wound on her lower leg that has not healed for the last two (2) weeks. Which disease process would the nurse suspect that the client has developed?
   1. Type 1 diabetes.
   2. Type 2 diabetes.
   3. Gestational diabetes.
   4. Acanthosis nigricans.

2. The client diagnosed with Type 1 diabetes has a glycosylated hemoglobin (A1$_c$) of 8.1%. Which interpretation should the nurse make based on this result?
   1. This result is below normal levels.
   2. This result is within acceptable levels.
   3. This result is above recommended levels.
   4. This result is dangerously high.

3. The nurse administered 28 units of Humulin N, an intermediate-acting insulin, to a client diagnosed with Type 1 diabetes at 1600. Which action should the nurse implement?
   1. Ensure the client eats the bedtime snack.
   2. Determine how much food the client ate at lunch.
   3. Perform a glucometer reading at 0700.
   4. Offer the client protein after administering insulin.

4. The client diagnosed with Type 1 diabetes is receiving Humalog, a rapid-acting insulin, by sliding scale. The order reads blood glucose level: <150, 0 units; 151–200, 3 units; 201–250, 6 units; >251, contact health-care provider. The unlicensed nursing assistant reports to the nurse that the client's glucometer reading is 189. How much insulin should the nurse administer to the client? _____

5. The nurse is discussing the importance of exercising to a client diagnosed with Type 2 diabetes whose diabetes is well controlled with diet and exercise. Which information should the nurse include in the teaching about diabetes?
   1. Eat a simple carbohydrate snack before exercising.
   2. Carry peanut butter crackers when exercising.
   3. Encourage the client to walk 20 minutes three (3) times a week.
   4. Perform warmup and cooldown exercises.

6. The nurse is caring for a client with long-term Type 2 diabetes and is assessing the feet. Which assessment data would warrant immediate intervention by the nurse?
   1. The client has crumbling toenails.
   2. The client has athlete's feet.
   3. The client has a necrotic big toe.
   4. The client has thickened toenails.

7. The home health nurse is completing the admission assessment for a 76-year-old client diagnosed with Type 2 diabetes that must be controlled with 70/30-combination insulin. Which intervention should be included in the plan of care?
   1. Assess the client's ability to read small print.
   2. Monitor the client's serum PT level.
   3. Teach the client how to perform a hemoglobin A1$_c$ test daily.
   4. Instruct the client to check the feet weekly.

8. The client with Type 2 diabetes controlled with biguanide oral diabetic medication is scheduled for a computed tomography (CT) with contrast of the abdomen to evaluate pancreatic function. Which intervention should the nurse implement?
   1. Provide a high-fat diet 24 hours prior to test.
   2. Hold the biguanide medication for 48 hours prior to test.
   3. Obtain an informed consent form for the test.
   4. Administer pancreatic enzymes prior to the test.

9. The diabetic educator is teaching a class on diabetes Type 1 and is discussing sick-day rules. Which interventions should the diabetes educator include in the discussion? Select all that apply.
   1. Take diabetic medication even if unable to eat the client's normal diabetic diet.
   2. If unable to eat, drink liquids that are equal to the client's normal caloric intake.
   3. It is not necessary to notify the health-care provider if ketones are in the urine.
   4. Test blood glucose levels and test urine ketones once a day and keep a record.
   5. Call the health-care provider if glucose levels are higher than 180 mg/dL.

10. The client received 10 units of Humulin R, a fast acting insulin, at 0700. At 1030 the unlicensed nursing assistant tells the nurse the client has a headache and is really acting "funny." Which action should the nurse implement first?
    1. Instruct the assistant to obtain blood glucose level.
    2. Have the client drink eight (8) ounces of orange juice.
    3. Go to the client's room and assess the client for hypoglycemia.
    4. Prepare to administer one amp 50% Dextrose intravenously.

11. The nurse at a freestanding health clinic is caring for a 56-year-old client who is homeless and is a Type 2 diabetic controlled with insulin. Which action is an example of client advocacy?
    1. Ask the client if he has somewhere he can go and live.
    2. Arrange for someone to give him his insulin at a local homeless shelter.
    3. Notify Adult Protective Services about the client's situation.
    4. Ask the health-care provider to take the client off insulin because he is homeless.

12. The nurse is developing a care plan for the client diagnosed with Type 1 diabetes. The nurse identifies the problem "high risk for hyperglycemia related to noncompliance with the medication regimen." Which statement would be an appropriate short-term goal for the client?
    1. The client will have a blood glucose level between 90 and 140 mg/dL.
    2. The client will demonstrate appropriate insulin injection technique.
    3. The nurse will monitor the client's blood glucose levels four times a day.
    4. The client will maintain normal kidney function with 30 mL/hr urine output.

13. The client diagnosed with Type 2 diabetes is admitted to the intensive care department with hyperosmolar hyperglycemic nonketonic state coma (HHS). Which assessment data would the nurse expect the client to exhibit?
    1. Kussmaul's respirations.
    2. Diarrhea and epigastric pain.
    3. Dry mucous membranes.
    4. Ketone breath odor.

14. The elderly client is admitted to the intensive care department diagnosed with severe HHS. Which collaborative intervention should the nurse include in the plan of care?
    1. Infuse 0.9% normal saline intravenously.
    2. Administer intermediate-acting insulin.
    3. Perform blood glucometer checks daily.
    4. Monitor arterial blood gas results.

15. Which electrolyte replacement should the nurse anticipate being ordered by the health-care provider in the client diagnosed with DKA who has just been admitted to the ICD?
    1. Glucose.
    2. Potassium.
    3. Calcium.
    4. Sodium.

16. The client diagnosed with HHS was admitted yesterday with a blood glucose level of 780 mg/dL. The client's blood glucose level is now 300 mg/dL. Which intervention should the nurse implement?
    1. Increase the regular insulin IV drip.
    2. Check the client's urine for urinary ketones.
    3. Provide the client with a therapeutic diabetic meal.
    4. Notify the HCP to obtain an order to decrease insulin therapy.

17. The client diagnosed with Type 1 diabetes is found lying unconscious on the floor of the bathroom. Which intervention should the nurse implement first?
    1. Administer 50% dextrose IVP.
    2. Notify the health-care provider.
    3. Move the client to the ICD.
    4. Check the serum glucose level.

18. Which assessment data indicate that the client diagnosed with diabetic ketoacidosis is responding to the medical treatment?
    1. The client has tented skin turgor and dry mucous membranes.
    2. The client is alert and oriented to date, time, and place.
    3. The client's ABGs results are pH 7.29, $PaCO_2$ 44, $HCO_3$ 15.
    4. The client's serum potassium level is 3.3 mEq/L.

19. The nursing assistant on the medical floor tells the primary nurse that the client diagnosed with DKA wants something else to eat for lunch. What action should the nurse implement?
    1. Instruct the assistant to get the client additional food.
    2. Notify the dietician about the client's request.
    3. Ask the assistant to obtain a glucometer reading.
    4. Tell the assistant that the client cannot have anything else.

20. The client diagnosed with Type 2 diabetes comes to the emergency department. The client's blood glucose is 680 mg/dL and the client is diagnosed with HHS. Which question should the nurse ask the client to determine the cause of this acute complication?
    1. When is the last time you took your insulin?
    2. When did you have your last meal?
    3. Have you had some type of infection lately?
    4. How long have you had diabetes?

21. The nurse is discussing ways to prevent diabetic ketoacidosis with the client diagnosed with Type 1 diabetes. Which instruction would be most important to discuss with the client?
    1. Refer the client to the American Diabetes Association.
    2. Do not take any over-the-counter medications.
    3. Take the prescribed insulin even when unable to eat because of illness.
    4. Be sure to get your annual flu and pneumonia vaccines.

22. The charge nurse is making client assignments in the intensive care department. Which client should be assigned to the most experienced nurse?
    1. The client with Type 2 diabetes who has a blood glucose level of 348 mg/dL.
    2. The client diagnosed with Type 1 diabetes who is experiencing hypoglycemia.
    3. The client with DKA who has multifocal premature ventricular contractions.
    4. The client with HHS who has a plasma osmolarity of 290 mOsm/L.

23. Which arterial blood gas would the nurse expect in the client diagnosed with diabetic ketoacidosis?
    1. pH 7.34, $PaO_2$ 99, $PaCO_2$ 48, $HCO_3$ 24.
    2. pH 7.38, $PaO_2$ 95, $PaCO_2$ 40, $HCO_3$ 22.
    3. pH 7.46, $PaO_2$ 85, $PaCO_2$ 30, $HCO_3$ 26.
    4. pH 7.30, $PaO_2$ 90, $PaCO_2$ 30, $HCO_3$ 18.

24. The client is admitted to the ICD diagnosed with DKA. Which interventions should the nurse implement? Select all that apply.
    1. Maintain adequate ventilation.
    2. Assess fluid volume status.
    3. Administer intravenous potassium.
    4. Check for urinary ketones.
    5. Monitor intake and output.

## Pancreatitis

25. The client is admitted to the medical department with a diagnosis of R/O acute pancreatitis. Which laboratory value should the nurse monitor to confirm this diagnosis?
    1. Creatinine and BUN.
    2. Troponin and CPK-MB.
    3. Serum amylase and lipase.
    4. Serum bilirubin and calcium.

26. Which client problem has priority for the client diagnosed with acute pancreatitis?
    1. Risk for fluid volume deficit.
    2. Alteration in comfort.
    3. Imbalanced nutrition: less than body requirements.
    4. Knowledge deficit.

27. The nurse is preparing to administer A.M. medications to the following clients. Which medication should the nurse question before administering?
    1. Pancreatic enzymes to the client who has finished breakfast.
    2. The pain medication, morphine, to the client who has a respiratory rate of 20.
    3. The loop diuretic to the client who has a serum potassium level of 3.9 mEq/L.
    4. The beta blocker to the client who has an apical pulse of 68 bpm.

28. The client is diagnosed with acute pancreatitis. Which health-care provider's admitting order should the nurse question?
    1. Bed rest with bathroom privileges.
    2. Initiate IV therapy at D5W 125 mL/hr.
    3. Weigh client daily.
    4. Low-fat, low-carbohydrate diet.

29. The nurse is completing discharge teaching to the client diagnosed with acute pancreatitis. Which instruction should the nurse discuss with the client?
    1. Instruct the client to decrease alcohol intake.
    2. Explain the need to avoid all stress.
    3. Discuss the importance of stopping smoking.
    4. Teach the correct way to take pancreatic enzymes.

30. The male client diagnosed with chronic pancreatitis calls and reports to the clinic nurse that he has been having a lot of "gas," along with frothy and very foul-smelling stools. Which action should the nurse take?
    1. Explain that this is common for chronic pancreatitis.
    2. Ask the client to bring in a stool specimen to the clinic.
    3. Arrange an appointment with the HCP for today.
    4. Discuss the need to decrease fat in the diet so that this won't happen.

31. The nurse is discussing complications of chronic pancreatitis with a client diagnosed with the disease. Which complication should the nurse discuss with the client?
    1. Diabetes insipidus.
    2. Crohn's disease.
    3. Narcotic addiction.
    4. Peritonitis.

32. The client has just had an endoscopic retrograde cholangiopancreatogram (ERCP). Which post-procedure intervention should the nurse implement?
    1. Assess for rectal bleeding.
    2. Increase fluid intake.
    3. Assess gag reflex.
    4. Keep in supine position.

33. The client diagnosed with acute pancreatitis is in pain. Which position should the nurse assist the client to assume to help decrease the pain?
    1. Recommend lying in the prone position with legs extended.
    2. Maintain a tripod position over the bedside table.
    3. Place in side-lying position with knees flexed.
    4. Encourage a supine position with a pillow under the knees.

34. The client with an acute exacerbation of chronic pancreatitis has a nasogastric tube and is NPO. Which interventions should the nurse implement? Select all that apply.
    1. Monitor the bowel sounds.
    2. Weigh the client daily.
    3. Assess the intravenous site.
    4. Provide oral and nasal care.
    5. Monitor the blood glucose.

35. The nurse is administering a pancreatic enzyme to the client diagnosed with chronic pancreatitis. Which statement best explains the rationale for administering this medication?
    1. It is an exogenous source of protease, amylase, and lipase.
    2. This enzyme increases the number of bowel movements.
    3. This medication breaks down in the stomach to help with digestion.
    4. Pancreatic enzymes help break down fat in the small intestine.

36. The client diagnosed with acute pancreatitis is being discharged home. Which statement by the client indicates the teaching has been effective?
    1. "I should decrease my intake of coffee, tea, and cola."
    2. "I will eat a low-fat diet and avoid spicy foods."
    3. "I will check my amylase and lipase levels daily."
    4. "I will return to work tomorrow but take it easy."

## Cancer of the Pancreas

37. The nurse is assessing a client with complaints of vague upper abdominal pain that is worse at night but is relieved by sitting up and leaning forward. Which assessment question should the nurse ask next?
    1. "Have you noticed a yellow haze when you look at things?"
    2. "Does the pain get worse when you eat a meal or snack?"
    3. "Have you had your amylase and lipase checked recently?"
    4. "How much weight have you gained since you saw the HCP?"

38. The nurse caring for a client diagnosed with cancer of the pancreas writes the collaborative problem of "altered nutrition." Which intervention should the nurse include in the plan of care?
    1. Continuous feedings via PEG tube.
    2. Have the family bring in foods from home.
    3. Assess for food preferences.
    4. Refer to the dietitian.

39. The nurse is planning a program for clients at a health fair regarding the prevention and early detection of cancer of the pancreas. Which self-care activity should the nurse teach that is an example of primary nursing care?
    1. Monitor for elevated blood glucose at random intervals.
    2. Inspect the skin and sclera of the eyes for a yellow tint.
    3. Limit meat in the diet and eat a diet that is low in fats.
    4. Instruct the client with hyperglycemia about insulin injections.

40. The nurse and an unlicensed nursing assistant are caring for clients on an oncology floor. Which intervention should the nurse delegate to the assistant?
    1. Assist the client with abdominal pain to turn to the side and flex the knees.
    2. Monitor the Jackson Pratt drainage tube to make sure it is draining properly.
    3. Check to see if the client is sleeping after pain medication is given.
    4. Empty the bedside commode of the client who has been having melena.

41. The client diagnosed with cancer of the pancreas is being discharged to start chemotherapy in the HCP's office. Which statement made by the client indicates the client understands the discharge instructions?
    1. "I will have to see the HCP every day for six (6) weeks for my treatments."
    2. "I should write down all my questions so I can ask them when I see the HCP."
    3. "I am sure that this is not going to be a serious problem for me to deal with."
    4. "The nurse will give me an injection in my leg and I will get to go home."

42. The client is being admitted to the outpatient department prior to an endoscopic retrograde cholangiopancreatogram (ERCP) to rule out cancer of the pancreas. Which pre-procedure instruction should the nurse teach?
    1. Prepare to be admitted to the hospital after the procedure for observation.
    2. If something happens during the procedure, then emergency surgery will be done.
    3. Do not eat or drink anything after midnight the night before the test.
    4. If done correctly, this procedure will correct the blockage of the stomach.

43. The client is diagnosed with cancer of the head of the pancreas. When assessing the patient, which signs and symptoms would the nurse expect to find?
    1. Clay-colored stools and dark urine.
    2. Night sweats and fever.
    3. Left lower abdominal cramps and tenesmus.
    4. Nausea and coffee-ground emesis.

44. The client diagnosed with cancer of the head of the pancreas is two (2) days post-pancreatoduodenectomy (Whipple's procedure). Which nursing problem has the highest priority?
    1. Anticipatory grieving.
    2. Fluid volume imbalance.
    3. Acute incisional pain.
    4. Altered nutrition.

45. The client has had a total pancreatectomy and splenectomy for cancer of the body of the pancreas. Which discharge instructions should the nurse teach? Select all that apply.
    1. Keep a careful record of intake and output.
    2. Use a stool softener or bulk laxative regularly.
    3. Use correct insulin injection technique.
    4. Take the pain medication before the pain gets too bad.
    5. Sleep with the head of the bed on blocks.

46. The client admitted to rule out pancreatic islet tumors complains of feeling weak, shaky, and sweaty. Which should be the first intervention implemented by the nurse?
    1. Start an IV with D5W.
    2. Notify the health-care provider.
    3. Perform a bedside glucose check.
    4. Give the client some orange juice.

47. The home health nurse is admitting a client diagnosed with cancer of the pancreas. Which information is the most important for the nurse to discuss with the client?
    1. Determine the client's food preferences.
    2. Ask the client if there is an advance directive.
    3. Find out about insurance/Medicare reimbursement.
    4. Explain that the client should eat as much as possible.

48. The nurse caring for a client diagnosed with cancer of the pancreas writes the nursing diagnosis of "risk for altered skin integrity related to pruritus." Which interventions should the nurse implement?
    1. Assess tissue turgor.
    2. Apply antifungal creams.
    3. Monitor bony prominences for breakdown.
    4. Have the client keep the fingernails short.

## Adrenal Disorders

49. The nurse is admitting a client diagnosed with primary adrenal cortex insufficiency (Addison's disease). When assessing the client, which clinical manifestations would the nurse expect to find?
    1. Moon face, buffalo hump, and hyperglycemia.
    2. Hirsutism, fever, and irritability.
    3. Bronze pigmentation, hypotension, and anorexia.
    4. Tachycardia, bulging eyes, and goiter.

50. The nurse is developing a plan of care for the client diagnosed with acquired immuno-deficiency syndrome (AIDS) who has developed an infection in the adrenal gland. Which problem would have the highest priority?
    1. Altered body image.
    2. Activity intolerance.
    3. Impaired coping.
    4. Fluid volume deficit.

51. The nurse is planning the care of a client diagnosed with Addison's disease. Which interventions should be included?
    1. Administer steroid medications.
    2. Place the client on fluid restriction.
    3. Provide frequent stimulation.
    4. Consult physical therapy for gait training.

52. The client is admitted to rule out Cushing's syndrome. Which laboratory tests would the nurse anticipate being ordered?
    1. Plasma drug levels of quinidine, digoxin, and hydralazine.
    2. Plasma levels of ACTH and cortisol.
    3. 24-hour urine for metanephrine and catecholamine.
    4. Spot urine for creatinine and white blood cells.

53. The client has developed iatrogenic Cushing's disease. Which is a scientific rationale for the development of this problem?
    1. The client has an autoimmune problem that causes the destruction of the adrenal cortex.
    2. The client has been taking steroid medications for an extended period for another disease process.
    3. The client has a pituitary gland tumor that causes the adrenal glands to produce too much cortisol.
    4. The client has developed an adrenal gland problem for which the health-care provider does not have an explanation.

54. The nurse is performing discharge teaching for a client diagnosed with Cushing's disease. Which statement made by the client demonstrates an understanding of the instructions?
    1. "I will be sure to notify my health-care provider if I start to run a fever."
    2. "Before I stop taking the prednisone, I will be taught how to taper it off."
    3. "If I get weak and shaky, I need to eat some hard candy or drink some juice."
    4. "It is fine if I continue to participate in weekend games of tackle football."

55. The charge nurse of an intensive care unit is making assignments for the night shift. Which client should be assigned to the most experienced intensive care nurse?
    1. The client diagnosed with respiratory failure who is on a ventilator and requires frequent sedation.
    2. The client diagnosed with lung cancer and iatrogenic Cushing's disease with ABGs of pH 7.35, $PaO_2$ 88, $PaCO_2$ 44, and $HCO_3$ 22.
    3. The client diagnosed with Addison's disease who is lethargic and has a BP of 80/45, P 124, and R 28.
    4. The client diagnosed with hyperthyroidism who has undergone a thyroidectomy two (2) days ago and has a negative Trousseau's sign.

56. The nurse writes a problem of "altered body image" for a 34-year-old client diagnosed with Cushing's disease. Which interventions should be implemented?
    1. Monitor blood glucose levels q.i.d before meals and at bedtime.
    2. Perform a head-to-toe assessment every shift.
    3. Use therapeutic communication to allow the client to discuss feelings.
    4. Assess bowel sounds and temperature every four (4) hours.

57. The client diagnosed with Addison's disease is admitted to the emergency department after a day at the lake. The client is lethargic, forgetful, and weak. Which intervention should be the emergency department nurse's first action?
    1. Start an IV with an 18-gauge needle and infuse NS rapidly.
    2. Have the client wait in the waiting room until a bed is available.
    3. Perform a complete head-to-toe assessment.
    4. Collect urinalysis and blood samples for a CBC and calcium level.

58. The client diagnosed with Cushing's disease has developed 1+ peripheral edema. The client has been receiving intravenous fluids at 100 mL per hour via IV pump for the past 79 hours. The client has also received IVPB medication in 50 mL of fluid every 6 hours for 15 doses. How many mL of fluid has the client received? _____

59. The nurse manager of a medical/surgical unit is asked to determine if the unit should adopt a new care delivery system. Which is an example of an autocratic style of leadership?
    1. Call a meeting and educate the staff on the new delivery system that will be used.
    2. Organize a committee of nurses to investigate the various types of delivery systems.
    3. Wait until another unit has implemented the new system and see if it works out.
    4. Discuss with the nursing staff if a new delivery system should be adopted.

60. The client diagnosed with Cushing's disease has undergone a unilateral adrenalectomy. Which discharge instructions should the nurse teach?
    1. Instruct the client to take the glucocorticosteroid and mineralcorticosteroid medications as prescribed.
    2. Teach the client regarding sexual functioning and androgen replacement therapy.
    3. Explain the signs and symptoms of infection and when to call the health-care provider.
    4. Demonstrate turn, cough, and deep-breathing exercises that the client should perform every (2) hours.

## Pituitary Disorders

61. The client diagnosed with a pituitary tumor has developed syndrome of inappropriate antidiuretic hormone (SIADH). Which interventions would the nurse implement?
    1. Assess for dehydration and monitor blood glucose levels.
    2. Assess for nausea and vomiting and weigh daily.
    3. Monitor potassium levels and encourage fluid intake.
    4. Administer vasopressin IV and conduct a fluid deprivation test.

62. The nurse is admitting a client to the neurological intensive care unit who is postoperative transsphenoidal hypophysectomy . Which data would warrant immediate intervention?
    1. The client is alert to name but is unable to tell the nurse the location.
    2. The client has an output of 2500 mL since surgery and an intake of 1000 mL.
    3. The client's vital signs are T 97.6, P 88, R 20, and BP 130/80.
    4. The client has a 3-cm amount of dark-red drainage on the turban dressing.

63. The client is diagnosed with diabetes insipidus. Which laboratory value should be monitored by the nurse?
    1. Serum sodium.
    2. Serum calcium.
    3. Urine glucose.
    4. Urine white blood cells.

64. The nurse is discharging a client diagnosed with diabetes insipidus. Which statement made by the client warrants further intervention?
    1. "I will keep a list of my medications in my wallet and wear a Medi bracelet."
    2. "I should take my medication in the morning and leave it refrigerated at home."
    3. "I should weigh myself every morning and record any weight gain."
    4. "If I develop a tightness in my chest, I will call my health-care provider."

65. The client is admitted to the medical unit with a diagnosis of rule out diabetes insipidus (DI). Which instructions should the nurse teach regarding a fluid deprivation test?
    1. The client will be asked to drink 100 mL of fluid as rapidly as possible and then will not be allowed fluid for 24 hours.
    2. The client will be given an injection of antidiuretic hormone, and urine output will be measured for four (4) to six (6) hours.
    3. The client will be NPO, and vital signs and weights will be done hourly until the end of the test.
    4. An IV will be started with normal saline, and the client will be asked to try and hold the urine in the bladder until a sonogram can be done.

66. The nurse is caring for clients on a medical floor. Which client should be assessed first?
    1. The client diagnosed with syndrome of inappropriate antidiuretic hormone (SIADH) who has a weight gain of 1.5 pounds since yesterday.
    2. The client diagnosed with a pituitary tumor who has developed diabetes insipidus (DI) and has an intake of 1500 mL and an output of 1600 mL in the last 8 hours.
    3. The client diagnosed with syndrome of inappropriate antidiuretic hormone (SIADH) who is having muscle twitching.
    4. The client diagnosed with diabetes insipidus (DI) who is complaining of feeling tired after having to get up at night.

67. The health-care provider has ordered 40 g/24 hours of intranasal vasopressin for a client diagnosed with diabetes insipidus. Each metered spray delivers 10 g. The client takes the medication every 12 hours. How many sprays are delivered at each dosing time? _____

68. The nurse is planning the care of a client diagnosed with syndrome of inappropriate antidiuretic hormone (SIADH). Which interventions should be implemented? Select all that apply.
    1. Restrict fluids per health-care provider order.
    2. Assess level of consciousness every two (2) hours.
    3. Provide atmosphere of stimulation.
    4. Monitor urine and serum osmolality.
    5. Weigh the client every three (3) days.

69. The nurse is caring for a client diagnosed with diabetes insipidus (DI). Which nursing intervention should be implemented?
    1. Monitor blood glucoses before meals and at bedtime.
    2. Restrict caffeinated beverages.
    3. Check urine ketones if blood glucose is >250.
    4. Assess tissue turgor every four (4) hours.

70. The unlicensed nursing assistant complains to the nurse that she has filled the water pitcher four (4) times during the shift for a client diagnosed with a closed head injury and the client has asked for the pitcher to be filled again. Which intervention should the nurse do first?
    1. Tell the unlicensed nursing assistant to fill the pitcher again.
    2. Instruct the unlicensed nursing assistant to start measuring I & O.
    3. Assess the client for polyuria and polydipsia.
    4. Check the client's BUN and creatinine levels.

71. The nurse is admitting a client diagnosed with syndrome of inappropriate antidiuretic hormone (SIADH). Which clinical manifestations should be reported to the health-care provider?
    1. Serum sodium of 112 mEq/L and a headache.
    2. Serum potassium of 5.0 mEq/L and a heightened awareness.
    3. Serum calcium of 10 mg/dL and tented tissue turgor.
    4. Serum magnesium of 1.2 mg/dL and large urinary output.

72. The male client diagnosed with syndrome of inappropriate antidiuretic hormone (SIADH) secondary to cancer of the lung tells the nurse that he would like to discontinue the fluid restriction and does not care if he dies. Which action by the nurse would be an example of the ethical principle of autonomy?
    1. Discuss the information the client told the nurse with the health-care provider and significant other.
    2. Explain that it is possible that the client would seize if he drank fluid beyond the restrictions.
    3. Notify the health-care provider of the client's wishes and give the client fluids as desired.
    4. Allow the client an extra drink of water and explain that the nurse could get into trouble if the client tells the health-care provider.

## Thyroid Disorders

73. The client is diagnosed with hypothyroidism. Which signs/symptoms would the nurse expect the client to exhibit?
    1. Complaints of extreme fatigue and hair loss.
    2. Exophthalmos and complaints of nervousness.
    3. Complaints of profuse sweating and flushed skin.
    4. Tetany and complaints of stiffness of the hands.

74. The nurse identifies the client problem "risk for imbalanced body temperature" for the client diagnosed with hypothyroidism. Which intervention would be included in the client problem?
    1. Encourage the use of an electric blanket.
    2. Protect from exposure to cold and drafts.
    3. Keep the room temperature cool.
    4. Space activities to promote rest.

75. The client diagnosed with hypothyroidism is prescribed the thyroid hormone levothyroxine (Synthroid). Which assessment data indicate the medication has been effective?
    1. The client has a three (3)-pound weight gain.
    2. The client has a decreased pulse rate.
    3. The client's temperature is WNL.
    4. The client denies any diaphoresis.

76. Which nursing intervention should be included in the plan of care for the client diagnosed with hyperthyroidism?
    1. Increase the amount of fiber in the diet.
    2. Encourage a low-calorie, low-protein diet.
    3. Decrease the client's fluid intake to 1000 mL day.
    4. Provide six (6) small, well-balanced meals a day.

77. The client with hypothyroidism is admitted to the intensive care department diagnosed with myxedema coma. Which assessment data would warrant immediate intervention by the nurse?
    1. Serum blood glucose level of 74 mg/dL.
    2. Pulse oximeter reading of 90%.
    3. Telemetry reading showing sinus bradycardia.
    4. The client is lethargic and sleeps all the time.

78. Which medication order would the nurse question in the client diagnosed with untreated hypothyroidism?
    1. Thyroid hormones.
    2. Oxygen.
    3. Sedatives.
    4. Laxatives.

79. Which statement made by the client would make the nurse suspect that the client is experiencing hyperthyroidism?
    1. "I just don't seem to have any appetite anymore."
    2. "I have a bowel movement about every 3 to 4 days."
    3. "My skin is really becoming dry and coarse."
    4. "I have noticed that all my collars are getting tighter."

80. The 68-year-old client diagnosed with hyperthyroidism is being treated with radioactive iodine therapy. Which interventions should the nurse discuss with the client?
    1. Explain that it will take up to a month for symptoms of hyperthyroidism to subside.
    2. Teach that the iodine therapy will have to be tapered slowly over one (1) week.
    3. Discuss that the client will have to be hospitalized during the radioactive therapy.
    4. Inform the client that after therapy the client will not have to take any medication.

81. The nurse is teaching the client diagnosed with hyperthyroidism. Which information should be taught to the client? Select all that apply.
    1. Notify the HCP if a three (3)-pound weight loss occurs in two (2) days.
    2. Discuss ways to cope with the emotional lability.
    3. Notify the HCP if taking over-the-counter medication.
    4. Carry a medical identification card or bracelet.
    5. Teach how to take antithyroid medications correctly.

82. The nurse is giving an in-service on thyroid disorders. One of the attendees asks the nurse, "Why don't the people in the United States get goiters as often?" Which statement by the nurse is the best response?
    1. "It is because of the screening techniques used in the United States."
    2. "It is a genetic predisposition that is rare in North Americans."
    3. "The medications available in the United States decrease goiters."
    4. "Iodized salt helps prevent the development of goiters in the United States."

83. The nurse is preparing to administer the following medications. Which medication should the nurse question administering?
    1. The thyroid hormone to the client that does not have a T3, T4 level.
    2. The regular insulin to the client with a blood glucose level of 210 mg/dL.
    3. The loop diuretic to the client with a potassium level of 3.3 mEq/L.
    4. The cardiac glycoside to the client who has a digoxin level of 1.4 mg/dL.

84. Which signs/symptoms would make the nurse suspect that the client is experiencing a thyroid storm?
    1. Obstipation and hypoactive bowel sounds.
    2. Hyperpyrexia and extreme tachycardia.
    3. Hypotension and bradycardia.
    4. Decreased respirations and hypoxia.

## Diabetes Mellitus

1. 1. Type 1 diabetes usually occurs in young clients who are underweight. In this disease, there is no production of insulin from the beta cells in the pancreas. People with Type 1 diabetes are insulin-dependent with a rapid onset of symptoms, including polyuria, polydipsia, and polyphagia.
   2. Type 2 diabetes is a disorder that usually occurs around the age of 40, but it is now being detected in children and young adults as a result of obesity and sedentary lifestyles. Wounds that do not heal are a hallmark sign of Type 2 diabetes. This client weighs 248.6 pounds and is short.
   3. Gestational diabetes is diabetes that occurs during pregnancy.
   4. Acanthosis nigricans (AN), dark pigmentation and skin creases in the neck, is a sign of hyperinsulinemia. The pancreas is secreting excess amounts of insulin as a result of excessive caloric intake. It is identified in young children and is a precursor to the development of Type 2 diabetes.

   **TEST-TAKING HINT: The test taker must be aware of kilogram and pounds; the stem is asking about a disease process and acanthosis nigricans is a clinical manifestation of a disease, not a disease itself. Therefore, the test taker should not select this as a correct answer.**

2. 1. The acceptable level for an $A1_c$ for a client with diabetes is between 6% and 7%, which corresponds to a 120–140 mg/dL average blood glucose level.
   2. This result is not within acceptable levels for the client with diabetes, which is 6% to 7%.
   3. This result parallels a serum blood glucose level of approximately 180 to 200 mg/dL. An $A1_c$ is a blood test that reflects average blood glucose levels over a period of 2–3 months; clients with elevated blood glucose levels are at risk for developing long-term complications.
   4. An $A1_c$ of 13% is dangerously high; it reflects a 300-mg/dL average blood glucose level over the past 3 months.

   **TEST-TAKING HINT: The test taker must know normal and abnormal diagnostic laboratory values. Lab values vary depending on which lab performs the test.**

3. 1. Humulin N peaks in 6–8 hours, making the client at risk for hypoglycemia around midnight, which is why the client should receive a bedtime snack. This snack will prevent nighttime hypoglycemia.
   2. The food intake at lunch will not affect the client's blood glucose level at midnight.
   3. The client's glucometer reading should be done around 2100 to assess the effectiveness of insulin at 1600.
   4. Humulin N is an intermediate-acting insulin that has an onset in 2–4 hours but does not peak until 6–8 hours.

   **TEST-TAKING HINT: Remember to look at the adjective or descriptor. Intermediate-acting insulin gives the reader a clue that anything intermediate, instead of longer-acting, action would be incorrect.**

4. **Three (3) units.** The client's result is 189, which is between 151 and 200, so the nurse should administer 3 units of Humalog insulin subcutaneously.

   **TEST-TAKING HINT: The test taker must be aware of the way the HCPs write medication orders. HCPs order insulin in a sliding scale according to a range of blood glucose levels.**

5. 1. The client diagnosed with Type 2 diabetes who is not taking insulin or oral agents does not need extra food before exercise.
   2. The client with diabetes who is at risk for hypoglycemia when exercising should carry a simple carbohydrate, but this client is not at risk for hypoglycemia.
   3. Clients with diabetes that is controlled by diet and exercise must exercise daily at the same time and in the same amount to control the glucose level.
   4. All clients who exercise should perform warmup and cooldown exercises to help prevent muscle strain and injury.

   **TEST-TAKING HINT: The "1" and "2" options apply directly to clients diagnosed with diabetes and "3" and "4" options do not directly address clients diagnosed with diabetes. The reader could narrow the choices by either eliminating or including the two similar options.**

6. 1. Crumbling toenails indicate tinea unguium, which is a fungus infection of the toenail.
   2. Athlete's foot is a fungal infection that is not life threatening.
   3. A necrotic big toe indicates "dead" tissue. The client does not feel pain in the lower extremity and does not realize there has been an injury and therefore does not seek treatment. Increased blood glucose levels decrease oxygen supply that is needed to

heal the wound and increase the risk for developing an infection.

4. Big, thick toenails are fungal infections and would not require immediate intervention by the nurse; 50% of the adult population has this.

**TEST-TAKING HINT: The test taker should select the option that indicates to the nurse that this is possibly a life-altering complication or some type of assessment data that the health-care provider should be informed of immediately. Remember "warrants immediate intervention."**

7. 1. Age-related visual changes and diabetic retinopathy occur that could lead to the client having difficulty in reading and drawing up insulin dosage accurately.
   2. The PT level is monitored for clients receiving Coumadin, an anticoagulant, which is not ordered for client with diabetes, Type 1 or 2.
   3. Glycosylated hemoglobin is a serum blood test usually performed in a laboratory, not in the client's home. The hemoglobin $Al_c$ is performed every three (3) months. Self-monitoring blood glucose (SMBG) should be taught to the client.
   4. The client's feet should be checked daily, not weekly. In a week the client could have developed gangrene from an injury that the client did not realize he or she had.

**TEST-TAKING HINT: Always notice the age of a client if it is given because this is often important when determining the correct answer for the question. Be sure to read the adjectives such as "weekly," instead of "daily."**

8. 1. High-fat diets are not recommended for clients diagnosed with diabetes, and food does not have an effect on a CT scan with contrast.
   2. Biguanide medication must be held for a test with contrast medium because it increases the risk of lactic acidosis, which leads to renal problems.
   3. Informed consent is not required for a CT scan. The admission consent covers routine diagnostic procedures.
   4. Pancreatic enzymes are administered when the pancreas cannot produce amylase and lipase, not when the beta cells cannot produce insulin.

**TEST-TAKING HINT: The test taker could eliminate option "1" because high-fat diets are not recommended for any client. Because the stem specifically refers to the biguanide medication and CT contrast, a good choice would address both of these. Option "2" discusses both the medication and the test.**

9. 1. The most important issue to teach clients is to take insulin even if they are unable to eat. Glucose levels are increased with illness and stress.
   2. The client should drink liquids such as regular cola, orange juice, or regular gelatin, which provide enough glucose to prevent hypoglycemia when receiving insulin.
   3. Ketones indicate a breakdown of fat and must be reported to the HCP because they can lead to metabolic acidosis.
   4. Blood glucose levels and ketones must be checked every three (3) to four (4) hours, not daily.
   5. The HCP should be notified if the blood glucose level is this high. Regular insulin may need to be prescribed to keep the blood glucose level within acceptable range.

**TEST-TAKING HINT: This is an alternate-type question that may have more than one correct answer. The test taker should read all options and determine if it is an intervention that is appropriate.**

10. 1. The blood glucose level should be obtained, but it is not the first intervention.
    2. If it is determined that the client is having a hypoglycemic reaction, orange juice would be appropriate.
    3. Regular insulin peaks in 2–4 hours. Therefore, the nurse should think about the possibility that the client is having a hypoglycemic reaction and should assess the client. The nurse should not delegate nursing tasks to an assistant if the client is unstable.
    4. Dextrose 50% is only administered if the client is unconscious and the nurse suspects hypoglycemia.

**TEST-TAKING HINT: When answering a question that requires the nurse to implement an intervention first, all four options will be interventions that are appropriate for the situation but only one answer should be implemented first. The test taker must apply the nursing process, which states assessment of the first intervention.**

11. 1. This is an example of interviewing the client; it is not an example of client advocacy.
    2. Client advocacy focuses support on the client's autonomy. Even if the nurse disagrees with his living on the street, it is the client's right. Arranging for someone to give him his insulin provides for his needs and allows his choices.
    3. Adult Protective Services is an organization

that investigates any actual or potential abuse in adults. This client is not being abused by anyone.

4. The client needs the insulin to control the diabetes and talking to the HCP about taking him off a needed medication is not an example of advocacy.

**TEST-TAKING HINT: Remember to make sure the test taker knows what the question is asking and the definition of the terms.**

12. 1. The short-term goal must address the response part of the nursing diagnosis, which is "high risk for hyperglycemia," and this blood glucose level is within acceptable ranges for a client who is noncompliant.
2. This is an appropriate goal for a knowledge-deficit nursing diagnosis. Noncompliance is not always the result of knowledge deficit.
3. Note that this is the nurse implementing an intervention and the question asks for a goal, which addresses the problem of "high risk for hyperglycemia."
4. The question asks for a short-term goal and this is an example of a long-term goal.

**TEST-TAKING HINT: Remember the nursing diagnosis consists of a problem related to an etiology. The goals must address the problem and the interventions must address the etiology. Always remember a short-term goal is usually a goal that can be met during the hospitalization, and the long-term goal may take weeks, months, or even years.**

13. 1. This occurs with diabetic ketoacidosis (DKA) as a result of the breakdown of fat, resulting in ketones.
2. Diarrhea and epigastric pain are not associated with HHS.
3. Dry mucous membranes are a result of the hyperglycemia and occur with both HHS and DKA.
4. This occurs with DKA as a result of the breakdown of fat, resulting in ketones.

**TEST-TAKING HINT: The test taker must be able to differentiate between HHS (Type 2) and DKA (Type 1), which primarily is the result of the breakdown of fat and results in an increase in ketones that causes a decrease in pH, resulting in metabolic acidosis.**

14. 1. The initial fluid replacement is 0.9% normal saline (an isotonic solution) intravenously, followed by 0.45% saline. The rate depends on the client's fluid volume status and physical health, especially that of the heart.

2. Regular insulin, not intermediate, is the insulin of choice because of its quick onset and peak in two (2) to four (4) hours.
3. Blood glucometer checks are done every one (1) hour or more often in clients with HHS who are receiving regular insulin drips.
4. Arterial blood gases are not affected in HHS because there is no breakdown of fat resulting in ketones that cause metabolic acidosis.

**TEST-TAKING HINT: The test taker should eliminate option "3" based on the word "daily." In the ICU with a client who is very ill, most checks would be more often than daily. Remember to look at adjectives; "intermediate" in option "2" is the word that eliminates this as a possible correct answer.**

15. 1. Glucose is elevated in DKA; therefore, the HCP would not be replacing glucose.
2. The client in DKA loses potassium from increased urinary output, acidosis, catabolic state, and vomiting. Replacement is essential for preventing cardiac dysrhythmias secondary to hypokalemia.
3. Calcium is not affected in the client with DKA.
4. The IV that is prescribed 0.9% normal saline has sodium, but it is not specifically ordered for sodium replacement. This is an isotonic solution.

**TEST-TAKING HINT: Option "1" should be eliminated because the problem with DKA is elevated glucose so the HCP would not be replacing it. The test taker should use physiology knowledge and realize potassium is in the cell.**

16. 1. The regular intravenous insulin is continued because ketosis is not present, as with DKA.
2. The client diagnosed with Type 2 diabetes does not excrete ketones in HHS because there is enough insulin to prevent fat breakdown but not enough to lower blood glucose.
3. The client may or may not feel like eating, but it is not the appropriate intervention when the blood glucose level is reduced to 300 mg/dL.
4. When the glucose level is decreased to around 300 mg/dL, the regular insulin infusion therapy is decreased. Subcutaneous insulin will be administered per sliding scale.

**TEST-TAKING HINT: When two (2) options are the opposite of each other, they can either be eliminated or they can help eliminate the other two options as incorrect answers. Options "2" and "3" do not have insulin in the answer; therefore they should be eliminated as possible answers.**

17. 1. The nurse should assume the client is hypoglycemic and administer IVP dextrose, which will rouse the client immediately. If the collapse is the result of hyperglycemia, this additional dextrose will not further injure the client.
2. The health-care provider may or may not need to be notified, but this would not be the first intervention.
3. The client should be left in the client's room, and 50% dextrose should be administered first.
4. The serum glucose level requires a venipuncture, which will take too long. A blood glucometer reading may be obtained, but the nurse should first treat the client, not the machine. The glucometer only reads "low" after a certain point, and a serum level would be needed to confirm exact glucose level.

**TEST-TAKING HINT:** The question is requesting the test taker to select which intervention should be implemented first. All four options could be possible interventions, but only one is first. The test taker should select the intervention that will directly treat the client; do not select a diagnostic test.

18. 1. This indicates the client is dehydrated, which does not indicate that the client is getting better.
2. The client's level of consciousness can be altered because of dehydration and acidosis. If the client's sensorium is intact, the client is getting better and responding to the medical treatment.
3. These ABGs indicate metabolic acidosis; therefore the client is not responding to treatment.
4. This potassium level is low and indicates hypokalemia, which shows the client is not responding to medical treatment.

**TEST-TAKING HINT:** Responding to medical treatment is asking the test taker to determine which data indicate the client is getting better. The correct answer will be normal data and the other three (3) options will be signs/symptoms of the disease process or condition.

19. 1. The client is on a special diet and should not have any additional food.
2. The client will not be compliant with the diet if he or she is still hungry. Therefore, the nurse should request the dietician to talk to the client to try and adjust the meals so that the client will adhere to the diet.
3. There is no need for the assistant to check the client's glucose level.
4. The client is on a special diet. The nurse needs to help the client maintain compliance with the

medical treatment and should refer the client to the dietician.

**TEST-TAKING HINT:** The test taker should select the option that attempts to ensure that the client maintains compliance. The test taker should remember to work with members of the multidisciplinary health-care team.

20. 1. A client with Type 2 diabetes usually is prescribed oral hypoglycemic medications, not insulin.
2. The client could not eat enough food to cause a 680 mg/dL blood glucose level; therefore this question does not need to be asked.
3. The most common precipitating factor is infection. The manifestations may be slow to appear, with onset ranging from 24 hours to 2 weeks.
4. This would not help determine the cause of this client's HHS.

**TEST-TAKING HINT:** If the test taker does not know the answer to this question, the test taker could possibly relate acute complication and realize that a medical problem might cause this and select infection, option "3."

21. 1. The American Diabetic Association is an excellent referral, but the nurse should discuss specific ways to prevent DKA.
2. The client should be careful with OTC medications, but this intervention would not help prevent the development of DKA.
3. Illness increases blood glucose levels; therefore the client must take insulin and drink high-carbohydrate fluids such as regular Jell-O, regular popsicles, and orange juice.
4. Vaccines are important to help prevent illness, but regardless of whether the client gets these vaccines, the client can still develop diabetic ketoacidosis.

**TEST-TAKING HINT:** The words "most important" in the stem of the question indicate that one or more option may be appropriate instructions but only one is the priority intervention.

22. 1. This blood glucose level is elevated, but not life threatening, in the client diagnosed with Type 2 diabetes. Therefore, a less experienced nurse could care for this client.
2. Hypoglycemia is an acute complication of Type 1 diabetes, but it can be managed by frequent monitoring, so a less experienced nurse could care for this client.
3. Multifocal PVCs, which are secondary to hypokalemia and which can occur in clients

with DKA, are an emergency and can be life threatening. This client needs an experienced nurse.

4. A plasma osmolarity of 280–300 mOsm/L is within normal limits; therefore, a less experienced nurse could care for this client.

**TEST-TAKING HINT:** The test taker must select the client that has an abnormal, unexpected, or life-threatening sign/symptom for the disease process and assign this client to the most experienced nurse.

23. 1. This ABG indicates respiratory acidosis, which would not be expected.
    2. This ABG is normal, which would not be expected.
    3. This ABG indicates respiratory alkalosis, which would not be expected.
    4. This ABG indicates metabolic acidosis, which is what is expected in a client that is in diabetic ketoacidosis.

**TEST-TAKING HINT:** The client must know normal ABGs to be able to correctly answer this question. Normal ABGs are pH 7.35–7.45; $PaO_2$ 80–100; $PaCO_2$ 35–45; $HCO_3$ 22–26.

24. 1. The nurse should always address the airway when a client is seriously ill.
    2. The client must be assessed for fluid volume deficit and then for fluid volume excess after fluid replacement is started.
    3. The electrolyte imbalance of primary concern is depletion of potassium.
    4. Ketones are excreted in the urine; levels are documented from negative to large amount. Ketones should be monitored frequently.
    5. The nurse must ensure that the client's fluid intake and output are equal.

**TEST-TAKING HINT:** The test taker must select all that apply. Do not try to outguess the item writer. In some instances all options are correct.

## Pancreatitis

25. 1. These laboratory values are monitored for clients in kidney failure.
    2. These laboratory values are elevated in clients with a myocardial infarction.
    3. Serum amylase increases within 2 to 12 hours of the onset of acute pancreatitis to 2 to 3 times normal and returns to normal in 3 to 4 days; lipase elevates and remains elevated for 7 to 14 days.
    4. Bilirubin may be elevated as a result of compression of common duct, and hypocalcemia

develops in up to 25% of clients with acute pancreatitis, but these laboratory values do not confirm the diagnosis.

**TEST-TAKING HINT:** The test taker must be able to identify at least two (2) laboratory values that reflect each organ function prior to taking the RN-NCLEX. There is really no Test-Taking Hint that can help select the correct answer; this is knowledge.

26. 1. The client will be NPO to help decrease pain, but it is not the priority problem because the client will have intravenous fluids.
    2. Autodigestion of the pancreas results in severe epigastric pain, accompanied by nausea, vomiting, abdominal tenderness, and muscle guarding.
    3. Nutritional imbalance would be a possible client problem, but it is not priority.
    4. Knowledge deficit is always a client problem, but it is not priority over pain.

**TEST-TAKING HINT:** The test taker should apply Maslow's Hierarchy of Needs when selecting the priority problem for a client. After airway, pain is usually priority.

27. 1. Pancreatic enzymes must be administered with meals to enhance the digestion of starches and fats in the gastrointestinal tract.
    2. The client's respiratory rate is within normal limits; therefore the morphine should be administered to the client who is having pain.
    3. This is a normal potassium level; therefore the nurse would not need to question administering this medication.
    4. The apical pulse is within normal limits; therefore the nurse should not question administering this medication.

**TEST-TAKING HINT:** The test taker must determine if the assessment data provided in the answer option are abnormal, unexpected, or life-threatening so that it warrants questioning the administration of the medication. The test taker should also think about whether the administration of the medication would create an abnormal or life-threatening situation.

28. 1. Bed rest will decrease metabolic rate, gastrointestinal secretion, pancreatic secretions, and pain; therefore this HCP's order should not be questioned.
    2. The client will be NPO; therefore, initiating IV therapy would be an appropriate order.
    3. Short-term weight gain changes reflect fluid balance because the client will be NPO and receiving IV fluids. Daily weighing would be an appropriate HCP's order.

4. The client will be NPO, which will decrease stimulation of the pancreatic enzymes, which will result in decreased autodigestion of the pancreas, therefore decreasing pain.

**TEST-TAKING HINT: The test taker must determine which HCP's order is not expected for the diagnosis. Sometimes if the test taker asks which order would be expected, it is easier to identify the unexpected or abnormal HCP order.**

29. 1. Alcohol must be avoided entirely because it can cause stones to form, blocking pancreatic ducts and the outflow of pancreatic juice, causing further inflammation and destruction of the pancreas.
2. Stress stimulates the pancreas and should be dealt with, but it is unrealistic to think that a client can avoid all stress. By definition, the absence of all stress is death.
3. Smoking stimulates the pancreas to release pancreatic enzymes and should be stopped.
4. The client has acute pancreatitis, and pancreatic enzymes are only needed for chronic pancreatitis.

**TEST-TAKING HINT: The test taker should eliminate "2" because of the word "all," which is an absolute and there are very few absolutes in health care. The test taker should note the adjective "acute" in the stem, which may help the test taker eliminate option "4" because enzymes are given for a chronic condition.**

30. 1. Any change in the client's stool should be a cause for concern to the clinic nurse.
2. This is not necessary because the nurse knows changes in stool occur as a complication of pancreatitis and the client needs to see the HCP.
3. Steatorrhea (fatty, frothy, foul-smelling stool) is caused by a decrease in pancreatic enzyme secretion and indicates impaired digestion and possibly an increase in the severity of the pancreatitis. The client should see the HCP.
4. Decreasing fat in the diet will not help stop this type of stool.

**TEST-TAKING HINT: This question requires the test taker to have knowledge of the disease process, but if the test taker knows that the exocrine function of the pancreas is part of the gastrointestinal system, the test taker might think that altered stool would be cause for concern.**

31. 1. The client is at risk for diabetes mellitus (destruction of beta cells), not diabetes insipidus, a disorder of the pituitary gland.

2. Crohn's disease is an inflammatory disorder of the lining of the gastrointestinal system, especially of the terminal ileum.
3. Narcotic addiction is related to the frequent, severe pain episodes that often occur with chronic pancreatitis and its complications and that require narcotics for relief.
4. Peritonitis, an inflammation of the lining of the abdomen, is not a common complication of chronic pancreatitis.

**TEST-TAKING HINT: The test taker may be able to delete options based on normal anatomical and physiological data. Diabetes insipidus is a complication of the pituitary gland; Crohn's disease is a disease of the GI tract; and the peritoneum is the lining of the abdomen. Therefore, options "1," "2," and "4" can be eliminated.**

32. 1. During this procedure a scope is placed down the client's mouth; therefore, assessing for rectal bleeding would not be a common intervention.
2. The client's throat has been anesthetized to insert the scope; therefore, fluid and food are withheld until the gag reflex has returned.
3. The gag reflex will be suppressed as a result of the local anesthesia applied to the throat to insert the endoscope into the esophagus; therefore, the gag reflex must be assessed prior to allowing the client to resume eating or drinking.
4. The client should be in a semi-Fowler's or side-lying position to prevent aspiration.

**TEST-TAKING HINT: The test taker should apply the nursing process and select an option that addresses assessment—either "1" or "3." The medical suffix "endo" should help the test taker select "3" as the correct answer.**

33. 1. Lying on the stomach will not help to decrease the client's pain.
2. This is a position used by clients with chronic obstructive pulmonary disease to help lung expansion.
3. This fetal position decreases pain caused by stretching of the peritoneum as a result of edema.
4. Laying supine causes the peritoneum to stretch, which increases the pain.

**TEST-TAKING HINT: The test taker should think about where the pancreas is located in the abdomen to help identify the correct answer. Prone or supine would cause the abdomen to be stretched, which would increase pain.**

34. 1. The return of bowel sounds indicates the return of peristalsis, and the nasogastric

suction is usually discontinued within 24 to 48 hours thereafter.
2. Daily weight gain reflects fluid gain.
3. The nurse should assess for signs of infection or infiltration.
4. Fasting and the N/G tube increase the client's risk for mucous membrane irritation and breakdown.
5. Blood glucose levels are monitored because clients with chronic pancreatitis can develop diabetes mellitus.

**TEST-TAKING HINT: This alternative-type question requires the test taker to select all interventions that are appropriate for the client's diagnosis. The test taker should not try to eliminate options because all options could be correct.**

35. 1. Pancreatic enzymes enhance the digestion of starches (carbohydrates) in the gastrointestinal tract by supplying an exogenous (outside) source of the pancreatic enzymes protease, amylase, and lipase.
2. Pancreatic enzymes decrease the number of bowel movements.
3. The enzymes are enteric coated and should not be crushed because the hydrochloric acid in the stomach will destroy the enzymes; these enzymes work in the small intestine.
4. Pancreatic enzymes help break down carbohydrates, and bile breaks down fat.

**TEST-TAKING HINT: Remember that enzymes break down other foods and end in "ase." The test taker must know the normal function of organs to identify correct answers.**

36. 1. Coffee, tea, and cola stimulate gastric and pancreatic secretions and may precipitate pain, so these foods should be avoided, not decreased.
2. High-fat and spicy foods stimulate gastric and pancreatic secretions and may precipitate an acute pancreatic attack.
3. Amylase and lipase levels must be checked via venipuncture with laboratory tests, and there are no daily tests the client can monitor at home.
4. The client will be fatigued as a result of decreased metabolic energy production and will need to rest and not return to work immediately.

**TEST-TAKING HINT: The test taker should be careful with words such as "decrease" because many times the client must avoid certain foods and situations completely, not decrease their intake of them. There are only a few blood studies that can be monitored at home on a**

daily basis—mainly glucose levels, which would cause the test taker to eliminate option "3."

## Cancer of the Pancreas

37. 1. A yellow haze is a sign of a toxic level of digoxin, with the client seeing through the yellow haze. Seeing a yellow haze is not the same as the client being jaundiced. In jaundice, the skin and sclera are yellow, signs of pancreatic cancer.
2. The abdominal pain is often made worse by eating and lying supine in clients diagnosed with cancer of the pancreas.
3. The client would not know these terms, and the HCP would be the one to check these laboratory values.
4. Clients diagnosed with cancer of the pancreas lose weight, not gain weight.

**TEST-TAKING HINT: The test taker could arrive at the correct answer by correlating words in the stem of the question and words in the answer options—the abdomen with eating and pain with pain.**

38. 1. Tube feedings are collaborative interventions, but the stem did not say the client had a feeding tube.
2. This is an independent intervention.
3. Assessment is an independent intervention and the first step in the nursing process. No one should have to tell the nurse to assess the client.
4. A collaborative intervention would be to refer to the nutrition expert, the dietitian.

**TEST-TAKING HINT: The key word in the stem is "collaborative." which means another health-care discipline must be involved. Only options "1" and "4" involve other members of the health-care team. The test taker could eliminate distracter "1" by rereading the stem and realizing that the stem did not say the client had a feeding tube.**

39. 1. Monitoring the blood glucose at random intervals, as would be done at a health fair, can pick up possible diabetes mellitus or the presence of a pancreatic tumor, but detecting a disease at an early stage is secondary screening, not primary prevention.
2. Inspecting the skin for jaundice would be a secondary nursing intervention.
3. Limiting the intake of meat and fats in the diet would be an example of primary interventions. Risk factors for the development of cancer of the pancreas are cigarette

smoking and eating a high-fat diet that is high in animal protein. By changing these behaviors the client could possibly prevent the development of cancer of the pancreas. Other risk factors include genetic predisposition and exposure to industrial chemicals.

4. Instructing a client with hyperglycemia (diabetes mellitus) is an example of tertiary nursing care.

**TEST-TAKING HINT: Even if the test taker was not sure of the definition of primary, secondary, or tertiary nursing care, primary means first. Only one answer option is preventive, and preventing something comes before treating it.**

40. 1. The nursing assistant can help a client to turn to the side and assume the fetal position, which would decrease some abdominal pain.
2. This is a high-level nursing intervention that the unlicensed nursing assistant is not qualified to implement,
3. Evaluation of the effectiveness of a PRN medication must be done by the nurse.
4. The nurse should empty the bedside commode to determine if the client is continuing to pass melena (blood in the stool).

**TEST-TAKING HINT: There are basic rules to delegation. The nurse cannot delegate assessment, evaluation, unstable clients, or situations requiring nursing judgment.**

41. 1. This would be the routine for radiation therapy, but chemotherapy is given one (1) to three (3) or four (4) days in a row and then a period of three (3) to four (4) weeks will elapse before the next treatment. This is called intermittent pulse therapy.
2. The most important person in the treatment of the cancer is the client. Research has proved that the more involved a client becomes in his or her care, the better the prognosis. Clients should have a chance to ask all the questions that they have.
3. Cancer of any kind is a serious problem.
4. Most antineoplastic medications are given intravenously. Many of the medications can cause severe complications if given intramuscularly.

**TEST-TAKING HINT: The test taker can eliminate option "3" on the basis that this statement is denial of the problem.**

42. 1. The client should stay in the outpatient department after the procedure for observa-

tion unless the HCP determines that a more extensive workup should be completed.
2. This is not the type of procedure where the results warrant an emergency surgery. A cardiac catheterization sometimes results in an emergency surgery and the client is prepared for this possibility, but this is not the case with an ERCP.
3. The client should be NPO after midnight to make sure the stomach is empty to reduce the risk of aspiration during the procedure.
4. The possible blockage would be of the duodenum, common bile duct, or pancreatic outlet.

**TEST-TAKING HINT: The nurse should never preface any instruction with "if done correctly" because this sets the nurse, HCP, and facility up for a lawsuit. The client is NPO for any procedure or surgery where the client will receive general or twilight sleep anesthesia.**

43. 1. The client will have jaundice, clay-colored stools, and tea-colored urine resulting from blockage of the bile drainage.
2. Night sweats and fevers are associated with lymphoma.
3. Left lower abdominal cramps are associated with diverticulitis, and tenesmus is straining when defecating.
4. Nausea and coffee-ground emesis are symptoms of gastric ulcers.

**TEST-TAKING HINT: The test taker should remember anatomical placement of organs. This would eliminate answer options "3" and "4." The pancreas empties pancreatic enzymes into the small bowel to aid in the digestion of carbohydrates and fats in close proximity to where the common bile duct enters the intestine.**

44. 1. Clients diagnosed with cancer of the pancreas have a poor prognosis, but this is not the priority problem at this time.
2. This is a major abdominal surgery, and there are massive fluid volume shifts that occur when this type of trauma is experienced by the body. Maintaining the circulatory system without overloading it requires extremely close monitoring.
3. Pain is a priority but not over fluid volume status.
4. Altered nutrition would be the next highest priority. The client will be NPO with a nasogastric tube to suction and will be receiving total parenteral nutrition.

**TEST-TAKING HINT:** The nurse should identify all of the problems, but one—fluid volume imbalance—has the greatest priority because if not addressed promptly and correctly, it could lead to severe complications.

45. 1. The client is being discharged. There is no need for the client to continue recording intake and outputs at home.
    2. The client has undergone a radical and extensive surgery and will need to be administered narcotic pain medication, and a bowel regimen should be in place to prevent constipation.
    3. Removal of the pancreas will create a diabetic state for the client. The client will need insulin and pancreatic enzyme replacement.
    4. Client should not allow pain to reach above a "5" before taking pain medication or it will be more difficult to get the pain under control.
    5. There is no reason for the client to sleep with the head of the bed elevated.

**TEST-TAKING HINT:** The test taker might choose option "3" by remembering that the pancreas secretes insulin. Option "4" is taught to all clients in pain.

46. 1. The client may need IV medication, but in this case if it is needed, it would be 50% dextrose.
    2. The HCP might be notified, but the nurse needs to assess the client first.
    3. These are symptoms of an insulin reaction (hypoglycemia). A bedside glucose check should be done. Pancreatic islet tumors can produce hyperinsulinemia or hypoglycemia.
    4. This would be done after the nurse knows the glucose reading.

**TEST-TAKING HINT:** The test taker should remember the function of the pancreas. This would lead the test taker to look for interventions for hypoglycemia.

47. 1. Food preferences are important for the caregiver to know because this will be the person preparing meals for the client.
    2. Cancer of the pancreas has a poor prognosis for most clients, and the nurse should determine if the client has executed an advance directive regarding their wishes.
    3. This is important because of payment issues, but it is not the highest priority.
    4. Clients diagnosed with cancer frequently have anorexia, and explaining that the client should eat does not mean the client will eat.

**TEST-TAKING HINT:** The test taker would need to know general information about the disease process to answer this question, but "2" is a good choice for many terminal diseases. Remember to read the questions carefully. The home health nurse is not arranging meals for the client.

48. 1. The client is at risk for poor nutrition and malabsorption syndrome for which tissue turgor assessment is appropriate, but the client problem here is pruritus, or itching.
    2. The itching is associated with the cancer and not a fungus.
    3. The client should be monitored for skin breakdown, but pruritus is itching and an intervention is needed to prevent skin problems from scratching.
    4. Keeping the fingernails short will reduce the chance of breaks in the skin from scratching.

**TEST-TAKING HINT:** The problem is "risk for skin breakdown." The etiology is "pruritus." Interventions address the etiology. Goals address the problem.

## Adrenal Disorders

49. 1. Moon face, buffalo hump, and hyperglycemia result from Cushing's syndrome, hyperfunction of the adrenal gland.
    2. Hirsutism is hair growth where it normally would not occur, such as facial hair on women. Fever and irritability, along with hirsutism, are clinical manifestations of Cushing's syndrome.
    3. Bronze pigmentation of the skin, particularly of the knuckles and other areas of skin creases, occurs in Addison's disease. Hypotension and anorexia also occur with Addison's.
    4. Tachycardia, bulging eyes, and goiter are clinical manifestations that occur with thyroid disorders.

**TEST-TAKING HINTS:** This question contains answer options referring to two opposite diseases, Addison's disease and Cushing's syndrome. If two options—in this case, "1" and "2"—are appropriate for one of the diseases, then these two can be ruled out as the correct answer.

50. 1. Altered body image is a psychosocial problem, not a priority over a potentially lethal physical complication, and physical changes occur over an extended period.

2. Activity intolerance will occur with adrenal gland hypofunction, but this is not a priority over dehydration.
3. Impaired coping can occur in clients with adrenal gland disorders, but it is not a priority over dehydration.
4. Fluid volume deficit (dehydration) can lead to circulatory impairment and hyperkalemia.

**TEST-TAKING HINTS: Assuming that all of the problems listed apply to the client diagnosed with Addison's disease, two are psychosocial problems and two are physiological. Applying Maslow's Hierarchy of Needs, the two psychological problems can be ruled out as the highest priority. Of the two that are left, activity intolerance is not life altering or threatening.**

51. 1. Clients diagnosed with Addison's disease have adrenal gland hypofunction. The hormones normally produced by the gland must be replaced. Steroids and androgens are produced by the adrenal gland.
2. The client will have decreased fluid volume, and fluid restriction would exacerbate a crisis.
3. The client requires a quiet, calm, relaxed atmosphere.
4. The client walks with a stooped posture from fatigue, but gait training is not needed.

**TEST-TAKING HINTS: To answer this question the test taker must have knowledge of adrenal gland function.**

52. 1. The drugs quinidine, digoxin, and hydralazine can interfere with adrenal gland secretions and cause hypofunction. Cushing's syndrome is adrenal gland hyperfunction.
2. The adrenal gland secretes cortisol and the pituitary gland secretes adrenocorticotropic hormone (ACTH), a hormone used by the body to stimulate the production of cortisol.
3. 24-hour urine specimens for 17 hydroxycorticosteroids and 17 ketosteroids may be collected. Metanephrines and catecholamines are urine collections for pheochromocytomas.
4. Spot urinalysis and white blood cell count will not provide information on adrenal gland functions.

**TEST-TAKING HINTS: If the test taker was aware that the adrenal gland produces cortisol, then there is only one answer option that refers to cortisol.**

53. 1. Cushing's disease is not an autoimmune problem.
2. Iatrogenic means that a problem has been caused by a medical treatment or procedure—in this case, treatment with steroids for another problem. Clients taking steroids over a period of time develop the clinical manifestations of Cushing's disease. Disease processes for which long-term steroids are prescribed include chronic obstructive pulmonary disease, cancer, and arthritis.
3. This could be a cause for primary Cushing's syndrome.
4. There is a known reason for the client to have iatrogenic Cushing's.

**TEST-TAKING HINTS: This question requires the test taker to know basic medical terminology.**

54. 1. Cushing's syndrome/disease predisposes the client to develop infections as a result of the immunosuppressive nature of the disease.
2. The client has too much cortisol; this client would not be receiving prednisone, a steroid medication.
3. These are symptoms of hypoglycemia, which would not be expected in this client because this client has high glucose levels.
4. The client is predisposed to osteoporosis and fractures. Contact sports should be avoided.

**TEST-TAKING HINTS: If the test taker is not aware of the disease problem, this question could be answered correctly because of common standard discharge instructions—namely, notify the health-care provider of a fever.**

55. 1. This client could be cared for by any nurse qualified to work in an intensive care unit.
2. These blood gases are within normal limits.
3. This client has a low blood pressure and tachycardia. This client could be about to go into an Addisonian crisis, a potentially life-threatening condition. The most experienced nurse should care for this client.
4. A negative Trousseau's sign is good for this client.

**TEST-TAKING HINTS: The answer options "1," "2," and "4" have expected or normal data. There is only one option with abnormal data. Even if the reader is unaware of Addisonian crisis, these are vital signs that indicate potential shock.**

56. 1. Blood glucose levels do not address the problem of altered body image.
2. Head-to-toe assessments are performed to detect a physiological problem, not a psychosocial one.

3. This is an intervention that will allow the client to discuss feelings of body image.
4. Bowel sounds and temperature are physical symptoms.

**TEST-TAKING HINTS: The intervention must match the problem.**

57. 1. This client has been exposed to wind and sun at the lake during the hours prior to being admitted to the emergency department. This predisposes the client to dehydration and an Addisonian crisis. Rapid IV fluid replacement is necessary.
2. Waiting in the waiting area could cause the client to go into a coma and die.
3. A head-to-toe assessment could be done after starting replacement fluid.
4. Laboratory specimens would not be priority and calcium is not a problem in clients with Addison's disease.

**TEST-TAKING HINTS: This client is weak, lethargic, and forgetful, indicating a diminished level of consciousness. The nurse should choose an action that will address the problem.**

58. The client has received 8650 mL of intravenous fluid.

**TEST-TAKING HINT: This is a basic addition problem. If the test taker has difficulty with this problem, then a math review course would be in order.**

59. 1. An autocratic style is one in which the person in charge makes the decision without consulting anyone else.
2. This is an example of a democratic style.
3. This is an example of laissez-faire.
4. This is an example of democratic leadership style.

**TEST-TAKING HINTS: The test taker could choose the correct answer if the test taker knew lay terms such as autocratic and democratic.**

60. 1. A unilateral adrenalectomy leaves one adrenal gland still functioning. No hormone replacement will be required.
2. The client can still have normal physiological functioning, including sexual functioning, with the remaining gland.
3. This is information given to all surgical clients on discharge.
4. This should be done prior to surgery, not at discharge.

**TEST-TAKING HINTS: The test taker must notice the adjectives; discharge tells the reader a time frame for the instructions. This rules out "4."**

## Pituitary Disorders

61. 1. The client has excess fluid and would not be dehydrated, and blood glucose levels are not affected.
2. Early signs and symptoms are nausea and vomiting. The client has a syndrome of the inappropriate secretion of the antidiuresis (against allowing the body to urinate) hormone. In other words, the client is producing a hormone that will not allow the client to urinate.
3. The client experiences dilutional hyponatremia and the body has too much fluid already.
4. Vasopressin is the name of the antidiuretic hormone. Giving more would increase the client's problem. Also, a water challenge test is performed, not a fluid deprivation test.

**TEST-TAKING HINTS: The syndrome's name is confusing with a double negative—"inappropriate" and "anti." It is helpful to put the situation in the reader's own words to remember which way the fluids are being shifted in the body.**

62. 1. Neurological status is monitored every one (1) to two (2) hours. This client's neurological status appears intact. Clients waking up in an intensive care area may not be aware of their surroundings.
2. The output is more than double the intake in a short time. This client could be developing diabetes insipidus, a complication of trauma to the head.
3. These vital signs are within normal limits.
4. A transphenoidal hypophysectomy is performed by surgical access above the gum line and through the nasal passage. There is no dressing. A drip pad is taped below the nares.

**TEST-TAKING HINTS: Two (2) of the answer options contain normal data and would not warrant immediate intervention. Option "4" does not match the type of surgery.**

63. 1. The client will have an elevated sodium level as a result of low circulating blood volume. The fluid is being lost through the urine. Diabetes means "to pass through" in Greek, indicating polyuria, a symptom shared with diabetes mellitus. Diabetes insipidus is a totally separate disease process.
2. Serum calcium is not affected by diabetes insipidus.
3. Urine glucose would be monitored for diabetes mellitus.
4. White blood cells in the urine indicate the presence of a urinary tract infection.

**TEST-TAKING HINTS: The test taker should not confuse diabetes insipidus and diabetes mellitus.**

64. 1. The client should keep a list of medication being taken and wear a Medic Alert bracelet.
    2. Medication taken for DI is usually every 8–12 hours, depending on the client. The client should keep the medication close at hand.
    3. The client is at risk for fluid shifts. Weighing every morning allows the client to follow the fluid shifts. Weight gain could indicate too much medication.
    4. Tightness in the chest could be an indicator that the medication is not being tolerated; if this occurs the client should call the healthcare provider.

**TEST-TAKING HINTS: This is an "except" question. This means that all answers except one will be actions that the client should do. If the reader missed interpreting this from the stem, then the reader could jump to the first action the client should do as the correct answer.**

65. 1. The client is not allowed to drink during the test at all.
    2. This test does not require any medications to be given, and vasopressin will treat the DI, not help diagnose it.
    3. The client is deprived of all fluids, and if the client has DI the urine production will not diminish. Vital signs and weights are taken every hour to determine circulatory status. If a marked decrease in weight or vital signs occurs, the test is immediately terminated.
    4. No fluid is allowed and a sonogram is not involved.

**TEST-TAKING HINTS: The name of the test is a fluid deprivation test. Two (2) of the options require the administration of some type of fluid.**

66. 1. Clients with SIADH have a problem with retaining fluid. This is expected.
    2. This client's intake and output are relatively the same.
    3. Muscle twitching is a sign of early sodium imbalance. If an immediate intervention is not made, the client could begin to seize.
    4. This is expected.

**TEST-TAKING HINTS: All of the answer options contain expected information except option "3".**

67. Two (2) sprays per dose. 40 g of medication every 24 hours is to be given in doses administered

every 12 hours. First, determine number of doses needed.

$$24 \div 12 = 2 \text{ doses}$$

Then, determine amount of medication to be given in each of those 2 doses:

$$40 \div 2 = 20 \text{ g of medication per dose}$$

Finally, determine how many sprays are needed to deliver the 20 mg when each spray delivers 10 g:

$$20 \div 10 = 2 \text{ sprays}$$

**TEST-TAKING HINT: The test taker should take each step of the problem one at a time and check the answer with the pull-down calculator if taking the exam on a computer.**

68. 1. Fluids are restricted to 500–600 mL per 24 hours.
    2. Orientation to person, place, and times should be assessed every two (2) hours or more often.
    3. A safe environment, not a stimulating one, is provided.
    4. Urine and serum osmolality are monitored to determine fluid volume status.
    5. The client should be weighed daily.

**TEST-TAKING HINTS: The test taker should notice numbers: Is assessing the client's level of consciousness every two (2) hours enough, or is weighing the client every three (3) days enough?**

69. 1. Diabetes insipidus is not diabetes mellitus; glucose levels are not monitored.
    2. There is no caffeine restriction for DI.
    3. Checking urine ketones is not indicated.
    4. The client is excreting large amounts of dilute urine. If the client is unable to take in enough fluids, the client will quickly become dehydrated, so tissue turgor should be assessed frequently.

**TEST-TAKING HINTS: Two (2) of the answer options would be appropriate for diabetes mellitus, not diabetes insipidus, and can be eliminated on this basis alone.**

70. 1. The client should have the water pitcher filled, but this is not the first action.
    2. This should be done but not before assessing the problem.
    3. The first action should be to determine if the client is experiencing polyuria and polydipsia as a result of developing diabetes insipidus, a complication of the head trauma.
    4. This could be done, but it will not give the nurse information about DI.

**TEST-TAKING HINTS: The nurse must apply a systematic approach to answering priority questions. Maslow's Hierarchy of Needs should be applied if it is a physiological problem and the nursing process if it is a question of this nature. Assessment is the first step in the nursing process.**

71. 1. A serum sodium level of 112 mEq/L is dangerously low, and the client is at risk for seizures. A headache is a symptom of a low sodium level.
    2. This is a normal potassium level, and a heightened level of awareness indicates drug usage.
    3. This is a normal calcium level and the client is fluid overloaded, not dehydrated, so there would not be tented tissue turgor.
    4. This is a normal magnesium level, and a large urinary output would be desired.

    **TEST-TAKING HINTS: The nurse must know common laboratory values.**

72. 1. Discussing the information with others is not allowing clients to decide what is best for themselves.
    2. This could be an example of beneficence (to do good) if the nurse did this so the client would have information on which to base a decision on whether to continue the fluid restriction.
    3. This is an example of autonomy (the client has the right to decide for himself).
    4. This is an example of dishonesty and should never be tolerated in a health-care setting.

    **TEST-TAKING HINTS: The stem asks the test taker about autonomy. Even if the test taker did not know the ethical principle, autonomy means the right of self-governance. Only one of the answer options could fit the definition of autonomy.**

## Thyroid Disorders

73. 1. A decrease in the thyroid hormone causes decreased metabolism, which leads to fatigue and hair loss.
    2. These are signs of hyperthyroidism.
    3. These are signs of hyperthyroidism.
    4. These are signs of parathyroidism.

    **TEST-TAKING HINT: Often if the test taker does not know the specific signs/symptoms of the disease but knows the function of the system that is affected by the disease, some possible answers can be ruled out. Tetany and stiffness of the hands are related to calcium, the level of which is influenced by the parathyroid gland,**

not the thyroid gland; therefore, option "4" can be ruled out. All of the other three options relate to metabolism, which is regulated by the thyroid gland. The test taker must decide which option lists symptoms of decreased thyroid function

74. 1. External heat sources (heating pads, electric or warming blankets) should be discouraged because they increase the risk of peripheral vasodilatation and vascular collapse.
    2. Decreased metabolism causes the client to be cold frequently; therefore, protecting the client from exposure to cold will help increase comfort and decrease further heat loss.
    3. The room temperature should be kept warm because the client will have complaints of being cold.
    4. The client is fatigued and this is an appropriate intervention, but it would not be applicable to the client problem of "risk for imbalanced body temperature."

    **TEST-TAKING HINT: The test taker must always know exactly what the question is asking. Option "4" can be ruled out because it does not address body temperature. If the test taker knows the normal function of the thyroid gland, this may help identify the answer; decreased metabolism will cause the client to be cold.**

75. 1. The medication will help increase the client's metabolism rate. A weight gain would indicate that not enough medication is being taken to put the client in a euthyroid (normal thyroid) state.
    2. A decreased pulse rate indicates that there is not enough thyroid hormone level; therefore the medication is not effective.
    3. The client with hypothyroidism frequently has a subnormal temperature, so a temperature WNL indicates the medication is effective.
    4. Diaphoresis (sweating) occurs with hyperthyroidism, not hypothyroidism.

    **TEST-TAKING HINT: One way of determining the effectiveness of medication is to determine if the signs/symptoms of the disease are no longer noticeable.**

76. 1. Fiber should be increased in the client diagnosed with hypothyroidism because the client experiences constipation secondary to decreased metabolism.
    2. The client with hyperthyroidism should have a high-calorie, high-protein diet.

3. The client's fluid intake should be increased to replace fluids that are lost through diarrhea and excessive sweating.
4. The client with hyperthyroidism has an increased appetite; therefore, well-balanced meals served several times throughout the day will help with the client's constant hunger.

**TEST-TAKING HINT: If the test taker knows that with hyperthyroidism the metabolism is increased, then increasing the food intake would be the most appropriate choice.**

77. 1. Hypoglycemia is expected in a client with myxedema; therefore a 74 blood glucose level would be expected.
2. **A pulse oximeter reading of less than 93% is significant. A 90% pulse oximeter reading indicates a PaO$_2$ of approximately 60 on an arterial blood gas; this is severe hypoxemia and requires immediate intervention.**
3. The client with myxedema coma is in an exaggerated hypothyroid state; a low pulse is expected in a client with hypothyroidism.
4. Lethargy is an expected symptom in a client diagnosed with myxedema; therefore this would not warrant immediate intervention.

**TEST-TAKING HINT: The words "warrants immediate intervention" mean the test taker should select an option that is abnormal for the disease process or a symptom that is life threatening or life altering.**

78. 1. Thyroid hormones are the treatment of choice for the client diagnosed with hypothyroidism; therefore, the nurse would not question this medication.
2. In untreated hypothyroidism, the medical management is aimed at supporting vital functions, so administering oxygen would be an appropriate medication.
3. Untreated hypothyroidism is characterized by an increased susceptibility to the effects of most hypnotic and sedative agents; therefore, the nurse would question this medication.
4. Clients with hypothyroidism become constipated as a result of decreased metabolism, so laxatives would not be questioned by the nurse.

**TEST-TAKING HINT: When a question asks which order the nurse would question, three of the options would be orders that the nurse would expect to administer to the client. Sometimes saying, "The nurse would administer this medication," may help the test taker select the correct answer.**

79. 1. Decreased appetite is a symptom of hypothyroidism, not hyperthyroidism.
2. Constipation is a symptom of hypothyroidism.
3. Dry, coarse skin is a sign of hypothyroidism.
4. **The thyroid gland (in the neck) enlarges as a result of the increased need for thyroid hormone production; an enlarged gland is called a goiter.**

**TEST-TAKING HINT: If the test taker does not know the answer, sometimes thinking about the location of the gland or organ that is causing the problem may help the test taker select or rule out specific options.**

80. 1. **Radioactive iodine therapy is used to destroy the overactive thyroid cells. After treatment the client is followed closely for three (3) to four (4) weeks until the euthyroid state is reached.**
2. A single dose of radioactive iodine therapy is administered; the dosage is based on the client's weight.
3. The colorless, tasteless radioiodine is administered by the radiologist, and the client may have to stay up to two (2) hours after the treatment in the office.
4. If too much of the thyroid gland is destroyed by the radioactive iodine therapy, the client may develop hypothyroidism and have to take thyroid hormone the rest of his or her life.

**TEST-TAKING HINT: Some questions require the test taker to be knowledgeable of the information, especially medical treatments, and there are no specific hints to help the test taker answer the question.**

81. 1. Weight loss indicates the medication may not be effective and will probably need to be increased.
2. **The client needs to know that emotional highs and lows are secondary to hyperthyroidism. With treatment this emotional liability will subside.**
3. **Any over-the-counter medications (for example, alcohol-based medications) may negatively affect the client's hyperthyroidism or medications being used for treatment.**
4. **This will help any HCP immediately know of the client's condition, especially if the client is unable to tell the HCP.**
5. **The client may be receiving antithyroid medications and should know how to take them properly.**

**TEST-TAKING HINT: This alternate-type question instructs the test taker to select all the**

interventions that apply. The test taker should not try to outguess the test writer; in some instances all the options are correct.

82. 1. There is no screening for thyroid disorders, just serum thyroid levels.
    2. This is not a true statement.
    3. Medications do not decrease the development of goiters.
    4. Almost all of the iodine that enters the body is retained in the thyroid gland. A deficiency in iodine will cause the thyroid gland to work hard and enlarge, which is called a goiter. Goiters are commonly seen in geographical regions that have an iodine deficiency. Most table salt in the United States has iodine added.

**TEST-TAKING HINT: The nurse must know about disease processes. There is no test-taking hint that will help determine the answer to the question.**

83. 1. The thyroid hormone must be given daily, and thyroid levels are drawn every six (6) months or so.
    2. A blood glucose level of 210 mg/dL requires insulin administration; therefore the nurse would not question giving this medication
    3. This potassium level is below normal, which is 3.5–5.5 mEq/L. Therefore, the nurse would question administering this

medication because loop diuretics cause potassium loss in the urine.

4. This digoxin level is within therapeutic range—0.8–2.0 mg/dL; therefore the nurse would administer this medication.

**TEST-TAKING HINT: When administering medication the nurse must know when to question the medication, how to know it is effective, and what must be taught to keep the client safe while taking the medication. The test taker may want to turn the question around and say, "I would give this medication."**

84. 1. These are signs of myxedema (hypothyroidism) coma. Obstipation is extreme constipation.
    2. Hyperpyrexia (high fever) and heart rate above 130 beats/minute are signs of thyroid storm, a severely exaggerated hyperthyroidism.
    3. Decreased blood pressure and slow heart rate are signs of myxedema coma.
    4. These are signs/symptoms of myxedema coma.

**TEST-TAKING HINT: If the test taker does not have the knowledge to answer the question, then the test taker should look at the options closely. Options "1," "3," and "4" all have signs/symptoms of "decrease"—hypoactive, hypotension, and hypoxia. The test taker should select the option that does not match.**

1. The nurse is teaching a community class to people with Type 2 diabetes mellitus. Which explanation would explain the development of Type 2 diabetes?
   1. The islet cells in the pancreas stop producing insulin.
   2. The client eats too many foods that are high in sugar.
   3. The pituitary gland does not produce vasopressin.
   4. The cells become resistant to the circulating insulin.

2. The nurse is teaching the client diagnosed with Type 2 diabetes mellitus about diet. Which diet selection indicates the client understands the teaching?
   1. A submarine sandwich, potato chips, and diet cola.
   2. Four (4) slices of a supreme thin-crust pizza and milk.
   3. Smoked turkey sandwich, celery sticks, and unsweetened tea.
   4. A roast beef sandwich, fried onion rings, and a cola.

3. The nurse is preparing to administer sliding scale insulin to a client with Type 2 diabetes. The Medication Administration Record is as follows:

| Client Name: ABCD | Client Number: 1234567 | Allergies: NKA | Diagnosis: Diabetes Mellitus |
|---|---|---|---|
| | Medication | Administration | Record |
| Medication Regular insulin subcutaneously ac and hs $0-60 = 1$ amp $D_{50}$ $61-150 = 0$ units $151-300 = 5$ units $301-450 = 10$ units $>450 =$ Call HCP | 0701–1500 0730 1130 | 1501–2300 1630 2100 | 2301–0700 |
| Metformin 500 mg po. b.i.d. | 0800 | 1700 | |

At 1130, the client has a blood glucometer level of 322. Which action should the nurse implement?
   1. Notify the health-care provider.
   2. Administer ten (10) units of regular insulin.
   3. Administer five (5) units of Humalog insulin.
   4. Administer ten (10) units of intermediate-acting insulin.

4. When assessing a 31-year-old client who has a sustained release of growth hormone (GH), what signs/symptoms would the nurse expect to find?
   1. An enlarged forehead, maxilla, and face.
   2. A six (6)-inch increase in height of the client.
   3. The client complaining of a severe headache.
   4. A systolic blood pressure of 200 to 300 mm Hg.

5. Which sign/symptom would indicate to the nurse that the client is experiencing hyperparathyroidism?
   1. A negative Trousseau's sign.
   2. A positive Chvostek's sign.
   3. Nocturnal muscle cramps.
   4. Tented skin turgor.

6. Which laboratory data would make the nurse suspect that the client with primary hyperparathyroidism is experiencing a complication?
   1. A serum creatinine level of 2.8 mg/dL.
   2. A calcium level of 9.2 mg/dL.
   3. A serum triglyceride level of 130 mg/dL.
   4. A sodium level of 135 mEq/L.

7. Which information is a risk factor for developing pheochromocytoma?
   1. A history of skin cancer.
   2. A history of high blood pressure.
   3. A family history of adrenal tumors.
   4. A family history of migraine headaches.

8. The client is three (3) days postoperative unilateral adrenalectomy. Which discharge instructions should the nurse teach?
   1. Discuss the need for lifelong steroid replacement.
   2. Instruct the client on administration of vasopressin.
   3. Teach the client to care for the suprapubic Foley catheter.
   4. Tell the client to notify the HCP of a temperature greater than 101°F.

9. Which psychosocial problem should be included in the plan of care for a female client diagnosed with Cushing's syndrome?
   1. Altered glucose metabolism.
   2. Body image disturbance.
   3. Risk for suicide.
   4. Impaired wound healing.

10. The nurse is admitting a client to rule out aldosteronism. Which assessment data should the nurse monitor that supports the client's diagnosis?
    1. Temperature.
    2. Pulse.
    3. Respirations.
    4. Blood pressure.

11. Which client history would be most significant in the development of symptoms for a client who has iatrogenic Cushing's disease?
    1. Long-term use of anabolic steroids.
    2. Extended use of inhaled steroids for asthma.
    3. History of long-term glucocorticoid use.
    4. Family history of increased cortisol production.

12. The client is one (1) hour postoperative thyroidectomy. Which intervention should the nurse implement?
    1. Check the posterior neck for bleeding.
    2. Assess the client for the Chvostek's sign.
    3. Monitor the client's serum calcium level.
    4. Change the client's surgical dressing.

13. Which signs/symptoms would indicate that the client with hypothyroidism is not taking enough thyroid hormone?
    1. Complaints of weight loss and fine tremors.
    2. Complaints of excessive thirst and urination.
    3. Complaints of constipation and being cold.
    4. Complaints of delayed wound healing and belching.

14. Which client problem is the nurse's priority concern for the client diagnosed with acute pancreatitis?
    1. Impaired nutrition.
    2. Skin integrity.
    3. Anxiety.
    4. Pain relief.

15. Which laboratory data indicate the client's pancreatitis is improving?
    1. The amylase and lipase serum levels are decreased.
    2. The white blood cell count (WBC) is decreased.
    3. The conjugated and unconjugated bilirubin levels are decreased.
    4. The blood urea nitrogen (BUN) serum level is decreased.

16. The client diagnosed with acute pancreatitis has developed a pseudocyst that ruptures. Which procedure should the nurse anticipate the HCP ordering?
    1. Paracentesis.
    2. Chest tube insertion.
    3. Lumbar puncture.
    4. Biopsy of the pancreas.

17. Which signs/symptoms would the nurse expect to find in the client diagnosed with an insulinoma?
    1. Nervousness, jitteriness, and diaphoresis.
    2. Flushed skin, dry mouth, and tented skin turgor.
    3. Polyuria, polydipsia, and polyphagia.
    4. Hypertension, tachycardia, and feeling hot.

18. Which risk factor would the nurse expect to find in the client diagnosed with pancreatic cancer?
    1. Chewing tobacco.
    2. Low-fat diet.
    3. Chronic alcoholism.
    4. Exposure to industrial chemicals.

19. The nurse is aware that epinephrine and norepinephrine are secreted by which endocrine gland?
    1. The pancreas.
    2. The adrenal cortex.
    3. The adrenal medulla.
    4. The anterior pituitary gland.

20. Which question should the nurse ask when assessing the client for an endocrine dysfunction?
    1. "Have you noticed any pain in your legs when walking?"
    2. "Have you had any unexplained weight loss?"
    3. "Have you noticed any change in your bowel movements?"
    4. "Have you experienced any joint pain or discomfort?"

21. Which nursing instruction should the nurse discuss with the client who is receiving glucocorticoids for Addison's disease?
    1. Discuss the importance of tapering medications when discontinuing medication.
    2. Explain that the dose will need to be decreased during times of stress or infection.
    3. Instruct the client to take medication on an empty stomach with a glass of water.
    4. Encourage the client to wear a Medic Alert bracelet and carry a card in the wallet.

22. The client with chronic alcoholism has chronic pancreatitis and hypomagnesemia. What should the nurse assess when administering magnesium sulfate to the client?
    1. Deep tendon reflexes.
    2. Arterial blood gases.
    3. Skin turgor.
    4. Capillary refill time.

23. Which endocrine disorder would the nurse assess for in the client who has a closed head injury with increased intracranial pressure?
    1. Pheochromocytoma.
    2. Diabetes insipidus.
    3. Hashimoto's disease.
    4. Gynecomastia.

24. Which sign/symptom would the nurse expect in the client diagnosed with syndrome of inappropriate antidiuretic hormone (SIADH)?
    1. Excessive thirst.
    2. Orthopnea.
    3. Ascites.
    4. Concentrated urine output.

25. In which area should the nurse administer the regular insulin to ensure the best absorption of the medication?
    1. A
    2. B
    3. C
    4. D

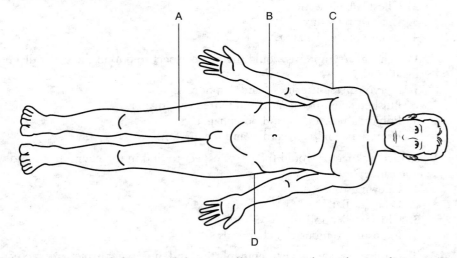

26. The client diagnosed with Type 1 diabetes mellitus received regular insulin two (2) hours ago. The client is complaining of being jittery and nervous. Which interventions should the nurse implement? List in order of priority.
    1. Call the laboratory to confirm blood glucose level.
    2. Administer a quick-acting carbohydrate.
    3. Have the client eat a bologna sandwich.
    4. Check the client's blood glucose level at the bedside.
    5. Determine if the client has had anything to eat.

1. 1. This is the cause of Type 1 diabetes mellitus.
   2. This may be a reason for obesity, which may lead to Type 2 diabetes, but eating too much sugar does not cause diabetes.
   3. This is the explanation for diabetes insipidus, which should not be confused with diabetes mellitus.
   4. **Normally insulin binds to special receptors sites on the cell and initiates a series of reactions involved in metabolism. In Type 2 diabetes these reactions are diminished primarily as a result of obesity and aging.**

2. 1. A submarine sandwich is on a bun-type bread and is usually 6 to 12 inches long and potato chips add fat and more carbohydrates to the meal.
   2. Four (4) slices of pizza would contain excessive numbers of carbohydrates, plus cheese and meats, and whole milk is high in fat.
   3. **Turkey is a low-fat meat. A sandwich usually means normal slices of bread and the client needs at least 50% carbohydrates in each meal. Celery sticks are not counted as carbohydrates.**
   4. The roast beef sandwich is high in carbohydrates, fried onion rings are high in fat, and a regular coke is high in carbohydrates.

3. 1. The client's blood glucose level does not warrant notifying the HCP.
   2. **According to the sliding scale, any blood glucose reading between 301 and 450 requires 10 units of regular insulin, which is fast-acting insulin.**
   3. Humalog is rapid-acting insulin, but the order reads regular insulin.
   4. Intermediate-acting insulin, NPH or Humulin N, is not regular insulin.

4. 1. **Acromegaly, enlarged extremities, occurs when sustained GH hypersecretion begins during adulthood, most commonly because of a pituitary tumor.**
   2. Gigantism occurs when GH hypersecretion begins before puberty when the closure of the epiphyseal plates occurs. Note the age of the client.
   3. This is not a symptom of acromegaly.
   4. This is a sign of pheochromocytoma.

5. 1. A carpopedal spasm occurs when the blood flow to the arm is decreased for three (3) minutes with a blood pressure cuff; a positive Trousseau's sign indicates hypocalcemia, which is a sign of hyperparathyroidism.

2. When a sharp tapping over the facial nerve elicits a spasm or twitching of the mouth, nose, or eyes, the client is hypocalcemic, which occurs in clients with hyperparathyroidism. This is known as a positive Chvostek's sign.
   3. This would make the nurse suspect hypokalemia (low potassium).
   4. This would make the nurse suspect dehydration that occurs with hypernatremia.

6. 1. **A serum creatinine level of 2.8 mg/dL would indicate the client is in renal failure, which is a complication of hyperparathyroidism. The formation of stones in the kidneys related to the increased urinary excretion of calcium and phosphorus occurs in about 55% of clients with primary hyperparathyroidism and can lead to renal failure.**
   2. This calcium level is within the normal range of 9.0–10.5 mg/dL.
   3. This serum triglyceride level is within the normal range of 40–150 mg/dL in males and 30–140 mg/dL for females.
   4. This sodium level is within the normal range of 135–145 mEq/L.

7. 1. A history of skin cancer is not a risk factor for pheochromocytoma.
   2. A history of high blood pressure is a sign of this disease, not a risk factor for developing it.
   3. **There is a high incidence of pheochromocytomas in family members with adrenal tumors, and the von Hippel-Lindau gene is thought to be a primary cause.**
   4. Headaches are a symptom of this disease but not a risk factor for it.

8. 1. Because the client has one adrenal gland remaining, the client may not need lifelong supplemental steroids.
   2. Vasopressin is administered to clients with diabetes insipidus.
   3. The client does not have a suprapubic catheter during this procedure.
   4. **Any temperature greater than 101°F would indicate an infection and the client will need to receive antibiotics, so the HCP must be notified.**

9. 1. This is not a psychosocial problem; it is a physiological problem that does occur in clients diagnosed with Cushing's syndrome.
   2. **The client with Cushing's syndrome has body changes, including moon face, buffalo hump, truncal obesity, hirsutism, and striae**

and bruising, all of which affect the client's body image.

3. This is a psychosocial problem, but it is not one that occurs commonly in clients diagnosed with Cushing's syndrome.

4. This is not a psychosocial problem; it is a physiological problem that does occur in clients diagnosed with Cushing's syndrome.

10. 1. The temperature is not affected by aldosteronism.

2. The pulse is not affected by this disorder.

3. The respirations are not affected by this disorder.

4. **Blood pressure is affected by aldosteronism, with hypertension being the most prominent and universal sign of aldosteronism.**

11. 1. Anabolic steroids are used by individuals to build muscle mass. Long-term use can lead to psychosis or heart attacks.

2. Inhaled steroids do not have systemic effects, which is described by iatrogenic Cushing's disease.

3. **Iatrogenic Cushing's disease is Cushing's disease caused by medical treatment—in this case, by taking excessive steroids that result in the symptoms of moon face, buffalo hump, and other associated symptoms.**

4. Family history does not cause iatrogenic problems.

12. 1. **The incision for a thyroidectomy allows the blood to drain dependently by gravity to the back of the client's neck. Therefore, the nurse should check this area for hemorrhaging, which is a possible complication of any surgery.**

2. The Chvostek's sign indicates hypocalcemia, which is too early to assess for in this client.

3. Accidental removal or damage to the parathyroid glands will not decrease calcium level for at least 24 hours.

4. Surgeons prefer to change the surgical dressing for the first time.

13. 1. **Weight loss and fine tremors would make the nurse suspect the client is taking too much thyroid hormone because these are symptoms of hyperthyroidism.**

2. Excessive thirst and urination are symptoms of diabetes.

3. If the client were not taking enough thyroid hormone, then the client would exhibit symptoms of hypothyroidism such as constipation and being cold.

4. This would indicate Cushing's disease.

14. 1. The client would be NPO and can live without food for a number of days as long as he or she receives fluids.

2. The client is not on strict bed rest and can move about in the bed; therefore, skin integrity would not be a priority problem. In pancreatitis, the tissue damage is internal.

3. The client may be anxious, but psychosocial problems are not priority.

4. **The client with pancreatitis is in excruciating pain because the enzymes are autodigesting the pancreas; severe abdominal pain is the hallmark symptom of pancreatitis.**

15. 1. **These laboratory data are used to diagnose and monitor pancreatitis because amylase and lipase are the enzymes produced by the pancreas.**

2. Pancreatitis is not an infection of the pancreas resulting from bacteria; such an infection would cause an elevation in the WBCs.

3. Bilirubin is used to monitor liver problems.

4. BUN monitors kidney function.

16. 1. A paracentesis is used to remove fluid from the abdominal cavity.

2. **The pancreas lies immediately below the diaphragm. When the cyst ruptures alkaline substances in the abdomen cause fluid leaks at the esophageal diaphragmatic opening into the thorax. The fluid must be removed to prevent lung collapse.**

3. Lumbar puncture is used to diagnose meningitis.

4. Biopsies are performed to confirm a diagnosis; they are not used for treatment.

17. 1. **Insulinoma is a tumor of the islet cells of the pancreas that produces insulin. The signs/symptoms of an insulinoma are signs of hypoglycemia.**

2. These are signs/symptoms of hyperglycemia.

3. These are signs/symptoms of hyperglycemia.

4. These are signs/symptoms of hyperthyroidism.

18. 1. A history of smoking cigarettes would be pertinent, but a history of chewing tobacco is not.

2. A diet high in fat, not low in fat, would be a risk factor.

3. Chronic alcoholism is not a risk factor, but chronic pancreatitis is a risk factor.

4. **Exposure to industrial chemicals or environmental toxins is a risk factor for pancreatic cancer.**

19. 1. The endocrine function of the pancreas is the secretion of insulin and amylin.

2. The adrenal cortex secretes mineralocorticoids, glucocorticoids, and gonadotrophins.

3. The adrenal medulla secretes the catecho-lamines epinephrine and norepinephrine.

4. The anterior pituitary gland secretes the growth hormone.

20. 1. Leg pain when walking would indicate intermittent claudication, which occurs with peripheral vascular disease.

2. Weight loss with normal appetite may indicate hyperthyroidism.

3. Changes in bowel movements may indicate colon cancer.

4. Joint pain would indicate a musculoskeletal or degenerative joint disease.

21. 1. The client will have to receive this medication the rest of his or her life so this should not be discussed with the client.

2. The dose will need to be increased, not decreased, in times of stress, infection, or dental work.

3. The medication should be taken with food to minimize its ulcerogenic effect.

4. If the client does not receive these medications consistently, death (from Addisonian crisis) can occur. The dose needs to be increased during times of physical and emotional stress. Because this medication masks infection and affects other medications, the client should wear a Medic Alert bracelet and carry a Medic Alert card to make sure all HCPs are aware of the client's condition and medications taken.

22. 1. If deep tendon reflexes are hypoactive or absent, the nurse should hold the magnesium and notify the health-care provider.

2. The arterial blood gases are not affected by the serum magnesium level.

3. The client's skin turgor will not be affected by the client's serum magnesium level.

4. The client's capillary refill time is not affected by the client's serum magnesium level.

23. 1. This is a tumor of the adrenal medulla.

2. Diabetes insipidus can be caused by brain tumors or infections, pituitary surgery, cerebrovascular accidents, or renal and organ failure, or it may be a complication of a closed head injury with increased intracranial pressure. Diabetes insipidus is a result of antidiuretic hormone (ADH) insufficiency.

3. Hashimoto's thyroiditis causes hypothyroidism.

4. Gynecomastia is abnormal enlargement of breast tissue in men.

24. 1. Excessive thirst is a symptom of diabetes insipidus, which is a deficiency of antidiuretic (ADH) hormone.

2. Orthopnea is difficulty breathing when in the supine position, which is not a sign/symptom of SIADH.

3. Ascites is excess fluid in the peritoneal cavity, which is not a sign/symptom of SIADH.

4. Excess antidiuretic hormone (ADH) causes SIADH, which causes increased water reabsorption and leads to increased fluid volume and scant, concentrated urine.

25. 1. The anterior thigh is an appropriate area, but it does not provide the best absorption.

2. The abdominal area allows for the most rapid absorption of insulin and is the recommended site.

3. The deltoid is an appropriate area, but it does not provide the most rapid absorption.

4. The gluteal buttocks area is primarily the best area for intramuscular injections.

26. In order of performance: 5, 4, 1, 2, 3

5. Regular insulin peaks in 2–4 hours; therefore the nurse should suspect a hypoglycemic reaction if the client has not eaten anything.

4. The nurse should obtain the client's blood glucose level as soon as possible; this can be done with a glucometer at the bedside.

1. Most hospitals require a confirmatory serum blood glucose level. Do not wait for results to give food.

2. The antidote for insulin is glucose; therefore the nurse should give the client some type of quick-acting food source.

3. A source of long-acting carbohydrate and protein should be given to prevent a reoccurrence of hypoglycemia.

*The possession of knowledge does not kill the sense of wonder and mystery. There is always more mystery.*—Anais Nin

# 9 Genitourinary Disorders

The genitourinary system includes the kidneys; ureters; bladder; urethra; and the associated organ, the prostate gland. The urinary system organs are subject to acute and chronic infections and functioning disorders/diseases and, for some organs, the formation of calculi (stones). These disorders can lead to fluid and electrolyte disorders that can have wide-ranging effects throughout the body. The prostate is also subject to disorders, a very common one being benign prostatic hypertrophy. (Cancer of the prostate is discussed in Chapter 10.) The nurse must know the normal laboratory values of the many tests used to assess the function of these organs and recognize what independent and collaborative interventions are necessary.

## KEYWORDS

anuria
azotemia
corrected output
creatinine
diffusion
hyperkalemia
intravesical
oliguria
osmolality
osmosis

## ABBREVIATIONS

Acute Renal Failure (ARF)
Benign Prostatic Hypertrophy (BPH)
Bicarbonate ($HCO_3$)
Blood Urea Nitrogen (BUN)
Computed Tomography (CT)
End-Stage Renal Disease (ESRD)
Gastrointestinal (GI)
Glomerular Filtration Rate (GFR)
Health-Care Provider (HCP)
Intensive Care Department (ICD)
Intravenous (IV)
Intravenous Push (IVP)
Intravenous Piggy Back (IVPB)
Licensed Practical Nurse (LPN)
Magnetic Resonance Imaging (MRI) scan
Nasogastric Tube (NGT)
Nothing By Mouth (NPO)
Nurse Practitioner (NP)
Nursing Assistant (NA)
Patient-Controlled Analgesia (PCA)
Prostate Specific Antigen (PSA)
Premature Ventricular Contraction (PVC)
Rule Out (R/O)
Transurethral Resection Of Prostate (TURP)
Unlicensed Assistive Personnel (UAP)
Urinary Tract Infection (UTI)
When Required, As Needed (PRN)
White Blood Cells (WBCs)

## Acute Renal Failure (ARF)

1. The nurse is admitting a client diagnosed with acute renal failure (ARF). Which question would be most important for the nurse to ask during the admission interview?
   1. "Have you recently traveled outside the United States?"
   2. "Did you recently begin a vigorous exercise program?"
   3. "Is there a chance you have been exposed to a virus?"
   4. "What over-the-counter medications do you take regularly?"

2. The client is diagnosed with ARF. Which laboratory values are most significant for diagnosing ARF?
   1. BUN and creatinine.
   2. WBC and hemoglobin.
   3. Potassium and sodium.
   4. Bilirubin and ammonia level.

3. The client is diagnosed with rule out ARF. Which condition would predispose the client to developing pre-renal failure?
   1. Diabetes mellitus.
   2. Hypotension.
   3. Aminoglycosides.
   4. Benign prostatic hypertrophy.

4. The client is diagnosed with ARF. Which signs/symptoms would indicate to the nurse that the client is in the recovery period? Select all that apply.
   1. Increased alertness and no seizure activity.
   2. Increase in hemoglobin and hematocrit.
   3. Denial of nausea and vomiting.
   4. Decreased urine-specific gravity.
   5. Increased serum creatinine level.

5. The client diagnosed with ARF has a serum potassium level of 6.8 mEq/L. Which collaborative treatment would the nurse anticipate for the client?
   1. Administer a phosphate binder.
   2. Type and cross-match for whole blood.
   3. Assess the client for leg cramps.
   4. Prepare the client for dialysis.

6. The nurse is developing a plan of care for a client diagnosed with ARF. Which statement would be an appropriate outcome for the client?
   1. Monitor intake and output every shift.
   2. Decrease of pain by 3 levels on a 1–10 scale.
   3. Electrolytes are within normal limits.
   4. Administer enemas to decrease hyperkalemia.

7. The client diagnosed with ARF is admitted to the intensive care department and placed on a therapeutic diet. Which diet would be most appropriate for the client?
   1. A high-potassium and low-calcium diet.
   2. A low-fat and low-cholesterol diet.
   3. A high-carbohydrate and restricted-protein diet.
   4. A regular diet with six (6) small feedings a day.

8. The client diagnosed with ARF is placed on bed rest. The client asks the nurse, "Why do I have to stay in bed, I don't feel that bad." Which scientific rationale would support the nurse's response?
   1. Bed rest helps increase the blood return to the renal circulation.
   2. Bed rest reduces the metabolic rate during the acute stage.
   3. Bed rest decreases the workload of the left side of the heart.
   4. Bed rest aids in reduction of peripheral and sacral edema.

9. The nurse and unlicensed nursing assistant are caring for clients on a medical floor. Which nursing task would be most appropriate for the nurse to delegate?
   1. Collect a clean voided midstream urine specimen.
   2. Evaluate the client's 8-hour intake and output.
   3. Assist in checking a unit of blood prior to hanging.
   4. Administer a cation-exchange resin enema.

10. The client is admitted to the emergency department after a gunshot wound to the abdomen. Which nursing intervention would the nurse implement first to prevent ARF?
    1. Administer normal saline IV.
    2. Take vital signs.
    3. Place client on telemetry.
    4. Assess abdominal dressing.

11. The unlicensed nursing assistant tells the nurse that the client with ARF has a white layer on top of the skin that looks like crystals. Which intervention should the nurse implement?
    1. Have the assistant apply a moisture barrier cream to the skin.
    2. Instruct the nursing assistant to bathe the client in cool water.
    3. Tell the nursing assistant not to turn the client in this condition.
    4. Explain that this is normal and do not do anything to the client.

12. The client diagnosed with ARF is experiencing hyperkalemia. Which medication should the nurse prepare to administer to help decrease the potassium level?
    1. Erythropoietin.
    2. Calcium gluconate.
    3. Regular insulin.
    4. Osmotic diuretic.

## Chronic Renal Failure

13. The client diagnosed with end-stage renal disease (ESRD) is experiencing metabolic acidosis. Which statement best describes the scientific rationale for metabolic acidosis in this client?
    1. There is an increased excretion of phosphates and organic acids, which leads to an increase in arterial blood pH.
    2. A shortened life span of red blood cells because of damage secondary to dialysis treatments. This, in turn, leads to metabolic acidosis.
    3. The kidney cannot excrete increased levels of acid because the kidneys cannot excrete ammonia or cannot reabsorb sodium bicarbonate.
    4. An increase in nausea and vomiting causes a loss of hydrochloric acid and the respiratory system cannot compensate adequately.

14. The nurse in the dialysis center is initiating the morning dialysis run. Which client should the nurse assess first?
    1. The client who has hemoglobin of 9.8 mg/dL and hematocrit of 30%.
    2. The client who does not have a palpable thrill or auscultated bruit.
    3. The client who is complaining of being exhausted and is sleeping.
    4. The client who did not take antihypertensive medication this morning.

15. The male client in ESRD has received the initial dose of erythropoietin, a biologic response modifier, 1 week ago. Which complaint by the client would indicate the need to notify the health-care provider?
    1. The client complains of flulike symptoms.
    2. The client complains of being tired all the time.
    3. The client reports an elevation in his blood pressure.
    4. The client reports discomfort in his legs and back.

16. The nurse is developing a nursing care plan for the client diagnosed with ESRD. Which nursing problem would have priority for the client?
    1. Low self-esteem.
    2. Knowledge deficit.
    3. Activity intolerance.
    4. Excess fluid volume.

17. The client with ESRD is placed on a fluid restriction of 1500 milliliters per day. On the 7 A.M. to 7 P.M. shift the client drank an eight (8)-ounce cup of coffee, 4 ounces of juice, 12 ounces of tea, and 2 ounces of water with medications. What amount of fluid can the 7 P.M. to 7 A.M. nurse give to the client? _____

18. The client diagnosed with ESRD has a new arteriovenous fistula in the left forearm. Which intervention should the nurse implement?
    1. Teach the client to carry heavy objects with the right arm.
    2. Perform all laboratory blood tests on the left arm.
    3. Instruct the client to lie on the left arm during the night.
    4. Discuss the importance of not performing any hand exercises.

19. The male client diagnosed with ESRD secondary to diabetes has been receiving dialysis for 12 years. The client is notified that he will not be placed on the kidney transplant list. The client tells the nurse he will not be back for any more dialysis treatments. Which response would be most therapeutic?
    1. "You cannot just quit your dialysis. This is not an option."
    2. "Are you angry at not being on the list, so you want to quit dialysis?"
    3. "I will call your nephrologist right now so you can talk to the HCP."
    4. "Make your funeral arrangements because you are going to die."

20. The nurse is discussing kidney transplants with clients at a dialysis center. Which population is less likely to participate in organ donation?
    1. Caucasian.
    2. African American.
    3. Asian.
    4. Hispanic.

21. The client receiving dialysis is complaining of being dizzy and light-headed. Which action should the nurse implement first?
    1. Place the client in the Trendelenburg position.
    2. Turn off the dialysis machine immediately.
    3. Bolus the client with 500 mL of normal saline.
    4. Notify the health-care provider as soon as possible.

22. The nurse caring for a client diagnosed with ESRD writes a client problem of "noncompliance of dietary restrictions." Which intervention should be included in the plan of care?
    1. Teach the client the proper diet to eat while undergoing dialysis.
    2. Refer the client and significant other to the dietician.
    3. Explain the importance of eating the proper foods.
    4. Determine the reason for the client not adhering to the diet.

23. The client diagnosed with ESRD is receiving peritoneal dialysis. Which assessment data warrant immediate intervention by the nurse?
    1. Inability to auscultate a bruit over the fistula.
    2. The client's abdomen is soft, is nontender, and has bowel sounds.
    3. The dialysate being removed from the client's abdomen is clear.
    4. The dialysate instilled into the client was 1500 mL and that removed was 1500 mL.

24. The client receiving hemodialysis is being discharged home from the dialysis center. Which instruction should the nurse teach the client?
    1. Notify the HCP if oral temperature is 102°F or greater.
    2. Apply ice to the access site if it starts bleeding at home.
    3. Keep fingernails short and try not to scratch the skin.
    4. Encourage significant other to make decisions for the client.

## Fluid and Electrolyte Disorders

25. The client is admitted to a nursing unit from a long-term care facility with a hematocrit of 56% and a serum sodium level of 152 mEq/L. Which condition would be a cause for these findings?
    1. Overhydration.
    2. Anemia.
    3. Dehydration.
    4. Renal failure.

26. The client who has undergone an exploratory laparotomy and subsequent removal of a large intestinal tumor has a nasogastric tube (NGT) in place and an IV running at 150 mL/hr via an IV pump. Which data should be reported to the HCP?
    1. The pump keeps sounding an alarm that the high pressure has been reached.
    2. Intake is 1800 mL, NGT output is 550 mL, and Foley output 950 mL.
    3. On auscultation, crackles and rales in all lung fields are noted.
    4. Client has negative pedal edema and an increasing level of consciousness.

27. The client diagnosed with diabetes insipidus weighed 180 pounds when the daily weight was taken yesterday. This morning's weight is 175.6 pounds. One liter of fluid weighs approximately 2.2 pounds. How much fluid has the client lost?_____

28. The nurse writes the nursing problem of "fluid volume excess" (FVE). Which intervention should be included in the plan of care?
    1. Change the IV fluid from 0.9% NS to D5W.
    2. Restrict the client's sodium in the diet.
    3. Monitor blood glucose levels.
    4. Prepare the client for hemodialysis.

29. The client is admitted with a serum sodium level of 110 mEq/L. Which nursing intervention should be implemented?
    1. Encourage fluids orally.
    2. Administer 10% saline solution IVPB.
    3. Administer antidiuretic hormone intranasally.
    4. Place on seizure precautions.

30. The telemetry monitor technician notifies the nurse of the morning telemetry readings. Which client should the nurse assess first?
    1. The client in normal sinus rhythm with a peaked T wave.
    2. The client diagnosed with atrial fibrillation with a rate of 100.
    3. The client diagnosed with a myocardial infarction who has occasional PVC.
    4. The client with a first-degree AV block and a rate of 92.

31. The client post-thyroidectomy complains of numbness and tingling around the mouth and the tips of the fingers. Which intervention should the implement first?
    1. Notify the health-care provider immediately.
    2. Tap the cheek about two (2) cm anterior to the ear lobe.
    3. Check the serum calcium and magnesium levels.
    4. Prepare to administer calcium gluconate IVP.

32. Which statement best explains the scientific rationale for Kussmaul's respirations in the client diagnosed with diabetic ketoacidosis (DKA)?
    1. The kidneys produce excess urine and the lungs try to compensate.
    2. The respirations increase the amount of carbon dioxide in the bloodstream.
    3. The lungs speed up to release carbon dioxide and increase the pH.
    4. The shallow and slow respirations will increase the $HCO_3$ in the serum.

33. The client is NPO and is receiving total parenteral nutrition (TPN) via a subclavian line. Which precautions should the nurse implement? Select all that apply.
    1. Place the solution on an IV pump at the prescribed rate.
    2. Monitor blood glucose every six (6) hours.
    3. Weigh the client weekly, first thing in the morning.
    4. Change the IV tubing every three (3) days.
    5. Monitor intake and output every shift.

34. The client has received IV solutions for three (3) days through a 20-gauge IV catheter placed in the left cephalic vein. On morning rounds the nurse notes the IV site is tender to palpation and a red streak has formed. Which action should the nurse implement first?
    1. Start a new IV in the right hand.
    2. Discontinue the intravenous line.
    3. Complete an incident record.
    4. Place a warm washrag over the site.

35. The nurse and an unlicensed nursing assistant are caring for a group of clients. Which nursing intervention should the nurse perform?
    1. Measure the client's output from the indwelling catheter.
    2. Record the client's intake and output on the I & O sheet.
    3. Instruct the client on appropriate fluid restrictions.
    4. Provide water for a client diagnosed with diabetes insipidus.

36. The client has been vomiting and has had numerous episodes of diarrhea. Which laboratory test should the nurse monitor?
    1. Serum calcium.
    2. Serum phosphorus.
    3. Serum potassium.
    4. Serum sodium.

## Urinary Tract Infection

37. The client from a long-term care facility is admitted with a fever, hot flushed skin, and clumps of white sediment in the indwelling catheter. Which intervention should the nurse implement first?
    1. Start an IV with a 20-gauge catheter.
    2. Initiate antibiotic therapy IVPB.
    3. Collect a urine specimen for culture.
    4. Change the indwelling catheter.

38. The nurse is inserting an indwelling catheter into a female client. Which interventions should be implemented? Select all that apply.
    1. Explain the procedure to the significant other.
    2. Set up the sterile field.
    3. Inflate the catheter bulb.
    4. Place absorbent pads under the client.
    5. Clean the perineum from clean to dirty with Betadine.

39. The nurse performs bladder irrigation through an indwelling catheter. The nurse instilled 90 mL of sterile normal saline. The catheter drained 710 mL. What is the client's output? _____

40. The nurse is examining a 15-year-old female who is complaining of pain, frequency, and urgency when urinating. After asking the parent to leave the room, which question should the nurse ask the client?
    1. "When was your last menstrual cycle?"
    2. "Have you noticed any change in the color of the urine?"
    3. "Are you sexually active?"
    4. "What have you taken for the pain?"

41. The client is reporting chills, fever, and left costovertebral pain. Which diagnostic test would the nurse expect the HCP to order first?
    1. A midstream urine for culture.
    2. A sonogram of the kidney.
    3. An intravenous pyelogram for renal calculi.
    4. A CT scan of the kidneys.

42. The client with chronic pyelonephritis is being admitted to a medical unit for intensive intravenous therapy. Which assessment data support the diagnosis of chronic pyelonephritis?
    1. The client has fever, chills, flank pain, and dysuria.
    2. The client complains of fatigue, headaches, and increased urination.
    3. The client had a group b beta hemolytic strep infection last week.
    4. The client has an acute viral pneumonia infection.

43. The female client in an outpatient clinic is being sent home with a diagnosis of urinary tract infection. Which instruction should the nurse teach to prevent a recurrence of a UTI?
    1. Clean the perineum from back to front after a bowel movement.
    2. Take warm tub baths instead of hot showers daily.
    3. Void immediately preceding sexual intercourse.
    4. Avoid coffee, tea, colas, and alcoholic beverages.

44. The pregnant client is admitted to a medical unit for the treatment of acute pyelonephritis. Which scientific rationale supports the client being hospitalized for this condition?
    1. The client must be treated aggressively to prevent maternal/fetal complications.
    2. The nurse can force the client to drink fluids and avoid nausea and vomiting.
    3. The client will be dehydrated and there won't be sufficient blood flow to the baby.
    4. Pregnant clients historically are afraid to take the antibiotics as ordered.

45. The nurse is discharging a client with a nosocomial urinary tract infection. Which information should the nurse include in the discharge teaching?
    1. Limit fluid intake so the urinary tract can heal.
    2. Collect a routine urine specimen for culture.
    3. Take all antibiotics as prescribed.
    4. Be sure to void every five (5) to six (6) hours.

46. The nurse is preparing a plan of care for the client diagnosed with acute glomerulonephritis. Which would be a long-term goal?
    1. The client will have a blood pressure within normal limits.
    2. The client will show no protein in the urine.
    3. The client will maintain renal function.
    4. The client will have clear lung sounds.

47. The elderly client is diagnosed with chronic glomerulonephritis. Which lab value indicates the condition has gotten worse?
    1. The BUN is 15 mg/dL.
    2. The creatinine level is 1.2 mg/dL.
    3. The glomerular filtration rate is 40 mL/minute.
    4. The 24-hour creatinine clearance is 100 mL/minute.

48. The client diagnosed with chronic pyelonephritis is given a prescription for Bactrim, trimethoprim sulfa, a sulfa antibiotic, twice a day for 90 days. Which statement is the scientific rationale for prescribing this medication?
    1. The antibiotic will treat the bladder spasms that accompany a urinary tract infection.
    2. If the urine cannot be made bacteria free, the Bactrim will suppress bacterial growth.
    3. In three (3) months the client should be rid of all bacteria in the urinary tract.
    4. The HCP is providing the client with enough medication to treat future infections.

## Benign Prostatic Hypertrophy

49. The nurse empted 2000 mL from the drainage bag of a continuous irrigation of a client who had a transurethral resection of the prostate (TURP). The amount of irrigation in the bag hanging was 3000 mL at the beginning of the shift. There was 1800 mL left in the bag eight (8) hours later. What is the correct urine output at the end of the eight (8) hours? _____

50. The nurse observes red urine and several large clots in the tubing of the normal saline continuous irrigation catheter for the client who is 1 day postoperative TURP. Which intervention should the nurse implement?
    1. Remove the indwelling catheter.
    2. Titrate the NS irrigation to run faster.
    3. Administer protamine sulfate IVP.
    4. Administer vitamin K slowly.

51. Which data would support the client's diagnosis of acute bacterial prostatitis?
    1. Terminal dribbling.
    2. Urinary frequency.
    3. Stress incontinence.
    4. Sudden fever and chills.

52. When preparing a teaching plan for the client with chronic prostatitis, which intervention should the nurse include?
    1. Sit in a warm sitz bath for 10 to 20 minutes several times daily.
    2. Sit in the chair with the feet elevated for two (2) hours daily.
    3. Drink at least 3000 mL of oral fluids, especially tea and coffee, daily.
    4. Stop broad-spectrum antibiotics as soon as the symptoms subside.

53. Which nursing diagnosis would be priority for the client who has undergone a TURP?
    1. Potential for sexual dysfunction.
    2. Potential for an altered body image.
    3. Potential for chronic infection.
    4. Potential for hemorrhage.

54. Which data would indicate that discharge teaching has been effective for the client who is postoperative TURP?
    1. "I will call the surgeon if I experience any difficulty urinating."
    2. "I will take my Proscar daily, the same as before my surgery."
    3. "I will continue restricting my oral fluid restriction."
    4. "I will need to take my pain medication routinely even if I do not hurt."

55. The client is one (1) day postoperative TURP. Which nursing task can be delegated to the unlicensed assistive personnel?
    1. Increase the irrigation fluid to clear clots from the tubing.
    2. Elevate the scrotum on a towel roll for support.
    3. Change the dressing on the first postoperative day.
    4. Teach the client how to care for the continuous irrigation catheter.

56. The client with a TURP who has a continuous irrigation catheter complains of the need to urinate. Which intervention should the nurse implement first?
    1. Call the surgeon to inform the HCP of the client's complaint.
    2. Give the client a narcotic medication for pain.
    3. Tell him that the sensation happens frequently.
    4. Assess the continuous irrigation catheter for patency.

57. The client who is postoperative TURP asks the nurse, "When will I know if I will be able to have sex after my TURP?" Which response would be most appropriate by the nurse?
    1. "You seem anxious about your surgery."
    2. "Tell me about your fears of impotency."
    3. "Potency can return in six (6) to eight (8) weeks."
    4. "Did you ask your doctor about your concern?"

58. The client asks, "What does an elevated PSA test mean?" On which scientific rationale would the nurse base the response?
    1. An elevated PSA can result from several different causes.
    2. An elevated PSA can be only from prostate cancer.
    3. An elevated PSA can be diagnostic for testicular cancer.
    4. An elevated PSA is the only test used to diagnose benign prostatic hypertrophy.

59. The client returned from surgery after having a TURP and has a P 110, R 24, B/P 90/40, and cool and clammy skin. Which interventions should the nurse implement? Select all that apply.
    1. Assess the red urine in the continuous irrigation drainage bag.
    2. Increase the irrigation fluid in the continuous irrigation catheter.
    3. Lower the head of the bed while raising the foot of the bed.
    4. Contact the surgeon to give an update in the client's condition.
    5. Monitor the client's postoperative hematocrit and hemoglobin.

60. Which expected outcome would indicate that the client's condition following a TURP is improving?
    1. The client is using the maximum amount allowed by the PCA pump.
    2. The client's bladder spasms are relieved by medication.
    3. The client's scrotum is swollen and tender with movement.
    4. The client has passed a large, hard, brown stool this morning.

## Renal Calculi

61. The laboratory data reveal a calcium phosphate renal stone for a client diagnosed with renal calculi. Which discharge teaching intervention should the nurse implement?
    1. Encourage the client to eat a low-purine diet and limit foods such as organ meats.
    2. Explain the importance of not drinking water two (2) hours before bedtime.
    3. Discuss the importance of limiting vitamin D–enriched foods.
    4. Prepare the client for extracorporeal shock wave lithotripsy (ESWL).

62. The client diagnosed with renal calculi is admitted to the medical unit. Which intervention should the nurse implement first?
    1. Monitor the client's urinary output.
    2. Assess the client's pain and rule out complications.
    3. Increase the client's oral fluid intake.
    4. Use a safety gait belt when walking the client.

63. The client with possible renal calculi is scheduled for a renal ultrasound. Which intervention should the nurse implement for this procedure?
    1. Ask if the client is allergic to shell fish or iodine.
    2. Keep the client NPO eight (8) hours prior to the ultrasound.
    3. Ensure the client has a signed informed consent form.
    4. Explain the test is noninvasive and there is no discomfort.

64. Which clinical manifestations would the nurse expect to assess for the client diagnosed with a ureteral renal stone?
    1. Dull, aching flank pain and microscopic hematuria.
    2. Nausea; vomiting; pallor; and cool, clammy skin.
    3. Gross hematuria and dull suprapubic pain with voiding.
    4. No symptoms.

65. The client diagnosed with renal calculi is scheduled for a 24-hour urine specimen collection. Which interventions should the nurse implement? Select all that apply.
    1. Check for the ordered diet and medication modifications.
    2. Instruct the client to urinate, and discard this urine when starting collection.
    3. Collect all urine during 24 hours and place in appropriate specimen container.
    4. Insert a Foley catheter in client after having the client empty the bladder.
    5. Post notices on the client's door to save all urine output.

66. The client is diagnosed with an acute episode of ureteral calculi. Which client problem is priority when caring for this client?
    1. Fluid volume loss.
    2. Knowledge deficit.
    3. Impaired urinary elimination.
    4. Pain.

67. The client diagnosed with renal calculi is scheduled for lithotripsy. Which postprocedure nursing task would be most appropriate to delegate to the unlicensed nursing assistant (NA)?
    1. Monitor the amount, color, and consistency of urine output.
    2. Teach the client about care of the indwelling Foley catheter.
    3. Assist the client to the car when being discharged home.
    4. Take the client's post-procedural vital signs.

68. Which statement indicates that the client diagnosed with calcium phosphate renal calculi understands the discharge teaching for ways to prevent future calculi formation?
    1. "I should increase my fluid intake, especially in warm weather."
    2. "I should eat foods that contain cocoa and chocolate."
    3. "I will walk about a mile every week and not exercise often."
    4. "I should take one vitamin a day that has extra calcium."

69. Which intervention is most important for the nurse to implement for the client diagnosed with rule out renal calculi?
    1. Assess the client's neurological status every 2 hours.
    2. Strain all urine and send any sediment to the laboratory.
    3. Monitor the client's creatinine and BUN levels.
    4. Take a 24-hour dietary recall during the client interview.

70. The client with a history of renal calculi calls the clinic and reports having burning on urination, chills, and an elevated temperature. Which instruction should the nurse discuss with the client?
    1. Increase water intake for the next 24 hours.
    2. Take two Tylenol to help decrease the temperature.
    3. Come to the clinic and give a urinalysis specimen.
    4. Use a sterile 4 × 4 gauze to strain the client's urine.

71. The client had surgery to remove a kidney stone. Which laboratory assessment data would warrant immediate intervention by the nurse?
    1. A serum potassium level of 3.8 mEq/L.
    2. A urinalysis that shows microscopic hematuria.
    3. A creatinine level of 0.8 mg/100 mL.
    4. A white blood cell count of 14,000 mm/dL.

72. The client is diagnosed with a uric acid stone. Which foods should the client eliminate from the diet to help prevent reoccurrence?
    1. Beer and colas.
    2. Asparagus and cabbage.
    3. Venison and sardines.
    4. Cheese and eggs.

## Cancer of the Bladder

73. The nurse is working on a renal surgery unit. After the afternoon report, which client should the nurse assess first?
    1. The male client who just returned from a CT scan and states that he left his glasses in the x-ray department.
    2. The client who is one (1) day post-op and has a moderate amount of serous drainage on the dressing.
    3. The client who is scheduled for surgery in the morning and wants an explanation of the operative procedure before signing the permit.
    4. The client who had ileal conduit surgery this morning and has not had any drainage in the drainage bag.

74. Which is a modifiable risk factor for the development of cancer of the bladder?
    1. Previous exposure to chemicals.
    2. Pelvic radiation therapy.
    3. Cigarette smoking.
    4. Parasitic infections of the bladder.

75. The client diagnosed with cancer of the bladder is scheduled to have a cutaneous urinary diversion procedure. Which preoperative teaching intervention specific to the procedure should be included?
    1. Demonstrate turn, cough, and deep breathing.
    2. Explain that a bag will drain the urine from now on.
    3. Instruct the client on the use of a PCA pump.
    4. Take the client to the ICD so that he or she can become familiar with it.

76. The client diagnosed with cancer of the bladder is undergoing intravesical chemotherapy. Which instruction should the nurse provide the client about the pre-therapy routine?
    1. Instruct the client to remain NPO after midnight before the procedure.
    2. Explain the use of chemotherapy in bladder cancer.
    3. Teach the client to administer Neupogen, a biologic response modifier.
    4. Have the client take Tylenol, an analgesic, before coming to the clinic.

77. The nurse is planning the care of a postoperative client with an ileal conduit. Which intervention should be included in the plan of care?
    1. Provide meticulous skin care and pouching.
    2. Apply sterile drainage bags daily.
    3. Monitor the pH of the urine weekly.
    4. Assess the stoma site every day.

78. The nurse and a licensed practical nurse (LPN) are caring for a group of clients. Which intervention should be assigned to the LPN?
    1. Assessment of the client who has had a Kock pouch procedure.
    2. Monitoring of the post-op client with a WBC of 22,000 mm/dL.
    3. Administration of the prescribed antineoplastic medications.
    4. Care for the client going for a MRI of the kidneys.

79. The male client diagnosed with metastatic cancer of the bladder is emaciated and refuses to eat. Which nursing action is an example of the ethical principle of paternalism?
    1. The nurse allows the client to talk about not wanting to eat.
    2. The nurse tells the client that if he does not eat, a feeding tube will be placed.
    3. The nurse consults the dietitian about the client's nutritional needs.
    4. The nurse asks the family to bring favorite foods for the client to eat.

80. The client diagnosed with cancer of the bladder states, "I have young children. I am too young to die." Which statement is the nurse's best response?
    1. "This cancer is treatable and you should not give up."
    2. "Cancer occurs at any age. It is just one of those things."
    3. "You are afraid of dying and what will happen to your children."
    4. "Have you talked to your children about your dying?"

81. The client with a continent urinary diversion is being discharged. Which discharge instructions should the nurse include in the teaching?
    1. Have the client demonstrate catheterizing the stoma.
    2. Instruct the client on how to pouch the stoma.
    3. Explain the use of a bedside drainage bag at night.
    4. Tell the client to call the HCP if the temperature is 99°F or less.

82. Which information regarding the care of a cutaneous ileal conduit should the nurse teach?
    1. Teach the client to instill a few drops of vinegar into the pouch.
    2. Tell the client that the stoma should be slightly dusky colored.
    3. Inform the client that large clumps of mucus are expected.
    4. Tell the client that it is normal for the urine to be pink or red in color.

83. The client is two (2) days post-ureterosigmoidostomy for cancer of the bladder. Which assessment data warrant notification of the HCP by the nurse?
    1. The client complains of pain at a "3," 30 minutes after being medicated.
    2. The client complains that it hurts to cough and deep breathe.
    3. The client ambulates to the end of the hall and back before lunch.
    4. The client is lying in a fetal position and has a rigid abdomen.

84. The female client diagnosed with bladder cancer with a cutaneous urinary diversion states, "Will I be able to have children now?" Which statement is the nurse's best response?
    1. "Cancer does not make you sterile, but sometimes the therapy can."
    2. "Are you concerned that you can't have children?"
    3. "You will be able to have as many children as you want."
    4. "Let me have the chaplain come to talk with you about this."

## Acute Renal Failure

1. 1. Usually there are no diseases or conditions that would warrant this question when discussing ARF.
   2. Vigorous exercise will not impede blood flow to the kidneys, leading to ARF.
   3. Usually viruses do not cause ARF.
   4. Medications such as nonsteroidal anti-inflammatory drugs (NSAIDs) and some herbal remedies are nephrotoxic; therefore, asking about medications is appropriate.

   **TEST-TAKING HINT: Asking about medications, especially over-the-counter and herbal remedies, during the admission interview is an important intervention because many of these are nephrotoxic and hepatotoxic.**

2. 1. Blood urea nitrogen (BUN) levels reflect the balance between the production and excretion of urea from the kidneys. Creatinine is a byproduct of the metabolism of the muscles and is excreted by the kidneys. Creatinine is the ideal substance for determining renal clearance because it is relatively constant in the body and is the laboratory value most significant in diagnosing renal failure.
   2. WBCs (white blood cells) are monitored for infection, and hemoglobin is monitored for blood loss.
   3. Potassium (intracellular) and sodium (interstitial) are electrolytes and are monitored for a variety of diseases or conditions not specific to renal function. Potassium levels will increase with renal failure, but the level is not a diagnostic indicator for renal failure.
   4. Bilirubin and ammonia levels are laboratory values that determine the functioning of the liver, not the kidneys.

   **TEST-TAKING HINT: The nurse must know specific laboratory tests for specific organ functioning or conditions. This is memorizing, but it must be done.**

3. 1. Diabetes mellitus is a disease that will lead to chronic renal failure.
   2. Hypotension, which causes a decreased blood supply to the kidney, is one of the most common causes of pre-renal failure (before the kidney).
   3. Nephrotoxic medications are a cause of intrarenal failure (directly to kidney).
   4. Benign prostatic hypertrophy (BPH) is a cause of post-renal failure (after the kidney).

   **TEST-TAKING HINT: The test taker must be cautious of adjectives, those words that describe**

something; "pre-renal" is the key to selecting the correct answer. The prefix means before.

4. 1. Renal failure affects almost every system in the body. Neurologically the client may have drowsiness, headache, muscle twitching, and seizures. In the recovery period, the client would be alert and not have seizures.
   2. In renal failure, levels of erythropoietin are decreased, leading to anemia. An increase in hemoglobin and hematocrit indicates the client is in the recovery period.
   3. Nausea, vomiting, and diarrhea are common in the client with ARF; therefore, an absence of these indicates the client is in the recovery period.
   4. The client in the recovery period would have increased urine-specific gravity.
   5. The client in the recovery period would have a decreased serum creatinine level.

   **TEST-TAKING HINT: This is an alternate-type question in which the test taker may choose as many correct answers as warranted. The test taker should not immediately assume that the option that says urine is the correct answer. The nurse must realize that renal failure affects every body system.**

5. 1. Phosphate binders are used to treat elevated phosphorus levels, not elevated potassium levels.
   2. Anemia is not the result of an elevated potassium level.
   3. Assessment is an independent nursing action, which would be appropriate for the elevated potassium level, but the question asks for a collaborative treatment.
   4. Normal potassium level is 3.5–5.5 mEq/L. A level of a 6.8 mEq/L is life threatening and could lead to cardiac dysrhythmias. Therefore, the client may be dialyzed to decrease the potassium level quickly. This would be done with an order from a health-care provider, so it is a collaborative intervention.

   **TEST-TAKING HINT: Adjectives must be noted when reading the stem of the intervention.**

6. 1. This is a nursing intervention, not a client outcome.
   2. This is a measurable client outcome, but acute renal failure does not cause pain.
   3. Renal failure causes an imbalance of electrolytes (potassium, sodium, calcium, phosphorus). Therefore the desired client outcome would be that all the electrolytes are within normal limits.

4. A Kayexalate resin enema may be administered to help decrease the potassium level, but this is an intervention, not a client outcome.

**TEST-TAKING HINT: The nurse must be knowledgeable of the nursing process. Client outcomes are used to evaluate the planning part of the nursing process. The outcomes must be measurable, client focused, and realistic.**

7. 1. The diet would be low potassium, and calcium is not restricted in ARF.
   2. This is a diet recommended for clients with cardiac disease and atherosclerosis.
   3. Carbohydrates are increased to provide for the client's caloric intake and protein is restricted to minimize protein breakdown and to prevent accumulation of toxic end products.
   4. The client must be on a therapeutic diet, and small feedings are not required.

**TEST-TAKING HINTS: The test taker must notice adjectives. A "therapeutic" diet should cause the test taker to eliminate option "4" because it is a regular diet.**

8. 1. Kidney function is improved about 40% when recumbent, but this is not the scientific rationale for bed rest in ARF.
   2. Bed rest reduces exertion and the metabolic rate, thereby reducing catabolism and subsequent release of potassium and accumulation of endogenous waste products (urea and creatinine).
   3. This is a scientific rationale for prescribing bed rest in clients with heart failure.
   4. This is not the scientific rationale for prescribing bed rest. The foot of the bed may be elevated to help decrease peripheral edema, and bed rest causes an increase in sacral edema.

**TEST-TAKING HINT: The test taker should not jump to conclusions and select the only option that has "renal" in the sentence. The nurse must know normal anatomy and physiology of the body and be aware that keeping someone in bed will not restore kidney function when the kidneys have failed.**

9. 1. The assistant can collect specimens. Collecting a midstream urine specimen requires the client to clean the perineal area, to urinate a little, and then collect the rest of the urine output in a sterile container.
   2. The assistant can obtain the client's intake and output, but the nurse must evaluate the data to determine if interventions are needed or if interventions are effective.
   3. Two registered nurses must check the unit of blood at the bedside prior to administering.

4. This is a medication enema and assistants cannot administer medications. Also, for this to be ordered, the client must be unstable with an excessively high serum potassium level.

**TEST-TAKING HINT: Nursing tasks that may not be delegated include any task that requires nursing judgment, medication administration, teaching, evaluating, or assessing.**

10. 1. Preventing and treating shock with blood and fluid replacement will prevent acute renal failure from hypoperfusion of the kidneys. Significant blood loss would be expected in the client with a gunshot wound.
    2. Taking and evaluating the client's vital signs is an appropriate action, but regardless of the results, this will not prevent ARF.
    3. Placing the client on telemetry is an appropriate action, but telemetry is an assessment tool for the nurse and will not prevent ARF.
    4. Assessment is often the first action, but assessing the abdominal dressing will not help prevent ARF.

**TEST-TAKING HINT: The test taker must read the stem carefully and understand what the question is asking. Options "2," "3," and "4" are all forms of assessment and would not help prevent ARF because they are not treatment.**

11. 1. Moisture barrier cream will keep the crystals on the skin.
    2. These crystals are uremic frost resulting from irritating toxins deposited in the client's tissues. Bathing in cool water will remove the crystals, promote client comfort, and decrease the itching that occurs from uremic frost.
    3. The client should be turned every two (2) hours or more frequently to prevent skin breakdown.
    4. This may occur with ARF, and it does require a nursing intervention.

**TEST-TAKING HINT: The nurse must know what is normal for specific disease processes, and something coming out of the skin would require some action even if the test taker was not familiar with the disease process. Option "4" could be eliminated based on this test-taking strategy. The test taker should also eliminate option "3" because there are very few instances in which the client is not turned or moved; turning and movement are necessary to prevent the development of pressure ulcers.**

12. 1. Erythropoietin is a chemical catalyst that is produced by the kidneys to stimulate red blood cell production; it does not affect potassium level.

2. Calcium gluconate helps protect the heart from the effects of high potassium levels.
3. Regular insulin, along with glucose, will drive potassium into the cells, thereby lowering serum potassium levels temporarily.
4. A loop diuretic, not an osmotic diuretic, may be ordered to help decrease the potassium level.

**TEST-TAKING HINT: The test taker must be familiar with medical terms such as hyperkalemia and know the rationale for administering medications.**

## Chronic Renal Failure

13. 1. There is a decrease in the excretion of phosphates and organic acids, not an increase.
    2. The red blood cell destruction does not affect the arterial blood gases pH.
    3. This is the correct scientific rationale for metabolic acidosis occurring in the client with ESRD.
    4. This is the compensatory mechanism that occurs to maintain an arterial blood pH between 7.35 and 7.45, but it does not occur as a result of ESRD.

    **TEST-TAKING HINT: In option "1" the test taker should note that it is "increased excretion"; ESRD would not have any type of increase in excretion so the test taker could eliminate the "1" option. Option "4" does not even mention the renal system and a loss of hydrochloric acid would result in a metabolic alkalosis, not acidosis, so the test taker can eliminate this option.**

14. 1. These laboratory findings are low but would not require a blood transfusion and often are expected in a client who is anemic secondary to ESRD.
    2. This client's dialysis access is compromised and should be assessed first.
    3. It is not uncommon for a client undergoing dialysis to be exhausted and sleep through the treatment.
    4. Clients are instructed not to take their antihypertensive medications before dialysis to help prevent episodes of hypotension.

    **TEST-TAKING HINT: The test taker must determine which client's situation is not normal or expected for the disease process, which in this question would be ESRD because all clients are in the dialysis unit.**

15. 1. Flulike symptoms are expected and tend to subside with repeated doses; the nurse would suggest Tylenol prior to the injections.

2. This medication takes up to two (2) to six (6) weeks to become effective in improving anemia and thereby reducing fatigue.
3. After the initial administration of erythropoietin, a client's antihypertensive medications may need to be adjusted. Therefore, this complaint requires notification of the HCP. Erythropoietin therapy is contraindicated in clients with hypertension that cannot be controlled.
4. Long bone and vertebral pain is an expected occurrence because the bone marrow is being stimulated to increase production of red blood cells.

**TEST-TAKING HINT: The test taker should select the option that is potentially life threatening or a complaint that would require the medication to be adjusted or discontinued. The nurse should notify the HCP if the medication is causing an adverse effect, not an expected side effect.**

16. 1. Low-self esteem, related to dependency, role changes, and changes in body image, is a pertinent client problem, but psychosocial problems are not priority over physiological problems.
    2. Teaching is always an important part of the care plan, but it is not priority over a physiological problem.
    3. Activity intolerance related to fatigue, anemia, and retention of waste products is a physiological problem, but it is not a life-threatening problem.
    4. Excess fluid volume is priority because of the stress placed on the heart and vessels, which could lead to heart failure, pulmonary edema, and death.

    **TEST-TAKING HINT: The test taker must read the stem of the question and understand what the question is asking. This is a priority question. This means that all the options are pertinent problems for ESRD, but only one is priority. Applying Maslow's Hierarchy of Needs is one way to determine priorities: physiological problems are always priority over psychosocial problems, and life-threatening conditions take priority.**

17. Answer: 720 mL. The nurse must add up how many milliliters of fluid the client drank on the 7 A.M. to 7 P.M. shift and then subtract that number from 1500 mL to determine how much fluid the client can receive on the 7 P.M. to 7 A.M. shift. One (1) ounce is equal to 30 mL. The client drank 26 ounces (8 + 4 + 12 + 2) of fluid, or 780 mL (26 × 30) of fluid. Therefore, the client can have 720 mL (1500 − 780) of fluid on the 7 P.M. to 7 A.M. shift.

**TEST-TAKING HINT: The nurse must be knowledgeable of basic conversion factors. Use the pull-down calculator on the computer exam to ensure accuracy in computations.**

18. 1. Carrying heavy objects in the left arm could cause the fistula to clot by putting undue stress on the site, so the client should carry objects in the right arm.
    2. The fistula should only be used for dialysis access, not for routine blood draws.
    3. The client should not lie on the left arm because this may cause clotting by putting pressure on the site.
    4. Hand exercises are recommended for new fistulas to help mature the fistula.

**TEST-TAKING HINT: The test taker must notice the adjectives, such as "left" and "right." Options "2" and "3" have the nurse doing something to the arm with the fistula.**

19. 1. The client does have the right to quit dialysis if he or she wants to.
    2. Reflecting the client's feelings and restating them are therapeutic responses that the nurse should use when addressing the client's issues.
    3. This is passing the buck; the nurse should address the client's issues.
    4. This may be true, but it is not therapeutic in attempting to get the client to verbalize feelings.

**TEST-TAKING HINTS: When asked to select a therapeutic response, the test taker should select an option that has some type of "feeling" in the response, such as "angry" in option "2."**

20. 1. Caucasians are composed of a multitude of cultures but for the most part organ donation is very likely, although individual preferences vary.
    2. The African American culture believes that the body must be kept intact after death, and organ donation is rare among African Americans. This is also why a client of African American descent will be on a transplant waiting list longer than people of other races. This is because of tissue-typing compatibility.
    3. Asians as a culture participate in organ donation.
    4. Hispanics as a culture participate in organ donation.

**TEST-TAKING HINT: The nurse must be aware of cultural differences in health care.**

21. 1. The nurse should place the client's chair with the head lower than the body, which will shunt blood to the brain; this is the Trendelenburg position.
    2. The blood in the dialysis machine must be infused back into the client before the machine is turned off.
    3. Normal saline infusion is a last resort because one of the purposes of dialysis is to remove excess fluid from the body.
    4. Hypotension is an expected occurrence in clients receiving dialysis; therefore the HCP does not need to be notified.

**TEST-TAKING HINT: The Trendelenburg position is often used as a distracter in questions and the nurse needs to know that it is only used in cases where blood needs to be shunted to the brain.**

22. 1. Teaching is an intervention for knowledge deficit, not noncompliance.
    2. Referring the client does not address the issue of noncompliance.
    3. Noncompliance is a client's choice, and explaining interventions will not necessarily make the client choose differently.
    4. Noncompliance is a choice the client has a right to make, but the nurse should determine the reason for the noncompliance and then take appropriate actions based on the client's rationale. For example, if the client has financial difficulties, the nurse may suggest how the client can afford the proper foods along with medications, or the nurse may be able to refer the client to a social worker.

**TEST-TAKING HINT: The test taker must always clarify and understand exactly what the question is asking the nurse to do. Answer options "1," "2," and "3" have the nurse doing the talking; only "4" is allowing the client to explain the lack of compliance.**

23. 1. Peritoneal dialysis is administered through a catheter inserted into the peritoneal cavity; a fistula is used for hemodialysis.
    2. Peritonitis, inflammation of the peritoneum, is a serious complication that would result in a hard, rigid abdomen. Therefore, a soft abdomen would not warrant immediate intervention.
    3. The dialysate return is normally colorless or straw-colored, but it should never be cloudy, which indicates an infection.
    4. Because the client is in ESRD, fluid must be removed from the body so the output

should be more than the amount instilled. These assessment data require intervention by the nurse.

**TEST-TAKING HINT: The words "warrants immediate intervention" should clue the test taker into selecting an option that is not normal or expected for the client.**

24. 1. The client should not wait until the temperature is 102°F to call the HCP; the client should call when the temperature is 100°F or greater.
    2. The client should apply direct pressure and notify the HCP if the access site starts to bleed, not apply ice to the site.
    3. Uremic frost, which results when the skin attempts to take over the function of the kidneys, causes itching, which can lead to scratching that results in a break in the skin.
    4. The nurse should encourage the client's independence, not foster dependence by encouraging the significant other to make the client's decision.

**TEST-TAKING HINT: The test taker must read the question carefully. A temperature of 102°F would never be acceptable in any client. Fostering dependence in any chronic illness is not encouraged by the nurse and so the test taker could eliminate option "4."**

## Fluid and Electrolyte Disorders

25. 1. Clients who are overhydrated or have fluid volume excess would experience dilutional values of sodium (135–145 mEq/L) and red blood cells (44% to 52%). The levels would be lower than normal, not higher.
    2. Anemia is a low red blood cell count for a variety of reasons.
    3. Dehydration results in concentrated serum that causes lab values to increase because the blood has normal constituents but not enough volume to dilute the values to within normal range or possibly lower.
    4. In renal failure, the kidneys cannot excrete, and this results in too much fluid in the body.

**TEST-TAKING HINT: The test taker must decide first if the values are high or low and then determine what is happening with body fluids in each process. Overhydration and renal failure result in the same fluid shift, so these two (2) options ("1" and "4") could be excluded.**

26. 1. The pump is alerting the nurse that there is resistance distal to the pump; this does not requiring notifying the HCP.

2. The client has an 1800 mL intake and total output of 1500 mL. The body has an insensible loss of approximately 400 mL per day through the skin, respirations, and other body functions. This would not warrant notifying the HCP.
3. Crackles and rales in all lung fields indicate that the body is not able to process the amounts of fluids being infused. This should be brought to the HCP's attention.
4. Negative pedal edema and an increasing level of consciousness indicate that the client is not experiencing a problem.

**TEST-TAKING HINT: The question requires the test taker to distinguish nursing problems from client problems. Option "1" is a nursing problem and options "2" and "4" are expected results, so the HCP does not need to be notified. Only one option—"3"—contains abnormal or life-threatening information.**

27. 2000 mL has been lost. First, determine how many pounds the client has lost:

$$180 - 175.6 = 4.4 \text{ pounds lost}$$

Then, based on the fact that 1 liter of fluid weighs 2.2 pounds, determine how many liters of fluid have been lost.

$$4.4 \div 2.2 = 2 \text{ liters lost}$$

Then, because the question asks for the answer in milliliters convert 2 liters into milliliters.

$$2 \times 1000 = 2000 \text{ mL}$$

**TEST-TAKING HINT: The test taker must be able to work basic math problems. This problem has several steps. Sometimes it is helpful to write out what is occurring at each step, such as 4.4 divided by 2.2 kg per pound. This can help the test taker realize if a step has been overlooked. Remember, on the RN-NCLEX use the pull-down calculator on the computer.**

28. 1. The nursing plan of care does not include changing the HCP's orders.
    2. Fluid volume excess refers to an isotonic expansion of the extracellular fluid by an abnormal expansion of water and sodium. Therefore sodium is restricted to allow the body to excrete the extra volume.
    3. High blood glucose levels result in viscous blood and cause the kidneys to try and fix the problem by excreting the glucose through increasing the urine output, which results in fluid volume deficits.
    4. If the FVE is the result of renal failure, then hemodialysis may be ordered, but this infor-

mation was not provided in the stem of the question.

**TEST-TAKING HINT:** Option "1" is not a nursing prerogative. The test taker should not read into the question.

29. 1. The client probably will be placed on fluid restriction. Fluids should not be encouraged for a client with a low sodium level (135–145 mEq/L).
    2. Hypertonic solutions of saline are 3% to 5%, not 10%, because of the extreme nature of hypertonic solutions. Hypertonic solutions of saline may be used but very cautiously because if the sodium levels are increased too rapidly, a massive fluid shift can occur in the body, resulting in neurological damage and heart failure.
    3. The antidiuretic hormone (vasopressin) would cause water retention in the body and increase the problem.
    4. Clients with sodium levels less than 120 mEq/L are at risk for seizures as a complication. The lower the sodium level, the greater the risk of a seizure.

**TEST-TAKING HINTS:** The test taker must memorize certain common lab values and understand how deviations in the electrolytes affect the body.

30. 1. A client with a peaked wave could be experiencing hyperkalemia. Changes in potassium levels can initiate cardiac dysrhythmias and instability.
    2. Fluctuations in rate are expected in clients diagnosed with atrial fibrillation, and a heart rate of 100 is at the edge of a normal rate.
    3. Most people experience an occasional premature ventricular contraction (PVC); this would not warrant the nurse assessing this client first.
    4. A first-degree block is not an immediate problem.

**TEST-TAKING HINT:** The test taker must know the normal data so that the abnormal will be apparent. Normal heart rate is 60–100. The nurse should assess the client who has an abnormal or life-threatening condition.

31. 1. The HCP may need to be notified, but the nurse should perform assessment first.
    2. These are signs and symptoms of hypocalcemia, and the nurse can confirm this by tapping the cheek to elicit the Chvostek's sign. If the muscles of the cheek begin to twitch, then the HCP should be notified immediately because hypocalcemia is a medical emergency.
    3. A positive Chvostek's sign can indicate a low calcium or magnesium level, but serum lab

levels may have been drawn hours previously or may not be available.
    4. If the client does have hypocalcemia, this may be ordered, but it is not implemented prior to assessment.

**TEST-TAKING HINT:** Assessment is the first step in the nursing process and is an appropriate option to select if the test taker has difficulty when trying to decide between two options.

32. 1. Kussmaul's respirations are the lung's attempt to maintain the narrow range of pH that is compatible with human life. The respiratory system reacts rapidly to changes in pH.
    2. Respiration is the act of moving oxygen and carbon dioxide. Kussmaul's respirations are rapid and deep and allow the client to exhale carbon dioxide.
    3. The lungs attempt to increase the blood pH level by blowing off the carbon dioxide (carbonic acid).
    4. $HCO_3$ (sodium bicarbonate) is an alkaline (base) substance that is a metabolic buffer system, not a respiratory system buffer. The excretion and retention of sodium bicarbonate is regulated by the kidneys; therefore, it is a metabolic buffer system. The excretion and retention of carbon dioxide ($CO_2$) are regulated by the lungs and therefore is a respiratory buffer system,

**TEST-TAKING HINT:** Homeostasis is a delicate balance between acids and bases. The test taker can discard option "1" by realizing that production of urine does not affect the respirations.

33. 1. TPN is a hypertonic solution that has enough calories, proteins, lipids, electrolytes, and trace elements to sustain life. It is administered via a pump to prevent too rapid infusion.
    2. TPN contains 50% dextrose solution; therefore, the client is monitored to ensure that the pancreas is adapting to the high glucose levels.
    3. The client is weighed daily, not weekly, to monitor for fluid overload.
    4. The IV tubing is changed with every bag because the high glucose level can cause bacterial growth.
    5. Intake and output are monitored to observe for fluid balance.

**TEST-TAKING HINT:** Options "3" and "5" refer to the same factor—namely, fluid level. The test taker should then determine if the time factors are appropriate. Weekly weighing is not appropriate so "3" can be eliminated.

34. 1. A new IV will be started in the right hand after the IV is discontinued.
    2. **The client has signs of phlebitis and the IV must be removed to prevent further complications.**
    3. Depending on the health-care facility, this may or may not be done, but client care comes before documentation.
    4. A warm washrag placed on an IV site sometimes provides comfort to the client. If this is done, it should be done for 20 minutes four (4) times a day.

    **TEST-TAKING HINT: The question is asking for a first action, which means all of the options may be actions the nurse would implement, but only one is priority. In general, priority actions are stop the problem, continue treatment, treat the problem, and then document.**

35. 1. An assistant can empty the catheter and measure the amount.
    2. The assistant can record intake and output on the I & O sheet.
    3. The nurse cannot delegate teaching.
    4. The client has a disease, but all the assistant is being asked to do is take water to the client.

    **TEST TAKNING HINT: This is an example of an "except" question. Frequently questions ask which tasks can be assigned to the assistant, but this question asks which action the nurse should implement. If the test taker does not read carefully, it is easy to jump to the first option for actions that the assistant can perform.**

36. 1. Serum calcium is decreased in conditions such as osteoporosis or post-thyroid surgery, but not in vomiting and diarrhea.
    2. Serum phosphorus levels are altered in acute and chronic renal failure or diabetic ketoacidosis, among other conditions, but not with acute fluid losses from the gastrointestinal tract.
    3. **Clients lose potassium from the GI tract or through the use of diuretic medications. Potassium imbalances can lead to cardiac arrhythmias.**
    4. The body is not at risk from losing sodium from these sources as it is with potassium.

    **TEST-TAKING HINT: The nurse must recognize basic fluids and electrolytes in the body and the implications of excess or loss. The body holds onto sodium and releases potassium.**

## Urinary Tract Infection (UTI)

37. 1. The first action is to get a viable urine culture so that the causative pathogen can be identi-

fied. An IV would be started, but this is not the first action.
    2. Initiating an IV antibiotic is priority, but obtaining a culture is done first to make sure that the HCP can treat the causative organism.
    3. This will be sent when the new catheter has been inserted.
    4. **Unless the nurse can determine that the catheter has been inserted within a few days, the nurse should replace the catheter and then get a specimen. This will provide the most accurate specimen for analysis.**

    **TEST-TAKING HINT: In a question that requires the test taker to choose a "first" action, the test taker usually can order the choices 1, 2, 3, 4. In this question, options "4," "3," "1," and "2" should be the order of interventions.**

38. 1. The procedure should be explained to the client, not to the significant other.
    2. **Inserting an indwelling catheter is a sterile procedure.**
    3. **The bulb of the catheter should be tested to make sure it will inflate and deflate prior to inserting the catheter into the client.**
    4. **Incontinence pads should be placed under the client before beginning the sterile part of the procedure.**
    5. **During the procedure the perineum is swiped with Betadine swabs from front to back and also down the middle, then side to side with new swabs (clean to dirty).**

    **TEST-TAKING HINT: This is an alternative-type question that requires the test taker to select more than one option as the correct answer. The test taker must be knowledgeable of skills performed by the nurse.**

39. **620 mL of urine.** The amount of sterile normal saline is subtracted from the total volume removed from the catheter.

    **TEST-TAKING HINT: This is a simple subtraction problem, but the test taker must understand that any fluid used to irrigate a body system must be subtracted from the total volume in the suction device or catheter bag to get accurate information of the client's fluid-balance status.**

40. 1. This could be asked with a parent in the room, and the nurse would receive a truthful answer.
    2. There is no reason that the client would not answer this question in the presence of the parent.
    3. These are symptoms of cystitis, a bladder infection that may be caused by sexual intercourse resulting from the introduction of bacteria into the urethra during the

physical act. A teenager may not want to divulge this information in front of the parent.

4. This information could be obtained in front of the parent.

**TEST-TAKING HINT: The test taker must analyze the client's age, 15, and determine which of the options might not be answered truthfully if the parents are present. In this question "asking the parent to leave the room" is the key to choosing the correct option.**

41. 1. Fever, chills, and costovertebral pain are symptoms of a urinary tract infection (acute pyelonephritis), which requires a urine culture first to confirm the diagnosis.
    2. A sonogram of the kidney might be ordered if the client has recurrent UTIs to determine if a physical obstruction is causing the recurrent infections but not as the first diagnostic procedure.
    3. An intravenous pyelogram (IVP) is rarely used to determine pyelonephritis because the results are negative 75% of the time in clients diagnosed with acute pyelonephritis.
    4. A CT scan might be ordered if other tests have not been conclusive.

**TEST-TAKING HINT: The question asks which test would be ordered first, and the test taker should determine what the symptoms might be indicating. Fever and chills indicate an infection. The anatomical position of the costovertebral angle (flank area between a rib and a vertebra) should alert the test taker to the kidney area of the body. A urine culture would most likely determine if a kidney infection is present.**

42. 1. Fever, chills, flank pain, and dysuria are symptoms of acute pyelonephritis, not chronic pyelonephritis.
    2. Fatigue, headache, and polyuria as well as loss of weight, anorexia, and excessive thirst are symptoms of chronic pyelonephritis.
    3. Group b beta hemolytic streptococcus infections cause acute glomerulonephritis.
    4. Acute viral pneumonia is a cause of acute glomerulonephritis.

**TEST-TAKING HINT: The key to this question is the adjective "chronic." The test taker must be aware that disease processes may change over time to produce different effects.**

43. 1. The perineum should be cleaned from front to back after a bowel movement to prevent fecal contamination of the urethral meatus.
    2. The temperature of the water does not matter,

but the client should take showers instead of baths to prevent bacteria in the bath water from entering the urethra.

3. Voiding immediately after, not before, sexual intercourse uses the action of the urine passing through the urethra to the outside of the body to flush bacteria from the urethra that might have been introduced during intercourse.

4. Coffee, tea, cola, and alcoholic beverages are urinary tract irritants.

**TEST-TAKING HINT: The test taker might jump to option "3" as the correct answer if the test taker did not read the word "preceding."**

44. 1. A pregnant client diagnosed with a UTI will be admitted for aggressive IV antibiotic therapy. After symptoms subside the client will be sent home to complete the course of treatment with oral medications. The mother and child need aggressive treatment to prevent systemic bacteremia.
    2. The nurse cannot "force" a client to drink, and forcing fluids could result in nausea and vomiting, not prevent it.
    3. The client may or may not be dehydrated.
    4. Pregnant clients have a right to be concerned about taking medications, but most are comfortable taking medications prescribed by the obstetrician.

**TEST-TAKING HINT: In option "2" the nurse is "forcing" a client to do something, which should be eliminated as a possible correct answer. Option "4" is a broad generalization about "all" pregnant clients and should be discarded as a possible correct answer.**

45. 1. The function of the urinary tract is to process fluids and wastes from the body. Limiting its functioning will increase the problem, not help the problem.
    2. A routine urine specimen is not a clean voided specimen and cannot be used for culture.
    3. The client should be taught to take all the prescribed medication any time a prescription is written for antibiotics.
    4. The client should be taught to void every two (2) to three (3) hours and to empty the bladder completely. This prevents overdistention of the bladder wall and resulting compromised blood supply, either of which predisposes the client to developing a UTI.

**TEST-TAKING HINT: Unless contraindicated by a disease process it is recommended for all clients to drink six (6) to eight (8) glasses of water each day; therefore, option "1" should be eliminated as a possible correct answer.**

Option "2" has the adjective "routine" urine specimen, and a clean voided specimen or catheterized specimen is needed for a culture.

46. 1. Blood pressure within normal limits would be a short-term goal.
    2. Lack of protein in the urine would be a short-term goal.
    3. A long-term complication of glomerulonephritis is that it can become chronic if unresponsive to treatment and this can lead to end-stage renal disease. Maintaining renal function would be an appropriate long-term goal.
    4. Clear lung sounds would indicate that the client has been able to process fluids and excrete them from the body. Preventing pulmonary edema would be a short-term goal.

    **TEST-TAKING HINT:** Answer options "1," "2," and "4" all refer to body processes that should be controlled or treated immediately on assessment of the problem. The stem is requesting a long-term goal.

47. 1. Normal blood urea nitrogen levels are 7–18 mg/dL or 8–20 mg/dL for clients older than age 60 years.
    2. Normal creatinine levels are 0.6–1.2 mg/dL.
    3. Glomerular filtration rate (GFR) is approximately 120 mL per minute. If the GFR is decreased to 40 mL per minute, the kidneys are functioning at about one-third filtration capacity.
    4. Normal creatinine clearance is 85–125 mL per minute for males and 75–115 mL per minute for females.

    **TEST-TAKING HINT:** The nurse must memorize common lab values. BUN and creatinine levels are common lab values used to determine status in a number of diseases. Options "1" and "2" are normal values and could be eliminated. Then, the test taker would have to choose from only two (2) options.

48. 1. Antibiotics may indirectly treat bladder spasms if the spasms are caused by an infection, but this is not the reason for prescribing the antibiotic in this manner.
    2. Some clients develop a chronic infection and must receive antibiotic therapy as a routine daily medication to suppress the bacterial growth. The prescription will be refilled after the 90 days and continued.
    3. Clients who develop chronic infections may never be free of the bacteria.
    4. HCPs do not usually give PRN prescriptions for antibiotics.

**TEST-TAKING HINT:** The question is asking why an HCP would prescribe long-term use of antibiotics for a client with a chronic infection. Antibiotics treat bacterial infections. Based on this, option "1" can be eliminated. Option "3" promises that "all" infection will be gone and can be eliminated. Option "4" describes future infections, but the client currently has an infection, so this option can be eliminated.

## Benign Prostatic Hypertrophy

49. 800 mL. First, determine the amount of irrigation fluid:

    3000 − 1800 = 1200 mL of irrigation fluid

    Then, subtract 1200 of irrigation fluid from the drainage of 2000 to determine the urine output:

    2000 − 1200 = 800 mL of urine output

    **TEST-TAKING HINT:** Be sure that you use the pull-down calculator for the NCLEX examination.

50. 1. The indwelling catheter should not be removed because doing so may result in edema, which, in turn, may obstruct the urethra and not allow the client to urinate.
    2. Increasing the irrigation fluid will flush out the clots and blood.
    3. Protamine is the reversal agent for heparin, an anticoagulant.
    4. Vitamin K is the reversal agent for the anticoagulant warfarin (Coumadin).

    **TEST-TAKING HINT:** The test taker should eliminate the options "3" and "4" because both are medications and the problem is with continuous irrigation, which would not require medications.

51. 1. Terminal dribbling is a symptom of BPH.
    2. Urinary frequency is a sign of a UTI.
    3. Stress incontinence occurs in women who urinate when coughing, running, or jumping.
    4. Clients with acute bacterial prostatitis will frequently experience a sudden onset of fever and chills. Clients with chronic prostatitis have milder symptoms.

    **TEST-TAKING HINTS:** The words "acute" and "bacterial" should cue the test taker into the specific symptoms of infection. Symptoms for any infection would be fever and chills.

52. 1. The client should sit in a warm sitz bath for 10–20 minutes several times each day to provide comfort and assist with healing.

2. Clients should avoid sitting for extended periods because it increases the pressure.
3. Oral fluids should be consumed to satisfy thirst but not to push fluids to dilute the medication levels in the bladder.
4. Broad-spectrum antibiotics are administered for 10–14 days and should be not stopped until all medications are taken by the client.

**TEST-TAKING HINT: The test taker must know basic concepts when answering questions; this includes the need to take all prescribed antibiotics. If the test taker is unsure of option "3," the portion that states to drink plenty of tea and coffee should indicate that this is an incorrect answer because these are high in caffeine.**

53. 1. TURPs can cause a sexual dysfunction, but if there were a sexual dysfunction, it would not be priority over a physiological problem such as hemorrhaging.
2. This is not a life-threatening problem.
3. This client has had this problem preoperative.
4. This is a potential life-threatening problem.

**TEST-TAKING HINT: A basic concept the test taker must know is that for most surgeries the highest priority problem is hemorrhaging. Hemorrhaging is life threatening.**

54. 1. This indicates that teaching is effective.
2. Clients do not need to take Proscar postoperatively.
3. There is no reason to restrict the client's fluid intake.
4. Pain medication should be taken as needed.

**TEST-TAKING HINT: If the test taker is not sure of the correct answer, selecting an option that addresses notifying a health-care provider is usually a good choice.**

55. 1. This intervention requires analysis and should not be delegated.
2. Elevating the scrotum on a towel for support is an intervention that can be delegated to the UAP.
3. The surgeon changes the first dressing; therefore, this cannot be delegated. A TURP does not have a dressing.
4. The nurse is responsible for teaching.

**TEST-TAKING HINT: Teaching, assessing, evaluating, and intervening for clients who are unstable cannot be delegated to an unlicensed nursing assistant.**

56. 1. The nurse should not call a surgeon until all assessment is completed.
2. A pain medication should not be administered until the cause of the problem is determined and all complications are ruled out.

3. Telling a client that what he is experiencing is expected without assessing the situation is dangerous.
4. The nurse should always assess any complaint before dismissing it as a commonly occurring problem.

**TEST-TAKING HINT: When the question requires the test taker to decide which intervention should be first, assessment is usually first. If the test taker has no idea which intervention is correct, choose assessment.**

57. 1. The client wants information and the nurse should provide facts.
2. The client wants information and the nurse should provide facts.
3. This is usually the length of time clients need to wait prior to having sexual intercourse; this is the information that the client wants to know.
4. The client may need to talk with his surgeon, but it should be after the nurse answers the client's question.

**TEST-TAKING HINT: The client is asking for factual information and the nurse should provide this information. Options "1" and "2" are therapeutic responses addressing feelings and "4" is passing the buck—the nurse can discuss this with the client.**

58. 1. An elevated PSA can be from urinary retention, BPH, prostate cancer, or prostate infarct.
2. An elevated PSA does not indicate only prostate cancer.
3. PSA does not diagnose testicular cancer.
4. An elevated PSA and digital examination are used in combination to diagnosis BPH or prostate cancer.

**TEST-TAKING HINT: Answer options "2" and "4" have the word "only," which is an absolute word that may cause the test taker to eliminate them as possible answers. Terms that are absolute such as "always," "never," and "only" are usually incorrect answers.**

59. 1. The nurse should assess the drain postoperative.
2. The nurse should increase the irrigation fluid to clear the red urine.
3. The head of the bed should be lowered and the foot should be elevated to protect the brain.
4. The surgeon needs to be notified of the change in condition.
5. These laboratory values should be assessed for bleeding.

**TEST-TAKING HINT:** When the test taker reads vital signs with the blood pressure decreased and the pulse and respiratory rate elevated, the test taker should recognize the signs and symptoms of shock.

60. 1. Using the maximum amount of medication does not indicate that the client is achieving pain management.
    2. Bladder spasms are common, but being relieved with medication indicates the condition is improving.
    3. Scrotal swelling and tenderness do not indicate improvement.
    4. Clients are given laxatives or stool softeners to prevent constipation, which could cause increased pressure.

**TEST-TAKING HINT:** The stem asks which option indicates the client is improving. Needing maximum medication "1" and scrotal swelling "3" would not indicate getting better. A bowel movement has nothing to do the prostate.

## Renal Calculi

61. 1. This would be appropriate for the client who has uric acid stones.
    2. The nurse should recommend drinking one to two glasses of water at night to prevent concentration of urine during sleep.
    3. Dietary changes for preventing renal stones include reducing the intake of the primary substance forming the calculi. In this case, limiting vitamin D will inhibit the absorption of calcium from the gastrointestinal tract.
    4. This is a treatment for an existing renal stone, not a discharge teaching intervention for a client who has successfully passed a renal calculus.

**TEST-TAKING HINT:** Remember to read the question carefully. The question asks for a "discharge teaching" intervention. This would rule out "4," which is a treatment, as a potential answer.

62. 1. The client's urinary output should be monitored, but it is not the first nursing intervention.
    2. Assessment is the first part of the nursing process and is always priority. The intensity of the renal colic pain can be so intense it can cause a vasovagal response, with resulting hypotension and syncope.
    3. Increased fluid increases urinary output, which will facilitate movement of the renal stone

through the ureter and help decrease pain, but it is not the first intervention.
    4. Ambulation will help facilitate movement of the renal stone through the ureter and safety is important, but it is not the first intervention.

**TEST-TAKING HINT:** Remember if the question asks which intervention is first, all 4 (four) options may be appropriate for the client's diagnosis but only one has priority. Assessment is the first part of the nursing process and it is the first intervention a nurse should implement.

63. 1. An ultrasound does not require administration of contrast dye.
    2. Food, fluids, and ordered medication are not restricted prior to this test.
    3. This is not an invasive procedure so a signed consent is not required.
    4. No special preparation is needed for this noninvasive, nonpainful test. A conductive gel is applied to the back or flank and then a transducer is applied that produces sound waves that produce a picture.

**TEST-TAKING HINT:** The nurse must be aware of pre-procedure and post-procedure teaching and care. The test taker must know the invasive and noninvasive diagnostic tests in general. Ultrasound, computed tomography (CT), and magnetic resonance imaging (MRI) are a few of the noninvasive diagnostic tests.

64. 1. Dull flank pain and microscopic hematuria are manifestations of a renal stone in the kidney.
    2. The severe flank pain associated with a stone in the ureter often causes a sympathetic response with associated nausea; vomiting; pallor; and cool, clammy skin.
    3. Gross hematuria and suprapubic pain when voiding are manifestations of a stone in the bladder.
    4. Kidney stones and bladder stones may produce no signs/symptoms, but a ureteral stone always causes pain on the affected side because a ureteral spasm occurs when the stone obstructs the ureter.

**TEST-TAKING HINT:** Note that options "1" and "3" both have assessment data that indicate bleeding. The test taker can usually eliminate these as possible answers or eliminate the other two options that do not address blood. Renal stones are painful; therefore "4" could be eliminated as a possible answer.

65. 1. The health-care provider may order certain foods and medications when obtaining 24-hour urine collection to evaluate for calcium oxalate or uric acid.

2. When the collection begins, the client should completely empty the bladder and discard that urine.

3. All urine for 24 hours should be saved and put in a container with preservative, refrigerated, or put on ice as indicated. Not following specific instructions will result in an inaccurate test result.

4. The urine is obtained in some type of urine collection device such as a bedpan, bedside commode, or commode hat. The client is not catheterized.

5. Posting signs will help ensure that all the urine is saved during the 24-hour period. If any urine is discarded, the test may result in inaccurate information or the need to start the test over.

**TEST-TAKING HINT:** This is an alternate-type question that may have more than one correct answer. The test taker must be knowledgeable of specific laboratory tests.

66. 1. The client's fluid volume is increased and there is usually not a fluid volume loss.

2. Knowledge deficit is important to help prevent future renal calculi, but this is not priority when the client is in pain, which will occur with an acute episode.

3. Impaired urinary elimination may occur, but it is not priority for the client with an acute episode of calculi.

4. Pain is priority. The pain can be so severe that a sympathetic response may occur, causing nausea; vomiting; pallor; and cool, clammy skin.

**TEST-TAKING HINT:** Remember Maslow's Hierarchy of Needs: airway and pain are priority. No option mentions possible airway problems, so pain is priority.

67. 1. The urine must be assessed for bleeding and cloudiness. Initially the urine is bright red, but the color soon diminishes and cloudiness may indicate an infection. This assessment should not be delegated to an NA.

2. Teaching cannot be delegated to an NA. The nurse should teach and evaluate the effectiveness of the teaching.

3. The NA could assist the client to the car once the discharge has been completed.

4. The kidney is highly vascular. Hemorrhaging and resulting shock are potential complications of lithotripsy, so the nurse should not delegate vital signs post-procedure.

**TEST-TAKING HINT:** There are some basic rules about delegation; the nurse should never delegate assessment, teaching, or any task that requires judgment.

68. 1. An increased fluid intake that ensures 2–3 L of urine a day prevents the stone-forming salts from becoming concentrated enough to precipitate.

2. Cocoa and chocolate are high in calcium and should be avoided or the amount should be decreased to help prevent formation of calcium phosphate renal stones.

3. Physical activity prevents bone absorption and possible hypercalciuria; therefore, the nurse should instruct the client to walk daily to help retain calcium in bone.

4. The renal calculi are caused by calcium; therefore, the client should not increase calcium intake.

**TEST-TAKING HINT:** This is a urinary problem and fluid is priority. Therefore the test taker should select an option that addresses fluid, and there is only one option that addresses oral intake.

69. 1. Assessment is important but the neurological system is not priority for a client with a urinary problem.

2. Passing a renal stone may negate the need for the client to have lithotripsy or a surgical procedure. Therefore, all urine must be strained, and a stone, if found, should be sent to the laboratory to determine what caused the stone.

3. These are laboratory studies that evaluate kidney function, but they are not pertinent when passing a renal stone. These values do not elevate until at least half the kidney function is lost.

4. A dietary recall can be done to determine what types of foods the client is eating that may contribute to the stone formation, but it is not the most important intervention.

**TEST-TAKING HINT:** Remember if the question asks for "most important," more than one of the options could be appropriate but only one is most important. Assessment is always priority, but make sure it is appropriate for the situation.

70. 1. The client needs to be evaluated for a possible urinary tract infection, which may accompany renal calculi. Therefore, the clinic nurse should not give advice without knowing what is wrong with the client.

2. The nurse should not prescribe medication (even Tylenol) unless the nurse is absolutely sure what is wrong with the client.

3. A urinalysis can assess for hematuria (red blood cells in the urine), the presence of white blood cells, crystal fragments, or all three, which can determine if the client has a urinary tract infection or possibly a renal stone, with accompanying signs/symptoms of UTI.

4. The client would need to strain the urine if there is a possibility of renal calculi, which these signs/symptoms do not support. Further diagnostic testing is needed to determine the presence of renal calculi.

**TEST-TAKING HINT: Fever, chills, and burning on urination require some type of assessment. Therefore the test taker should select an option that helps determine what is wrong with the client and "3" is the only option.**

71. 1. This potassium level is within normal limits, 3.5 to 5.5 mEq/L.
    2. Hematuria is not uncommon after removal of a kidney stone.
    3. A normal creatinine level is 0.8 to 1.2 mg/100 mL.
    4. This white blood cell count is elevated; normal is 5,000–10,000 mm.

**TEST-TAKING HINT: The nurse must know normal laboratory data and be able to apply the normal and abnormal results to specific diseases and disorders.**

72. 1. Beer and colas are foods high in oxalate, which can cause calcium oxalate stones.
    2. Asparagus and cabbage are foods high in oxalate, which can cause calcium oxalate stones.
    3. Venison, sardines, goose, organ meats, and herrings are high purine foods, which should be eliminated from the diet to help prevent uric acid stones.
    4. Cheese and eggs are foods that help acidify the urine and do not cause the development of uric acid stones.

**TEST-TAKING HINT: The nurse has to be knowledgeable of foods included in specific diets. This is memorizing, but the reader must have this knowledge to answer questions evaluating types of diets for specific diseases and disorders.**

## Cancer of Bladder

73. 1. This client does not need to be assessed first. The NA or ward secretary can call the department and check on the glasses.
    2. A moderate amount of serous drainage is expected after a surgery. Serous is pale-yellow

body fluid. Sanguineous is the term used to describe bloody drainage.

3. The nurse is not responsible for informing the client about operative procedures. The surgeon should be notified to see this client and provide the explanation.

4. An ileal conduit is a procedure that diverts urine from the bladder and provides an alternate cutaneous pathway for urine to exit the body. Urinary output should always be at least 30 mL per hour. This client should be assessed to make sure that the stents placed in the ureters have not become dislodged or to ensure that edema of the ureters is not occurring.

**TEST-TAKING HINT: Basic care of any post-op client is to ensure urinary output. Two of the options involve tasks that can be delegated or are not in the realm of the nurse.**

74. 1. The client has already been exposed; this cannot be undone.
    2. Pelvic radiation is prescribed for cancer in the abdomen. It is a life-saving procedure, but one of the risks of radiation therapy is the development of a secondary cancer.
    3. Cigarette smoke contains more than 400 chemicals, 17 of which are known to cause cancer. The risk is directly proportional to the amount of smoking.
    4. Clients may be unaware of a parasitic infection of the bladder for some time prior to diagnosis, but it is not a risk factor for cancer of the bladder.

**TEST-TAKING HINT: The question asks for a modifiable risk factor. Modifiable factors involve lifestyle changes, weight loss, tobacco use, and eating habits.**

75. 1. Any client undergoing general anesthesia should be taught to turn, cough, and deep breathe to prevent pulmonary complications. This is not specific to a urinary diversion procedure.
    2. A urinary diversion procedure involves the removal of the bladder. In a cutaneous procedure the ureters are implanted in some way to allow for stoma formation on the abdominal wall, and the urine then drains into a pouch. There are numerous methods used for creating the stoma.
    3. Many clients with multiple types of procedures use PCA pumps to control pain after surgery.
    4. This should be done for any client who is expected to need intensive care postoperatively.

**TEST-TAKING HINT: The test taker must notice the phrase "specific to the surgery" to be able to correctly answer this question. All of the options are standard procedures for major surgeries but only one is specific to the procedure.**

76. 1. The client will have medication instilled in the bladder that must remain in the bladder for a prescribed length of time. For this reason, the client must remain NPO before the procedure.
    2. This is important to do when informing the client about chemotherapy so the client can give informed consent, but this is done when the client gives consent to receiving intravesical chemotherapy, not as part of the pre-therapy routine.
    3. The advantage of administering chemotherapy intravesically is that systemic side effects of bone marrow suppression are avoided. Neupogen is used to stimulate the production of white blood cells so a client is not at risk for developing an infection.
    4. The procedure is not painful so an analgesic is not needed.

**TEST-TAKING HINT: If the test taker is not aware of the term intravesical, then dividing the word into its components may be useful. "Intra" means "into" and "vesical" means "bladder." The test taker should choose an option that would have a direct effect on urine production.**

77. 1. Urine is acidic and the abdominal wall tissue is not designed to tolerate acidic environments. The stoma is pouched so that urine will not touch the skin.
    2. Urinary diversion drainage bags are changed every four (4) to five (5) days so that the skin can remain intact; the bags should be clean but not sterile.
    3. The urine will have the normal pH of all urine; it is not necessary to monitor the pH.
    4. The stoma should be assessed a minimum of every two (2) hours initially, then every four (4) hours.

**TEST-TAKING HINT: The test taker should look at time frames—daily and weekly. If the time frame is not sufficient, then the option can be eliminated as a possible correct answer.**

78. 1. Assessment cannot be assigned to an LPN, no matter how knowledgeable the LPN.
    2. This client has the laboratory symptoms of an infection; therefore, the nurse should assess and care for this client.

3. Antineoplastic medication is administered only by a qualified registered nurse.
4. It is in the scope of practice for the LPN to care for this client.

**TEST-TAKING HINT: The client who is the least ill or the client having the least invasive procedure is the one that should be assigned to the LPN.**

79. 1. This is therapeutic communication and is allowing the client autonomy, but it is not an example of paternalism.
    2. Paternalism is deciding for the client what is best, such as a parent making decisions for a child. Feeding a client, as with a feeding tube, without the client wishing to eat is paternalism.
    3. Consulting with a dietitian about the nutritional needs of a client is an appropriate nursing intervention, but it does not represent any ethical principle.
    4. This is an excellent intervention, but it does not represent any ethical principle.

**TEST-TAKING HINT: The question asks for an ethical principle, and only two of the options could be considered ethical principles. Option "1" is allowing the client a voice in the situation; the term "paternal" would eliminate this option.**

80. 1. This is advising the client, a nontherapeutic technique.
    2. This statement does not address the client's feelings.
    3. This is an example of restating, a therapeutic technique used to clarify the client's feelings and encourage a discussion of those feelings.
    4. The stem did not say the client was dying. The stem said the client thinks that the client is too young to die. A conversation to discuss the client's death with the children may be premature.

**TEST-TAKING HINT: When the question requires a therapeutic response the test taker should be careful not to choose any answer that does not acknowledge the client's feelings. Any option that contains a nontherapeutic technique could be eliminated.**

81. 1. A continent urinary diversion is a surgical procedure in which a reservoir is created that will hold urine until the client can self-catheterize the stoma. The nurse should observe the client's technique before discharge.

2. The purpose of creating a continent diversion is so the client will not need a pouch.

3. Clients with cutaneous diversions that drain constantly use bedside drainage bags at night, not those with continent diversions.

4. The client should be taught to notify the HCP if the temperature is 100°F or greater.

**TEST-TAKING HINT: Options "1" and "2" are related to continuous drainage and could be eliminated on this basis. The word "continent" in the stem should key the test taker in to the fact that this diversion is a procedure in which there is no continuous drainage of urine.**

82. 1. Vinegar will act as a deodorizing agent in the pouch and help prevent a strong urine smell.

2. The stoma should be pink and moist at all times. A dusky color indicates a compromised blood supply to the stoma and the HCP should be notified immediately.

3. There will be mucus in the urine because of the tissue used to create the diversion, but large clumps of mucus could occlude the stoma or ureters.

4. Urinary drainage should be a pale yellow to amber color. The procedure does not change the color of the urine.

**TEST-TAKING HINT: A dusky color is never normal when discussing body functioning. There are very few procedures for which bloody urine is a normal expectation.**

83. 1. A complaint of a three (3) on a one (1) to ten (10) pain scale is expected after medication and does not warrant notifying the HCP.

2. Pain on coughing and deep breathing after surgery is expected.

3. This indicates that the client is able to ambulate and is doing the things needed to recover.

4. The client is drawn up in a position that takes pressure off the abdomen; a rigid abdomen is an indicator of peritonitis, a medical emergency.

**TEST-TAKING HINT: When the test taker is deciding on a priority question, the test taker should decide if the situation is expected or if it is life threatening.**

84. 1. This client is asking for information and should be given factual information. The surgery will not make the client sterile, but chemotherapy can induce menopause and radiation therapy to the pelvis can render a client sterile.

2. This is a therapeutic response, but the client asked for information.

3. This is a false statement and lying to the client.

4. This is outside the realm of a chaplain.

**TEST-TAKING HINT: When the stem has the client asking for specific information, then the nurse should provide the correct information. It is easy to confuse these questions with ones requiring therapeutic responses.**

1. The elderly client being seen in the clinic has complaints of urinary frequency, urgency, and "leaking." Which intervention should the nurse implement?
   1. Ensure communication is nonjudgmental and respectful.
   2. Set the temperature for comfort in the examination room.
   3. Speak loudly to ensure the client understands the nurse.
   4. Discuss incontinence problems with female clients only.

2. The client is experiencing urinary incontinence. Which intervention should the nurse implement?
   1. Teach the client to drink prune juice weekly.
   2. Encourage the client to eat a high-fiber diet.
   3. Discuss the need to urinate every six (6) hours.
   4. Administer diuretics at 2100 every day.

3. Which information would indicate to the nurse that teaching about treatment of urinary incontinence has been effective?
   1. The client prepares a scheduled voiding plan.
   2. The client verbalizes the need to increase fluid intake.
   3. The client explains how to perform pelvic floor exercises.
   4. The client attempts to retain the vaginal cone in place the entire day.

4. Which intervention should the nurse implement first for the client diagnosed with urinary incontinence?
   1. Palpate the bladder after an incontinent episode to assess for urinary retention.
   2. Administer oxybutynin, an anticholinergic agent, to decrease bladder contractions.
   3. Prepare the client for surgical intervention to repair the problem.
   4. Administer a cognitive function examination to determine abilities to function.

5. The client recovering from a prostatectomy has been experiencing stress incontinence. Which independent nursing intervention should the nurse discuss with the client?
   1. Establish a set voiding frequency of every two (2) hours while awake.
   2. Encourage a family member to check every two (2) hours and assist the client to void.
   3. Apply a transurethral electrical stimulator to relieve symptoms of urinary urgency.
   4. Discuss the use of a "bladder drill," including a timed voiding schedule.

6. The nurse is preparing the plan of care for the client diagnosed with a neurogenic flaccid bladder. Which expected outcome would be appropriate for this client?
   1. The client has conscious control over bladder activity.
   2. The client's bladder does not become overdistended.
   3. The client has bladder sensation and no discomfort.
   4. The client is able to check for bladder location in relation to the umbilicus.

7. Which intervention would be the most important before attempting to catheterize a client?
   1. Determine the client's history of catheter use.
   2. Evaluate the level of anxiety of the client.
   3. Verify that the client is not allergic to latex.
   4. Assess the client's sensation level and ability to void.

8. Which client should not be assigned to an unlicensed nursing assistant (NA) working on a surgical floor?
   1. The client with a suprapubic catheter inserted yesterday.
   2. The client who has had an indwelling catheter for the past week.
   3. The client who is on a bladder-training regimen.
   4. The client who had a catheter removed this morning and is being discharged.

Genitourinary

9. The nurse is caring for an elderly client who has an indwelling catheter. Which data warrant further investigation?
   1. The client's temperature is 98.0°F.
   2. The client has become confused and irritable.
   3. The client's urine is clear and light yellow.
   4. The client has no discomfort or pain.

10. The nurse is observing the unlicensed nursing assistant (NA) provide direct care to a client with a Foley catheter. Which data warrant immediate intervention by the nurse?
    1. The NA secures the tubing to the client's leg with tape.
    2. The NA provides catheter care with the client's bath.
    3. The NA positions the collection bag on the client's bed.
    4. The NA cares for the catheter after washing the hands.

11. Which intervention should the nurse implement when caring for the client with a nephrostomy tube?
    1. Change the dressing only if soiled by urine.
    2. Clean the end of the tubing and the connecting tube with Betadine.
    3. Clean the drainage system every day with bleach and water.
    4. Assess the tube for kinks to prevent obstruction.

12. The client is 12 hours postoperative renal surgery. Which data warrant immediate intervention by the nurse?
    1. The abdomen is soft, nontender, and rounded.
    2. Pain is not felt with dorsal flexion of the foot.
    3. The urine output is 60 mL for the past two hours.
    4. The trough vancomycin level is 24 mcg/mL.

13. The nurse is teaching the client diagnosed with tuberculosis of the urinary tract prior to discharge. Which information should the nurse include specific to this diagnosis?
    1. Instruct the client to take the medication with food.
    2. Explain that condoms should be used during treatment.
    3. Discuss the need for follow-up chest x-rays.
    4. Encourage a well-balanced diet and fluid intake.

14. The nurse is assessing a client diagnosed with urethral strictures. Which data support the diagnosis?
    1. Complaints of frequency and urgency.
    2. Clear yellow drainage from the urethra.
    3. Complaints of burning during urination.
    4. A diminished force and stream during voiding.

15. The nurse is providing discharge teaching to the client diagnosed with polycystic kidney disease. Which statement made by the client indicates that the teaching has been effective?
    1. "I need to avoid any activity that may pose a risk for injury to my kidney."
    2. "I should avoid taking medications that treat high blood pressure."
    3. "When I urinate there may be normal blood streaks in my urine."
    4. "I don't need to report any burning during urination or frequency."

16. Which intervention should the nurse include when assessing the client for urinary retention? Select all that apply.
    1. Inquire if the client has the sensation of fullness.
    2. Percuss the suprapubic region for a dull sound.
    3. Scan the bladder with the ultrasound scanner.
    4. Palpate from the umbilicus to the suprapubic area.
    5. Insert an indwelling catheter in the bladder.

17. The nurse has been assigned to train the unlicensed nursing assistant about prioritizing care. Which client should the nurse instruct the unlicensed nursing assistant to see first?
    1. The client who needs both sequential compression devices removed.
    2. The elderly woman who needs assistance ambulating to the bathroom.
    3. The surgical client who needs help changing the gown after bathing.
    4. The male client who needs the intravenous fluid discontinued.

18. The nurse is caring for the client recovering from a percutaneous renal biopsy. Which data indicate that the client is complying with client teaching?
    1. The client lies flat in the supine position for 12 hours.
    2. The client continues oral fluids restriction while on bed rest.
    3. The client's family changed the dressing on return to the room.
    4. The family activates the patient-controlled analgesia pump.

19. Which intervention should the nurse implement for the client who has had an ileal conduit?
    1. Pouch the stoma with a one (1)-inch margin around the stoma.
    2. Refer the client to the United Ostomy Association for discharge teaching.
    3. Report to the health-care provider any decrease in urinary output.
    4. Monitor the stoma for signs and symptoms of infection every shift.

20. The nurse is preparing the plan of care for a client with fluid volume deficit. Which interventions should the nurse include in the plan of care? Select all that apply.
    1. Monitor vital signs every two (2) hours until stable.
    2. Measure the client's oral intake and urinary output daily.
    3. Administer mouth care every eight (8) hours.
    4. Weigh the client in the same clothing at the same time daily.
    5. Assess skin turgor and mucous membranes every shift.

21. Which outcome should the nurse identify for the client diagnosed with fluid volume excess?
    1. The client will void a minimum of 30 mL per hour.
    2. The client will have elastic skin turgor.
    3. The client will have no adventitious breath sounds.
    4. The client will have a serum creatinine of 1.4 mg/dL.

22. The nurse is caring for a client diagnosed with rule out nephrotic syndrome. Which intervention should be included in the plan of care?
    1. Monitor the urine for bright-red bleeding.
    2. Evaluate the calorie count of the 500-mg protein diet.
    3. Assess the client's sacrum for dependent edema.
    4. Monitor for a high serum albumin level.

23. The nurse is preparing a teaching care plan for the client diagnosed with nephrotic syndrome. Which intervention should the nurse include?
    1. Discontinue the use of steroid therapy immediately if symptoms develop.
    2. Take diuretics as needed to treat the dependent edema in ankles.
    3. Increase the intake of dietary sodium every day to decrease fluid retention.
    4. Report any decrease in daily weight during treatment to the HCP.

24. Which intervention would be the most important for the nurse to implement for the client with a left nephrectomy?
    1. Assess the intravenous fluids for rate and volume.
    2. Change surgical dressing every day at the same time.
    3. Monitor the client's medication levels daily.
    4. Monitor the percentage of each meal eaten.

25. The nurse is preparing the discharge teaching plan for the male client with a left-sided nephrectomy. Which data indicate that the teaching was effective?
    1. The client informs the nurse he is returning to work on a loading dock of a factory.
    2. The client reports that he will notify the HCP if there is a decrease in urine output.
    3. The client says that there is no reason to keep track of the amount of urinary output.
    4. The client tells the nurse he is glad to be able to eat and drink what he pleases now.

26. The client on the medical unit is exhibiting peaked T waves on the electrocardiogram. Which interventions should the nurse implement? List in order of priority.
    1. Assess the client for leg and muscle cramps.
    2. Check the serum potassium level.
    3. Notify the health-care provider.
    4. Arrange for a transfer to the telemetry floor.
    5. Administer Kayexalate, a cation resin.

1.  1. Clients who have urinary incontinence are hesitant to discuss this problem because they may be embarrassed. Many clients will try to hide this condition from others, so it is the responsibility of the nurse to approach this subject with respect and consideration.
    2. The temperature of the room is not pertinent to the client's physical examination.
    3. The nurse should not assume that elderly clients have hearing difficulty. If the client is "hard of hearing," the nurse should speak clearly and concisely but should not shout.
    4. Incontinence is experienced by both sexes and by all ages. All adult clients may experience this and should be questioned at least initially.

2.  1. Prune juice is given to prevent constipation but should be taken daily, not weekly.
    2. Clients experiencing incontinence should eat a high-fiber diet to avoid constipation.
    3. Bladder training is used to assist with urinary incontinence by voiding every two (2) to three (3) hours, not every six (6) hours.
    4. Diuretics should be taken in the morning to allow for rest during the night.

3.  1. There are several plans for training the bladder to decrease frequency and incontinence. One plan is to schedule each voiding two (2) to three (3) hours apart, and when the client has remained consistently dry, the interval is increased by about 15 minutes.
    2. Managing the fluid intake is an important part of assisting the client with incontinence. The daily fluid intake is usually limited to 1500 mL, the majority of which should be drunk early in the day to prevent nocturia.
    3. Pelvic floor exercises (Kegel) should be performed two (2) to three (3) times daily with repetitions of 10 to 30 each session, but this is recommended for stress incontinence, not urinary incontinence.
    4. A series of vaginal weights can be used to increase the muscle tone. The time is usually only 15 minutes, not all day.

4.  1. The nurse should assess first to determine the etiology of the incontinence before the treatment plan can be formulated. By palpating the bladder after voiding, the nurse can determine if the incontinence was the result of overdistention of the bladder.
    2. Medications—for instance, anticholinergic agents such as oxybutynin—can cause adverse effects. Nonpharmacologic methods of treatment are preferred before medications are administered.
    3. Surgery would pose many risks for clients, so it would not be the first treatment choice.
    4. The nurse should assess the client's abilities to sense, interpret, and act on the need to void, but it is not the first intervention.

5.  1. Timed voiding is more helpful with neurogenic disorders, such as those related to diabetes.
    2. A prompted voiding is useful with a client who does not have the cognitive ability to recognize the need.
    3. The use of transvaginal or transurethral electrical stimulation to stimulate the pelvic floor muscles to contract is a collaborative intervention.
    4. Use of the bladder training drill is helpful in stress incontinence. The client is instructed to void at scheduled intervals. After consistently being dry, the interval is increased by 15 minutes until the client reaches an acceptable interval.

6.  1. In the flaccid neurogenic bladder, the client has lost the ability to recognize the need to void; therefore, this is not a realistic expected outcome.
    2. The treatment goal of the flaccid bladder would be to prevent overdistention.
    3. The sensation has been lost as a result of a lower motor neuron problem; therefore, there is no sensation to maintain and no discomfort, so this is not a realistic goal.
    4. The client does not have to assess the bladder; this is a nursing intervention.

7.  1. To determine if the client has had a catheter in place previously would assist with teaching and alleviating anxiety, but it is not the most important intervention.
    2. Assessing the level of anxiety would be helpful in assisting the client, but it would not endanger the client; therefore it is not the most important intervention.
    3. The nurse should always assess for allergies for latex prior to inserting a latex catheter or using a drainage system because if the client is allergic to latex, use of it could cause a life-threatening reaction. This is the most important intervention.
    4. There are many reasons that the client would be catheterized regardless of the sensation and ability to void. The nurse would not need to assess this until the catheter is removed.

8. 1. This client would require the most skill and knowledge because this client has the greatest potential for an infection; therefore the client should not be assigned to an NA.
2. The NA could care for a client with an indwelling Foley catheter because adherence to Standard Precautions is the only requirement for safe client care.
3. The NA cannot teach bladder training but can implement the strategies for the client on a bladder-training program.
4. The NA could care for this client because noting if the client voided after removal of the catheter is within the realm of the NA's ability.

9. 1. This temperature, 98.0°F, is within normal limits and would not require further investigation.
2. When an elderly client's mental status changes to confused and irritable, the nurse should seek the etiology, which may be a UTI secondary to an indwelling catheter. Elderly clients often do not present with classic signs and symptoms of infection.
3. The client's urine should be clear and light yellow; therefore, this would not warrant further investigation.
4. The client should have no discomfort and pain; therefore, this would not warrant further investigation.

10. 1. The client's catheter should be secured on the leg to prevent manipulation, which increases the risk for a urinary tract infection.
2. The client with an indwelling catheter should receive catheter care with the bath and as needed.
3. The drainage bag should be kept below the level of the bladder to prevent reflux of urine into the renal system; it should not be placed on the bed.
4. Hand hygiene is important before and after handling any portion of the drainage system.

11. 1. The dressing should be routinely changed as often as daily or weekly.
2. When connecting the tubing to the drainage bags, both ends should be cleaned with alcohol, not Betadine.
3. The drainage system can be cleaned daily with soap and water.
4. The nephrostomy tube should never be clamped or have kinks because an obstruction can cause pyelonephritis.

12. 1. The client who has renal surgery is at risk for paralytic ileus from the manipulation of the

colon. A soft, rounded, and nontender abdomen does not require intervention.
2. Pain felt with the dorsal flexion of the foot indicates a deep vein thrombosis; therefore, no pain does not require intervention.
3. The minimum of 30 mL per hour does not require intervention by the nurse.
4. The client who has restricted kidney function from surgery should be monitored for damage as a result of the use of aminoglycoside antibiotics, such as vancomycin, which are nephrotoxic.

13. 1. Antitubercular medications (rifampin and INH) should be taken one (1) hour before or two (2) two hours after a meal.
2. Clients who have been diagnosed with tuberculosis of the renal tract should use condoms to prevent transmission of the mycobacterium. If the infection is located in the penis or urethra, abstaining from sexual activity is recommended.
3. Follow up chest x-rays are important for the client with tuberculosis of the lung.
4. Maintaining a well-balanced diet and fluid intake is important for recovery from any illness and for a healthy lifestyle, but it is not specifically for this diagnosis.

14. 1. Frequency and urgency are signs and symptoms of a urinary tract infection.
2. Urethral drainage that is clear yellow is urine.
3. A complaint of burning during voiding is a sign and symptom of urinary tract infection.
4. The client with urethral strictures will report a decrease in force and stream during voiding. The stricture is treated by dilation using small filiform bougies.

15. 1. Polycystic kidney disease poses an increased risk for rupture of the kidney, and therefore sports activities or occupations that have risks for trauma should be avoided.
2. Antihypertensive medications should be taken to protect the kidneys from further damage.
3. Blood should always be reported to the healthcare provider, and hematuria is a sign of polycystic kidney disease. Further evaluation is needed.
4. Burning during urination or frequency are signs of a urinary tract infection that should be treated to prevent further damage to the kidneys and renal system.

16. 1. The nurse needs to assess the client's sensation of needing to void or feeling of fullness.

2. A dull sound heard when percussing the bladder indicates it is filled with urine.

3. A portable bladder scan is used to assess for the presence of urine, rather than using a straight catheter.

4. A distended bladder can be palpated.

5. Inserting a straight catheter or an in-and-out catheter is used to assess for residual urine, but not an indwelling catheter.

17. 1. The client who needs a sequential compression device removed is not urgent.

2. The elderly woman has age-related changes that can cause this request to be met as soon as possible. The elderly female client has a decreased bladder capacity, can be incontinent if not emptied frequently, has weakened urinary sphincter muscles, and has shortened urethras. The client is at risk for falling while attempting to get to the bathroom.

3. Changing a gown does not have a high priority.

4. The client will not be harmed if the intravenous fluid infuses for a short time, and this task should not be delegated to an NA.

18. 1. The client needs to lie flat on the back to apply pressure that prevents bleeding.

2. The client has oral intake withheld prior to the biopsy but not after the client is awake.

3. The client will have a pressure dressing on to maintain pressure that prevents bleeding. Clients and their families would not change this dressing.

4. Family members should be taught not to medicate the client. The client can become too sedated and develop respiratory distress.

19. 1. The nurse should maintain the drainage bag with a one-eighth–inch border around the stoma.

2. The United Ostomy Association would be an excellent referral for information. The nurse retains the responsibility to teach information that the client needs to know prior to discharge.

3. The output should be monitored to detect a decreased amount that may indicate an obstruction from edema or ureteral stenosis. Any decrease should be reported to the health-care provider.

4. The stoma should be monitored much more frequently than once a shift.

20. 1. Vital signs should be monitored every two (2) hours until stable and more frequently if the client is unstable.

2. Intake and output should be monitored more frequently than every 24 hours. Depending on the client's condition, frequency may vary from every hour to every four (4) hours.

3. Mouth care should be given as often as needed. A minimum of care should be every eight (8) hours.

4. The client should be weighed daily at the same time wearing the same clothing to ensure the reliability of this indicator.

5. Skin turgor and mucous membranes should be assessed every shift or more often depending on the client's condition.

21. 1. Voiding a minimum of 30 mL of urine each hour would be appropriate for a client with fluid volume deficit.

2. Elastic skin turgor would indicate that the client has adequate fluid volume status. This would be an expected output for the client with fluid volume deficit.

3. The client with fluid volume excess has too much fluid. Excess fluid would be reflected by adventitious breath sounds. Therefore an expected outcome would be to have no excess fluid, as evidenced by normal, clear breath sounds.

4. The creatinine would be elevated in a client who is dehydrated. The normal male should have a creatinine of 0.6–1.2 mg/dL, and a female client's normal creatinine is between 0.5 and 1.1 mg/dL.

22. 1. Hematuria is not a symptom of nephrotic syndrome.

2. A calorie count may be helpful in the treatment of this client, but a calorie count monitors just what the name implies—calories. The dietitian can calculate the amount of protein the client consumes, but this would be a protein count.

3. The classic sign and symptom of nephritic syndrome is dependent edema located on the client's sacrum and ankles.

4. A low serum level is expected for a client diagnosed with nephrotic syndrome.

23. 1. Long-term steroid therapy should not be stopped abruptly because it may result in adrenal insufficiency.

2. Treatment includes diuretics to eliminate dependent edema, usually in the ankles and sacrum.

3. Sodium is restricted to prevent fluid retention.

4. A decrease in weight would be expected if a diuretic is administered; this indicates that the medication is effective.

24. 1. Assessing the rate and volume of intravenous fluid is the most important intervention for clients who have one (1) kidney because an overload of fluids can result in pulmonary edema.
    2. Changing a daily dressing can be performed at any time and is not the priority intervention.
    3. The level of use of medication would not be the most important intervention because the nurse is administering all medications.
    4. The nurse would assess the amount of food eaten, but it is not the most important intervention.

25. 1. The client recovering from a nephrectomy needs to refrain from strenuous or heavy activities, and normal activities should not be resumed until the client is given permission by the surgeon.
    2. The client or family needs to contact the surgeon if the client develops chills, flank pain, decreased urinary output, or fever.
    3. The client needs to be informed of how to monitor the urinary output and which parameters should be reported to the surgeon.
    4. The client needs to follow any dietary or fluid restriction that the surgeon prescribes.

26. In order of priority: 1, 2, 3, 5, 4
    1. The nurse should assess to determine if the client is symptomatic of hyperkalemia.
    2. A peaked T wave is indicative of hyperkalemia; therefore, the nurse should obtain a potassium level.
    3. Hyperkalemia is a life-threatening situation because of the risk of cardiac dysrhythmias; therefore the nurse should notify the health-care provider.
    5. Kayexalate is a medication that will help remove potassium through the gastrointestinal system and should be administered to decrease the potassium level.
    4. The client should be monitored continuously for cardiac dysrhythmias so a transfer to the telemetry unit is warranted.

*The aim of education is the knowledge not of fact, but of values.*—Dean William R. Inge

# Reproductive Disorders

The organs of the male and female reproductive systems are subject to many disorders/ diseases. Some are hereditary, some are related to the endocrine system and may involve an underproduction or overproduction of hormones, and still others may be the result of infections or neoplastic growths. Whatever the etiology, the nurse must be well informed about all the possible disorders/diseases and how to monitor and treat them, both independently when allowed or under the direction of an HCP.

## KEYWORDS

aneuploid
brachytherapy
chancre
colporrhaphy
DNA ploidy
dysmenorrhea
dyspareunia
nulliparity
pessary
phimosis

## ABBREVIATIONS

Absolute Neutrophil Count (ANC)
Acute Respiratory Distress Syndrome (ARDS)
Anterior and Posterior Repair (A & P Repair)
Blood Pressure (BP)
Breast Self Examination (BSE)
Deoxyribonucleic Acid (DNA)
Digital Rectal Examination (DRE)
Deep Vein Thrombosis (DVT)
Health-Care Provider (HCP)
Human Chorionic Gonadotropin (HCG)
Human Immunodeficiency Virus (HIV)
Human Papillomavirus (HPV)
Hormone Replacement Therapy (HRT)
Incision and Drainage (I & D)
International Normalized Ratio (INR)
Intravenous (IV)
Intravenous Piggy Back (IVPB)
Low Malignancy Potential (LMP)
Luteinizing Hormone–Releasing Hormone (LHRH)
Nursing Assistant (NA)
Pelvic Inflammatory Disease (PID)
Prostate-Specific Antigen (PSA)
Prothrombin Time (PT)
Rule Out (R/O)
Sexually Transmitted Disease (STD)
Unlicensed Assistive Personnel (UAP)
Urinary Tract Infection (URI)
White Blood Cells (WBCs)

### Breast Disorders

1. The client frequently finds lumps in her breasts, especially around her menstrual period. Which information should the nurse teach the client regarding breast self-care?
   1. This is a benign process that does not need follow-up.
   2. The client should eliminate chocolate and caffeine from the diet.
   3. The client should practice breast self-examination monthly.
   4. This is the way that breast cancer begins and the client needs surgery.

2. The client is diagnosed with breast cancer and is considering whether to have a lumpectomy or a more invasive procedure, a modified radical mastectomy. Which information should the nurse discuss with the client?
   1. Ask if the client is afraid of having general anesthesia.
   2. Determine how the client feels about radiation and chemotherapy.
   3. Tell the client that she will need reconstruction with either procedure.
   4. Find out if the client has any history of breast cancer in her family.

3. The client has undergone a wedge resection for cancer of the left breast. Which discharge instruction should the nurse teach?
   1. Don't lift more than five (5) pounds with the left hand until released by the HCP.
   2. The cancer has been totally removed and no follow-up therapy will be required.
   3. The client should empty the Hemovac drain about every 12 hours.
   4. The client should arrange an appointment with a plastic surgeon for reconstruction.

4. Which recommendation is the American Cancer Society's (ACS) guideline for the early detection of breast cancer?
   1. Beginning at age 18 years, have a biannual clinical breast examination by an HCP.
   2. Beginning at age 30, perform monthly breast self-exams.
   3. Beginning at age 40, receive a yearly mammogram.
   4. Beginning at age 50, have a breast sonogram every five (5) years.

5. The client has had a mastectomy for cancer of the breast and asks the nurse about a Tram Flap procedure. Which information should the nurse explain to the client?
   1. The surgeon will insert a saline-filled sac under the skin to simulate a breast.
   2. The surgeon will pull the client's own tissue under the skin to create a breast.
   3. The surgeon will use tissue from inside the mouth to make a nipple.
   4. The surgeon can make the breast any size the client wants the breast to be.

6. The nurse is teaching a class on breast health to a group of ladies at a senior citizen's center. Which is the most important risk factor to emphasize to this group of ladies?
   1. The clients should find out about their family history of breast cancer.
   2. Men at this age can get breast cancer also and should be screened.
   3. Monthly breast self-examination is the key to early detection.
   4. The older a woman gets, the greater the chance of developing breast cancer.

7. The client who is scheduled to have a breast biopsy with sentinel node dissection states, "I don't understand. What does a sentinel node biopsy do?" Which scientific rationale should the nurse use to base the response?
   1. A dye is injected into the tumor and traced to determine spread of cells.
   2. The surgeon removes the nodes that drain the diseased portion of the breast.
   3. The nodes that can be felt manually will be removed and sent to pathology.
   4. A visual inspection of the lymph nodes will be made while the client is sleeping.

8. The client who is four (4) months pregnant finds a lump in her breast and the biopsy is positive for stage II cancer of the breast. Which treatment would the nurse anticipate the HCP recommending to the client?
   1. A lumpectomy to be performed after the baby is born.
   2. A modified radical mastectomy.
   3. Radiation therapy to the chest wall only.
   4. Chemotherapy only until the baby is born.

9. The client who had a right modified radical mastectomy four (4) years before is being admitted for a cardiac workup for chest pain. Which intervention would be most important for the nurse to implement?
    1. Determine when the client had chemotherapy last.
    2. Ask the client if she received Adriamycin, an antineoplastic agent.
    3. Post a message at the head of the bed to not use the right arm.
    4. Examine the chest wall for cancer sites.

10. The client is being discharged after a left modified radical mastectomy. Which discharge instructions should the nurse include? Select all that apply.
    1. Notify the HCP of a temperature of 100°F.
    2. Carry large purses and bundles with the right hand.
    3. Do not go to church or anywhere with crowds.
    4. Try to keep the arm as still as possible until seen by the HCP.
    5. Have a mammogram of the right and left breast yearly.

11. The client who has had a mastectomy tells the nurse, "My husband will leave me now that I am not a whole woman anymore." Which response by the nurse would be most therapeutic?
    1. "Are you afraid that your husband will not find you sexually appealing?"
    2. "Your husband should be grateful that you will be able to live and be with him."
    3. "Maybe your husband would like to attend a support group for spouses."
    4. "You don't know that is true. You need to give him a chance."

12. The client has been diagnosed with cancer of the breast. Which would be the most appropriate referral for the nurse to make?
    1. The hospital social worker.
    2. CanSurmount.
    3. Reach to Recovery.
    4. I CanCope.

## Pelvic Floor Relaxation Disorders

13. Which question would be most important for the nurse to ask the client with a cystocele who is scheduled to have a pessary inserted?
    1. "Do you know if you are allergic to latex?"
    2. "When did you start having incontinence?"
    3. "When was your last bowel movement?"
    4. "Are you experiencing any pelvic pressure?"

14. Which intervention should the nurse include when teaching the client who is having an anterior colporrhaphy to repair a cystocele?
    1. Discuss the need to perform perineal care every four (4) hours.
    2. Teach the client to expect to have a Foley catheter for at least one (1) month.
    3. Instruct the client how to care for the pessary inserted in surgery.
    4. Teach the client how to perform Kegel exercises.

15. The nurse is assessing the client diagnosed with a rectocele. Which signs and symptoms would the nurse expect? Select all that apply.
    1. Rectal pressure.
    2. Flatus.
    3. Fecal incontinence.
    4. Constipation.
    5. Urinary frequency.

16. What intervention should the nurse implement for a client diagnosed with a rectocele?
    1. Limit oral intake to decrease voiding.
    2. Encourage a low-residue diet.
    3. Administer a stool softener daily.
    4. Arrange for the client to take sitz baths.

17. Which statement would indicate that further instruction is needed for the client with a cystocele?
    1. "I need to have a sonogram to diagnose this problem."
    2. "I need to practice Kegel exercises to help strengthen my muscles."
    3. "I lose my urine when I sneeze because of my cystocele."
    4. "I can never have sexual intercourse again."

18. Which specific complication would the nurse assess for in the client with a uterine prolapse recovering from an anterior and posterior repair?
    1. Orthostatic hypotension.
    2. Atelectasis
    3. Allen sign.
    4. Homans' sign.

19. Which information should the nurse include in the discharge teaching for the client recovering from an abdominal hysterectomy?
    1. The client should report any persistent vaginal bleeding or cramping to the surgeon.
    2. The client should start a vigorous exercise routine to restore her muscle tone.
    3. The client should continue sitting in the bedside chair at least six (6) hours daily.
    4. The client should soak in a warm bathtub each night for one (1) hour.

20. Which nursing task could be delegated to the unlicensed assistive personnel (UAP) for the client who had a total vaginal hysterectomy?
    1. Observe the color and amount of drainage on the client's perineal pad.
    2. Maintain a current intake and output for the client each shift.
    3. Provide the client with a plan of pharmacological pain management.
    4. Prepare the client for her discharge scheduled for the next day.

21. The nurse is formulating a care plan for a client who has had an abdominal hysterectomy. Which nursing diagnosis would be appropriate for the client who has developed a complication?
    1. Potential for urinary retention.
    2. Potential for nerve damage.
    3. Potential for intestinal obstruction.
    4. Potential for fluid imbalance.

22. The nurse is teaching the client diagnosed with uterine prolapse. Which information should the nurse include in the discussion?
    1. Increase fluids and daily exercise to prevent constipation.
    2. Explain that there is only one acceptable treatment for uterine prolapse.
    3. Instruct the client to visually check the uterine prolapse daily.
    4. Discuss limiting coughing and lifting heavy objects.

23. The nurse is preparing the client for an insertion of a pessary. Which information should the nurse teach the client?
    1. The pessary does not need to be changed.
    2. The client should clean the pessary routinely.
    3. The pessary must be inserted in surgery.
    4. Estrogen cream is necessary for effective use of a pessary.

24. An elderly woman is diagnosed with pelvic relaxation disorder secondary to age-related changes. Which medication would the nurse expect to administer?
    1. Estrogen, a hormone.
    2. Cervidil, a cervical ripening agent.
    3. Progesterone, a hormone.
    4. Pitocin, an oxytocic agent.

## Uterine Disorders

25. The nurse is caring for a 30-year-old nulliparous client who is complaining of severe dysmenorrhea. Which diagnostic test should the nurse prepare the client to undergo to determine a diagnosis?
    1. A bimanual vaginal exam.
    2. A pregnancy test.
    3. An exploratory laparoscopy.
    4. An ovarian biopsy.

26. The client in the gynecology clinic asks the nurse, "What are the risk factors for developing cancer of the cervix?" Which statement would be the nurse's best response?
    1. "The earlier the age of sexual activity and the more partners, the greater the risk."
    2. "Eating fast foods that are high in fat and taking birth control pills are risk factors."
    3. "A *Chlamydia trachomatis* infection can cause cancer of the cervix."
    4. "Having yearly Pap smears will protect the client from developing cancer."

27. The nurse is admitting a client diagnosed with stage Ia cancer of the cervix to an outpatient surgery center for a conization. Which data would the client report?
    1. Diffuse watery discharge.
    2. No symptoms.
    3. Dyspareunia.
    4. Intense itching.

28. The client diagnosed with cancer of the uterus is scheduled to have radiation brachytherapy. Which precautions should the nurse implement? Select all that apply.
    1. Place the client in a private room.
    2. Wear a dosimeter when entering the room.
    3. Encourage visitors to come and stay with the client.
    4. Plan to spend extended time with the client.
    5. Notify the nuclear medicine technician.

29. The postmenopausal client reveals that it has been several years since her last gynecological examination and states, "Oh, I don't need that anymore. I am beyond having children." Which statement should be the nurse's response?
    1. "As long as you are not sexually active, you don't have to worry."
    2. "You should be taking hormone replacement therapy now."
    3. "You are beyond bearing children. How does that make you feel?"
    4. "There are situations other than pregnancy that should be checked."

30. The client has had a total abdominal hysterectomy for cancer of the uterus. Which discharge instruction should the nurse teach?
    1. The client should take HRT every day to prevent bone loss.
    2. The client should practice pelvic rest until seen by the HCP.
    3. The client can drive a car as soon as she is discharged from the hospital.
    4. The client should expect some bleeding after this procedure.

31. The client diagnosed with uterine cancer is complaining of lower back pain and unilateral leg edema. Which statement best explains the scientific rationale for these signs/symptoms?
    1. This is expected pain for this type of cancer.
    2. This means that the cancer has spread to other areas of the pelvis.
    3. The pain is a result of the treatment of uterine cancer.
    4. Radiation treatment always causes some type of pain in the region.

Reproductive

32. The client diagnosed with endometriosis experiences pain rated a five (5) on a 1–10 pain scale during her menses. Which intervention should the nurse teach the client?
    1. Teach the client to take a stool softener when taking morphine, a narcotic.
    2. Instruct the client to soak in a tepid bath for 30–45 minutes when the pain occurs.
    3. Explain the need to take the nonsteroidal anti-inflammatory drugs with food.
    4. Discuss the possibility of a hysterectomy to help relieve the pain.

33. The client is diagnosed with benign uterine fibroid tumors. Which question should the nurse ask to determine if the client is experiencing a complication?
    1. "How many periods have you missed?"
    2. "Do you get short of breath easily?"
    3. "How many times have you been pregnant?"
    4. "Where is the location of the pain you are having?"

34. The HCP has prescribed two (2) IV antibiotics for the female client diagnosed with diabetes and pneumonia. Which order should the nurse request from the HCP?
    1. Request written information on antibiotic-caused vaginal infections.
    2. Request yogurt to be served on the client's meal trays.
    3. Request a change of one of the antibiotics to an oral route.
    4. Request lactic acidophilus, a yeast preparation, three (3) times a day.

35. The nurse and an unlicensed nursing assistant are caring for clients on a gynecology surgery floor. Which intervention cannot be delegated to the unlicensed nursing assistant?
    1. Empty the indwelling catheter on the three (3)-hour postop client.
    2. Assist the two (2)-day postop client who has had a hysterectomy to the bathroom.
    3. Monitor the peri-pad count on a client diagnosed with fibroid tumors.
    4. Encourage the client who is refusing to get out of bed to walk in the hall.

36. The nurse is caring for a client diagnosed with uterine cancer who has been receiving systemic therapy for six (6) months. Which intervention should the nurse implement first?
    1. Check to determine which antineoplastic medication the client has received.
    2. Ask the client if she has had any problems with mouth ulcers at home.
    3. Administer the biologic response modifier filgrastim (Neupogen).
    4. Encourage the client to discuss feelings about having cancer.

## Ovarian Disorders

37. The 24-year-old female client presents to the clinic with lower abdominal pain on the left side that she rates a "9" on a 1–10 scale. Which diagnostic procedure should the nurse prepare the client for?
    1. A computed tomography scan.
    2. A lumbar puncture.
    3. An appendectomy.
    4. A pelvic sonogram.

38. The nurse is caring for a client newly diagnosed with stage IV ovarian cancer. What is the scientific rationale for detecting the tumors at this stage?
    1. The client's ovaries lie deep within the pelvis and early symptoms are vague.
    2. The client has regular gynecological examinations and this helps with detection.
    3. The client had a history of dysmenorrhea and benign ovarian cysts.
    4. The client had a family history of breast cancer and was being checked regularly.

39. The female client presents to the gynecologist's office for the fifth time with an ovarian cyst and is scheduled for an exploratory laparoscopy. The client asks the nurse. "Why do I need to have another surgery? The other cysts have all been benign." Which statement is the nurse's best response?
    1. "Because eventually the cysts will become cancerous."
    2. "All abnormal findings in the ovary should be checked out."
    3. "The surgery will not be painful and you will have peace of mind."
    4. "Are you afraid of having surgery? Would you like to talk about it?"

40. The client has had an exploratory laparotomy to remove an ovarian tumor. The pathology report classifies the tumor as a "low malignancy potential" (LMP) tumor. Which statement explains the scientific rationale for this pathology report?
    1. The client does not have cancer but will need adjuvant therapy.
    2. The client would have developed cancer if the tumor had not been removed.
    3. These borderline tumors resemble ovarian cancer but have better outcomes.
    4. The client has a very poor prognosis and has less than six (6) months to live.

41. The 50-year-old female client complains of bloating and indigestion and tells the nurse that she has gained two (2) inches in her waist recently. Which question should the nurse ask the client?
    1. "What do you eat before you feel bloated?"
    2. "Have you had your ovaries removed?"
    3. "Are your stools darker in color lately?"
    4. "Is the indigestion worse when you lie down?"

42. The nurse writes a problem of "anticipatory grieving" for a client diagnosed with ovarian cancer. Which nursing intervention would be priority for this client?
    1. Request the HCP to order an antidepressant medication.
    2. Refer the client to a CanSurmount volunteer for counseling.
    3. Encourage the client to verbalize feelings about having cancer.
    4. Give the client an advance directive form to fill out.

43. The client diagnosed with ovarian cancer has had eight (8) courses of chemotherapy. Which laboratory data warrant immediate intervention by the nurse?
    1. Absolute neutrophil count (ANC) of 3500 mm/dL.
    2. Platelet count of $150 \times 10^3$.
    3. Red blood cell count of $5.0 \times 10^6$.
    4. Urinalysis report of 100 WBC.

44. The client diagnosed with ovarian cancer is prescribed radiation therapy for regional control of the disease. Which statement indicates the client requires further teaching?
    1. "I will not wash the marks off my abdomen."
    2. "I will have a treatment every day for six (6) weeks."
    3. "Nausea caused by radiation therapy cannot be controlled."
    4. "I need to drink a nutritional shake if I don't feel like eating."

45. The female client has a mother who died from ovarian cancer and a sister diagnosed with ovarian cancer. Which recommendations should the nurse make regarding early detection of ovarian cancer?
    1. The client should consider having a prophylactic bilateral oophorectomy.
    2. The client should have a transvaginal ultrasound and a CA-125 laboratory test every six (6) months.
    3. The client should have yearly magnetic resonance imaging (MRI) scans.
    4. The client should have a biannual gynecological examination with flexible sigmoidoscopy.

46. The client has had a total abdominal hysterectomy for cancer of the ovary. Which diet should the nurse discuss when providing discharge instructions?
    1. A low-residue diet without seeds.
    2. A low-sodium, low-fat diet with skim milk.
    3. A regular diet with fruits and vegetables.
    4. A full liquid-only diet with milkshake supplements.

47. The nurse is preparing an in-service for women in the community. Which teaching would be a primary nursing intervention regarding the development of ovarian cancer?
    1. Instruct the clients not to use talcum powder on the perineum.
    2. Encourage the clients to consume diets with a high fat content.
    3. Teach the women to have a lower pelvic sonogram yearly.
    4. Discuss the need to be aware of the family history of cancer.

48. The nurse is caring for a client who has had a hysterectomy for cancer of the ovary. Which nursing interventions should the nurse implement? Select all that apply.
    1. Assess for calf enlargement and tenderness.
    2. Turn, cough, and deep breathe every six (6) hours.
    3. Assess pain on a one (1) to ten (10) pain scale.
    4. Apply sequential compression devices to legs.
    5. Assess bowel sounds every four (4) hours.

## Prostate Disorders

49. Which is the American Cancer Society's recommendation for the early detection of cancer of the prostate?
    1. A yearly PSA level and DRE beginning at age 50.
    2. A biannual rectal examination beginning at age 40.
    3. A semi-annual alkaline phosphatase level beginning at age 45.
    4. A yearly urinalysis to determine the presence of prostatic fluid.

50. The client is diagnosed with early cancer of the prostate. Which assessment data would the client report?
    1. Urinary urgency and frequency.
    2. Retrograde ejaculation during intercourse.
    3. Low back and hip pain.
    4. States that he has not had any problems.

51. The 80-year-old male client has been diagnosed with cancer of the prostate. Which treatment would the nurse discuss with the client?
    1. Radiation therapy every day for four (4) weeks.
    2. Radical prostatectomy with lymph node dissection.
    3. Diethylstilbestrol (DES), an estrogen, daily.
    4. Penile implants to maintain sexual functioning.

52. The nurse writes a client problem of urinary retention for a client diagnosed with stage IV cancer of the prostate. Which intervention should the nurse implement first?
    1. Catheterize the client to determine the amount of residual.
    2. Encourage the client to assume a normal position for urinating.
    3. Teach the client to use the Valsalva maneuver to empty the bladder.
    4. Determine the client's normal voiding pattern.

53. The client has undergone a bilateral orchiectomy for cancer of the prostate. Which intervention should the nurse implement?
    1. Support the scrotal sac with a towel and apply ice.
    2. Administer testosterone replacement hormone orally.
    3. Encourage the client to place sperm in a sperm bank.
    4. Have the client talk to another man with ejaculation dysfunction.

54. The client diagnosed with cancer of the prostate has been placed on an LHRH agonist (luteinizing hormone–releasing hormone) therapy. Which statement indicates that the client understands the treatment?
    1. "I will be able to function sexually as always."
    2. "I may have hot flashes while taking this drug."
    3. "This medication will cure the prostate cancer."
    4. "There are no side effects with these medications."

55. The client is diagnosed with metastatic prostate cancer to the bones. Which nursing intervention should the nurse implement?
    1. Prepare for a transurethral resection of the prostate.
    2. Keep the foot of the bed elevated at all times.
    3. Place the client on a scheduled bowel regimen.
    4. Discuss the client's altered sexual functioning.

56. Which could be a complication of cryotherapy surgery for cancer of the prostate?
    1. The urethra could become scarred and cause retention.
    2. The client could have ejaculation difficulties and be impotent.
    3. Bone marrow depression could occur from the chemotherapy.
    4. Chronic vomiting and diarrhea causing electrolyte imbalance could occur.

57. The client is eight (8) hours post-transurethral prostatectomy for cancer of the prostate. Which nursing intervention is priority at this time?
    1. Control postoperative pain.
    2. Assess abdominal dressing.
    3. Encourage early ambulation to prevent DVT.
    4. Monitor fluid and electrolyte balance.

58. The client scheduled for a radical prostatectomy surgical procedure has an intravenous antibiotic medication ordered on call to surgery. The antibiotic is prepared in 100 mL of sterile normal saline. At what rate should the nurse infuse via the IV pump when notified by the operating room nurse?_____

59. The client diagnosed with cancer of the prostate tells the nurse, "I caused this by being promiscuous when I was young and now I have to pay for my sins." Which statement would be the most therapeutic response?
    1. "Why would you think that prostate cancer is caused by sex?"
    2. "Do you feel guilty about some of your actions when you were young?"
    3. "Well, there is nothing you can do about that behavior now."
    4. "Have you told the HCP and been checked for an AIDS infection?"

60. The nurse is preparing the care plan for a 45-year-old client who has had a radical prostatectomy. Which psychosocial and physiological problem should be included in the plan?
    1. Altered coping.
    2. High risk for hemorrhage.
    3. Sexual impotence.
    4. Risk for electrolyte imbalance.

## Testicular Disorders

61. The school nurse is preparing a class on testicular cancer for male high school seniors. Which information regarding testicular self-examination should the nurse include?
    1. Perform the examination in a cool room under a fan.
    2. Any lump should be examined by an HCP as soon as possible.
    3. Discuss having a second person confirm a negative result.
    4. The procedure will cause a mild discomfort if done correctly.

62. The nurse enters the room of a 24-year-old client diagnosed with testicular cancer. The fiancée of the client asks the nurse, "Will we be able to have children?" Which is the nurse's best response?
    1. "Your fiancée will be able to father children like always."
    2. "You will have to adopt children because he will be sterile."
    3. "You and he should consider sperm banking prior to treatment."
    4. "Have you discussed this with the client? I can't discuss this with you."

63. The client diagnosed with testicular cancer is scheduled for a unilateral orchiectomy. Which information is important to teach regarding sexual functioning?
    1. The client will have ejaculation difficulties after the surgery.
    2. The client will be prescribed male hormones following the surgery.
    3. The client may need to have a penile implant to be able to have intercourse.
    4. Libido and orgasm usually are unimpaired after this surgery.

64. Which client has the highest risk for developing cancer of the testicles?
    1. The client diagnosed with epididymitis.
    2. The client born with cryptorchidism.
    3. The client with an enlarged prostate.
    4. The client diagnosed with hypospadias.

65. The nurse is caring for a client who is eight (8) hours postoperative unilateral orchiectomy for cancer of the testes. Which intervention should the nurse implement?
    1. Provide an athletic supporter before ambulating.
    2. Encourage the client to delay use of pain medications.
    3. Place client on a clear liquid diet for the first 48 hours.
    4. Monitor the PT/INR levels and have vitamin K ready.

66. The nurse and unlicensed assistive personnel (UAP) are caring for clients on a genitourinary floor. Which nursing task can be delegated to the UAP?
    1. Increase the drip rate on the Murphy drip irrigation set.
    2. Check the suprapubic catheter insertion site for infection.
    3. Encourage the two (2) hour postoperative client to turn and cough.
    4. Document the amount of red drainage in the catheter.

67. The nurse is caring for a client with epididymitis secondary to a chlamydia infection. Which discharge instruction should the nurse discuss?
    1. The sexual partner must be prescribed antibiotics.
    2. Delay sexual intercourse for a minimum of three (3) months.
    3. Expect the urine to have white clumps for one (1) to two (2) months.
    4. Drainage from the scrotum is fine as long as there is no fever.

68. The nurse is assessing a client with rule out testicular cancer. Which assessment data would support that the client has testicular cancer?
    1. The client complains of pain when urinating.
    2. There is a chancre sore on the shaft of the penis.
    3. The patient complains of heaviness in the scrotum.
    4. There is a red, raised rash on the testes.

69. The 30-year-old male client diagnosed with germinal cell carcinoma of the testes asks the nurse, "What chance do I have? Should I end it all now?" Which response by the nurse indicates an understanding of the disease process?
    1. "God would not want you to give up hope and end it all now."
    2. "There is a good chance for survival with standard treatment options."
    3. "There may be little hope, but ending it all is not the answer."
    4. "You have a 50/50 chance of living for at least 5 years."

70. Which tumor marker information is used to follow the progress of a client diagnosed with testicular cancer?
    1. CA-125.
    2. Carcinogenic embryonic antigen (CEA).
    3. DNA ploidy test.
    4. Human chorionic gonadotropin (HCG).

71. The client diagnosed with cancer of the testes calls and tells the nurse that he is having low back pain that does not go away with acetaminophen, a nonnarcotic analgesic. Which action should the nurse implement?
    1. Ask the client to come in to see the HCP for an examination.
    2. Tell the client to use a nonsteroidal anti-inflammatory drug instead.
    3. Inform the client that this means the cancer has metastasized.
    4. Encourage the client to perform lower back–strengthening exercises.

72. The charge nurse is making rounds on the genitourinary surgery floor. Which action by the primary nurse warrants immediate intervention?
    1. The nurse elevates the scrotum of a client who has had an orchiectomy.
    2. The nurse encourages the client to cough although he complains of pain.
    3. The nurse empties the client's J-P drain and leaves it rounded.
    4. The nurse asks the unlicensed nursing assistant to empty a catheter drainage bag.

## Sexually Transmitted Diseases

73. The occupational health nurse is preparing a class regarding sexually transmitted diseases (STDs) for employees at a manufacturing plant. Which high-risk behavior information should be included in the class information?
    1. Engaging in oral or anal sex decreases the risk of getting an STD.
    2. Using a sterile needle guarantees that the client will not get an STD.
    3. The more sexual partners, the greater the chance of developing an STD.
    4. If a condom is used, the client will not get a sexually transmitted disease.

74. The female client diagnosed with human papillomavirus (HPV) asks the nurse, "What other problems can HPV lead to?" Which statement is the most appropriate response by the nurse?
    1. "HPV is transmitted during sexual intercourse."
    2. "HPV infection can cause cancer of the cervix."
    3. "It has been known to lead to ovarian problems."
    4. "Regular Pap smears can help prevent problems."

75. The male client presents to the public health clinic complaining of joint pain and malaise. On assessment the nurse notes a rash on the trunk, palms of the hands, and soles of the feet. Which action should the nurse implement next?
    1. Determine if the client has had a chancre sore within the last two (2) months.
    2. Ask the client how many sexual partners he has had in the past year.
    3. Refer the client to a dermatologist for a diagnostic workup.
    4. Have the client provide a clean voided midstream urine specimen.

76. The nurse is caring for a young adult client who has been diagnosed with gonorrhea. Which statement reflects an understanding of the transmission of sexually transmitted diseases?
    1. Only lower socioeconomic income people are at risk for gonorrhea and syphilis.
    2. The longer a client waits to become sexually active, the greater the risk for an STD.
    3. Females can transmit infectious diseases more rapidly than males.
    4. If a client is diagnosed with an STD, they should be evaluated for other STDs.

77. The young female client is admitted with pelvic inflammatory disease secondary to a chlamydia infection. Which discharge instruction should be taught to the client?
    1. The client will develop antibodies to protect against a future infection.
    2. This infection will not have any long-term effects for the client.
    3. Both the client and the sexual partner must be treated simultaneously.
    4. Once the infection subsides, the pain will go away and not be a problem.

78. The nurse is assessing a male client for symptoms of gonorrhea. Which data support the diagnosis?
    1. Presence of a chancre sore on the penis.
    2. No symptoms.
    3. A CD4 count of less than 200.
    4. Pain in the testes and scrotal edema.

79. The nurse is working in a health clinic. Which disease is required to be reported to the public health department?
    1. Pelvic inflammatory disease.
    2. Epididymitis.
    3. Syphilis.
    4. Ectopic pregnancy.

80. The nurse is planning the care of a client diagnosed with pelvic inflammatory disease secondary to an STD. Which collaborative diagnosis is appropriate for this client?
    1. Risk for infertility.
    2. Knowledge deficit.
    3. Fluid volume deficit.
    4. Noncompliance.

81. Which laboratory test would the nurse expect for the client to rule out the diagnosis of syphilis?
    1. Vaginal cultures.
    2. Rapid plasma reagin card test (RPR-CT).
    3. Gram stain specimen of the urethral meatus.
    4. Immunologic assay.

82. The client is diagnosed with tertiary syphilis. Which signs and symptoms would the nurse observe?
    1. Lymphadenopathy and hair loss.
    2. Warts in the genital area.
    3. Dementia and psychosis.
    4. Raised rash covering the body.

83. Which statement best describes the responsibility of the public health nurse regarding sexually transmitted diseases?
    1. Notify the sexual partners of clients diagnosed with an STD.
    2. Determine the course of treatment for clients diagnosed with an STD.
    3. Explain the legal aspects of STD reporting to a client diagnosed with an STD.
    4. Analyze the statistics regarding STD transmission and reporting the findings.

84. The nurse is admitting a client diagnosed with trichomonas. Which assessment data support this diagnosis?
    1. Odorless, white, curdlike vaginal discharge.
    2. Strawberry spots on the vaginal surface and itching.
    3. Scant white vaginal discharge and dyspareunia.
    4. Purulent discharge from the endocervix and pelvic pain.

## Breast Disorders

1. 1. This is symptomatic of benign fibrocystic disease, but follow-up is always needed if the lumps do not go away when the hormone levels change.
   2. Some practitioners suggest eliminating caffeine and chocolate from the diet if the breasts become tender from the changes, but there is no research that supports this to be effective in controlling the discomfort associated with fibrocystic breasts.
   3. The American Cancer Society no longer recommends breast self-examination (BSE) for all women, but it is advisable that women with known breast conditions perform BSE monthly to detect potential cancer.
   4. The client may need a breast biopsy for potential breast cancer at some point, but breast cancer develops when there is an alteration in the DNA of a cell.

   **TEST-TAKING HINT: The test taker could eliminate option "1" because of the clause "does not need follow-up." The question is asking about self-care and only two (2) options—"2" and "3"— involve the client doing something. The test taker should choose between these.**

2. 1. General anesthesia would be used for either procedure.
   2. **The client should understand the treatment regimen for follow-up care. A lumpectomy requires follow-up with radiation therapy to the breast and then systemic chemotherapy. If the cancer is in its early stages, this regimen has results that are equal to those with a modified radical mastectomy.**
   3. A lumpectomy removes only the tumor and a small amount of tissue surrounding the tumor; reconstruction is not needed.
   4. A history of breast cancer in the family is immaterial because this client has breast cancer.

   **TEST-TAKING HINT: The test taker should use the nursing process to answer this question and select an assessment intervention, which would eliminate option "3" as a correct answer. Option "1" uses the word "afraid," which is an assumption; therefore this option could be eliminated.**

3. 1. The client has had surgery on this side of the body. Pressure on the incision should be limited until released by the HCP to perform normal daily activities.
   2. This is giving the client false hope. Cancer cells characteristically move easily in the

lymph or bloodstream to other parts of the body. Microscopic disease cannot be determined by the naked eye.
   3. A client who has a mastectomy might be discharged with a Hemovac, but a wedge resection should not require one.
   4. The breast has not been removed; reconstruction is not needed.

   **TEST-TAKING HINT: If the test taker did not know this answer, option "1" is information that could be provided to any client who has had surgery on the upper chest or arm.**

4. 1. Unless there is a personal history of breast cancer or a strong family history, clinical breast exams should begin at age 30 years and should be performed yearly.
   2. If the client is going to perform breast self-exam (BSE), it should begin at age 18. The ACS no longer includes monthly BSE as part of its guidelines.
   3. **The ACS recommends a yearly mammogram for the early detection of breast cancer. A mammogram can detect disease that will not be large enough to feel.**
   4. Breast sonograms are performed to diagnose specific breast disease when a screening mammogram has shown a suspicious area.

   **TEST-TAKING HINT: This is a knowledge-based question. The test taker might be swayed by the option about BSE, but the age must be considered.**

5. 1. This is done for reconstruction of a breast or augmentation of breast size, but it is not a Tram Flap procedure, which uses the client's own tissue.
   2. **The Tram Flap procedure is one in which the client's own tissue is used to form the new breast. Tissue and fat are pulled under the skin with one end left attached to the body to provide circulation until the body builds collateral circulation in the area.**
   3. The plastic surgeon can rebuild a nipple from pigmented skin donor sites or can tattoo the nipple in place.
   4. This is true of saline implants but not of Tram Flaps.

   **TEST-TAKING HINT: If the test taker is taking a standard pencil and paper test and was not familiar with this procedure, then skipping the question and returning to it at a later time would be advisable. Another question might give a clue about the procedure. This is not possible on the RN-NCLEX computerized examination.**

Reproductive

6. 1. Most women who develop breast cancer do not have a family history of the disease. Specific genes—BRCA-1 and BRCA-2—that are implicated in the development of breast cancer have been identified, but most women with breast cancer do not have these genes.
2. Approximately 1000 men are diagnosed every year with breast cancer, but, as with women, it can occur at any age. Breast cancer in men frequently goes undetected because the men consider this a woman's disease.
3. Mammograms can detect breast cancer earlier than breast self-examination and are the current recommendation by the American Cancer Society.
4. **The greatest risk factor for developing breast cancer is being female. The second greatest risk factor is being elderly. By age 80, one (1) in every eight (8) women develop breast cancer.**

**TEST-TAKING HINT: The test taker cannot overlook the age when it is given in a question. "Senior citizen's center" should alert the test taker to the older age group. The test taker should decide what the age has to do with the answer.**

7. 1. **A sentinel node biopsy is a procedure in which a radioactive dye is injected into the tumor and then traced by instrumentation and color to try to identify the exact lymph nodes that the tumor could have shed into.**
2. This is the older procedure in which the surgeon removed the nodes that were thought to drain the tumor. There was no way of knowing that the surgeon was actually removing the affected nodes.
3. The purpose of the procedure is not to rely on guesswork in determining the extent of tumor involvement.
4. Microscopic disease cannot be seen by the naked eye.

**TEST-TAKING HINT: The test taker would eliminate options "3" and "4" if they were aware of the definition of "sentinel," which means "to watch over as a sentry." This might lead the test taker to determine that specific areas would have to be determined.**

8. 1. Waiting until the baby is born would allow the cancer to continue to develop and spread. This might be an option if the client was in the third trimester, but not at this early stage.
2. **A modified radical mastectomy would be recommended for this client because the client would not be able to begin radiation or chemotherapy, which are part of the regimen for a lumpectomy or wedge resec-**

tion. Many breast cancers that develop during pregnancy are hormone sensitive and would have the ideal grounds for growth. The tumor should be removed as soon as possible.
3. Radiation therapy cannot be delivered to a pregnant client because of possible harm to the fetus.
4. Chemotherapy would not be given to the client while she is pregnant because of potential harm to the fetus.

**TEST-TAKING HINT: The test taker should eliminate options "3" and "4" because of potential harm to the fetus, but each option has the word "only." There are very few "onlys" in health care.**

9. 1. A client four (4) years post-mastectomy should be finished with adjuvant therapy, which lasts from six (6) months to one (1) year.
2. The client may have received Adriamycin, which is a cardiotoxic medication, but knowing this will not change the tests that will be performed or preparation for the tests.
3. **The nurse should post a message at the head of the client's bed to not use the right arm for blood pressures or lab draws. This client is at risk for lymphedema, and this is a lymphedema precaution.**
4. The chest wall is sometimes involved in breast cancer, but the most important intervention is to prevent harm to the client.

**TEST-TAKING HINT: The question is asking for an intervention that is common in the healthcare industry. There are many breast cancer survivors who go on to develop unrelated problems, but the nurse must still be aware of the lingering needs of the client.**

10. 1. **It is a common instruction for any client who has had surgery to notify the HCP if a fever develops. This could indicate a postoperative infection.**
2. **The client who has had a mastectomy is at risk for lymphedema in the affected arm because the lymph nodes are removed during the surgery. The client should protect the arm from injury and carry heavy objects with the opposite arm.**
3. The client can attend church services and large gatherings. This client had surgery, not chemotherapy that would increase the potential for developing an infection if exposed to an infected individual.
4. The client should be taught arm-climbing exercises before leaving the hospital to facilitate maintaining range of motion.
5. The client has developed a malignancy in

one breast and is at a higher risk for developing another tumor in the remaining breast area.

**TEST-TAKING HINT: The test taker must determine if the option of keeping the arm still would be recommended. Most postoperative recommendations require the client to move as much as possible.**

11. 1. This is restating the client's feelings and is a therapeutic response.
    2. This is not recognizing the client's concerns and putting the nurse's expectations on the spouse.
    3. This is problem-solving and could be offered, but the therapeutic response is to restate the client's feeling and encourage a conversation.
    4. The client may know this is true. The nurse is telling the client that she has no reason for her feelings. Feelings are what they are and should be accepted as such.

**TEST-TAKING HINT: When the question asks for a therapeutic response, the test taker should choose an option that encourages the client to discuss his or her feelings.**

12. 1. The social worker assists clients in finding nursing home placement and financial arrangements, and some work with clients to discuss feelings, but this is not the best referral.
    2. CanSurmount volunteers work with all types of clients diagnosed with cancer, not just clients with breast cancer.
    3. Reach to Recovery is a specific referral program for clients diagnosed with breast cancer.
    4. I CanCope is a cancer education program for all clients diagnosed with cancer and their significant others.

**TEST-TAKING HINT: The question asks for the most appropriate, and the test taker should choose the one specific to breast cancer.**

## Pelvic Floor Relaxation Disorders

13. 1. The client should be assessed for allergies to latex as a result of the composition of the pessary.
    2. These clients frequently have incontinence, but that would have been assessed prior to the plan for the pessary.
    3. A pessary is manually inserted to keep a prolapsed uterus in place. Asking about a bowel movement would not be an appropriate question.
    4. This is a symptom experienced by a client with a cystocele.

**TEST-TAKING HINT: If the test taker has no idea what the answer is, then apply Maslow's Hierarchy of Needs, which in this question would be safety. Only option "1" addresses a safety issue. Allergies are a safety issue.**

14. 1. Perineal care is given every shift or as needed.
    2. The client may have a Foley catheter for two (2) to four (4) days postoperative but not for a month.
    3. A pessary would be used in place of surgery.
    4. A client should be taught how to perform Kegel exercises to strengthen the muscles.

**TEST-TAKING HINT: When selecting a correct answer, the test taker should always look at the adjectives, especially numbers such as four (4) in option "1" or one (1) in option "2."**

15. 1. A rectocele causes the rectum to be pouched upward, causing rectal pressure.
    2. When the rectum pushes against the posterior wall of the vagina, the result is flatus.
    3. Clients with a rectocele experience fecal incontinence.
    4. Clients with a rectocele frequently are constipated.
    5. A client who has a rectocele does not experience urinary frequency.

**TEST-TAKING HINT: The test taker should learn the terms. If the test taker does not know the answers, the test taker can eliminate urinary frequency because it is different from the other options. It refers to the urinary tract, whereas the others refer to bowel elimination.**

16. 1. There is no reason to limit oral intake or to decrease voiding.
    2. Client should be eating a high-fiber diet to prevent constipation.
    3. Stool softeners and laxatives are used to prevent and treat constipation, which is common with a rectocele. Because of the positioning of the rectum, stool can stay in the rectal pouch, causing constipation.
    4. Sitz baths are not used to treat a rectocele.

**TEST-TAKING HINT: The test taker who is knowledgeable of medical terminology could eliminate option "1," which has the word "voiding," and "rectocele" refers to the rectum.**

17. 1. Sonograms and pelvic examinations are used to diagnose cystoceles.
    2. Kegel exercises strengthen the pelvic floor muscles.
    3. Clients with cystoceles frequently have urinary incontinence when they cough, sneeze, laugh, lift heavy items, or make sudden jarring motions.

4. Clients with cystoceles may have sexual intercourse unless contraindicated by another medical reason.

**TEST-TAKING HINT:** This type of question is confusing to test takers because the correct option provides incorrect information. Most of the time absolutes such as "never," "only," and "always" make the option incorrect. Option "4" has an absolute—"never"—but it is the correct answer because all of the other answer options contain correct information that the client has learned.

18. 1. A surgery-specific complication would not be orthostatic hypotension.
    2. Atelectasis would be a complication of general anesthesia, not an A & P repair.
    3. An Allen test is a physical examination that tests the arterial blood supply to the radial and ulnar arteries.
    4. Assessing for DVT is performed on all clients having a vaginal hysterectomy. Any surgery that requires the client to be placed in the lithotomy position should be assessed for deep vein thrombosis (DVT). These clients are at a higher risk for this complication.

**TEST-TAKING HINT:** The test taker must have knowledge of this surgical procedure to be able to answer this question. It would be a good choice to choose an option that is performed for most clients who are immobile.

19. 1. The client should report any persistent vaginal bleeding or gastrointestinal changes such as distention, cramping, or changes in bowel habits.
    2. Clients should rest and not start a vigorous exercise program until the surgeon gives permission.
    3. Clients should avoid activities that increase pelvic congestion such as dancing, horseback riding, and sitting for long periods.
    4. Clients should avoid taking baths to help prevent infection of the incision site.

**TEST-TAKING HINT:** When the test taker is selecting possible correct answers, carefully consider the descriptive words. In option "1," the adjective "vigorous" should cause the test taker to eliminate it, and in option "3" the words "six (6) hours" should help eliminate it.

20. 1. Observation is assessment, which cannot be delegated.
    2. This nursing task can be delegated, but evaluation is the responsibility of the nurse.
    3. Teaching cannot be delegated.
    4. Teaching cannot be delegated.

**TEST-TAKING HINT:** The nurse cannot delegate assessing, planning, teaching, and evaluating.

21. 1. Urinary retention is a complication of a vaginal hysterectomy.
    2. Nerve damage is a possible complication of improper positioning in surgery, but the stem of the question does not state that this occurred.
    3. Clients who have had a total abdominal hysterectomy are at risk for intestinal obstruction.
    4. An imbalance of fluid is a complication of several surgeries, not specifically a total abdominal hysterectomy.

**TEST-TAKING HINT:** When the test taker does not know the answer, the test taker should consider the similarities and the differences in surgeries. A total abdominal hysterectomy would have complications, as do other abdominal surgeries.

22. 1. A uterine prolapse is not caused by constipation; it is caused by a weakening of the pelvic muscles. It is a protrusion of the uterus through the vagina. It can pull on the vaginal wall, bladder, and rectum.
    2. There are multiple treatment modalities for uterine prolapse. The selection of treatment is determined by the degree of the prolapse and the medical history of the client.
    3. The protraction can be seen from the vagina in some cases but this is not with all clients.
    4. Symptoms can be aggravated by coughing, sneezing, lifting heavy objects, standing for prolonged periods, and climbing stairs.

**TEST-TAKING HINTS:** The test taker should eliminate options that contain words like "only," "never," "always," "all," or "most of the time." If the test taker does not have a clue, uterine is not in the same body system as constipation, so option "1" can be eliminated.

23. 1. Pessaries need to be changed to prevent complications.
    2. Clients do need to clean the pessary routinely.
    3. Pessaries are inserted in areas other than surgery, such as in health-care provider's offices.
    4. Hormone cream may be used, but usually an oral estrogen is prescribed.

**TEST-TAKING HINTS:** The test taker should realize that any removable device inserted into the body would require routine changing at some time; therefore option "1" can be eliminated. Option "4" is a medication and a pessary is a device, so "4" can be eliminated.

24. 1. Estrogen changes the pelvic floor muscles and lining of the uterus and may help improve a pelvic relaxation disorder.
    2. Cervidil is used to prepare the cervix for delivery of a baby. It causes the cervix to shorten, soften, and dilate.
    3. Progesterone is given for implantation of a fertilized ovum.
    4. Pitocin causes the uterus to contract. It is used during the labor and delivery process.

    **TEST-TAKING HINT: Options "2," "3," and "4" are similar in that they are all used during a pregnancy or delivery. If the test taker doesn't have a clue what is the correct answer, the test taker should attempt to find what answer is different from all the others.**

## Uterine Disorders

25. 1. A vaginal exam would not provide a definitive diagnosis to determine the cause of the pain.
    2. A pregnancy test is not usually ordered unless the client has a reason to think she may be pregnant. Pregnancy would temporarily alleviate the symptoms of endometriosis because neither ovulation nor menses occur during pregnancy.
    3. There is a high incidence of endometriosis among women who have never had children (nulliparity) and those who have children later in life. The most common way to diagnose this condition is through an exploratory laparoscopy.
    4. The ovaries lie deep within the pelvic cavity. To reach the ovaries would require some form of abdominal procedure, such as a laparoscopy. However, the symptoms are not those of an ovarian cyst.

    **TEST-TAKING HINT: The test taker could eliminate answer option "1" because "diagnosis" is in the stem. The stem is asking for a procedure that will provide a definitive diagnosis. Option "2" could be eliminated because, if the client is menstruating ("dysmenorrhea" means "painful menstruation"), then the client is usually not pregnant.**

26. 1. Risk factors for cancer of the cervix include sexual activity before the age of 20 years; multiple sexual partners; early childbearing; exposure to the human papillomavirus; HIV infection; smoking; and nutritional deficits of folates, beta carotene, and vitamin C.
    2. High-fat diets place clients at risk for some cancers but not for cervical cancer. The use of birth control pills may allow increased sexual freedom because of the protection from pregnancy, but it does not increase the risk for cancer of the cervix.
    3. Infections with the human papillomavirus are a risk factor for cancer of the cervix.
    4. Having a yearly Pap smear increases the chance of detecting cellular changes early, but it does not increase the risk for developing cancer.

    **TEST-TAKING HINT: The test taker could discard "4" as a possible answer because it is a yearly test for the early detection of cervical cancer, not a risk factor.**

27. 1. Diffuse watery foul-smelling discharge would occur at a much later stage.
    2. At this stage the client is asymptomatic and the cancer has been determined by a Pap smear.
    3. Dyspareunia is painful sexual intercourse; the client is asymptomatic.
    4. Intense itching occurs with vaginal yeast infections.

    **TEST-TAKING HINT: The test taker could either choose answer option "2" because it is the least presenting symptom or discard it. Staging for all cancers start with "0" or "1" indicating the least detectable cancer.**

28. 1. Brachytherapy is the direct implantation of radioactive seeds through the vagina into the uterus. The client should be in a private room at the end of the hall to prevent radiation exposure to the rest of the unit.
    2. Nurses wear a dosimeter that registers the amount of radiation the nurse has been exposed to. When a certain level is reached, the nurse is no longer allowed to care for clients undergoing internal radiation therapy.
    3. Visitors are limited while the radiation is in place.
    4. In this case spending extra time with a client is not done. The nurse does only what must be done and leaves the room.
    5. The nuclear medicine technician will be the one that assists with the placement of the implants and will deliver the implants in a lead-lined container. The technician will also come and scan any items (linens and wastes) leaving the room for radiation contamination.

    **TEST-TAKING HINT: This is an alternate-type question, which requires the test taker to select more than one correct answer. The test taker must select all the correct answers to receive credit for the question.**

29. 1. This client is at risk for cancer of the ovary and uterus because of advancing age, regardless of sexual activity, and should see an HCP yearly.
    2. Hormone replacement therapy (HRT) is not recommended for most postmenopausal clients because research has shown that HRT increases the risk of myocardial infarctions and cerebrovascular accidents (strokes).
    3. This is a therapeutic response and the client did not state a feeling.
    4. The client should have a yearly clinical examination of the breasts and pelvic area for the detection of cancer.

    **TEST-TAKING HINT: If the stem was not asking for a therapeutic response, then factual information should be provided to the client. This would eliminate answer option "3."**

30. 1. Clients who are diagnosed with cancer of the uterus have the ovaries removed to reduce hormone production. The client will not be taking HRT.
    2. Pelvic rest means that nothing is placed in the vagina. The client would not need a tampon at this time, but sexual intercourse should be avoided until the vaginal area has healed.
    3. The sitting position a client assumes when driving a vehicle places stress on the lower abdomen. The client should wait until the HCP releases her to drive.
    4. The client should not have any vaginal bleeding.

    **TEST-TAKING HINT: The test taker should apply basic postoperative concepts when answering questions and realize that bleeding is not expected postoperatively and safety should always be addressed.**

31. 1. This pain indicates metastasis to the retroperitoneal region. If caught early, a complete hysterectomy is usually the only therapy recommended. This type of pain indicates that the cancer is advanced and the prognosis is poor.
    2. This pain indicates that the cancer is in the retroperitoneal region and the prognosis is poor.
    3. Pain is not part of the treatment of cancer. Surgery may cause pain, but most treatments do not.
    4. Radiation therapy does not always result in pain; that depends on the area irradiated.

    **TEST-TAKING HINT: Answer option "4" has the absolute word "always" and should be eliminated as a correct answer. The stem is describing symptoms in regions other than the**

lower pelvis, so an educated choice would be option "2."

32. 1. The client taking a narcotic medication should be placed on a bowel regimen, but this client would not be prescribed narcotic medication.
    2. A tepid bath for 30–45 minutes would not be appropriate because the lukewarm water would get cold. A heating pad to the abdomen sometimes helps with the pain.
    3. The medication of choice for mild to moderate dysmenorrhea is an NSAID. NSAIDs cause gastrointestinal upset and should be taken with food.
    4. This may be an option eventually, but the stem did not give an age or say that the client has decided that she does not want to get pregnant.

    **TEST-TAKING HINT: The test taker should not read into the question. Option "4" is only correct when more information is provided. The test taker must know about the scales used to rate pain, nausea, or depression. The client's report of midrange symptoms would not indicate the need for routine narcotic administration.**

33. 1. Benign fibroid tumors in the uterus cause the client to bleed longer with a heavier flow, not miss periods.
    2. Many women delay surgery until anemia has occurred from the heavy menstrual flow. A symptom of anemia is shortness of breath.
    3. The number of pregnancies does not matter at this time; the client has a different problem.
    4. The pain is in the pelvic region to low back, where the uterus lies.

    **TEST-TAKING HINT: This is a high-level question requiring the test taker to make several judgments before arriving at the answer. First, the test taker must decide what happens when a client has fibroid tumors and then what symptom that is likely to produce.**

34. 1. The nurse does not require an order to teach. Teaching is an independent nursing function.
    2. The nurse can request the dietitian to include yogurt in the client's calorie restrictions without an order.
    3. If the HCP has ordered an IV antibiotic, then there is no reason to request a change to an oral route.
    4. Female clients on antibiotics are at risk for killing the good bacteria, which keep yeast infections in check. This is especially true in clients diagnosed with diabetes. Lactic acidophilus is a yeast replacement medication.

TEST-TAKING HINT: **The test taker must be aware of independent nursing functions. This would eliminate options "1" and "2."**

35. 1. The unlicensed nursing assistant can empty the indwelling catheter and record the output.
2. This is an appropriate assignment.
3. Monitoring a peri-pad count is done to determine if the client is bleeding excessively; the nurse should do this as part of the assessment.
4. All personnel should encourage the client to ambulate.

TEST-TAKING HINT: **The nurse cannot delegate assessment. "Monitor" is a word that can be interpreted as "assess." This is an except question so the test taker should not jump to option "1" as the correct answer because the UAP can perform this task.**

36. 1. This can be done to determine specific problems resulting from the specific side effects of the medication, but it is not the first action. The nurse can ask general assessment questions to determine how the client is tolerating the treatments.
2. **The systemic side effects of chemotherapy are not always apparent, and the development of stomatitis can be extremely distressing for the client. The nurse should assess the client's tolerance to treatments.**
3. This is done if the white blood cell count is low. The nurse would have to assess the WBC count and then have an order from an HCP.
4. This is an appropriate action but not before assessing physical problems.

TEST-TAKING HINT: **When prioritizing nursing interventions the test taker should apply the nursing process, and assess is the first step.**

## Ovarian Disorders

37. 1. The client has symptoms of an ovarian cyst, usually diagnosed by a pelvic sonogram.
2. The client has abdominal pain, not back or neurological pain, which is when a lumbar puncture would be performed.
3. The appendix is in the right lower abdomen, not the left.
4. **Ovarian cysts are fluid-filled sacs located on the surface of the ovary. A lower pelvic sonogram is the preferred diagnostic tool. It is not invasive and usually not painful.**

TEST-TAKING HINT: **The test taker could eliminate options "2" and "3" by using knowledge of basic anatomy and physiology. The age of**

the client places this client in the typical age range for a benign ovarian cyst; before age 29 years, 98% of ovarian cysts are benign.

38. 1. **The ovaries are anatomically positioned deep within the pelvis, and because of this, signs and symptoms of cancer are vague and nonspecific. Symptoms include increased abdominal girth, pelvic pressure, indigestion, bloating, flatulence, and pelvic and leg pain. Increasing abdomen size as a result of accumulation of fluid is the most common sign. Many women ignore the symptoms because they are so nonspecific.**
2. Regular gynecological examinations are recommended, but this is advanced disease.
3. Dysmenorrhea is not a risk factor for developing ovarian cancer. Any enlarged ovary should be evaluated, especially if the client is postmenopausal when the ovaries shrink in size.
4. A family history of breast cancer is a cause for the client to be assessed regularly for breast and ovarian cancer, but this is late disease.

TEST-TAKING HINT: **Stage IV should help the test taker to eliminate options "2" and "4" because this client has advanced disease and it is hoped regular checkups find problems early.**

39. 1. All cysts do not become cancerous; 98% of ovarian cysts in clients younger than age 29 are benign, whereas in women older than age 50, about half are benign.
2. **Any abnormal ovary that cannot be diagnosed with a transvaginal ultrasound should be examined laparoscopically.**
3. Any time the client has surgery she should be prepared to experience some pain. This is a false statement and could cause a breach in the nurse–client relationship.
4. This is a therapeutic statement and the client is asking for information.

TEST-TAKING HINT: **The test taker should read the stem of the question carefully. Option "1" has a form of absolute, "eventually will become," so it can be eliminated. Option "3" is a false statement. Option "4" is a therapeutic response and the stem asks the nurse to provide information.**

40. 1. The client has a low-grade cancer that occurs in approximately 15% of ovarian tumors. The affected ovary usually is removed, and the woman may or may not require adjuvant therapy. Women with this type of tumor are usually younger than age 40 years.
2. The tumor is classified as cancer. The follow-up care is not as extensive because of the characteristics that the tumor displays.

3. These tumors are low-grade cancers that have fewer propensities for metastasis than most ovarian cancers.

4. This client has a better prognosis than 85% of clients diagnosed with ovarian cancer.

**TEST-TAKING HINT:** The test taker could eliminate option "4" because low malignancy potential and poor prognosis do not match. The statement in option "1" says the client does not have cancer but will need therapy for cancer, so the test taker could eliminate this option.

41. 1. This statement would be appropriate if not for the abdominal girth change. This should alert the nurse to some internal reason for the change in girth. Ascites causes a change in abdominal girth.

2. Ovarian cancer has vague symptoms of abdominal discomfort, but increasing abdominal girth is the most common symptom. If the client has had the ovaries removed, then the nurse could assess for another cause.

3. This could be assessing for a peptic ulcer, but ulcers do not cause increasing abdominal girth.

4. This is a question to determine if the client has gastroesophageal reflux, but this would not cause increased waist size.

**TEST-TAKING HINT:** The test taker must notice all the symptoms the client is reporting. Flatulence and bloating could be associated with a number of problems, but these symptoms, along with increased waist size, narrow the possibilities.

42. 1. An antidepressant may be needed at some time, but at this point the nurse should offer his or her time and interest and encourage the client to discuss the feeling of having cancer.

2. CanSurmount volunteers are extremely helpful in talking about having cancer with the client, but they do not provide counseling. The programs work on the basis of the fact that someone who has had cancer and gone through treatment can relate to the client about to begin treatment.

3. The nurse should plan to spend time with the client and allow the client to discuss the feelings of having cancer, dying, fear of the treatments, and any other concerns.

4. The client will need to complete an advance directive, but this action does not address the client's grieving process.

**TEST-TAKING HINT:** The test taker could eliminate option "2" because a volunteer is not referred to for counseling. Only one (1) option

directly addresses the problem and requires the nurse to interact with the client.

43. 1. An absolute neutrophils count of 3500 indicates the client has sufficient mature white blood cells or granulocytes to act as a defense against infections.

2. A platelet count of 150,000 is within normal range. Thrombocytopenia is less than 100,000 ($150 \times 10^3$ [1000] = 150,000)

3. A red blood cell count of 5,000,000 is within normal limits. ($5.0 \times 10^6$ [1,000,000] = 5,000,000)

4. A normal urinalysis contains one (1) to two (2) WBCs. A report of 100 WBCs indicates the presence of an infection. A clean voided specimen should be obtained and a urine culture should be done. This client should be prescribed antibiotics immediately.

**TEST-TAKING HINT:** The test taker should memorize normal values for common laboratory tests. Urine will not have a large number of white blood cells unless there is a pathological process occurring. The kidneys filter the blood but do not process the destruction of blood cells.

44. 1. The radiation markings on a client are there to guide the technician to irradiate only the area within the marks. The marks remain until the client has completed the treatments.

2. Radiation therapy is administered in fractionated (divided) doses to allow for regeneration of normal cells. Cancer cells do not regenerate as rapidly as normal cells.

3. There are many medications that can be prescribed for cancer or treatment-induced nausea. The client should notify the HCP if adequate relief is not obtained.

4. Cancer treatments frequently interfere with the client's appetite, but supporting the nutritional status of the client is important.

**TEST-TAKING HINT:** The question is an "except" question. All options except one (1) will be statements indicating the client does understand the teaching. If the test taker missed the information making this an "except" question, finding two (2) options with correct answers might clue the test taker to reread the stem.

45. 1. This is appropriate information if the client is in her mid-to-late 30s and has completed her family, but this is not discussing early detection of ovarian cancer.

2. A transvaginal ultrasound is a sonogram in which the sonogram probe is inserted into the vagina and sound waves are directed toward the ovaries. This positioning of the

probe is the closest that the probe can be made to the ovaries without surgical intervention. The CA-125 tumor marker is elevated in several cancers. It is nonspecific but coupled with the sonogram can provide information about ovarian cancer for early diagnosis.

3. Yearly MRI scans will not provide the information that the two (2) tests will and every 12 months is too long an interval.

4. A flexible sigmoidoscopy provides the HCP with a visual examination of the sigmoid colon, not the ovaries.

**TEST-TAKING HINT: The test taker could eliminate option "4" because of anatomical site and option "3" because of the time factor. The test taker should ask, "If looking for early detection, at what interval should the client see the HCP?"**

46. 1. This diet would be appropriate for a client diagnosed with diverticulitis.
    2. This diet would apply to a client with coronary artery disease and hypertension.
    3. The client is not placed on a specific diet, but it is always a good recommendation to include fruits and vegetables in the diet.
    4. There is no reason to limit the consistency of the foods consumed to full liquids.

**TEST-TAKING HINT: The test taker should recognize option "3" as a recommended diet for all clients without a specific disease process limiting the types of foods consumed.**

47. 1. Research has shown that the use of talcum powder perineally increases the risk for developing ovarian cancer, although there is no explanation known for this occurrence. Other risk factors include a high-fat diet, nulliparity, infertility, older age (70–80 years) has the greatest incidence), mumps before menarche, and family history of ovarian cancer.
    2. Nurses should never encourage a high-fat diet.
    3. Only clients in a high-risk category should have routine sonograms. The time frame for the high-risk group of clients is six (6) months. This is not primary intervention; early detection is secondary intervention.
    4. This would alert the client to participate in activities that would detect cancer early, a secondary intervention.

**TEST-TAKING HINT: The test taker could eliminate options "3" and "4" because of the word primary in the stem. Option "2" could be eliminated because of the recommendation of a high-fat diet.**

48. 1. All clients who have had surgery are at risk for developing deep vein thrombosis, and an enlarged, tender calf would be a sign of DVT.
    2. The client should be turned and encouraged to cough and deep breathe at least every two (2) hours.
    3. Clients who have had surgery should be assessed for pain on a pain scale and by observing for physiologic markers indicating pain.
    4. Sequential compression hose are used prophylactically to prevent deep vein thrombosis.
    5. The client should be assessed for the return of bowel sounds.

**TEST-TAKING HINT: Option "2" has a time frame in it, and the test taker should ask if the time frame is correct for the intervention.**

## Prostate Disorders

49. 1. The American Cancer Society recommends that all men have a yearly prostate specific antigen (PSA) blood level, followed by a digital rectal examination (DRE) beginning at age 50. Men in the high-risk group, including all African American men, should begin at age 45.
    2. A biannual (6 months) examination is not recommended.
    3. Alkaline phosphatase levels are performed on men with known prostate cancer to determine bone involvement. This is not a screening test.
    4. This test is done if the client has signs and symptoms of prostatitis.

**TEST-TAKING HINT: The nurse must be aware of recommended screening guidelines for a number of diseases. The test taker should carefully look at the time frame for the tests and the age of the client.**

50. 1. Urgency and frequency are obstructive symptoms and are late signs.
    2. Retrograde ejaculation occurs when the sperm is ejaculated into the urine; it occurs in some cases of male infertility.
    3. Low back pain and hip pain are symptoms of metastasis to the bone and are late symptoms.
    4. In early-stage prostate cancer, the man will not be aware of the disease. Early detection is achieved by screening for the cancer.

**TEST-TAKING HINT: The test taker should notice the word "early" in the stem of the question and choose the option with the least amount of symptoms.**

51. 1. Radiation therapy is considered aggressive therapy and would not be recommended for the elderly client unless needed to alleviate pain from bony metastasis.
    2. A radical prostatectomy with lymph node dissection is extensive surgery and only recommended for clients with a life expectancy of greater than ten (10) years.
    3. DES is a hormone preparation that suppresses the male hormones and slows the growth of the tumor. Some men with a life expectancy of less than ten (10) years choose not to treat the cancer at all and will die from causes other than prostate cancer.
    4. Penile implants do not treat prostate cancer. Sexual functioning may or may not be impaired, depending on whether the client is treated surgically by a radical prostatectomy. If so, then the client may be prescribed Viagra or Cialis. Eighty-year-old men would not be candidates for a radical prostatectomy.

    TEST-TAKING HINT: The test taker should notice the age of the client. When an age is provided in the question, it is significant. The elderly do not tolerate many treatments well, so the test taker should choose the least invasive treatment.

52. 1. The nurse should assess the client's normal voiding pattern before taking any action.
    2. This is a good intervention, but it comes after assessment.
    3. The Valsalva maneuver will help the client to empty the bladder, but assessment comes before teaching.
    4. Determining the client's normal voiding patterns provides a baseline for the nurse and client to use when setting goals.

    TEST-TAKING HINT: Assessment is the first step of the nursing process. In any question that requires the test taker to choose the first action, an answer option that says check, assess, or determine should be considered as a possible answer.

53. 1. Elevating a surgical site and applying ice will reduce edema to the area.
    2. The testes have been excised to remove the majority of male hormones. Replacing the hormones negates the purpose of the surgery.
    3. Sperm banking is encouraged for younger men who would like to father children. Prostate cancer is a cancer diagnosed in older men, and sperm banking is not normally recommended.
    4. Bilateral orchiectomy will render the client impotent but not with ejaculation dysfunction.

    TEST-TAKING HINT: The test taker should try to match the procedure to the answer option.

The procedure removes hormone-producing ability, so option "2" could be eliminated because it reverses the effects of the procedure.

54. 1. This hormone will suppress the production of male hormones, and the client will not function sexually as always.
    2. The client may have hot flashes because these drugs increase hypothalamic activity, which stimulates the thermoregulatory centers of the body.
    3. The medication decreases the growth rate of the cancer, but it does not cure the cancer.
    4. There are side effects with all medications. These medications can cause gynecomastia, hot flashes, cardiovascular effects, and decreased sexual functioning. The LHRH agonists have fewer side effects than the estrogens.

    TEST-TAKING HINT: The test taker could eliminate options "3" and "4" because of the promise of no side effects or a cure.

55. 1. This intervention addresses the prostate cancer but not the metastatic process of bony involvement.
    2. There is no reason to keep the foot of the bed elevated.
    3. Bone metastasis is very painful, and the client should be placed on a scheduled regimen of pain medication. Pain medication slows peristalsis and causes constipation. The client should be placed on a routine bowel management program to prevent impactions.
    4. This does not address the metastasis to the bone.

    TEST-TAKING HINT: The test taker must decide which intervention addresses both the cancer and the metastasis to the bone. Only one (1) option does this.

56. 1. Cryotherapy involves placing freezing probes into the prostate to freeze the cancer cells. An indwelling catheter is placed into the urethra, and warm water is circulated through the catheter to try to prevent the urethra from freezing. If the urethra scars, then the lumen will constrict, causing retention of urine.
    2. Ejaculation difficulties would be caused by obstruction from tumor growth.
    3. Bone marrow suppression is caused by radiation or chemotherapy.
    4. Cryotherapy does not cause chronic vomiting or diarrhea.

    TEST-TAKING HINT: The test taker should dissect the word cryotherapy. "Cryo" means "to freeze" so cryotherapy would indicate some form of cold therapy. Then decide what cold therapy could cause to happen in the area that is being treated.

57. 1. Pain does not have priority over a fluid and electrolyte imbalance.
    2. There is no dressing for a transurethral resection. The body cavity is entered through the penis.
    3. Early ambulation prevents several complications, but the immediate complication is electrolyte imbalance and fluid overload.
    4. With irrigation of the surgical site through the indwelling three (3)-way catheter to prevent blood clots, fluids may be absorbed through the open surgical site and retained. This can lead to fluid volume overload and electrolyte imbalance (hyponatremia).

    **TEST-TAKING HINT: This client is eight (8) hours postoperative, so the test taker could eliminate preventing DVT option "3." Option "2" could be eliminated if the test taker looks at the surgical approach described in the procedure. Pain is a priority, but the test taker should read to see if another option has a higher priority.**

58. 200 mL/hour. IV pumps work on the principle of number of milliliters per hour to infuse, and, unless otherwise specified, IVPB medications are infused over a 30-minute time frame. Sixty (60) minutes in one (1) hour divided by 30 = 2. Two (2) times the volume of 100 mL = 200 mL, the rate the nurse should set the pump

    **TEST-TAKING HINT: The test taker must know basic rules for medication administration and be able to compute simple math equations.**

59. 1. The nurse should never ask "why." The client does not owe the nurse an explanation.
    2. The question asks for a therapeutic response from the nurse. This response is restating and clarifying.
    3. This is dismissive to the client's feelings and appears to agree with the client. There is no evidence that cancer of the prostate is caused by promiscuous behavior.
    4. This is a problem-solving statement and does not address the client's feelings.

    **TEST-TAKING HINT: Because the question is asking for a therapeutic response, the test taker should address the client's feelings. However, the test taker should not use this test-taking hint as an absolute because each question should be answered on its own merit.**

60. 1. This is a psychosocial problem.

2. This is a physiological problem.
3. This problem has both physiological and psychosocial implications.
4. This is a physiological problem.

**TEST-TAKING HINT: The test taker should read the stem carefully. The stem asks for a physiological and psychosocial problem. Options "1," "2," and "4" can be sorted into only one of the categories.**

## Testicular Disorders

61. 1. The body temperature should be warm for the scrotum to relax. The best place to perform testicular self-examination is in a warm to hot shower.
    2. The client may note a cordlike structure; this is the spermatic cord and is normal. Any lump or mass felt is abnormal and should be checked by an HCP as soon as possible.
    3. The client can confirm his own negative result; a negative result is no masses felt.
    4. The procedure is painless. If pain is elicited, then an HCP should examine the client. Cancer is usually painless; the presence of pain may indicate an infection.

    **TEST-TAKING HINT: The test taker might choose option "2" as an answer because any abnormality should be examined by an HCP.**

62. 1. The usual treatment for testicular cancer is removal of the involved testicle followed by radiation to the area and chemotherapy. Every attempt is made to shield the remaining testicle from the radiation, but sterility sometimes occurs.
    2. With artificial insemination the client may be able to father children, if the client has banked his sperm.
    3. Sperm banking will allow the client to father children through artificial insemination with the client's sperm.
    4. The nurse is in the client's room. The client's presence implies consent for the nurse to discuss his case with the fiancée.

    **TEST-TAKING HINT: The nurse must abide by HIPAA rules. It is important for the nurse to know and understand the confidentiality laws. The answer options "1" and "2" are opposites so only one could be correct or neither may be correct. Option "3" actually gives an option that lies between the extremes.**

63. 1. The client usually will be able to maintain normal sexual functioning with the remaining

testicle. If not, testosterone may be prescribed to improve functioning. Ejaculation is not the problem. It would be impotence (erectile dysfunction).

2. This will not be done until the HCP determines that the remaining testicle is not able to maintain adequate hormone production.

3. The client will be able to function sexually with the remaining testicle alone or with prescribed male hormones.

4. Sex drive (libido) and orgasms usually are unimpaired because the client still has one testicle.

**TEST-TAKING HINT:** The key to this question is unilateral. The client will still have one testicle that should function and preserve the client's sexual functioning.

64. 1. Epididymitis is inflammation of the epididymis, usually caused by bacteria descending from the prostate or bladder. This does not increase the risk of developing cancer of the testes.

2. Cryptorchidism is the medical term for undescended testicle. The testicles may be in the abdomen or inguinal canal at birth. This condition places the client at high risk for testicular cancer.

3. Prostate enlargement occurs as men age, whereas the most common age range for testicular cancer is age 15–35.

4. Hypospadias is a congenital abnormality in which the urethral meatus is on the underside of the penis. This does not increase the risk for cancer.

**TEST-TAKING HINT:** This is a knowledge-based question, but answer options "3" and "4" could be eliminated based on anatomical position.

65. 1. The scrotum will require support during ambulation. An athletic supporter is designed to provide support in this area.

2. The client should be encouraged to take pain medications before the pain is at a high level to help the pain medication be more effective.

3. The client can be on a regular diet as soon as the client is not nauseated from the anesthesia.

4. This surgery does not increase bleeding times.

**TEST-TAKING HINT:** Answer option "2" can be eliminated because it states the opposite of the instructions given to clients about pain medication.

66. 1. Increasing the drip rate on a continuous bladder (Murphy) irrigation requires nursing judgment and cannot be delegated.

2. In this situation, checking for infection is an assessment situation. The nurse cannot delegate assessment.

3. The unlicensed assistive personnel can be asked to help a client turn, cough, and deep breathe. This requires the assistant to perform an action only, not to use judgment or assess.

4. Red drainage in the catheter implies bleeding. The nurse should assess the amount of bleeding that is occurring.

**TEST-TAKING HINT:** The test taker should choose the lowest level activity when choosing an action to have unlicensed personnel to perform. Blood should always be assessed.

67. 1. Chlamydia is a sexually transmitted disease that is usually silent in the male partner but can cause epididymitis. If both sexual partners are not treated, then the partner can reinfect the client.

2. Sexual intercourse can be resumed within a couple of weeks as long as both partners have been treated for the infection.

3. This would indicate a urinary tract infection, one that has not resolved. A UTI is another cause of epididymitis.

4. The scrotum is a closed cavity. There should not be any drainage from the scrotum. If there is drainage, this could indicate a fistula and require immediate notification of the HCP.

**TEST-TAKING HINT:** The test taker should always look at the time frame provided in either the stem or the answer option as a clue to answering the question correctly. The test taker should look very closely at any option that has a "month" time frame.

68. 1. Pain when urinating indicates a urinary tract infection.

2. A chancre sore on the shaft of the penis indicates syphilis, a sexually transmitted disease.

3. Classic signs of cancer of the testes are a mass on the testicle, painless enlargement of the testes, and heaviness of the scrotum or lower abdomen.

4. There is no rash associated with cancer of the testes.

**TEST-TAKING HINT:** The test taker could eliminate option "2" because the penis and testes are separate body parts. The testicles lie within the scrotum. Only one (1) option concerns that part of the body.

69. 1. The nurse should not impose any personal religious beliefs on the client.

2. Testicular cancers have very good prog-

noses, and even if the tumor returns, there is a good prognosis for extended survival.
3. There is a great deal of hope to offer these clients.
4. This is giving the client incorrect information.

**TEST-TAKING HINT: This is a question in which the test taker must know the information. Rarely would a nurse give a specific percentage of survival.**

70. 1. CA-125 is a tumor marker that is used for a number of cancers but not for testicular cancer.
2. CEA is a nonspecific tumor marker that is used for a number of cancers, but it does not apply to testicular cancer.
3. The DNA ploidy test is used to determine the number of chromosomes and arrangement of chromosomes in a tumor cell. It is used for prognosis in some cancers, such as breast cancer, but not as a tumor marker to determine response to treatment.
4. **Tumor markers are substances synthesized by the tumor and released into the bloodstream. They can be used to follow the progress of the disease. Testicular cancers secrete HCG and alpha-fetoprotein.**

**TEST-TAKING HINT: This is a knowledge-based question. If the test taker were aware of what the test tells the HCP, then the DNA ploidy test could be eliminated. The other options are all tumor markers.**

71. 1. **This information could signal the onset of symptoms of metastasis to the retroperitoneum. The HCP should see the client and discuss follow-up diagnostic tests.**
2. This information should be investigated and not put off.
3. This may or may not have occurred. Only diagnostic tests can confirm metastasis.
4. Low back exercises will not help the client if this is metastatic cancer, and they could increase the pain.

**TEST-TAKING HINT: The nurse cannot diagnose the client with metastasis, so option "3" can be eliminated. As a rule, any pain unrelieved with pain medication would require the client to see the HCP.**

72. 1. This should be done for clients who have had scrotal surgery.
2. Postoperative clients do not want to perform deep breathing and coughing exercises because it hurts, but they should be encouraged to do so to prevent complications.
3. The Jackson-Pratt (J-P) drain is a drain attached to a bulb, and the bulb should

remain compressed to apply gentle suction to the surgical site.
4. This is appropriate delegation.

**TEST-TAKING HINT: The test taker could eliminate "4" by knowing the rules of delegation. The nurse did not ask the assistant to perform anything that requires nursing judgment or assessment. Option "2" is just good nursing practice and could be eliminated. The charge nurse would not need to stop this action.**

## Sexually Transmitted Diseases

73. 1. **Engaging in oral and anal sex increases the risk of contracting an STD.**
2. Using a sterile needle for drug abuse does ensure that the client will not get an STD from needle sharing, but the client can still contract an STD from other risky behaviors.
3. **The more sexual partners, the greater the risk for contracting an STD.**
4. Condom use provides a barrier to contracting an STD, but it is not a guarantee. The condom can break or come off during intercourse.

**TEST-TAKING HINT: In answer option "2" the word "guarantees" appears, and the nurse cannot guarantee anything in dealing with health-care issues. Option "4" is an absolute statement—"will not get"—and can be eliminated on this basis.**

74. 1. This is a true statement, but it does not answer the client's question.
2. **Untreated HPV infection is a cause for developing cancer of the cervix.**
3. HPV infection does not invade the abdominal cavity and therefore would not cause ovarian cancer.
4. The Pap test was developed to note early cell changes in the cervix. It indirectly monitors the effects of HPV, but it does not help prevent problems.

**TEST-TAKING HINT: The test taker should choose the answer for the question that the client is asking. Option "1" discusses transmission and option "4" discusses prevention; therefore, these two (2) options could be eliminated based on the stem of the question.**

75. 1. **These are signs of second-stage syphilis. The nurse should ask about the development of a chancre sore, one of the first signs of a syphilis infection.**
2. This may be required of the public health nurse for notification of the partners, but it is not required to assess this problem.

3. This client does not need a dermatologist to determine an STD infection. The HCP can treat this infection.

4. A urine culture will not diagnose this disease.

**TEST-TAKING HINT: If the test taker was aware that the symptoms are those of an STD, options "3" and "4" can be eliminated.**

76. 1. All socioeconomic levels of clients contract STDs.

2. The longer the client abstains from sexual activity and the fewer partners the client has, the less the risk of an STD.

3. Females and males can spread STDs equally. Specific diseases may be asymptomatic in the sexes (in females, gonorrhea; in males, chlamydia) and they can transmit them unknowingly.

4. If the client has one STD, there is a great likelihood that the client has another disease also. If one STD is found, the client should be monitored for others.

**TEST-TAKING HINT: Answer option "2" does not make sense: if sexual activity is put off, there cannot be an increased risk. Socioeconomic reasons may be a reason for delaying treatment of a disease but diseases are not financially based and occur in all socioeconomic levels.**

77. 1. Chlamydia does not cause an antigen/antibody reaction.

2. There are long-term problems associated with any STD. Chlamydia may have the long-term effects of chronic pain and increased risk for ectopic pregnancy, postpartum endometritis, and infertility.

3. If both the client and the sexual partner are not treated simultaneously, the sexual partner can reinfect the client.

4. The client may develop chronic pelvic pain as a result of the infection.

**TEST-TAKING HINT: Options "2" and "4" have a form of absolute. The words "any," "will," or "will not" are absolutes and in health care, there are very few absolutes.**

78. 1. A chancre sore is a symptom of syphilis, not gonorrhea.

2. Gonorrhea is more likely to be asymptomatic in females.

3. A CD4 count of less than 200 is a diagnostic indictor for acquired immune deficiency syndrome (AIDS).

4. Pain in the testes and scrotal edema can indicate epididymitis, an inflammatory process of the epididymis. This and urethritis are the most common presenting symptoms of a male with gonorrhea.

**TEST-TAKING HINT: Two (2) answer options mention male anatomy. If the test taker did not know the information, then choosing between these two (2) options might be the appropriate method of elimination.**

79. 1. Pelvic inflammatory disease (PID) does not have to be reported, but the cause of the PID may need to be reported.

2. There are causes for epididymitis other than an STD.

3. Syphilis is an STD and therefore must be reported to the appropriate health department.

4. An ectopic pregnancy may have numerous causes.

**TEST-TAKING HINT: Only one (1) answer option is an STD. The other diseases/conditions may be caused by STDs, but they all have other causes as well.**

80. 1. Determining and diagnosing the risk for infertility problems requires collaboration between the nurse and the HCP.

2. The nurse is required to teach a client. This is an independent action.

3. Fluid volume deficit is not an appropriate nursing diagnosis for the client.

4. Noncompliance is an independent nursing problem.

**TEST-TAKING HINT: The question requires the test taker to determine which are autonomous functions of the nurse. The nurse does not have the capability to prescribe fertility medications or treatments.**

81. 1. Vaginal cultures are obtained to assess for gonorrhea and chlamydia.

2. The RPR test and the Venereal Disease Research Laboratory (VDRL) test are diagnostic tests for syphilis.

3. Gram stains of the vagina or urethral meatus of a male may be done for gonorrhea but not for syphilis.

4. An immunologic assay may be done for chlamydia but not for syphilis.

**TEST-TAKING HINT: The test taker must memorize the tests used to diagnose specific STDs and the symptoms that differentiate one STD from another.**

82. 1. Lymphadenopathy and hair loss are symptoms of secondary syphilis, not tertiary syphilis.

2. Genital warts are not signs of tertiary syphilis.
3. Aortitis and neurosyphilis (dementia, psychosis, stroke, paresis, and meningitis) are the most common manifestations of tertiary syphilis.
4. A rash covering the body is a symptom of gonorrhea.

**TEST-TAKING HINT:** The key word in this question is "tertiary." The test taker must decide which disease has three (3) distinct phases and then which symptoms accompany each phase.

83. 1. The public health nurse is responsible for attempting to notify sexual partners of a client diagnosed with an STD of a potential infection and urging the partner to be tested for the disease and to receive treatment. Health departments offer confidential testing and treatment.
2. An HCP will determine the course of treatment for a client diagnosed with an STD.
3. The nurse can teach some information about reporting, but the nurse is not qualified to discuss all the legal aspects of reporting an STD.

4. The nurse is not responsible for analyzing statistics.

**TEST-TAKING HINT: Answer options "2," "3," and "4" ask the nurse to take on roles that are not within the nurse's expertise. The nurse must know the Nursing Practice Act of the state where the nurse practices. No state allows the nurse to give legal or medical advice.**

84. 1. An odorless, white, curdlike vaginal discharge is a symptom of *Candida albicans*, a vaginal yeast infection.
2. A strawberry spot on the vaginal wall or cervix, a fishy-smelling vaginal discharge, and itching are symptoms of trichomonas.
3. Scant white vaginal discharge and dyspareunia are symptoms of atrophic vaginitis.
4. Purulent discharge from the endocervix and pelvic pain are symptoms of cervicitis.

**TEST-TAKING HINT: When studying for a test that covers similar diseases, the test taker should concentrate on the information that makes one different from another. Only one STD has a characteristic strawberry spot.**

Reproductive

1. The nurse is reviewing the lab data on a male client. Which interpretation should the nurse make regarding the prostate-specific antigen (PSA)?
   1. The client has early-stage prostate cancer.
   2. The client should have more tests.
   3. The client does not have prostate cancer.
   4. The client has benign prostatic hypertrophy.

| Laboratory Test | Client Value | Normal Value |
| --- | --- | --- |
| Prostate-specific antigen | 6 mcg/L | Male <4 mcg/L<br>Female <0.5 mcg/L |

2. The nurse is performing the admission assessment on a 78-year-old female client and observes bilateral pendulous breasts with a stringy appearance. Which intervention should the nurse implement?
   1. Request a mammogram.
   2. Notify the HCP of the finding.
   3. Continue with the examination.
   4. Assess for *peau d'orange* skin.

3. The client is scheduled for a right breast biopsy for a mass found in the tail of Spence. While the client is waiting in the holding area, the client asks the nurse, "Which lymph nodes will my surgeon take from my body?" Which area should the nurse identify?
   1. A
   2. B
   3. C
   4. D

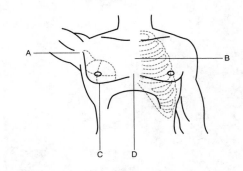

4. The client is diagnosed with left mastitis. Which assessment findings would the nurse observe?
   1. Dimpling of the left breast when the client raises the arm.
   2. A round lump in the left breast that is tender during menses.
   3. A dull pain in the left breast and tough, doughy-feeling skin.
   4. Bloody discharge from the nipple and a hard palpable mass.

5. The client has a diagnosis of rule out Paget's disease. Which test provides a definitive diagnosis of the disease?
   1. A breast biopsy.
   2. A diagnostic mammogram.
   3. Ultrasound of the breast.
   4. Magnetic resonance imaging (MRI).

6. The nurse in the gynecology clinic is assessing the 50-year-old client who has had four (4) children and is complaining of having lower abdominal pressure and fatigue along with some urinary incontinence. Which instruction should the nurse teach the client?
   1. Wear a peri-pad to keep from having an accident.
   2. Try not to laugh or sneeze unless at home.
   3. Discuss the pros and cons of a vaginal hysterectomy.
   4. Instruct to perform Kegel exercises.

7. The client is diagnosed with a rectovaginal fistula that is to be managed medically. Which information would the nurse teach the client prior to discharge?
   1. Douche with normal saline.
   2. Eat a low-residue diet.
   3. Keep ice packs to the area.
   4. Use an abdominal binder.

8. The client has an infected Bartholin's cyst and the HCP has performed an incision and drainage (I & D) of the area. Which discharge instructions should the nurse teach the client?
   1. Complete all antibiotics as ordered.
   2. Report any drainage immediately.
   3. Keep all water away from the area.
   4. Lie prone as much as possible.

9. The client is diagnosed with vulvar cancer. Which are the most common symptoms of cancer of the vulva?
   1. Red, painful lesions.
   2. Vulvar itching.
   3. Thin, white vulvar skin.
   4. Vaginal dryness.

10. The nurse is teaching a class to older women concerning cancer of the uterus. Which situation is a risk factor for developing endometrial cancer?
    1. Age 40 years or younger.
    2. Perimenopausal bleeding.
    3. Progesterone given with estrogen.
    4. Truncal obesity.

11. The nurse is caring for a client diagnosed with uterine cancer who has received after-load intracavitary radiation. Which precaution should the nurse implement?
    1. Wear rubber gloves to prevent the nurse from all exposure.
    2. Allow any visitor that the client wishes to see.
    3. Minimize the amount of time spent with the client.
    4. Encourage the client to ambulate in the hallway.

12. The nurse is caring for client A, who is postoperative after a breast biopsy. The pathology report is posted on the chart. Which statement is the interpretation of the DNA ploidy pathology report?
    1. This is stage IV breast cancer with a poor prognosis.
    2. The cancer will respond to hormonal therapy.
    3. The chromosomes do not resemble normal human DNA.
    4. The client should have a mastectomy as soon as possible.

---

**Client A**                                **Client Number 001234567**

---

A 0.5- × 1.2-cm specimen of tissue from the right breast was examined under a microscope. Margins were not clear. Tissue sample indicates high-grade invasive ductal cell carcinoma. DNA ploidy by flow cytometry reveals aneuploid characteristics.

Findings: Invasive ductal cell carcinoma of the right breast with aneuploid findings.

---

13. The nurse is discharging a client diagnosed with pelvic inflammatory disease (PID). Which statement by the client indicates an understanding of the discharge instructions?
    1. "I should expect pelvic pain after intercourse."
    2. "I need to douche every day to prevent PID."
    3. "I will have a vaginal exam every two (2) years."
    4. "My partner should use a condom if he is infectious."

14. The client has failed to conceive after many attempts over a three (3)-year time period and asks the nurse, "I have tried everything. What should I do now?" Which statement is the nurse's best response?
    1. "By 'everything' do you mean you have consulted an infertility specialist?"
    2. "You have tried everything. This must be hard for you. Would you like to talk?"
    3. "You should get on an adoption list because it can take a long time."
    4. "You need to relax and not try so hard. It is your nerves preventing conception."

15. The nurse writes a problem of "potential for complications related to ovarian hyper-stimulation" for a client who is taking clomiphene (Clomid), an ovarian stimulant. Which intervention should be included in the plan of care?
    1. Instruct the client to delay intercourse until menses.
    2. Schedule the client for frequent pelvic sonograms.
    3. Explain that the infusion therapy will take 21 days.
    4. Discuss that this may cause an ectopic pregnancy.

16. The HCP care provider orders cultures of the urethral urine, bladder urine, and prostatic fluid. Which instructions would the nurse teach to achieve the first two (2) specimens?
    1. Collect the first 15 mL in one jar and then the next 50 mL in another.
    2. Collect three (3) early-morning, clean voided urine specimens.
    3. Collect the specimens after the HCP massages the prostate.
    4. Collect a routine urine specimen for analysis.

17. The nurse writes a client problem of "anxiety related to potential sexual dysfunction" for a client diagnosed with cancer of the prostate. Which intervention should the nurse implement?
    1. Tell the client to discuss his fears with the HCP.
    2. Talk to the wife about the client's concerns.
    3. Inform the client that sexual functioning will not be altered.
    4. Provide a private area for the client to discuss his concerns.

18. The male client is considering a vasectomy for birth control. Which information should the nurse teach the client?
    1. Instruct the client to use hot packs to relieve scrotal edema after the surgery.
    2. Tell the client to wear loose-fitting boxer underwear after the surgery.
    3. Explain that initially an alternate form of birth control will be required.
    4. Discuss that potency will be diminished about 20% after a vasectomy.

19. The 45-year-old male client has had a circumcision secondary to phimosis. Which intervention should the nurse include in the plan of care?
    1. Teach how to care for the glans to prevent recurrence of the phimosis.
    2. Assess for pain on a scale of one (1) to ten (10).
    3. Perform wet to dry dressing changes daily.
    4. Instruct client to perform a monthly penis check for cancer.

20. Which vaccination would the nurse recommend to the postpubertal male to prevent orchitis?
    1. Yearly flu injections.
    2. Herpes varicella inoculations.
    3. Mumps vaccination.
    4. Rubella injections.

21. The nurse is instructing a group of workers at an industrial plant regarding the trans-mission of sexually transmitted diseases (STDs). Which information should be included in the presentation?
    1. The same behaviors that cause one STD could lead to another.
    2. Once clients have had an STD, they develop immunity to it.
    3. An infection with syphilis protects the client from being infected with HIV.
    4. Herpes simplex I is a totally different disease from herpes simplex II.

22. The male client complains of mucuslike drainage from the rectum accompanied by rectal pain and diarrhea. Which interview question should the nurse ask the client?
    1. "Do you have difficulty trying to urinate?"
    2. "Have you had rectal sexual intercourse?"
    3. "Do you eat a high-fiber diet and drink lots of fluids?"
    4. "Does the diarrhea alternate with constipation?"

23. The client is diagnosed with primary syphilis. Which symptoms would the nurse observe?
    1. A chancre sore in the perineal area.
    2. A rash on the trunk and extremities.
    3. Blistering of the palms of the hands.
    4. Confusion and disorientation.

24. The nurse is discussing pelvic floor exercises with a client. Which information should the nurse teach?
    1. Perform the exercises four (4) times per day.
    2. The exercises will prevent stress incontinence.
    3. Contract the perineal muscles and hold for ten (10) seconds.
    4. Contract the abdominal and buttock muscles to increase strength.

25. The county health department nurse is reviewing a client record and notes the RPR laboratory results. Which question should the nurse ask the client?
    1. "When was your last tetanus shot?"
    2. "Have you had a cold recently?'
    3. "Do you have diabetes mellitus?"
    4. "Are you allergic to penicillin?"

| Laboratory Test | Client Result | Normal Finding |
|---|---|---|
| Rapid plasma reagin (RPR) | Reactive for *Treponema pallidum* | Nonreactive |

26. The nurse is teaching a class on Breast Health Awareness. Which are the American Cancer Society's recommended guidelines for the performance of self-breast examination (BSE)? List in order of recommended performance.
    1. Visualize the breast from the front while standing before a mirror.
    2. Gently squeeze the nipple to express any fluid.
    3. Turn to each side and view each breast in the mirror.
    4. Palpate each breast in a circular motion while lying on the back.
    5. Palpate each breast in a circular motion while in the shower.

1. 1. The client may have cancer of the prostate, but this test does not provide conclusive results. There are several reasons for the PSA to be elevated, not just cancer.
   2. The PSA is elevated and more tests should be completed to determine the cause. PSA levels are increased in benign prostatic hypertrophy, urinary retention, prostatic infarct, and prostate cancer.
   3. Cancer cannot be eliminated as a diagnosis until other tests have been completed.
   4. This may be the actual diagnosis, but the client should undergo more tests to confirm a diagnosis.

2. 1. These are normal findings in a postmenopausal breast and would not require a mammogram. The woman should have a mammogram yearly.
   2. These are normal findings in the postmenopausal breast so there is no need to notify the HCP.
   3. These are normal findings in the postmenopausal breast. Glandular tissue is replaced with fibrous tissue, the breasts become pendulous, and the Cooper's ligaments become prominent.
   4. *Peau d'orange* skin occurs in advanced breast cancer.

3. 1. The tail of Spence is the upper outermost part of the breast, which would extend toward the arm. The most likely lymph nodes to biopsy are the axillary nodes.
   2. This is the mediastinal node area, which is on the opposite side of the breast.
   3. The internal mammary nodes are under the breast, and the tail of Spence is at the top of the breast.
   4. The parasternal nodes are on the opposite side of the breast from the tail of Spence.

4. 1. Dimpling of the breast indicates a tumor that has attached itself to the chest wall.
   2. This would indicate fibrocystic changes in the left breast.
   3. Mastitis is an infection of the breast occurring most often in women who are lactating. The breast becomes red and warm to touch. The skin becomes doughy and tough in consistency, and the client develops a dull pain in the affected breast.
   4. Bloody discharge indicates a tumor, benign or malignant.

5. 1. Biopsy of the lesion is the only definitive test for Paget's disease, a form of breast cancer that accounts for about 1% of all breast cancers.
   2. Mammography is the only diagnostic test that routinely screens for breast cancer, but a definitive diagnosis is made by tissue identification.
   3. Ultrasound of the breasts can diagnose fluid-filled cysts.
   4. MRIs can be done to determine the extent of tumor involvement, but tissue identification is the definitive test for tumor diagnosis.

6. 1. The client would have determined the need for protection without the nurse having to tell her to do so.
   2. It is unrealistic to tell a client not to laugh or sneeze.
   3. The client probably has a cystocele resulting from childbirth. The corrective surgical repair would be a bladder suspension.
   4. Kegel exercises help to strengthen the pelvic muscles. They are recommended for all women and should be performed 30–80 times per day.

7. 1. Cleansing douches are prescribed with tepid water, not normal saline.
   2. Measures to assist the client to heal without surgical interventions include proper nutrition with a low-residue diet to minimize contamination of the tissues with feces, cleansing douches, enemas, and rest.
   3. Warm perineal irrigations and controlled heat-lamp applications promote healing; ice would vasoconstrict the area and delay wound healing.
   4. The client should wear perineal pads but not an abdominal binder.

8. 1. The client has an infection and should complete the ordered antibiotics.
   2. The client should be taught to expect some drainage from the area because the area has been opened to allow for exudate to escape the body.
   3. Routine hygiene is encouraged.
   4. The client can assume any position of comfort.

9. 1. Red, painful lesions are symptoms of lichen planus, which is a benign, although uncomfortable, lesion.
   2. Cancer of the vulva may be asymptomatic, but the client usually presents with persistent long-term itching.
   3. Thin, white vulvar skin indicates lichen sclerosis.
   4. Vaginal dryness is not associated with cancer of the vulva.

10. 1. Clients at risk for uterine cancer are usually 55 years old or older.
    2. Postmenopausal bleeding places the client at risk, but perimenopausal bleeding is expected as the ovaries begin to slow production of eggs.
    3. Unopposed estrogen replacement therapy predisposes women to developing uterine cancer, but progesterone offsets the risk.
    4. **Truncal obesity is one of the risk factors for developing endometrial cancer, although it has not been determined how this occurs.**

11. 1. Rubber gloves should be worn to dispose of any soiled material, but they will not protect the nurse from sealed radiation sources.
    2. Visitors who may be pregnant or who are younger than 18 years old should not be allowed in the client's room.
    3. **Afterload intracavitary radiation therapy treatments are completed in the client's room after prepared applicators are placed in surgery. This minimizes exposure of the health-care workers to radiation. The nurse should plan care to minimize exposure to the client and the radiation.**
    4. The client is placed in a room at the far end of the hallway, and in some facilities clients on either side of the client's room may have to be moved to limit exposure to radiation. The client is not allowed to leave the room until the radiation safety department clears the client for discharge.

12. 1. Staging for breast cancer is completed using a variety of measurements, including size of the tumor and metastasis sites, but staging does not involve the DNA characteristics.
    2. The DNA ploidy tests are performed to determine the response to all types of treatments. The more the cell represents normal human DNA pairings (euploid), the better the prognosis for the client.
    3. **Aneuploid means the cells do not have human pairing characteristics. This finding indicates that the cells cannot be expected to respond as normal human cells would respond and the prognosis is not good for the client.**
    4. The choice of surgical approach is determined between the client and HCP. The tumor should be removed with enough tissue to have clear margins. Whether the client chooses a modified radical mastectomy, lumpectomy, or wedge resection depends on the choice of follow-up treatment.

13. 1. Any pelvic pain after sexual exposure, childbirth, or pelvic surgery should be evaluated as soon as possible.
    2. Douching reduces the natural flora that combats infecting organisms and may help infecting bacteria move upward into the uterus, but douching will not prevent PID.
    3. The client should have a vaginal exam at least once a year.
    4. **The client and partner should consistently use a condom if there is any chance of transmission of any organism.**

14. 1. **The nurse should investigate which fertility measures have been attempted. There are many reasons for infertility, and only a specialist in the area can identify the cause.**
    2. This is a therapeutic response, but the client is asking for information.
    3. This is advising and not answering the client's question.
    4. The nurse cannot know this to be true, and this does not address the client's concern.

15. 1. Clomid is begun on the fifth day of the menstrual cycle and is taken for five (5) days; ovulation should occur four (4) to eight (8) days after that—approximately from day nine (9) to day 13 of the cycle. Intercourse should be planned for the optimum chance of conception.
    2. **Frequent sonograms are needed to monitor follicular stimulation. The ovaries are monitored to prevent overstimulation, which can cause ascites, pleural effusions, and acute respiratory distress syndrome (ARDS).**
    3. Clomid is not given by infusion. GnRH, gonadotropin-releasing hormone, is given by infusion.
    4. Ovarian stimulation does not cause ectopic pregnancy.

16. 1. **After cleansing the penis and retracting the foreskin (if present) the client voids the first 15 mL in a sterile specimen cup; this is the urethral urine specimen. Then, the client voids the next 50–75 mL into another sterile specimen cup; this is the bladder urine. If the client does not have acute prostatitis, the HCP can massage the prostate and collect prostate fluid for culture, but if fluid is not expressed with massage, the next urine is sent for analysis.**
    2. Early morning has no bearing on collecting prostatitis specimens.
    3. This would be the third specimen and is obtained by the HCP.

4. A routine specimen will not provide the information needed.

17. 1. This is not an appropriate referral. The nurse should discuss the client's fears.
    2. The wife may need to be encouraged to talk about her concerns, but this does not address the client's concerns.
    3. The client's sexual functioning may be impaired depending on the treatment options chosen.
    4. **Because the client may be sensitive and embarrassed about discussing problems related to genitalia and sexual functioning, the nurse should provide a private area in which to discuss these concerns.**

18. 1. Ice packs, not hot packs, should be applied after surgery to reduce edema.
    2. The client should wear cotton, jockey-type underwear to provide support and added comfort.
    3. **The client will not be sterile until the sperm stored distal to the surgery site in the tubules have been ejaculated or reabsorbed by the body. Therefore, an alternate form of birth control is needed for a certain period of time following the vasectomy.**
    4. There is no effect on the client's potency after a bilateral vasectomy.

19. 1. Phimosis is a tightness of the prepuce of the penis that prevents retraction of the foreskin over the glans. Once the foreskin has been surgically removed, this is not a problem.
    2. **There is considerable pain after an adult circumcision, and the nurse should assess for the pain.**
    3. A petroleum-saturated gauze is wrapped around the penis, not a wet to dry dressing.
    4. Circumcision in infancy may prevent cancer of the penis. The older client who has a circumcision should be aware of the potential for cellular changes, but the risk is greatly reduced after the surgery.

20. 1. The flu vaccine will not prevent orchitis.
    2. This is the chickenpox vaccine and will not prevent orchitis.
    3. **When postpubertal males contract mumps, one (1) in five (5) develops some form of orchitis (infection of the testes) within four (4) to seven (7) days after the neck and jaw swell. The testes may show atrophy after the infection, and the client may become sterile.**
    4. Rubella, measles, does not cause orchitis.

21. 1. **The behaviors that led to the development of one STD could also lead to the development of another.**
    2. There is no antigen/antibody reaction development with STDs. A client can be reinfected multiple times.
    3. There is no protection provided by one STD from developing another, and frequently clients will have more than one STD simultaneously.
    4. Herpes simplex I and herpes simplex II are the same virus; I is transmitted to the genitalia through oral sex; II is transmitted through sexual intercourse.

22. 1. The client has rectal symptoms, not urinary tract symptoms.
    2. **The client has described symptoms of proctitis, inflammation of the rectum. Proctitis is commonly associated with anal-receptive intercourse with an infected partner. The pathogens most frequently associated with proctitis are gonorrhea, chlamydia, herpes simplex, and *Treponema pallidum*.**
    3. A high-fiber diet would not cause these symptoms.
    4. Diarrhea alternating with constipation would indicate a possible rectal tumor and would not cause these symptoms

23. 1. **A chancre sore on the perineal area is a symptom of primary syphilis.**
    2. A rash on the trunk and extremities occurs in secondary syphilis.
    3. Blistering of the palms of the hand occurs in secondary syphilis.
    4. Tertiary syphilis occurs over a prolonged period and includes symptoms of dementia, psychosis, paresis, stroke, and meningitis.

24. 1. Pelvic floor exercises (Kegel) should be performed 30–80 times per day.
    2. The exercises will help reduce stress incontinence, but they may not relieve all stress incontinence.
    3. **Perineal muscles should be contracted and held for ten (10) seconds followed by ten (10) seconds of rest.**
    4. The pelvic floor muscles are contracted without contracting the abdominal, buttock, or inner-thigh muscles.

25. 1. This is a test for syphilis and does not require a tetanus injection.
    2. Having a cold does not affect the diagnosis of syphilis.
    3. Diabetes places a client at risk for many ill-

nesses, but sexual behavior would place the client at risk for a sexually transmitted disease.

4. The test is positive for syphilis, and the nurse would anticipate the HCP ordering an antibiotic; penicillin is the antibiotic of choice for syphilis. Syphilis is caused by the *Treponema pallidum* bacteria.

26. The order should be: 1, 3, 5, 4, 2.

1. The first step in BSE is to visualize the breasts for symmetry while looking at a frontal view before the mirror.

3. The next step is to turn from side to side, looking for any dimpling, puckering, or asymmetry, in front of a mirror.

5. The client should palpate the breasts in a warm shower with the breasts soaped to allow for the fingers to glide over the breast tissue.

4. After the shower the client should lie on the bed with a towel rolled up and placed under the shoulder to flatten the breast tissue and palpate the breast.

2. The last step in BSE is to gently squeeze the nipple to determine if there is fluid that can be expressed.

# 11

# Musculoskeletal Disorders

Musculoskeletal injuries and disorders are common. Many, such as fractures, result from accidents; others, such as osteoarthritis, osteoporosis, and joint replacement, are often associated with the aging process; and still others, such as amputation, may result as a complication of a specific disease process such as diabetes. Nurses must know how to assess these clients, when to notify the health-care providers, and how to carry out the proper procedures and administer the medications ordered.

## KEYWORDS

abduction
avulsion
collaborative
comminuted
compound
degenerative
epiphyseal
greenstick
herniated nucleus pulposus
impacted
laminectomy
oblique
paresthesia
pathologic
primary care
prostheses
rhinitis
secondary care
tertiary care

## ABBREVIATIONS

Above the Knee Amputation (AKA)
Activated Partial Thromboplastin Time (aPTT)
Activities of Daily Living (ADL)
Below the Knee Amputation (BKA)
Blood Pressure (BP)
Computed Tomography (CT)
Continuous Passive Motion (CPM)
Erythrocyte Sedimentation Rate (ESR)
Health-Care Provider (HCP)
Immediately (STAT)
Intravenous (IV)
Intravenous Pyelogram (IVP)
Magnetic Resonance Imaging (MRI)
Nonsteroidal Anti-Inflammatory Drugs (NSAIDs)
Nursing Assistant (NA)
Osteoarthritis (OA)
Patient Controlled Analgesic (PAC)
Rule Out (R/O)
Total Hip Replacement (THR)
Total Knee Replacement (TKR)
When Required, As Needed (PRN)

### Degenerative/Herniated Disc Disease

1. The nurse is caring for an elderly client diagnosed with a herniated nucleus pulposus of L4-L5. Which scientific rationale explains the incidence of a ruptured disc in the elderly?
   1. The client did not use good body mechanics when lifting an object.
   2. There is an increased blood supply to the back as the body ages.
   3. Older clients develop atherosclerotic joint disease as a result of fat deposits.
   4. Clients develop intervertebral disc degeneration as they age.

2. The 34-year-old male client presents to the outpatient clinic complaining of numbness and pain radiating down the left leg. Which further data would the nurse assess?
   1. Posture and gait.
   2. Bending and stooping.
   3. Leg lifts and arm swing.
   4. Waist twists and neck mobility.

3. The occupational health nurse is preparing an in-service for a group of workers in a warehouse. Which information should be included to help prevent on-the job-injuries?
   1. Increase sodium and potassium in the diet during the winter months.
   2. Use the large thigh muscles when lifting and hold the weight near the body.
   3. Use soft-cushioned chairs when performing desk duties.
   4. Have the employee arrange for assistance with household chores.

4. The occupational health nurse is planning health promotion activities for a group of factory workers. Which activity would be an example of primary prevention for clients at risk for low back pain?
   1. Teach back exercises to workers after returning from an injury.
   2. Place signs in the work area about how to perform first aid.
   3. Start a weight-reduction group that would meet at lunchtime.
   4. Administer a nonnarcotic analgesic to a client complaining of back pain.

5. The client with a cervical neck injury as a result of a motor-vehicle injury is complaining of unrelieved pain after administration of a narcotic analgesic. Which alternative method of pain control would be an independent nursing action?
   1. Medicate the client with a muscle relaxant.
   2. Heat alternating with ice applied by a physical therapist.
   3. Watch television or listen to music.
   4. Discuss surgical options with the health-care provider.

6. The client diagnosed with cervical neck disc degeneration has undergone a laminectomy. Which interventions should the nurse implement?
   1. Position the client prone with the knees slightly elevated.
   2. Assess the client for difficulty speaking or breathing.
   3. Measure the drainage in the Jackson-Pratt bulb every day.
   4. Encourage the client to postpone the use of narcotic medications.

7. The client is 12-hours post-lumbar laminectomy. Which nursing interventions should be implemented?
   1. Assess ability to void and log roll every two (2) hours.
   2. Medicate with IV steroids and keep the bed in a Trendelenburg position.
   3. Place sand bags on each side of the head and give cathartic medications.
   4. Administer IV anticoagulants and place on $O_2$ at eight (8) L/min.

8. The nurse is working with an unlicensed nursing assistant. Which action by the assistant warrants immediate intervention?
   1. The assistant feeds a client 2 days postoperative cervical laminectomy a regular diet.
   2. The assistant calls for help when turning to the side a client who is post-lumbar laminectomy.
   3. The assistant is helping the client who weighs 300 pounds and diagnosed with back pain to the chair.
   4. The assistant places the call light within reach of the client who had a disc fusion.

9. The nurse is caring for clients on an orthopedic floor. Which client should be assessed first?
   1. The client diagnosed with back pain who is complaining of a "4" on a 1–10 scale.
   2. The client who has undergone a myelogram who is complaining of a slight headache.
   3. The client 2 days postop disc fusion that has a T 100.4, P 96, R 24, and BP 138/78.
   4. The client diagnosed with back pain who is being discharged and whose ride is here.

10. The nurse is administering 0730 medications to clients on a medical orthopedic unit. Which medication would be administered first?
    1. The daily cardiac glycoside to a client diagnosed with back pain and heart failure.
    2. The routine insulin to a client diagnosed with neck strain and Type 1 diabetes.
    3. The oral proton pump inhibitor to a client scheduled for a laminectomy this A.M.
    4. The fourth dose of IV antibiotic for a client diagnosed with a surgical infection.

11. The nurse writes the problem of "pain" for a client diagnosed with lumbar strain. Which nursing interventions should be included in the plan of care? Select all that apply.
    1. Assess pain on a 1–10 scale.
    2. Administer pain medication PRN.
    3. Provide a regular bed pan for elimination.
    4. Assess surgical dressing every four (4) hours.
    5. Perform a position change by the log roll method every two (2) hours.

12. The nurse working on a medical-surgical floor feels a pulling in the back when lifting a client up in the bed. Which should be the first action taken by the nurse?
    1. Continue working until the shift is over and then try to sleep on a heating pad.
    2. Go immediately to the emergency department for treatment and muscle relaxants.
    3. Inform the charge nurse and nurse manager on duty and document the occurrence.
    4. See a private health-care provider on the nurse's off time but charge the hospital.

## Osteoarthritis

13. The occupational health nurse is teaching a class on the risk factors for developing osteoarthritisoa (OA). Which is a modifiable risk factor for developing OA?
    1. Being overweight.
    2. Increasing age.
    3. Previous joint damage.
    4. Genetic susceptibility.

14. The client is diagnosed with osteoarthritis. Which sign/symptom would the nurse expect the client to exhibit?
    1. Severe bone deformity.
    2. Joint stiffness.
    3. Waddling gait.
    4. Swan neck fingers.

15. The client diagnosed with OA is a resident in a long-term care facility. The resident is refusing to bathe because she is hurting. Which instruction should the nurse give the unlicensed nursing assistant?
    1. Allow the client to stay in bed until the pain becomes bearable.
    2. Tell the assistant to give the client a bed bath this morning.
    3. Try to encourage the client to get up and go to the shower.
    4. Notify the family that the client is refusing to be bathed.

Musculoskeletal

16. The client has been diagnosed with OA for the last seven (7) years and has tried multiple medical treatments and alternative treatments but still has significant joint pain. Which psychosocial client problem would the nurse identify?
    1. Severe pain.
    2. Body-image disturbance.
    3. Knowledge deficit
    4. Depression.

17. The client diagnosed with OA is prescribed a nonsteroidal anti-inflammatory drug (NSAID). Which instruction should the nurse teach the client?
    1. Take the medication on an empty stomach.
    2. Make sure the client tapers the medication when discontinuing.
    3. Apply the medication topically over the affected joints.
    4. Notify the health-care provider if vomiting blood.

18. Which client goal would be most appropriate for a client diagnosed with OA?
    1. Perform passive range-of-motion exercises.
    2. Maintain optimal functional ability.
    3. Client will walk three (3) miles every day.
    4. Client will join a health club.

19. Which member of the health-care team should the nurse refer the client diagnosed with OA who is complaining of not being able to get in and out of the bathtub?
    1. Physiatrist.
    2. Social worker.
    3. Physical therapist.
    4. Counselor.

20. The nurse is discussing the importance of an exercise program for pain control to a client diagnosed with OA. Which intervention should the nurse include in the teaching?
    1. Wear supportive tennis shoes with white socks when walking.
    2. Carry a complex carbohydrate while exercising.
    3. Alternate walking briskly and jogging when exercising.
    4. Walk at least 30 minutes three (3) times a week.

21. The HCP prescribes glucosamine and chondroitin for a client diagnosed with OA. What is the scientific rationale for prescribing this medication?
    1. It will help decrease the inflammation in the joints.
    2. It improves tissue function and retards breakdown of cartilage.
    3. It is a potent medication that decreases the client's joint pain.
    4. It increases the production of synovial fluid in the joint.

22. The nurse is admitting the client with OA to the medical floor. Which statement by the client indicates an alternative form of treatment for OA?
    1. "I take medication every two (2) hours for my pain."
    2. "I use a heating pad when I go to bed at night."
    3. "I wear a copper bracelet to help with my OA."
    4. "I always wear my ankle splints when I sleep."

23. The client is complaining of joint stiffness, especially in the morning. Which diagnostic tests would the nurse expect the health-care provider to order to R/O osteoarthritis?
    1. Full body magnetic resonance imaging scan.
    2. Serum studies for synovial fluid amount.
    3. X-ray of the affected joints.
    4. Serum erythrocyte sedimentation rate (ESR).

24. The nurse is caring for the following clients. After receiving the shift report, which client should the nurse assess first?
    1. The client with a total knee replacement who is complaining of a cold foot.
    2. The client diagnosed with osteoarthritis who is complaining of stiff joints.
    3. The client who needs to receive a scheduled intravenous antibiotic.
    4. The client diagnosed with back pain who is scheduled for a lumbar myelogram.

## Osteoporosis

25. The nurse is discussing osteoporosis with a group of women. Which factor will the nurse identify as a nonmodifiable risk factor?
    1. Calcium deficiency.
    2. Tobacco use.
    3. Female gender.
    4. High alcohol intake.

26. The client diagnosed with osteoporosis asks the nurse, "Why does smoking cigarettes cause my bones to be brittle?" Which response by the nurse would be most appropriate?
    1. "Smoking causes nutritional deficiencies that contribute to osteoporosis."
    2. "Tobacco causes an increase in blood supply to the bones, causing osteoporosis."
    3. "Smoking low-tar cigarettes will not cause your bones to become brittle."
    4. "Nicotine impairs the absorption of calcium, causing decreased bone strength."

27. Which signs/symptoms would make the nurse suspect that the client has developed osteoporosis?
    1. The client has lost one (1) inch in height.
    2. The client has lost 12 pounds in the last year.
    3. The client's hands are painful to the touch.
    4. The client's serum uric acid level is elevated.

28. The client is being evaluated for osteoporosis. Which diagnostic test is the most accurate when diagnosing osteoporosis?
    1. X-ray of the femur.
    2. Serum alkaline phosphatase.
    3. Dual-energy x-ray absorptiometry (DEXA).
    4. Serum bone Gla-protein test.

29. Which foods should the nurse recommend to a client when discussing sources of dietary calcium?
    1. Yogurt and dark-green, leafy vegetables.
    2. Oranges and citrus fruits.
    3. Bananas and dried apricots.
    4. Wheat bread and bran.

30. Which intervention is an example of a secondary nursing intervention when discussing osteoporosis?
    1. Obtain a bone density evaluation test.
    2. Perform non–weight-bearing exercises regularly.
    3. Increase the intake of dietary calcium.
    4. Refer clients to a smoking cessation program.

31. The female client diagnosed with osteoporosis tells the nurse that she is going to perform swim aerobics for 30 minutes every day. Which response would be most appropriate by the nurse?
    1. Praise the client for committing to do this activity.
    2. Explain that walking 30 minutes a day is a better activity.
    3. Encourage the client to swim every other day instead of daily.
    4. Discuss that sedentary activities help prevent osteoporosis.

Musculoskeletal

32. The client newly diagnosed with osteoporosis is prescribed calcitonin by nasal spray. Which assessment data would indicate an adverse effect of the medication?
    1. The client complains of nausea and vomiting.
    2. The client is drinking two (2) glasses of milk a day.
    3. The client has a runny nose and nasal itching.
    4. The client has had numerous episodes of nosebleeds.

33. The nurse is teaching a class to pregnant teenagers. Which information is most important when discussing ways to prevent osteoporosis?
    1. Take at least 1200 mg of calcium supplements a day.
    2. Eat foods low in calcium and high in phosphorus.
    3. Osteoporosis does not occur until around age 50 years.
    4. Remain as active as possible until the baby is born.

34. The 84-year-old client is a resident in a long-term care facility. Which intervention should be implemented to help prevent complications secondary to osteoporosis?
    1. Keep the bed in the high position.
    2. Perform passive range-of-motion exercises.
    3. Turn the client every two (2) hours.
    4. Provide nighttime lights in the room.

35. The client is taking calcium carbonate (Tums) to help prevent further development of osteoporosis. Which teaching should the nurse implement?
    1. Encourage the client to take Tums with at least eight (8) ounces of water.
    2. Teach the client to take Tums with the breakfast meal only.
    3. Instruct the client to take Tums 30 to 60 minutes before a meal.
    4. Discuss the need to get a monthly serum calcium level.

36. The client must take three (3) grams of calcium supplement a day. The medication comes in 500 mg/tablets. How many tablets will the client need to take daily?_____

## Amputation

37. The nurse instructs the client with a right BKA to lie on the stomach for at least 30 minutes a day. The client asks the nurse, "Why do I need to lie on my stomach?" Which statement would be the most appropriate statement by the nurse?
    1. "This position will help your lungs expand better."
    2. "Lying on your stomach will help prevent contractures."
    3. "Many times this will help decrease pain in the limb."
    4. "The position will take pressure off your backside."

38. The recovery room nurse is caring for a client that has just had a left BKA. Which intervention should the nurse implement?
    1. Assess the client's surgical dressing every two (2) hours.
    2. Do not allow the client to see the residual limb.
    3. Keep a large tourniquet at the client's bedside.
    4. Perform passive range-of-motion exercises to the right leg.

39. The 62-year-old client diagnosed with Type 2 diabetes who has a gangrenous right toe is being admitted for a BKA amputation. Which nursing intervention should the nurse implement?
    1. Assess the client's nutritional status.
    2. Refer the client to an occupational therapist.
    3. Determine if the client is allergic to IVP dye.
    4. Start a 22-gauge Angiocath in the right arm.

40. The male nurse is helping his friend cut wood with an electric saw. His friend cut two fingers of his left hand off with the saw. Which action should the nurse implement first?
    1. Wrap the left hand with towels and apply pressure.
    2. Instruct the neighbor to hold his hand above his head.
    3. Apply pressure to the radial artery of the left hand.
    4. Go into the neighbor's house and call 911.

41. A person's right thumb was accidentally severed with an axe. The amputated right thumb was recovered. Which action would preserve the thumb so that it could possibly be reattached in surgery?
    1. Place the right thumb directly on some ice.
    2. Put the right thumb in a glass of warm water.
    3. Wrap the thumb in a clean piece of material.
    4. Secure the thumb in a plastic bag and place on ice.

42. The Jewish client with peripheral vascular disease is scheduled for a left AKA. Which question would be most important for the operating room nurse to ask the client?
    1. "Have you made any special arrangements for your amputated limb?"
    2. "What types of food would you like to eat while you're in the hospital?"
    3. "Would like the rabbi to visit you while you are in the recovery room?"
    4. "Will you start checking your other foot at least once a day for cuts?"

43. The client is three (3) hours postoperative left AKA. The client tells the nurse, "My left foot is killing me. Please do something." Which intervention should the nurse implement?
    1. Explain to the client that his left leg has been amputated.
    2. Medicate the client with a narcotic analgesic immediately.
    3. Instruct the client on how to perform biofeedback exercises.
    4. Place the client's residual limb in the dependent position.

44. The nurse is caring for a client with a right below the knee amputation. There is a large amount of bright red blood on the client's residual limb dressing. Which intervention should the nurse implement first?
    1. Notify the client's surgeon immediately.
    2. Assess the client's blood pressure and pulse.
    3. Reinforce the dressing with additional dressing.
    4. Check the client's last hemoglobin and hematocrit level.

45. The nurse is caring for clients on a surgical unit. Which nursing task would be most appropriate for the nurse to delegate to an unlicensed nursing assistant?
    1. Help the client with a 2-day postop amputation put on the prosthesis.
    2. Request the assistant double-check a unit of blood that is being hung.
    3. Change the surgical dressing on the client with a Syme amputation.
    4. Ask the assistant to take the client to the physical therapy department.

46. The client with a right AKA is being taught how to toughen the residual limb. Which intervention should the nurse implement?
    1. Instruct the client to push the residual limb against a pillow.
    2. Demonstrate how to apply an elastic bandage around the residual limb.
    3. Encourage the client to apply vitamin $B_{12}$ to the surgical incision.
    4. Teach the client to elevate the residual limb at least three times a day.

47. The 27-year-old client has a right above-the-elbow amputation secondary to a boating accident. Which statement by the rehabilitation nurse indicates the client has accepted the amputation?
    1. "I am going to sue the guy that hit my boat."
    2. "The therapist is going to help me get retrained for another job."
    3. "I decided not to get a prosthesis. I don't think I need it."
    4. "My wife is so worried about me and I wish she wouldn't."

Musculoskeletal

48. The 32-year old male client with a traumatic left AKA is being discharged from the rehabilitation department. Which discharge instructions should be included in the teaching? Select all that apply.
    1. Report any pain that is not relieved with analgesics.
    2. Eat a well-balanced diet and increase protein intake.
    3. Be sure to attend all outpatient rehabilitation appointments.
    4. Encourage the client to attend a support group for amputations.
    5. Stay at home as much as possible for the first couple of months.

## Fractures

49. The client is taken to the emergency department with an injury to the left arm. Which action should the nurse take first?
    1. Assess the nail beds for capillary refill time.
    2. Remove the client's clothing from the arm.
    3. Call radiology for a STAT x-ray of the extremity.
    4. Prepare the client for the application of a cast.

50. The nurse is preparing the plan of care for the client with an open fracture of the right arm. Which problem has the highest priority?
    1. Anger related to the inability to perform ADLs.
    2. Sleep disturbances related to loss of work.
    3. Infection related to exposed tissue.
    4. Altered body image related to scarring.

51. Which interventions should the nurse implement for the client diagnosed with an open fracture of the left ankle? Select all that apply.
    1. Apply an immobilizer snugly to prevent edema.
    2. Apply an ice pack for 10 minutes and remove for 20 minutes.
    3. Place the extremity in the dependent position to allow drainage.
    4. Obtain an x-ray of the ankle after applying the immobilizer.
    5. Administer tetanus, 0.5 mL intramuscularly, in the deltoid.

52. When assessing a client with a fractured left tibia and fibula, which data should the nurse report to the health-care provider immediately?
    1. Localized edema and discoloration occurring hours after the injury.
    2. Generalized weakness and increasing sensitivity to touch.
    3. Capillary refill time of nine (9) seconds and increasing pain.
    4. Pain relieved after taking four (4) mg hydromorphone, a narcotic analgesic.

53. The unlicensed nursing assistant (NA) notifies the nurse of the vital signs of a 28-year-old male client admitted the previous day with a fractured femur. The NA reports a temperature of 101°F; pulse 115; respiratory rate 28; copious amounts of thick, white sputum; and "globs" floating in the urinal. What intervention should the nurse implement first?
    1. Assess the client for dyspnea, breath sounds, and altered mental status.
    2. Draw blood for arterial blood gases and order a portable chest x-ray.
    3. Call the health-care provider for an order to administer an antibiotic.
    4. Instruct the assistant to encourage the client to deep breathe.

54. During the morning assessment, the nurse determines that the 80-year-old client admitted with a fractured right femoral neck is confused. Which action should the nurse implement first?
    1. Check for a positive Homans' sign.
    2. Encourage the client to take deep breaths and cough.
    3. Assess the left pedal pulse.
    4. Monitor the client's Buck's traction.

55. The client admitted with a diagnosis of a fractured hip is complaining of severe pain. Which pain management technique would be best for the nurse to implement for this client?
    1. Adjust the patient-controlled analgesia (PCA) machine for a lower dose.
    2. Ensure that the weights of the Buck's traction are off the floor and hang freely.
    3. Raise the head of the bed to 45 degrees and the foot to 15 degrees.
    4. Turn the client to the affected leg using pillows to support the other leg.

56. When preparing the discharge teaching for the 12-year-old with a fractured humerus, which information should the nurse include regarding cast care?
    1. Keep the arm at heart level.
    2. Handle the cast with the tips of the fingers only.
    3. Apply an ice pack to any area that itches.
    4. Foul smells are expected occurrences.

57. Which statement by the client diagnosed with a fractured ulna would indicate that the nurse needs to do further teaching?
    1. "I need to eat a high-protein diet to ensure healing."
    2. "I need to wiggle my fingers every hour to increase circulation."
    3. "I need to take my pain medication before my pain is too bad."
    4. "I need to keep this immobilizer on when lying down only."

58. When preparing the nursing care plan for a client with a fractured lower extremity, which would be the most appropriate treatment outcome for the nurse to include?
    1. The client will maintain function of the leg.
    2. The client will ambulate with assistance.
    3. The client will be turned every two (2) hours.
    4. The client will have no infection.

59. While caring for a client diagnosed with a fracture of the right distal humerus, what data would the nurse assess that would indicate a complication? Select all that apply.
    1. Numbness and mottled cyanosis.
    2. Paresthesia and paralysis.
    3. Proximal pulses and point tenderness.
    4. Coldness of the extremity and crepitus.
    5. Palpable radial pulse and functional movement.

60. An 88-year-old client is admitted to the orthopedic floor with the diagnosis of fractured pelvis. What intervention should the nurse implement first?
    1. Insert an indwelling catheter.
    2. Administer a Fleet's enema.
    3. Assess abdomen for bowel sounds.
    4. Apply Buck's traction.

## Joint Replacements

61. The nurse is preparing the preoperative client for a total hip replacement (THR). Which information should the nurse include concerning postoperative care?
    1. Keep abduction pillow in place between legs at all times.
    2. Cough and deep breathe at least every four (4) to five (5) hours.
    3. Turn to both sides every two (2) hours to prevent pressure ulcers.
    4. Sit in a high-seated chair for a flexion of less than 90 degrees.

62. The client that is one (1) day postoperative total hip replacement complains of hearing a "popping sound" when turning. What assessment data should the nurse report immediately to the surgeon?
    1. Dark red–purple discoloration.
    2. Equal length of lower extremities.
    3. Groin pain in the affected leg.
    4. Edema at the incision site.

63. The nurse is preparing the client who received a total hip replacement for discharge. Which statement would indicate that further teaching is needed?
    1. "I should not cross my legs because my hip may come out of the socket."
    2. "I will call my HCP if I have a sudden increase in pain."
    3. "I will sit on a chair with arms and a firm seat."
    4. "After three (3) weeks, I don't have to worry about infection."

64. When assessing the wound of a client who had a total hip replacement, the nurse finds small, fluid-filled lesions on the right side of the dressing. What explanation is the most probable rationale for this occurrence?
    1. These were caused by the cautery unit in the operating room.
    2. These are papular wheals from herpes zoster.
    3. These are blisters from the tape used to anchor the dressing.
    4. These macular lesions are from a latex allergy.

65. Which topics should the nurse include in the discharge teaching plan for a client after having a total hip replacement? Select all that apply.
    1. Weight-bearing limits.
    2. Use of assistive devices.
    3. Gradual increase in activity.
    4. Medication therapy.
    5. Periods of rest.

66. The nurse is preparing a plan of care for the client who has had a total hip replacement. Which outcome would be most appropriate for this client?
    1. The client has limited amount of pain relief.
    2. The client will have limited ability to ambulate.
    3. The client will have hip instability for several months.
    4. The client will have adequate hip joint motion.

67. When assessing the client six (6) hours after having a right total knee replacement, which data should the nurse report to the surgeon?
    1. A total of 100 mL of red drainage in the autotransfusion drainage system.
    2. Pain relief after using the patient-controlled analgesia (PCA) pump.
    3. Cool toes, distal pulses palpable, and pale nail beds bilaterally.
    4. Urinary output of 60 mL of clear yellow urine in three (3) hours.

68. When preparing the client for the transition to home rehabilitation after having a total knee replacement, which information regarding discharge teaching would the nurse include?
    1. Deep breathe and cough every two (2) hours.
    2. Procedure for emptying Jackson-Pratt drainage.
    3. Burning or frequency of urination is expected.
    4. Modify the home for altered mobility.

69. When developing the plan of care for the client having a total knee repair, which of the expected outcomes would the nurse include? Select all that apply.
    1. The client has effective pain management.
    2. The client does not smoke or use tobacco products.
    3. The client ambulates within the weight-bearing limits.
    4. The client participates in activities of daily living.
    5. The client is able to return to his or her previous lifestyle.

70. The nurse is caring for the client who had a total knee replacement (TKR). Which data would the nurse observe to determine if the nursing interventions are effective?
    1. The client's lungs have bilateral crackles.
    2. The client's knee has flexion of 45 degrees.
    3. The client participates in self-care activities.
    4. The client has reduced pain using a single approach.

71. The nurse is assessing the client who is immediately postoperative from a total knee replacement. Which assessment data would warrant immediate intervention?
    1. T 99°F, HR 80, RR 20, and BP 128/76.
    2. Pain in the unaffected leg during dorsiflexion of the ankle.
    3. Bowel sounds heard intermittently in four quadrants.
    4. Diffuse, crampy abdominal pain.

72. The nurse is working on an orthopedic floor. Which client should the nurse assess first after the change of shift report?
    1. The 84-year-old female with a fractured right femoral neck in Buck's traction.
    2. The 64-year-old female who had a left total knee replacement with confusion.
    3. The 88-year-old male who had a right total hip replacement with an abduction pillow.
    4. The 50-year-old postoperative client who has a continuous passive motion (CPM) device.

## Degenerative/Herniated Disc Disease

1. 1. Back pain occurs in 80% to 90% of the population at different times in their lives. Although not using good body mechanics when lifting an object may be a reason for younger clients to develop a herniated disc, it is not the reason that most elderly people develop back pain.
   2. There is a decreased blood supply as the body ages.
   3. Older clients develop degenerative joint disease. Fat does not deposit itself in the nucleus pulposus.
   4. **Less blood supply, degeneration of the disc, and arthritis are reasons elderly people develop back problems.**

   **TEST-TAKING HINT: The clue in this question is "elderly." The answer must address a problem that would occur as a result of aging.**

2. 1. **Posture and gait will be affected if the client is experiencing sciatica, pain radiating down a leg resulting from pressure on the sciatic nerve.**
   2. The client with pain and numbness would not be able to bend or stoop and should not be asked to do so.
   3. Leg lifts will not give the nurse the needed information and would cause this client pain; also, it is the lower extremity, not the upper extremity, that is being assessed.
   4. Waist twists will not assess the mobility of the lower extremity, and neck mobility would be assessed if a cervical neck problem were suspected.

   **TEST-TAKING HINT: Anatomical positioning and the function of spinal nerves would rule out options "3" and "4."**

3. 1. Increased calcium, not potassium or sodium, is helpful in preventing orthopedic injuries. Increasing sodium intake could prevent water loss in a non–air-conditioned warehouse in the summer months, not the winter months.
   2. **These are instructions to prevent back injuries as a result of poor body mechanics.**
   3. Soft-cushioned chairs are not ergonomically designed. Soft-cushioned chairs promote poor body posture.
   4. This might help the client prevent back injuries at home, but it would not prevent job-related injuries.

   **TEST-TAKING HINT: The question is asking for information that will prevent on-the-job back injuries. Option "4" can be ruled out because of this. The two (2) electrolytes in option "1"**

are not associated with orthopedic injuries or bones, thus ruling out this option.

4. 1. Teaching back exercises to a client who has already experienced a problem is tertiary care.
   2. Placing signs with instructions about how to render first aid is a secondary intervention, not primary prevention.
   3. **Excess weight increases the workload on the vertebrae. Weight-loss activities would help to prevent back injury.**
   4. Administering a nonnarcotic analgesic to a client with back pain is an example of secondary or tertiary care, depending on whether the client has a one-time problem or a chronic problem with back pain.

   **TEST-TAKING HINT: Primary care is any activity that prevents an illness or injury.**

5. 1. This is an example of collaborative care.
   2. This is an example of collaborative care.
   3. **This is distraction and is an alternative method often recommended for the promotion of client comfort.**
   4. Surgery is collaborative care.

   **TEST-TAKING HINT: The question asks for an alternative type of care. Options "1," "2," and "4" are all collaborative care. If the test taker can find a common thread among three of the options, then the correct answer will be the other option.**

6. 1. "Prone" means on the abdomen. On the abdomen with the knees flexed would be an uncomfortable position, placing the spine in an unnatural position.
   2. **The surgical position of the wound places the client at risk for edema of tissues in the neck. Difficulty speaking or breathing would alert the nurse to a potentially life-threatening problem.**
   3. The drainage from a J-P drain should be emptied and monitored every shift.
   4. The client should be kept as comfortable as possible.

   **TEST-TAKING HINT: The nurse must know the meaning of the common medical term "prone" and realize that this would be uncomfortable for the client, thus eliminating option "1." The time frame of "every day" makes option "3" wrong.**

7. 1. **The lumbar nerves innervate the lower abdomen. The bladder is in the lower abdomen. The client will be required to lie flat, and this is a difficult position for many clients, especially males, to be in to void. Clients are log rolled every 2 hours.**

2. The client would be receiving IV pain medication, not steroids. A Trendelenburg position is head down.
3. Sand bags would keep the neck still, but the surgical area is in the lumbar region, so there is no reason the client cannot turn the head; also, cathartic medications are harsh laxatives.
4. The client will be receiving subcutaneous anticoagulant medications to prevent deep vein thromboses, but IV anticoagulant therapy is not warranted. Eight (8) L/min of oxygen is high-flow oxygen that would be used for a client in respiratory distress who does not have carbon dioxide narcosis.

**TEST-TAKING HINT: The test taker must note the adjective "lumbar"; this can rule out option "3." Knowledge of medication classifications would rule out options "2" and "4."**

8. 1. Clients that are two (2) days postop laminectomy should be eating a regular diet.
   2. The client who has undergone a lumbar laminectomy is log rolled. It requires four (4) people or more to log roll a client.
   3. **The legs of any client diagnosed with back pain can give out and collapse at any time, but a large client diagnosed with back pain would be at increased risk of injuring the assistant as well as the client. The nurse should intervene before the client or assistant become injured.**
   4. This action helps ensures safety for the client.

**TEST-TAKING HINT: This question is an "except" question. All the options but one contain information that should be done.**

9. 1. Mild back pain is expected with this client.
   2. Lumbar myelograms require access into the spinal column. A small amount of cerebrospinal fluid may be lost, causing a mild headache. The client should stay flat in bed to prevent this from occurring.
   3. This client is postop and now has a fever. This client should be assessed and the health-care provider should be notified.
   4. A discharged client does not have priority over a surgical infection.

**TEST-TAKING HINT: Options "1" and "2" contain assessment data that are expected for the procedure.**

10. 1. This could be administered after breakfast if necessary. There is nothing in the action of the medication that requires a before-breakfast medication administration.
    2. **Clients with Type 1 diabetes are insulin dependent. This medication should be administered before the client eats.**

3. This medication should be held until after surgery.
4. The client has already received three (3) doses of IV antibiotic. This medication could be given after the insulin.

**TEST-TAKING HINT: The nurse must decide which medication has priority by determining the action of the medication, the route of administration, and the diagnosis of the client.**

11. 1. An objective method of quantifying the client's pain should be used.
    2. Once the nurse has determined that the client is stable and not experiencing complications, the nurse can medicate the client.
    3. A regular bed pan is high and could cause pain for a client diagnosed with back pain. The client should be given a fracture pan.
    4. There is no surgical dressing.
    5. The client has not been to surgery, so log rolling is not necessary.

**TEST-TAKING HINT: Two of the options—"4" and "5"—apply to post-surgical cases and could be eliminated.**

12. 1. The nurse should not continue working, and this is self-diagnosing and treating.
    2. The nurse may go to the emergency department, but this is not the first action.
    3. **The first action is to notify the charge nurse so that a replacement can be arranged to take over care of the clients. The nurse should notify the nurse manager or house supervisor. An occurrence report should be completed documenting the situation. This provides the nurse with the required documentation to begin a worker's compensation case for payment of medical bills.**
    4. The nurse has the right to see a private health-care provider in most states, but this is not the first action.

**TEST-TAKING HINT: When the test taker is determining a priority, then all of the answers may be appropriate interventions, but only one is implemented first. The test taker should read the full stem, identifying the important words and making sure that he or she understands what the question is asking.**

## Osteoarthritis

13. 1. Obesity is a well-recognized risk factor for the development of OA and it is modifiable in that the client can lose weight.
    2. Increasing age is a risk factor, but there is nothing the client can do about getting older, except to die.

3. Previous joint damage is a risk factor, but it is not modifiable, which means the client cannot do anything to change it.

4. Genetic susceptibility is a result of family genes, which the client cannot change; it is a nonmodifiable risk factor.

**TEST-TAKING HINT: The adjective "modifiable" is the key to selecting the correct answer. Only one option "1" contains anything the client has control over changing or modifying.**

14. 1. Severe bone deformity is seen in clients diagnosed with rheumatoid arthritis.

2. **Pain, stiffness, and functional impairment are the primary clinical manifestations of OA. Stiffness of the joints is commonly experienced after resting but usually lasts less than 30 minutes and decreases with movement.**

3. A waddling gait is usually seen in women in their third trimester of pregnancy or in older children with congenital hip dysplasia.

4. Swan neck fingers are seen in clients with rheumatoid arthritis.

**TEST-TAKING HINT: The test taker can have difficulty distinguishing clinical manifestations of two similar-sounding diseases, osteoarthritis and rheumatoid arthritis. Both diseases involve the joints and cause pain and stiffness. Remember that rheumatoid arthritis can permanently disfigure the client, leading to "bone deformity" and "swan neck fingers."**

15. 1. Clients with OA should be encouraged to move, which will decrease the pain.

2. A bed bath does not require as much movement from the client as getting up and walking to the shower.

3. **Pain will decrease with movement, and warm or hot water will help decrease the pain. The worse thing the client can do is not move.**

4. Notifying the family will not address the client's pain and the client has a right to refuse a bath, but the nursing staff must explain why moving and bathing will help decrease the pain.

**TEST-TAKING HINT: Allowing clients to stay in bed only increases complications of immobility and will increase the client's pain secondary to OA. Clients with chronic illnesses should be encouraged to be as independent as possible. The family should only be notified if a significant situation has occurred.**

16. 1. Pain is a physiological problem, not a psychosocial problem.

2. A client with OA does not have bone deformi-

ties; therefore body-image disturbance would not be appropriate.

3. After seven (7) years of OA and multiple treatment modalities, knowledge deficit would not be appropriate for this client.

4. **The client experiencing chronic pain often experiences depression and hopelessness.**

**TEST-TAKING HINT: The adjective "psychosocial" should help the test taker rule out option "1." The test taker needs to read the stem carefully. This client has had a problem for years and therefore "3" could be ruled out as a correct answer.**

17. 1. This medication should be taken with food to prevent gastrointestinal distress.

2. Glucocorticoids, not NSAIDs, must be tapered when discontinuing.

3. Topical analgesics are applied to the skin; NSAIDs are oral or intravenous medications.

4. **NSAIDs are well known for causing gastric upset and increasing the risk for peptic ulcer disease, which could cause the client to vomit blood.**

**TEST-TAKING HINT: The worse scenario option is "4," which has blood in the answer. If the test taker did not know the answer, then selecting an option with blood in it would be most appropriate.**

18. 1. This is an intervention, not a goal, and "passive" means the nurse performs the range of motion, which should not be encouraged.

2. **The two main goals of treatment for OA are pain management and optimizing functional ability of the joints to ensure movement of the joints.**

3. Most clients with OA are elderly, are overweight, and have a sedentary lifestyle so walking three (3) miles every day is not a realistic or safe goal.

4. Joining a gym is an intervention and just because the client joins the gym doesn't mean the client will exercise.

**TEST-TAKING HINT: The test taker must remember a goal is the measurable outcome of nursing interventions based on the client problem/diagnosis. Interventions are not goals; therefore the test taker could eliminate "1" and "4" as possible answers.**

19. 1. A physiatrist is a physician who specializes in physical medicine and rehabilitation, but the nurse would not refer the client to this person just because the client is having difficulty with transfers.

2. The social worker does not address this type of

physical problem. Social workers address issues concerning finances, placement, and acquiring assistive devices.

3. The physical therapist is able to help the client with transferring, ambulation, and other lower-extremity difficulties.

4. A counselor is not able to help the client learn how to get in and out of the bathtub.

**TEST-TAKING HINT: The nurse must know the role of all the health-care team members.**

20. 1. Safety should always be discussed when teaching about exercises. Supportive shoes will prevent shin splints. Colored socks have dye that may cause athlete's foot, which is why white socks are recommended.

2. Clients with diabetes mellitus should carry complex carbohydrates with them.

3. OA occurs most often in weight-bearing joints. Exercise is encouraged, but jogging increases stress on these joints.

4. For exercising to help pain control, the client must walk daily, not three (3) times a week. Walking at least 30 minutes 3 times a week would be appropriate for weight loss.

**TEST-TAKING HINT: The test taker can rule out "3" as an answer because the stem says pain control; "1" is correct for any exercise program.**

21. 1. NSAIDs or glucocorticoids help decrease inflammation of the joints.

2. This is the rationale for administering these medications.

3. Narcotic and nonnarcotic analgesics would help decrease the client's pain.

4. There is no medication at this time that helps increase synovial fluid production, but surgery can increase the viscosupplementation in the joint.

**TEST-TAKING HINT: There are some questions that require the test taker to have the knowledge and there are no Test-Taking Hints to help with selecting the right answer.**

22. 1. Medication is a standard therapy and is not considered an alternative therapy.

2. A heating pad is an accepted medical recommendation for the treatment of pain for clients with OA.

3. Alternative forms of treatment have not been proved efficacious in the treatment of a disease. The nurse should be nonjudgmental and open to discussions about alternative treatment, unless it interferes with the medical regimen.

4. Conservative treatment measures for OA include splints and braces to support inflamed joints.

**TEST-TAKING HINTS: The test taker needs to read the stem carefully to be able to determine what the question is asking; there is only one option with alternative-type treatment, which is option "3"; options "1," "2," and "4" these are accepted treatment options that would be listed in a textbook.**

23. 1. MRIs are not routinely ordered for diagnosing OA.

2. There is no serum lab test that measures synovial fluid in the joints.

3. X-rays reveal loss of joint cartilage, which appears as a narrowing of the joint space in clients diagnosed with OA.

4. An ESR is a diagnostic laboratory test for rheumatoid arthritis, not osteoarthritis.

**TEST-TAKING HINT: If the test taker is guessing which answer is correct and knows that "osteo" means bone, the only option that has any specific connection to bones is an x-ray. This selection would be an educated guess.**

24. 1. A cold foot on a client who has had surgery may indicate a neurovascular compromise and must be assessed first.

2. A client with osteoarthritis is expected to have stiff joints.

3. A routine medication is not priority over a potential complication of surgery.

4. A routine diagnostic procedure does not have priority over a complication of surgery.

**TEST-TAKING HINT: The test taker must take a systematic approach when answering prioritizing questions. First, the test taker must determine if any client is experiencing a life-threatening or life-altering complication such as "loss of limb." The test taker must determine if the sign/symptom is expected for the disease or condition.**

## Osteoporosis

25. 1. Calcium deficiency is a modifiable risk factor, which means the client can do something about this factor—namely, increase the intake of calcium—to help prevent the development of osteoporosis.

2. Smoking is a modifiable risk factor because the client can quit smoking.

3. A nonmodifiable risk factor is a factor that the client cannot do anything to alter or change. Approximately 50% of all women

will experience an osteoporosis-related fracture in their lifetime.

4. The client can quit drinking alcohol; therefore, this is a modifiable risk factor.

**TEST-TAKING HINT: The key word to answering this question is "nonmodifiable," which means the client cannot do anything to modify or change behavior that will help prevent developing osteoporosis.**

26. 1. This would be the rationale for heavy alcohol use leading to the development of osteoporosis.
    2. Smoking decreases, not increases, blood supply to the bone.
    3. Cigarette smoking has long been identified as a risk factor for osteoporosis, and it doesn't matter if it is low tar.
    4. **Nicotine slows the production of osteoblasts and impairs the absorption of calcium, contributing to decreased bone density.**

**TEST-TAKING HINT: The test taker must always be aware of the words "increase" and "decrease" when selecting a correct answer.**

27. 1. **The loss of height occurs as vertebral bodies collapse.**
    2. Weight loss is not a sign of osteoporosis.
    3. This may indicate rheumatoid arthritis but not osteoporosis.
    4. This would be a sign of gout.

**TEST-TAKING HINT: If the test taker is not sure of the answer and knows that "osteo" means bone, the only answer that is related to bones is the height of the client, the spine.**

28. 1. Osteoporotic changes do not occur in the bone until more than 30% of the bone mass has been lost.
    2. This serum blood study may be elevated after a fracture, but it does not help diagnose osteoporosis.
    3. **This test measures bone density in the lumbar spine or hip and is considered to be highly accurate.**
    4. This test is most useful to evaluate the effects of treatment, rather than as an indicator of the severity of bone disease.

**TEST-TAKING HINT: The option "2" does not have bone or x-ray in it; therefore, if the test taker did not know the correct answer, eliminating this option would be appropriate. If the test taker knew osteoporosis was secondary to poor absorption of calcium, "3" would be an appropriate selection for the correct answer.**

29. 1. **The best dietary sources of calcium are milk and other dairy products. Other sources include oysters; canned sardines or**

salmon; beans; cauliflower; and dark-green, leafy vegetables.

2. These foods are high in vitamin C.
3. These foods are high in potassium.
4. These foods are recommended for a high-fiber diet.

**TEST-TAKING HINT: A question about special diets is a knowledge-based question, and the test taker must know which foods are in which type of diets. Foods high in calcium should be associated with milk products such as yogurt.**

30. 1. This is an example of a secondary nursing intervention, which includes screening for early detection.
    2. **The client should perform weight-bearing exercises, which promote osteoblast activity that helps maintain bone strength and integrity. This is a primary nursing intervention.**
    3. Increasing dietary calcium may be a primary intervention to help prevent osteoporosis or a tertiary intervention, which helps treat osteoporosis.
    4. Smoking cessation is a primary intervention, which will help prevent the development of osteoporosis.

**TEST-TAKING HINT: The nurse must be knowledgeable of primary, secondary, and tertiary nursing interventions. Primary interventions are those that help prevent the disease; secondary interventions are interventions such as screening the client for the disease with the goal of detecting it early; tertiary interventions are interventions implemented when the client has the disease.**

31. 1. Swimming is not as beneficial as walking in maintaining bone density because of the lack of weight-bearing activity.
    2. **Weight-bearing activity, such as walking, is beneficial in preventing or slowing bone loss. The mechanical force of weight-bearing exercises promotes bone growth.**
    3. Swimming is not as beneficial in maintaining bone density because of the lack of weight-bearing activity.
    4. A sedentary lifestyle is a risk factor for the development of osteoporosis.

**TEST-TAKING HINT: Sedentary activities include sitting and very low-activity exercises, which are risk factors in developing many diseases and disorders; therefore, option "4" can be eliminated.**

32. 1. Nausea and vomiting may occur during initial stages of therapy, but they will disappear as treatment continues.
    2. The client should be sure to consume adequate

amounts of calcium and vitamin D while taking calcitonin.
3. Rhinitis, runny nose, is the most common side effect with calcitonin nasal spray along with itching, sores, and other nasal symptoms.
4. Nosebleeds are adverse effects and should be reported to the client's HCP.

**TEST-TAKING HINT: If the test taker has no idea of the answer, an appropriate option to select would be an option that has bleeding in it; bleeding is abnormal and would indicate an adverse effect.**

33. 1. The National Institutes of Health (NIH) recommend a daily calcium intake of 1200 to 1500 mg per day for adolescents, young adults, and pregnant and lactating women.
2. The pregnant teenager should eat foods high in calcium.
3. Osteoporosis may not occur before age 50 years, but taking calcium throughout the life span will help prevent it. Remember, teenagers tend to focus on the present, not the future, so the most important intervention to teach them is to take calcium supplements.
4. Activity will not help prevent osteoporosis in the teenager; the teenager must take calcium supplements.

**TEST-TAKING HINT: The age of the client is important when answering questions; developmental stages will help rule out or help select the correct answer.**

34. 1. The bed should be kept in the low position. Preventing falls is a priority for a client diagnosed with osteoporosis.
2. Range-of-motion exercises will help prevent deep vein thrombosis or contractures, but they do not help prevent osteoporosis.
3. Turning the client will help prevent pressure ulcers, but that does not help prevent osteoporosis.
4. Nighttime lights will help prevent the client from falling; fractures are the number-one complication of osteoporosis.

**TEST-TAKING HINT: The test taker should realize that the bed should be kept in a low position at all times and should eliminate this as a possible answer; ROM exercises and turning will help prevent complications of immobility, not osteoporosis.**

35. 1. There is no reason to take Tums with eight (8) ounces of water. Tums are usually chewed.
2. Tums should not be taken with meals.
3. Free hydrochloric acid is needed for calcium absorption; therefore Tums should be taken on an empty stomach.

4. To determine the effectives of calcium supplements the client must have a bone density test, not a serum calcium level measurement.

**TEST-TAKING HINT: If unsure of the answer, the test taker should not select an option that has an absolute-type word such as "only," "always," or "never." There are very few absolutes in health care.**

36. Six (6) tablets. 1000 mg is equal to one (1) gram. Therefore three (3) grams is equal to 3000 mg. If one (1) tablet is 500 mg, the client will need six (6) tablets to get the total amount of calcium needed daily:

$$3000 \div 500 = 6$$

**TEST-TAKING HINT: The test taker must know how to perform math calculations and must be knowledgeable of conversions. Remember to use the drop-down calculator on the RN-NCLEX exam.**

## Amputation

37. 1. This position will decrease lung expansion.
2. The prone position will help stretch the hamstring muscle, which will help prevent flexion contractures that may lead to problems when fitting the client for a prosthesis.
3. Lying on the back will not help decrease actual or phantom pain.
4. This will help take pressure off the client's buttocks area, but that is not why it is recommended for a client with a lower-extremity amputation.

**TEST-TAKING HINT: The test taker can eliminate option "1" if visualizing the client in a prone position. This position will limit expansion of the lung more than increase it. Clients are placed with the head elevated, a position the client in a prone position cannot achieve, when trying to allow for expansion of the lungs.**

38. 1. The client is in the recovery room, and the dressing must be assessed more frequently than every two (2) hours.
2. The client must come to terms with the amputation; therefore the nurse should encourage the client to look at the residual limb.
3. The large tourniquet can be used if the residual limb begins to hemorrhage either internally or externally.
4. The nurse should encourage active, not passive, range-of-motion exercises.

**TEST-TAKING HINTS: Remember to look at the adjectives that describe the intervention such as "every two (2) hours" and "passive."**

39. 1. For wound healing, a balanced diet with adequate protein and vitamins is essential, along with meals appropriate for Type 2 diabetes.
   2. An occupational therapist addresses activities of daily living and usually addresses upper-extremity amputations. A referral to a physical therapist would be more appropriate to address ambulating and transfer concerns.
   3. There is no type of intravenous dye used in this surgical procedure so this question is not appropriate.
   4. An 18-gauge catheter should be started because the client is going to surgery; the client may need a blood transfusion, which should be administered through an 18-gauge catheter.

   TEST-TAKING HINT: The nurse must take into account all the client's comorbid conditions (diabetes Type 2) when selecting the correct answer.

40. 1. Wrapping the hand with towels would be appropriate, but it is not the first intervention.
   2. Holding the arm above the head will help decrease the bleeding, but it is not the first intervention.
   3. Applying direct pressure to the artery above the amputated parts will help decrease the bleeding immediately and is the first intervention the nurse should implement. Then the nurse should instruct the client to hold the hand above the head, apply towels, and call 911.
   4. Calling 911 should be done, but it is not the first intervention.

   TEST-TAKING HINT: Remember that when the stem asks the test taker to identify the first intervention, all four options will be probable interventions, but only one is the first intervention.

41. 1. Placing the amputated part directly on ice will cause vasoconstriction and necrosis of viable tissue.
   2. Warm water will cause the amputated part to disintegrate and lose viable tissue.
   3. Wrapping the amputated part in a piece of material will not help preserve the thumb so that it can be reconnected.
   4. Placing the thumb in a plastic bag will protect it and then placing the plastic bag on ice will help preserve the thumb so that it may be reconnected in surgery. Do not place the amputated part directly on ice because this will cause necrosis of viable tissue.

   TEST-TAKING HINT: Make sure the test taker knows what the question is asking before selecting the option. The question is asking "what will help preserve the thumb?"—that is the key to answering this question.

42. 1. The Jewish faith believes that all body parts must be buried together. Therefore many synagogues will keep amputated limbs until death occurs.
   2. Specific foods are important, but not while the client is in the operating room.
   3. Spiritual issues are important for the nurse to discuss with the client, but the operating room should be concerned with disposition of the amputated limb.
   4. Addressing teaching issues is important, but the most important concern is disposition of the amputated limb.

   TEST-TAKING HINT: The nurse must always address the cultural needs of the client, and when the test taker sees a specific culture in the stem of a question, it is a prompt that this will be important when selecting the answer.

43. 1. The client is three (3) hours postoperative and needs medical intervention.
   2. Phantom pain is caused by severing the peripheral nerves. The pain is real to the client, and the nurse needs to medicate the client immediately.
   3. Biofeedback exercises will not help address the client's postoperative surgical pain.
   4. Placing the residual limb below the heart (dependent) will not help address the client's pain and could actually increase the pain.

   TEST-TAKING HINT: The test taker needs to be aware of adjectives such as "dependent." The nurse must know medical terms for positioning a client.

44. 1. If the client is hemorrhaging, the surgeon would need to be notified, but that has not been determined.
   2. Determining if the client is hemorrhaging would be the first intervention. The nurse should check for signs of hypovolemic shock, decreased BP, and increased pulse.
   3. Reinforcing the dressing would help decrease bleeding, but the nurse must assess first.
   4. Checking client's laboratory results is an appropriate intervention, but it is not the first intervention.

   TEST-TAKING HINT: Remember that when the stem asks the test taker to identify the first intervention, all four options will be probable interventions but only one is the first intervention. Also, the nurse should always assess first. Remember the nursing process.

45. 1. A client who is only two (2) days postop amputation would not be putting on a prosthesis.
    2. Two (2) registered nurses must double-check a unit of blood prior to infusing the blood.
    3. The surgical dressing is changed by the surgeon or the nurse; Syme amputation is above the ankle, just removing the foot.
    4. The nursing assistant could take a client to another department in the hospital.

    **TEST-TAKING HINT: Remember teaching, assessing, and evaluating cannot be delegated.**

46. 1. Applying pressure to the end of the residual limb will help toughen the limb. Gradually pushing the residual limb against harder and harder surfaces is done in preparation for prosthesis training.
    2. An Ace bandage applied distal to proximal will help decrease edema and help shape the residual limb into a conical shape.
    3. Vitamin E oil will help decrease the angriness of the scar, but it will not help with residual limb toughening.
    4. Elevating the residual limb will help decrease edema, but it will also cause a contracture if the residual limb is elevated after the first 24 hours.

    **TEST-TAKING HINT: The stem of the question asks the test taker to choose a method of toughening the residual limb. Demonstrating how to apply an elastic bandage or elevating the limb would not accomplish this, so these options could be eliminated from consideration.**

47. 1. This statement does not indicate acceptance; the client is still in the anger stage of grieving.
    2. Looking toward the future and problem-solving indicate that the client is accepting the loss.
    3. At this young age, a client with an upper-extremity prosthesis needs to be thinking about obtaining employment and living a full life. Getting a prosthesis is important to pursue this goal.
    4. This statement does not indicate acceptance; his wife will worry about his life that has been changed dramatically.

    **TEST-TAKING HINT: Always notice when the age is given for the client. This will help guide the test taker to the correct answer.**

48. 1. Pain not relieved with analgesics could indicate complications or could be phantom pain.
    2. A well-balanced diet promotes wound healing, especially a diet high in protein.
    3. The client must keep appointments in out-

patient rehabilitation to continue to improve physically and emotionally.
    4. A support group may help the client adjust to life with an amputation.
    5. The client should be encouraged to get out as much as possible and live as normal a life as possible.

    **TEST-TAKING HINT: The test taker needs to select all options that are appropriate.**

## Fractures

49. 1. The nurse should assess the nail beds for the capillary refill time. A prolonged time (greater than three [3] seconds) indicates impaired circulation to the extremity.
    2. Clothing may need to be removed but not before assessment.
    3. An x-ray will be done, but is not the highest priority action.
    4. A cast may or may not be applied, depending on the type and location of the fracture.

    **TEST-TAKING HINT: When the question asks to prioritize nursing care, usually assessment is first. Assessment is an independent nursing intervention.**

50. 1. The client may feel anger when unable to perform self-care, but physical problems have a higher priority than psychosocial problems.
    2. Sleep disturbances are physical problems but would not be life threatening.
    3. The definition of an open fracture is a bone that has penetrated the skin. The highest-priority problem is infection because the skin is the barrier that keeps bacteria from entering the surrounding tissue.
    4. Body image is a psychosocial problem that has a lower ranking than physical problems.

    **TEST-TAKING HINT: Physiological problems always have priority when the problem is applicable to the condition. Anger, sleep, and body image would not have priority over an infection.**

51. 1. An immobilizer should not be applied snugly. There should be enough room to allow for edema and adequate perfusion of the tissues.
    2. Ice packs should be applied ten (10) minutes on and twenty (20) minutes off. This allows for vasoconstriction and decreases edema. Ice is a nonpharmacological pain management technique.
    3. An injured extremity should be elevated above the level of the heart to decrease edema and pain.

Musculoskeletal

4. An x-ray should be done before the immobilizer is in place, not after.
5. Any time trauma occurs, tetanus should be considered. In an open fracture, this is an appropriate treatment.

**TEST-TAKING HINT: This is an alternative-type question. When selecting all that are correct, it is important to consider the descriptive words that make the options incorrect. Read adjectives and adverbs carefully. The terms "snugly," "dependent," and "after" make options "1," "3," and "4" incorrect.**

52. 1. Localized edema and discoloration hours after the injury are normal occurrences after a fracture.
2. Generalized weakness and increasing tenderness are common and not life threatening.
3. The normal capillary refill time (CRT) is less than three (3) seconds. A prolonged refill time and increasing pain indicate circulation impairment. This needs to be reported before compartment syndrome occurs.
4. Pain management is a desired outcome demonstrated by pain relieved after medication administration.

**TEST-TAKING HINT: The nurse should notify the health-care provider of abnormal or unexpected assessment data; increased capillary refill time indicates a neurovascular complication. All the other options contain normal or expected data.**

53. 1. The nurse should assess the client for signs of hypoxia from a fat embolism. The symptoms listed in this question indicate a fat embolism. Dyspnea, adventitious breath sounds, and confusion indicate hypoxia. Young males are more likely to suffer from a fat embolism, especially from fractured femurs.
2. Arterial blood gases and portable chest x-ray will be done, but they will not be done first.
3. An antibiotic is not the highest-priority medication for this client. Oxygenation is first.
4. Deep breathing is an important intervention in an immobile client, but it is not the first action. The client is unstable. The nurse cannot delegate an unstable client.

**TEST-TAKING HINT: If the test taker is unsure of the correct answer, always apply the nursing process. Assessment is the first part of the nursing process.**

54. 1. Assessing for a positive Homans' sign is an appropriate intervention, but it is not the best action indicated by the symptoms.

2. Encouraging the client to take deep breaths and cough would aid in the exchange of gases. Mental changes are early signs of hypoxia in the elderly client.
3. The client's right hip is fractured so assessing the left pedal pulse would not be priority.
4. Checking the client's Buck's traction will not address the problem of confusion.

**TEST-TAKING HINT: The test taker needs to understand what the question is asking. Although the client has a fractured hip, the confusion is the problem. Decreased oxygenation should be the first thought the test taker has when seeing the word "confusion."**

55. 1. The health-care provider orders the dosage on a PCA. Unless a range of dosages or new order is obtained, a lower dose will not help pain.
2. Weights from traction should be off the floor and hanging freely. Buck's traction is used to reduce muscle spasms preoperatively in clients who have fractured hips.
3. Raising the head of the bed or the foot will alter the traction.
4. Turning the client to the affected side would increase pain rather than relieve it.

**TEST-TAKING HINT: This intervention is a form of assessment, assessing the equipment being used for the client's condition. Remember to apply the nursing process.**

56. 1. The arm should be elevated above the heart, not at the level.
2. Handling drying casts with fingertips can create pressure spots that impair circulation and create pressure ulcers.
3. Applying ice packs to the cast will relieve itching and nothing should be placed down a cast to scratch. Skin becomes fragile inside the cast and is torn easily. Alteration in the skin's integrity can become infected.
4. Smells indicate infection and should be reported to the HCP.

**TEST-TAKING HINT: A concept for any injury is elevating it above the heart to decrease edema. Many times the test taker must apply basic concepts to a variety of client conditions. Any foul smell is not expected in any disease or condition.**

57. 1. Protein is necessary for healing.
2. By wiggling the fingers of the affected arm, the client can improve the circulation.
3. Pain medication should be taken prior to perception of severe pain. Pain relief will require more medication if allowed to become severe.
4. The immobilizer should be kept on at all

times. This indicates that the client does not understand the teaching and needs the nurse to provide more instruction.

**TEST-TAKING HINT: When selecting an answer for questions like this, the test taker should remember to look for an untrue statement. This indicates that teaching is needed.**

58. 1. The expected outcome for a client with a fracture is maintaining the function of the extremity.
    2. Ambulation with assistance is not the best goal.
    3. This is a nursing intervention, not a client goal.
    4. Infection is not the highest-priority problem for a client with a fracture.

**TEST-TAKING HINT: The test taker must note the word "most appropriate" and look at the client as a whole entity. With musculoskeletal problems, maintaining normal function or anatomical function is the desired outcome. Remember that independence is priority for the client.**

59. 1. The nurse should assess for numbness and mottled cyanosis, which might indicate nerve damage.
    2. The presence of paresthesia and paralysis indicate impaired circulation.
    3. Pulses should be assessed but not proximal to the fracture. Pulses distal to the fracture should be assessed. Point tenderness should be expected.
    4. Coldness indicates decreased blood supply. Crepitus indicates air in subcutaneous tissue and is not expected.
    5. Palpable radial pulses and functional movement do not indicate a complication has occurred.

**TEST-TAKING HINT: This is an alternate-type question in which the test taker must select all options that apply. The test taker should remember the neuromuscular assessment, which includes the 6 Ps—pulse, pain, paresthesia, paralysis, pallor, polar (cold).**

60. 1. Inserting an indwelling catheter would be a good intervention, but it would not be the first intervention. A tear or injury to the bladder should be suspected.
    2. Administering a Fleet's enema should not be implemented until internal bleeding has been ruled out.
    3. Assessing the bowel sounds should be the first intervention to determine if an ileus has occurred. This is a common complication of a fractured pelvis.
    4. Buck's traction is not used to treat a fractured pelvis. It is used to treat a fractured hip.

**TEST-TAKING HINT: When prioritizing two equal options, usually assessing is the answer.**

## Joint Replacements

61. 1. The abduction pillow should be kept between the legs while in bed to maintain a neutral position and prevent internal rotation.
    2. The client should deep breathe and cough at least every two (2) hours to prevent atelectasis and pneumonia.
    3. The client will need to turn every two (2) hours but should not turn to the affected side.
    4. Using a high-seated toilet and chair will help prevent dislocation by limiting the flexion to less than 90 degrees.

**TEST-TAKING HINT: Option "1" has the word "all"; an absolute word such as this usually eliminates the option as a possible correct answer. Nursing usually does not have situations that have absolutes.**

62. 1. Bruising is common after a total hip replacement.
    2. When a dislocation occurs, the affected extremity will be shorter.
    3. Groin pain or increasing discomfort in the affected leg and the "popping sound" indicate that the leg has dislocated and should be reported immediately to the HCP for a possible closed reduction.
    4. Edema at the incision site is common, but an increase in edema or redness should be reported.

**TEST-TAKING HINT: The nurse should notify the surgeon of abnormal, unexpected, or life-threatening assessment data; if the test taker did not have an idea of the answer, pain is always a good choice because pain means something is wrong—it may be expected pain, but it may mean a complication.**

63. 1. Clients should not cross their legs because the position increases the risk for dislocation.
    2. If the client experiences a sudden increase in pain, redness, edema, or stiffness in the joint or surrounding area, the client should notify the HCP.
    3. Clients should sleep on firm mattresses and sit on chairs with firm seats and high arms. These will decrease the risk of dislocating the hip joint.
    4. Infections are possible months after surgery. Clients should monitor temperatures and report any signs of infection.

**TEST-TAKING HINT: Note the stem is asking about the need for "further teaching." This**

means the test taker is looking for an option that is not expected. This is an "except" question. Sometimes if the test taker will change the question and say "the client understands the teaching," then the option that is incorrect is the answer.

64. 1. These are not burns from the cautery unit. Such burns would be located in or near the incision site and are usually black.
   2. These are not caused by herpes simplex, the lesions of which occur in a linear pattern along a dermatome.
   3. Fluid-filled blisters are from a reaction to the tape and usually occur along the edge of the tape.
   4. Skin reactions to latex are local irritations or generalized dermatitis, not blisters.

**TEST-TAKING HINT:** If the test taker does not know the answer, the test taker might think about the dressing because the lesions are on the side of the dressing. How is a dressing anchored to the skin? Answer: with tape. The test taker would choose the option that has the word "tape."

65. 1. Clients need to understand the amount of weight bearing to prevent injury.
   2. Teaching the safe use of assistive devices is necessary prior to discharge.
   3. Increases in activity should occur slowly to prevent complications.
   4. Using medication therapy, including analgesics, anti-inflammatory agents, or muscle relaxants, should be taught so that client is comfortable while ambulating.
   5. The client should be encouraged to rest periodically to promote healing and increase energy.

**TEST-TAKING HINT:** The test taker should apply basic concepts to all surgeries. Many times the test taker may not be familiar with the specific surgery, but by using discharge teaching that is applicable to all clients, a choice can be made.

66. 1. The expected outcome for the client who has had a total hip replacement should be pain free or almost pain free.
   2. The client should be able to ambulate with almost full mobility.
   3. The hip joint should be stable.
   4. The hip should have functional motion.

**TEST-TAKING HINT:** With musculoskeletal problems functional movement is priority. Also note that options "1" and "2" have the word "limited" and "3" has "instability," all of

which are negative outcomes, so the test taker could eliminate these options.

67. 1. Drainage in the first 24 hours can be expected to be 200–400 mL. When using an autotransfusion drainage system, the client's blood will be filtered and returned to the client.
   2. Pain relief with the PCA does not require notifying the surgeon.
   3. Coolness of toes is concerning but because there were other indicators of adequate circulation, the HCP should not be notified. Circulation is not restricted if pulses are present. Seeing pale pink indicates blood loss during surgery.
   4. The urinary output is not adequate; therefore the surgeon needs to be notified. This is only 20 mL per hour. The minimum should be 30 mL per hour.

**TEST-TAKING HINT:** A concept that the test taker will see throughout testing and throughout the nurse's practice is that 30 mL of urine output per hour is necessary. Remember this indicates that the kidneys are being adequately perfused and that the heart is pumping effectively.

68. 1. The client should continue to perform respiratory exercises such as incentive spirometry and deep breathing and coughing, but this is not needed every two (2) hours.
   2. The client will not be discharged with a J-P drain; it will be removed prior to discharge.
   3. Any client who experiences the symptoms of urinary tract infection should report these to the health-care provider.
   4. Modification of the home is essential to the rehabilitation of the client using assistive devices for ambulation. The postoperative goals for this client are to maximize mobility and promote health.

**TEST-TAKING HINT:** The nurse should always think about safety; therefore the test taker should select options that address safety issues. Note that option "1" is doing an intervention every two (2) hours and that would not be appropriate for discharge.

69. 1. The client needs to have the pain managed so that the client can be as active as possible. This will help avoid complications of immobility.
   2. Clients should not be able to smoke after surgery because smoking increases the risk for pulmonary complications. Most hospitals do provide smoking areas outside the building.

3. The client must ambulate within the weight-bearing restrictions so that the knee will not be injured, which may delay healing.
4. All clients should be encouraged to do as much self-care as possible to assist with self-esteem.
5. Not all clients will able to return to their previous life roles and activities but it is the goal. They should be assisted with coping skills so that they will be able to adapt to any changes.

**TEST-TAKING HINTS:** The test taker must select more than one option in these alternate-type questions. Options "1," "2," and "4" are interventions that are applicable to any client having a surgical procedure. Option "3" is the only option that addresses ambulation; therefore, because the client had knee surgery, this would be an appropriate selection for the correct answer.

70. 1. Effective deep breathing and coughing would be demonstrated by the absence of adventitious sounds.
    2. Knee flexion should be at 90 degrees.
    3. Clients should participate in care, in decision-making, and in activities that promote mobility and adaptation to the life changes postoperatively.
    4. Pain relief should involve multiple approaches.

**TEST-TAKING HINTS:** When evaluating interventions, the correct answer should be a desired outcome specific to that client.

71. 1. These vital signs are within normal limits.
    2. Pain with dorsiflexion of the ankle indicates deep vein thrombosis. This can be from immobility or surgery; therefore pain should be assessed on both legs.
    3. Bowel sounds are normally intermittent.
    4. This type of pain would make the nurse suspect the client has flatus, which is not a life-threatening complication and would not warrant immediate intervention.

**TEST-TAKING HINT:** "Warrants immediate intervention" means life threatening, abnormal, or unexpected for the client's condition. Pain with dorsiflexion of the ankle, the Homans' sign, may be life threatening if not treated immediately.

72. 1. This is a normal treatment of a fractured femoral neck.
    2. This is an abnormal occurrence from this information. This client should be seen first because confusion is a symptom of hypoxia.
    3. This is a common treatment of a total hip replacement.
    4. This is a treatment used for total knee replacement.

**TEST-TAKING HINT:** When deciding the answer for this type of question, the test taker who does not know the answer should realize that three (3) choices have normal treatments for the disease process and one (1) option contains different information, such as a symptom, and choose the option that is different.

Musculoskeletal

1. The 50-year-old client came to the health-care provider's office for an annual physical examination. Which information should the nurse assess to rule out osteoporosis? Select all that apply.
   1. Family history of osteoporosis.
   2. Estrogen or androgen deficit.
   3. Use of tobacco products.
   4. Level and amount of exercise.
   5. Alcohol intake.

2. In preparing a plan of care for a client diagnosed with carpal tunnel syndrome, which intervention should the nurse include?
   1. Teach hyperextension exercises to increase flexibility.
   2. Monitor safety during occupational hazards.
   3. Prepare for the insertions of pins or screws.
   4. Monitor dressing and drain after the fasciotomy.

3. When the manager is completing the client assignments for the next shift, which nurse should the manager assign to the client recovering from a repair of the hallux valgus?
   1. A new graduate nurse.
   2. An experienced nurse.
   3. A nurse practitioner.
   4. An unlicensed nursing assistant.

4. The client has been scheduled for a computed tomography (CT) scan. Which information is most important for the nurse to obtain before the procedure?
   1. The assessment of the client's pain.
   2. Vital signs are within normal limits.
   3. Whether client has allergies to seafood.
   4. Type of intravenous fluid being administered.

5. The student nurse asks the emergency department nurse why the nurse is careful to maintain asepsis when caring for the client with an open fracture of the right humerus. Which rationale explains the nurse's actions?
   1. It is a policy to prevent the transmission of blood borne pathogens.
   2. Clients who have open fractures are at a high risk for osteomyelitis.
   3. Failure to maintain asepsis may result in a malpractice lawsuit.
   4. The client has compromised immunity based on the laboratory values.

6. While working in the day surgery department, the nurse is caring for the client two (2) hours after having a right knee arthroscopy. Which intervention should the nurse implement?
   1. Encourage the client to perform range-of-motion exercises.
   2. Monitor the amount and color of the urinary output hourly.
   3. Check the client's pulses distally and assess the toes.
   4. Monitor the client's vital signs every eight (8) hours.

7. The nurse is responsible for teaching the client to take Fosamax, a bisphosphonate. Which information should the nurse include?
   1. Take this medication with a full glass of water.
   2. Take with breakfast to prevent gastrointestinal upset.
   3. Use sunscreen to prevent sensitivity to sunlight.
   4. This medication increases calcium reabsorption.

8. The school nurse is completing spinal screenings. Which data would require a referral to an HCP?
   1. Bilateral arm lengthens while bending over at the waist.
   2. A deformity that resolves when the head is raised.
   3. Equal spacing of the arms and body at the waist.
   4. A right arm lower than the left while bending over at the waist.

9. The nurse is working in the clinic and assesses the client with complaints of pain and numbness in the left hand and fingers. What data should the nurse look for when assessing this client to determine the cause of the complaints?
   1. Symmetric movements of elbows and shoulders.
   2. A capillary refill time of less than three (3) seconds.
   3. A history of any repetitive movements during work or leisure.
   4. Bilateral anterior and posterior deep-tendon reflexes.

10. The nurse is teaching the client diagnosed with osteoporosis about the medication calcitonin, a thyroid hormone. Which data would indicate that the teaching has been effective?
    1. The client states, "I should change nostrils from day to day."
    2. The client states, "I need to drink a lot of water when I take my medicine."
    3. The client demonstrates how to dilute the medication with vitamin D.
    4. The client states, "This will help the calcium leave my bones."

11. The client asks the nurse, "Why am I having this bone scan?" Which statement would be the nurse's best response?
    1. "You seem anxious. Tell me about your anxieties."
    2. "Why are you concerned? Your HCP ordered it."
    3. "I'll have the radiologist come back to explain it again."
    4. "A bone scan looks for cancer or infection inside the bones."

12. The client is scheduled for a magnetic resonance imaging (MRI) scan. Which intervention should the nurse delegate to the unlicensed nursing assistant?
    1. Prepare the client by removing all metal objects.
    2. Inject the contrast into the intravenous site.
    3. Administer a sedative to the client to decrease anxiety.
    4. Explain why the client cannot have any breakfast.

13. A client is admitted to the orthopedic floor after having sustained a fractured femur in a motor-vehicle accident. Which data would require immediate intervention by the nurse? Select all that apply.
    1. The client becomes restless and irritable.
    2. The client has tachypnea and tachycardia.
    3. The client has petechiae over the neck and chest.
    4. The client has a high arterial oxygen level.
    5. The client has yellow globules floating in the urine.

14. The nurse is caring for the client diagnosed with fat embolism syndrome. Which HCP order would the nurse question?
    1. Administer intravenous heparin.
    2. Administer intravenous fluids.
    3. Keep the $O_2$ saturation higher than 93%.
    4. Administer a loop diuretic.

15. The client has been admitted to the hospital for repair of a fractured femoral neck. Which would be the expected short-term goal for this client?
    1. The client will be turned every two (2) hours to prevent skin breakdown.
    2. The client will have a decrease in muscle spasms and pain in the affected leg.
    3. The client will have no objective or subjective signs or symptoms of infection.
    4. The client will be able to ambulate down the hallway to the nurse's station.

16. The nurse is preparing to administer subcutaneous Lovenox, a low molecular weight heparin. Which intervention should the nurse implement?
    1. Monitor the client's serum aPTT.
    2. Encourage oral and intravenous fluids.
    3. Give with food to protect the stomach.
    4. Administer in the "love handles."

Musculoskeletal

17. When caring for the client with a fractured right hip who has Buck's traction, which intervention should the nurse include in the plan of care?
    1. Assess the insertion sites for signs and symptoms of infection.
    2. Monitor for drainage or odor from under the plaster covering the pins.
    3. Monitor the condition of the skin beneath the Velcro™ boot every eight (8) hours.
    4. Take weights off for one (1) hour every eight (8) hours and as needed.

18. When caring for a client with a spica cast for a hip injury, what intervention should the nurse include in the plan of care?
    1. Assess client's popliteal pulses every shift.
    2. Elevate the leg on pillows and apply ice packs.
    3. Teach the client how to ambulate with a tripod walker.
    4. Assess the client for distention and vomiting.

19. When preparing the client in a short leg cast for discharge, which data indicate that the client needs further teaching?
    1. "I need to keep my leg elevated on two pillows for the first 24 hours."
    2. "I should apply ice packs for one (1) hour and remove them for one (1) hour."
    3. "I need to contact the health-care provider if I have any numbness or pale toenails."
    4. "I can put a coat hanger down the cast to scratch gently if I have severe itching."

20. Which psychosocial client problem would be most likely in a client with an external fixator device?
    1. Ineffective coping.
    2. Alteration in body image.
    3. Grieving.
    4. Social isolation.

21. A client recovering from a total hip replacement has developed a deep vein thrombosis. The health-care provider has ordered a continuous infusion of heparin, an anticoagulant, to infuse at 1200 units per hour. The bag comes with 20,000 unit of heparin in 500 mL of 0.9% normal saline. At what rate should the nurse set the pump?_____

22. When conducting rounds at change of shift, the nurse assesses the client with a fractured humerus. Which data would warrant immediate intervention by the nurse?
    1. Capillary refill time of that arm is less than three (3) seconds.
    2. Pain relieved by the patient-controlled anesthesia machine.
    3. Edema under the dressing that caused the nails to be white.
    4. Warm and dry skin on the fingers distally to the elastic bandage.

23. The client with a right open fractured elbow has a long arm cast and is complaining of unrelenting severe pain and feeling as if the fingers are asleep. Which complication should the nurse suspect that the client is experiencing?
    1. Fat embolism.
    2. Compartment syndrome.
    3. Pressure ulcer under cast.
    4. Surgical incision infection.

24. The elderly client is admitted to the hospital for severe back pain. Which data should the nurse assess first during the admission assessment?
    1. The client's use of herbs.
    2. The client's current pain level.
    3. The client's sexual orientation.
    4. The client's ability to care for self.

25. Which information should the nurse teach the client regarding sports injuries?
    1. Apply heat intermittently for the first 48 hours.
    2. An injury is not serious if the extremity can be moved.
    3. Only return to health-care provider if the foot becomes cold.
    4. Keep the injury immobilized and elevated for 24 to 48 hours.

**26.** The emergency department nurse is caring for a client with a compound fracture of the right ulna. Which interventions should the nurse implement? List in order of priority.
1. Apply a sterile, normal, saline-soaked gauze to the arm.
2. Send the client to radiology for an x-ray of the arm.
3. Assess the fingers of the client's right hand.
4. Stabilize the arm at the wrist and the elbow.
5. Administer a tetanus toxoid injection.

1. 1. Clients are more prone to have osteoporosis if there is a genetic predisposition.
   2. Clients who are deficient in either estrogen or androgen are at risk for osteoporosis.
   3. Clients who smoke are more at risk for osteoporosis.
   4. Regular, weight-bearing exercise promotes healthy bones.
   5. Clients who consume alcohol and have diets low in calcium are at a higher risk for osteoporosis.

2. 1. Treatment for carpal tunnel syndrome does not include hyperextension of the wrist.
   2. The nurse should monitor for potential injuries resulting from the alterations in motor, sensory, and autonomic function of the first three digits of the hand and palmar surface of the fourth. These alterations can interfere with pinching or grasping, which, in turn, increases the risk for injury in clients whose occupations require the use of equipment such as jackhammers and computers.
   3. Surgery may be needed to release the compression of the medial nerve, but pins and screws are used to hold the position.
   4. A fasciotomy is used to repair Dupuytren's contracture, not carpal tunnel syndrome. "Fascia" refers to the connective tissue. "Fasciectomy" refers to the surgical excision of strips of connective tissue.

3. 1. A new graduate is the best choice for this client. The client's surgery is not a high-risk procedure but would require assessment and pain management.
   2. This client does not need a more experienced nurse.
   3. A nurse practitioner would not be assigned this client.
   4. The unlicensed nursing assistant (NA) is not assigned the responsibility of managing the care of a client; the NA works under the guidance of the nurse.

4. 1. The assessment of the pain would be important so that the client will be able to tolerate the procedure. Pain would not be a life-threatening problem but would be a quality-of-care issue.
   2. Vital signs should be taken prior to transport to the radiology department. This intervention would not prevent a complication of the diagnostic examination.

   3. This is the most important information the nurse should obtain. Any client who is allergic to seafood cannot be injected with the iodine-based contrast. This contrast would cause an allergic response that could endanger the client's life.
   4. This would be important to determine if the fluid is compatible with the iodine-based contrast, but it is not the most important.

5. 1. This would explain a policy for all clients, not specific to the client to whom the question refers.
   2. The open skin and exposure of the bone is a direct pathway for infection and osteomyelitis.
   3. Failure to meet standards of care may result in malpractice legal action, but this is not the reason for maintaining aseptic technique.
   4. The question does not indicate that the client has a compromised immunity.

6. 1. The nurse should not encourage range of motion until the surgeon gives permission for flexion of the knee.
   2. Urinary output is important postoperatively, but monitoring it is not needed hourly for a client in day surgery. However, the nurse should make sure the client urinates before discharge.
   3. Pulses and circulation checks should be done every one (1) to two (2) hours postoperatively.
   4. Vital signs are assessed more frequently than every eight (8) hours.

7. 1. The client needs to take this medication with a full glass of water and remain upright for at least 30 minutes to reduce the risk of esophagitis.
   2. This medication should be taken before breakfast on an empty stomach.
   3. This medication does not cause photosensitivity.
   4. This medication decreases calcium reabsorption by decreasing the activity of osteoclasts.

8. 1. This is normal data that would not require intervention.
   2. If the screener suspects the client has scoliosis while the client is bending over, the screener asks the client to raise the head. An abnormality caused by scoliosis will not resolve.
   3. This indicates a normal occurrence and does not need to be referred.

4. Unequal arm length may indicate scoliosis, and further assessment is needed by an HCP.

9. 1. This would not be the cause of hand pain and numbness.
   2. This is normal data that would not cause pain or numbness.
   3. This information would assist with the diagnosis of carpal tunnel syndrome. Clients with this disorder experience pain and numbness.
   4. Bilateral deep tendon reflexes are normal data and would not cause hand pain and numbness.

10. 1. This should be taught so that when the client takes the medication intranasally it will decrease irritation from administration.
   2. This intervention should be implemented for Fosamax, a bisphosphonate, not calcitonin, thyroid hormone.
   3. This medication should not be diluted with vitamin D.
   4. Calcium should be retained in the bone to maintain bone strength; medications are not administered to encourage loss from the bone.

11. 1. This is a therapeutic technique, but the client is asking for information. When a client seeks information, the nurse should give that information first. Discussion of feelings should follow.
   2. This is a nontherapuetic technique that will block communication between the client and the nurse. The nurse should avoid a response with the word "why," which asks the client to explain or justify feelings to the nurse.
   3. When the client requests information, the nurse needs to provide accurate information, not pass the buck.
   4. This statement simply answers the client's question.

12. 1. Metal objects such as jewelry and zippers can interfere with the magnetic imaging and pose a danger to the client as a result of the magnetic properties of the equipment. Clients with pacemakers should not have an MRI because the magnet will disrupt the unit's program. This intervention can be delegated to the unlicensed nursing assistant.
   2. Injection of contrast is given in the radiology department.
   3. Unlicensed nursing assistants are unable to administer medications in hospitals.

4. The nurse cannot delegate teaching to unlicensed nursing assistants.

13. 1. The first sign of a fat embolism syndrome is an altered mental status. This requires an immediate response to save this client's life. The health-care provider should be notified.
   2. The client will experience rapid heart rate and rapid respiratory rates as a compensatory response to hypoxia. The nurse should recognize this situation and intervene. The health-care provider should be notified.
   3. Petechiae are macular, red–purple pinpoint bleeding under the skin. The appearance of petechiae is a classic sign of fat embolism syndrome.
   4. The arterial oxygen level would be low, not elevated. This sign would not warrant immediate intervention.
   5. Yellow globules in the urine are fat globules released from the bone as it breaks. This should be reported immediately.

14. 1. The HCP would prescribe heparin in treating a fat embolism.
   2. This client should be hydrated to prevent platelet aggregation.
   3. The nurse should monitor oxygen levels and administer oxygen as needed to prevent further complications.
   4. The nurse should question this order. This will decrease the client's hydration and may result in further embolism.

15. 1. This is not an outcome. This is a nursing intervention with rationale.
   2. This is an expected outcome for a preoperative client with a fractured femoral neck. This injury causes painful muscle spasms. Buck's traction is applied to decrease or prevent spasms by maintaining the position and alignment of the bone fragments.
   3. There is no break in the skin from the fracture so this would not be the best expected outcome for this client.
   4. Increased mobility would be an expected outcome for a postoperative client.

16. 1. An aPTT is used to determine therapeutic levels of unfractionated heparin. Laboratory studies such as aPTT are not monitored when administering subcutaneous Lovenox, a low molecular weight heparin. A therapeutic level will not be achieved as a result of a short life.
   2. Oral fluids would not need to be increased because of this medication.

3. This medication is administered parenterally, not orally. Food intake has no bearing on this medication.

4. **Administering this medication in the prescribed areas would ensure safety and decrease the risk of abdominal trauma.**

17. 1. Skeletal traction has a pin, screws, tongs, or wires inserted into the bone. There is no insertion site in skin traction.

    2. Plaster traction is a combination of skeletal traction using pins and a plaster brace to maintain alignment of any deformities.

    3. **In Buck's traction a Velcro boot is used to attach the ropes to weights to maintain alignment. Skin covered by the boot can become irritated and break down. The nurse should monitor the skin around the boot for redness and breakdown at least once every eight (8) hours while maintaining traction to the leg manually.**

    4. Buck's traction is applied preoperatively to prevent muscle spasms and maintain alignment, and the weights should not be removed unless assessing for skin breakdown.

18. 1. The client's popliteal pulse will be under the cast and cannot be assessed by the nurse; circulation is assessed by the 6 Ps of the neurovascular assessment.

    2. Elevation should be used with an arm cast or leg cast, but this is not possible with a spica cast.

    3. Clients with spica casts will not be able to ambulate because the cast covers the entire lower half of the body.

    4. **The nurse should assess the client for signs and symptoms of cast syndrome—vomiting after meals, epigastric pain, and abdominal distention. This is caused by a partial bowel obstruction from compression and can lead to complete obstruction. The client may still have bowel sounds present with this syndrome.**

19. 1. This is a correct intervention. The leg should be elevated for at least the first 24 hours. If edema is present, the client needs to keep it elevated longer.

    2. Ice packs should be applied to the cast for the first 24 hours, to help with itching and edema.

    3. The client needs to understand that severe complications can occur if edema impairs the circulation to the extremity. If there is pallor, numbness, paresthesia, coldness, or foul odor, the health-care provider should be notified.

    4. **Clients should be taught that putting objects down the cast to scratch an itch can cause breaks in skin integrity that may become infected.**

20. 1. This client problem ineffective coping is usually not indicated for a client with an external fixator device unless the stem provides more information about the client.

    2. **Many clients with an external fixator have alterations in body image because of the large bulky frame that makes dressing difficult and because of the scarring that occurs from the trauma and treatment. The length of healing is prolonged, so returning to the client's normal routine is delayed.**

    3. The client problem of grieving is usually not indicated for a client with an external fixator device, unless the stem of the question provides more information about the client.

    4. This client problem of social isolation is usually not indicated for a client with an external fixator device, unless the stem provides more information about the client.

21. 30 mL per hour. Divide the amount of heparin by the volume of fluid to get the concentration. Divide the dose ordered by the concentration for the amount of milliliters per hour to set the pump.

$$\frac{20000 \text{ units}}{500 \text{ mL}} = 40 \text{ units of heparin per 1 mL}$$

$$\frac{1200 \text{ units}}{40 \text{ units}} = 30 \text{ mL per hour}$$

22. 1. This is a normal assessment finding and would not require immediate action.

    2. Pain relieved by the patient-controlled anesthesia pump is an expected outcome that would not require intervention.

    3. **Cool, white nails indicate impaired circulation to the arm from edema. Without immediate intervention, the client could develop compartment syndrome.**

    4. The fingers distal to the Ace bandage indicate adequate circulation and would require no intervention.

23. 1. These are not signs/symptoms of a fat embolism.

    2. **These are the classic signs/symptoms of compartment syndrome.**

    3. Clients in casts rarely develop pressure ulcers and usually they are not painful.

    4. Hot spots on the cast usually indicate a surgical incision under the cast.

24. 1. This is a question that the admitting nurse would ask all clients, but it is not the most important.

    2. **Pain assessment and management are**

the most important issues if the client is breathing and has circulation. Lack of pain management decreases the attention of the client during the admission process. Pain is called the fifth vital sign.

3. Sexual practices are included in the admission forms, but they are not as important as pain management.

4. Assessing the client's ability to perform activities of daily living and self-care is important to prepare this client for discharge, which begins on admission, but this is not the most important at this time.

25. 1. Ice should be applied intermittently for the first 48 hours. Heat can be used later in the recovery process.

2. Severe injury can be present even with some range of motion.

3. The client needs to return if the injury does not improve and if the foot gets cold.

4. The leg should be iced, elevated, and immobilized for 48 hours.

26. The order should be 4, 1, 3, 2, 5.

4. The nurse first should stabilize the arm to prevent further injury.

1. A compound fracture is one in which the bone protrudes through the skin. The nurse should apply sterile, saline-soaked gauze to protect the area from the intrusion of bacteria.

3. The nurse should assess the client's circulation to the part distal to the injury. This is done after the first two interventions because life-threatening complications could occur if stabilization and protection from infection are not addressed first.

2. An x-ray will be needed to determine the extent of the injury.

5. A tetanus toxoid injection should be administered, but this can be done last.

Musculoskeletal

# 12

# Integumentary Disorders

The integument, or skin, the largest organ in the body, is subject to many disorders. Some, like the diseases/disorders that affect other body systems, are infectious; included are bacterial, viral, and fungal infections of the skin. Burns and pressure ulcers also affect the skin. This chapter discusses these disorders and other problems, including psoriasis, seborrheic dermatosis, and contact dermatitis.

## KEYWORDS

escharotomy
keloid
paraplegia
quadriplegia

## ABBREVIATIONS

Acquired Immunodeficiency Syndrome (AIDS)
Arterial Blood Gases (ABG)
Cerebrovascular Accident (CVA)
Emergency Department (ED)
Fluid Volume Deficit (FVD)
Health-Care Provider (HCP)
Intravenous (IV)
Intravenous Push (IVP)
Over-The-Counter (OTC)
Sun Protection Factor (SPF)
Ultraviolet Light (UVL)
Unlicensed Assistive Personnel (UAP)
Within Normal Limits (WNL)

## Burns

1. The client comes into the emergency room in severe pain and reports that a boiling pot of hot water accidentally spilled on his lower legs. The assessment reveals blistered, mottled red skin, and both feet are edematous. Which depth of burn should the nurse document?
   1. Superficial partial thickness.
   2. Deep partial thickness.
   3. Full thickness.
   4. First degree.

2. The client with full-thickness burns to 40% of the body, including both legs, is being transferred from a community hospital to a burn center. Which measure should be instituted before the transfer?
   1. A 22-gauge intravenous line with normal saline infusing.
   2. Wounds covered with moist sterile dressings.
   3. No intravenous pain medication.
   4. Adequate peripheral circulation to both feet ensured.

3. The client has full-thickness burns to 65% of the body, including the chest area. After establishing a patent airway, which collaborative intervention is priority for the client?
   1. Replace fluids and electrolytes.
   2. Prevent contractures of extremities.
   3. Monitor urine output hourly.
   4. Prepare to assist with an escharotomy.

4. The nurse is applying mafenide acetate, Sulfamylon, a sulfa antibiotic cream, to a client's lower-extremity burn. Which assessment data would require immediate attention by the nurse?
   1. The client complains of pain when the medication is administered.
   2. The client's potassium level is 3.9 mEq/L and sodium level is 137 mEq/L.
   3. The client's ABGs are pH 7.34, $PaO_2$ 98, $PaCO_2$ 38, and $HCO_3$ 20.
   4. The client is able to perform active range-of-motion exercises.

5. The client is scheduled to have a xenograft to a left lower-leg burn. The client asks the nurse, "What is a xenograft?" Which statement by the nurse would be the best response?
   1. "The doctor will graft skin from your back to your leg."
   2. "The skin from a donor will be used to cover your burn."
   3. "The graft will come from an animal, probably a pig."
   4. "I think you should ask your doctor about the graft."

6. The intensive care burn nurse is developing a nursing care plan for a client with severe full-thickness and deep-partial thickness burns over half the body. Which client problem has priority?
   1. High risk for infection.
   2. Ineffective coping.
   3. Impaired physical mobility.
   4. Knowledge deficit.

7. The nurse writes the nursing diagnosis "impaired skin integrity related to open burn wounds." Which intervention would be appropriate for this nursing diagnosis?
   1. Provide analgesia before pain becomes severe.
   2. Clean the client's wounds, body, and hair daily.
   3. Screen visitors for respiratory infections.
   4. Encourage visitors to bring plants and flowers.

8. Which nursing interventions should be included for the client who has full-thickness and deep-partial thickness burns to 50% of the body? Select all that apply.
   1. Perform meticulous hand hygiene.
   2. Use sterile gloves for wound care.
   3. Wear gown and mask during procedures.
   4. Change invasive lines once a week.
   5. Administer antibiotics as prescribed.

9. The nurse is caring for a client with deep partial-thickness and full-thickness burns to the chest area. Which assessment data would warrant notifying the health-care provider?
   1. The client is complaining of severe pain.
   2. The client's pulse oximeter reading is 95%.
   3. The client has a T 100.4°F, P 100, R 24, and BP 102/60.
   4. The client's urinary output is 50 mL in two (2) hours.

10. The client is admitted with full-thickness and partial-thickness burns to more than 30% of the body. The nurse is concerned with the client's nutritional status. Which intervention should the nurse implement?
    1. Encourage the client's family to bring favorite foods.
    2. Provide a low-fat, low-cholesterol diet for the client.
    3. Monitor the client's weight weekly in the same clothes.
    4. Make a referral to the hospital social worker.

11. The client sustained a hot grease burn to the right hand and calls the emergency room for advice. Which information should the nurse provide to the client?
    1. Apply an ice pack to the right hand.
    2. Place the hand in cool water.
    3. Be sure to rupture any blister formation.
    4. Go immediately to the doctor's office.

12. The client is being discharged after being in the burn unit for six (6) weeks. Which strategies should the nurse identify to promote the client's mental health?
    1. Encourage the client to stay at home as much as possible.
    2. Discuss the importance of not relying on the family for needs.
    3. Tell the client to remember that changes in lifestyle take time.
    4. Instruct the client to discuss feelings only with the therapist.

## Pressure Ulcers

13. The nurse in a long-term care facility is teaching a group of new unlicensed assistive personnel. Which information regarding skin care should the nurse emphasize?
    1. Keep the skin moist by leaving the skin damp after the bath.
    2. Do not rub any lotion into the skin.
    3. Turn clients who are immobile at least every two (2) hours.
    4. Only the licensed nursing staff may care for the client's skin.

14. The nurse is caring for a client who has developed stage IV pressure ulcers on the left trochanter and coccyx. Which collaborative problem has the highest priority?
    1. Impaired cognition.
    2. Altered nutrition.
    3. Self-care deficit.
    4. Altered coping.

15. The nurse is caring for clients in a long-term care facility. Which is a modifiable risk factor for the development of pressure ulcers?
    1. Constant perineal moisture.
    2. Ability of the clients to reposition themselves.
    3. Decreased elasticity of the skin.
    4. Impaired cardiovascular perfusion of the periphery.

Integumentary

16. What is the scientific rationale for placing lift pads under an immobile client?
    1. The pads will absorb any urinary incontinence and contain stool.
    2. The pads will prevent the client from being diaphoretic.
    3. The pads will keep the staff from workplace injuries such as a pulled muscle.
    4. The pads will help prevent friction shearing when repositioning the client.

17. The paraplegic client is being admitted to a medical unit from home with a stage IV pressure ulcer over the right ischium. Which assessment tool should be completed on admission to the hospital?
    1. Complete the Braden Scale.
    2. Monitor the client on a Glasgow Coma Scale.
    3. Assess for a Babinski sign.
    4. Initiate a Brudzinski flow sheet.

18. The wound care nurse documented a client's pressure ulcers on admission as 3.3 cm × 4.0 cm stage II on the coccyx. Which information would alert the nurse that the client's pressure ulcer is getting worse?
    1. The skin is not broken and is 2.5cm × 3.5 cm with erythema that does not blanch.
    2. There is a 3.2-cm × 4.1-cm blister that is red and drains occasionally.
    3. The skin covering the coccyx is intact but the client complains of pain in the area.
    4. The coccyx wound extends to the subcutaneous layer and there is drainage.

19. The nurse and unlicensed assistive personnel on a medical floor are caring for clients who are elderly and immobile. Which action by the assistant warrants immediate intervention by the nurse?
    1. The assistant elevates the head of the bed of a client that can feed himself with minimal assistance.
    2. The assistant asks to take a meal break before turning the clients at the two (2)-hour time limit.
    3. The assistant restocks the rooms that need unsterile gloves before clocking out for the shift.
    4. The assistant mixes Thick-It® into the glass of water for a client who has difficulty swallowing.

20. The nurse is caring for clients on a medical unit. After the shift report which client should the nurse assess first?
    1. The 34-year-old client who is quadriplegic and cannot move his arms.
    2. The elderly client diagnosed with a CVA who is weak on the right side.
    3. The 78-year-old client with pressure ulcers who has a temperature of 102.3°F.
    4. The young adult who is unhappy with the care that was provided last shift.

21. The nurse is developing a plan of care for a client diagnosed with left-sided paralysis secondary to a right-sided cerebrovascular accident (stroke). Which should be included in the interventions?
    1. Use a pillow to keep the heels off the bed when supine.
    2. Order a low air loss therapy bed immediately.
    3. Prepare to insert a nasogastric feeding tube.
    4. Order an occupational therapy consult for strength training.

22. The client who is debilitated and has developed multiple pressure ulcers complains to the nurse during a dressing change that he is "tired of it all." Which is the nurse's best therapeutic response?
    1. "These wound can heal if we get enough protein into you."
    2. "Are you tired of the treatments and needing to be cared for?"
    3. "Why would you say that? We are doing our best."
    4. "Have you made out an advance directive to let the HCP know your wishes?"

23. The nurse writes the problem "impaired skin integrity" for a client with stage IV pressure ulcers. Which interventions should be included in the plan of care? Select all that apply.
    1. Turn the client every three (3) to four (4) hours.
    2. Ask the dietician to consult.
    3. Have the client sign a consent for pictures of the wounds.
    4. Obtain an order for a low air loss bed.
    5. Elevate the head of the bed at all times.

24. The client diagnosed with stage IV infected pressure ulcers on the coccyx is scheduled for a fecal diversion operation. The nurse knows that client teaching has been effective when the client makes which statement?
    1. "This surgery will create a skin flap to cover my wounds."
    2. "This surgery will get all the old black tissue out of the wound so it can heal."
    3. "The surgery is important to allow oxygen to get to the tissue for healing to occur."
    4. "Stool will come out an opening in my abdomen so it won't get in the sore."

## Skin Cancer

25. The school nurse is preparing to teach a health promotion class to high school seniors. Which information regarding self-care should be included in the teaching?
    1. Wear a sunscreen with a protection factor of ten (10) or less when in the sun.
    2. Try to stay out of the sun between 0300 and 0500 daily.
    3. Perform a thorough skin check monthly.
    4. Remember that caps and long sleeves do not help prevent skin cancer.

26. The female client admitted for an unrelated diagnosis asks the nurse to check her back because "it itches all the time in that one spot." When the nurse assesses the client's back, the nurse notes an irregular-shaped lesion with some scabbed-over areas surrounding the lesion. Which action should the nurse implement first?
    1. Notify the HCP to check the lesion on rounds.
    2. Measure the lesion and note the color.
    3. Apply lotion to the lesion.
    4. Instruct the client to make sure the HCP checks the lesion.

27. The nurse is caring for clients in an outpatient surgery clinic. Which client should be assessed first?
    1. The client scheduled for a skin biopsy who is crying.
    2. The client who had surgery three (3) hours ago and is sleeping.
    3. The client who needs to void prior to discharge.
    4. The client who has received discharge instructions and is ready to go home.

28. Which client is at the greatest risk for the development of skin cancer?
    1. The African American male who lives in the northeast.
    2. The elderly Hispanic female who moved from Mexico as a child.
    3. The client who has a family history of basal cell carcinoma.
    4. The client with fair complexion who cannot get a tan.

29. The middle-aged client has had two (2) lesions diagnosed as basal cell carcinoma removed. Which discharge instruction should the nurse include?
    1. Teach the client that there is no more risk for cancer.
    2. Refer the client to a prosthesis specialist for prosthesis.
    3. Instruct the client how to apply sunscreen to the area.
    4. Demonstrate care of the surgical site.

30. The nurse is caring for a client diagnosed with squamous cell skin cancer and writes a psychosocial problem of "fear." Which nursing interventions should be included in the plan of care?
    1. Explain to the client that the fears are unfounded.
    2. Encourage the client to verbalize the feeling of being afraid.
    3. Have the HCP discuss the client's fear with the client.
    4. Instruct the client regarding all planned procedures.

31. The nurse and an unlicensed assistive personnel are caring for clients in a dermatology clinic. Which task should not be delegated to the unlicensed assistant?
    1. Stock the rooms with the equipment needed.
    2. Weigh the clients and position the clients for the examination.
    3. Discuss problems the client has experienced since the previous visit.
    4. Take the biopsy specimens to the laboratory.

32. The client is admitted to the outpatient surgery center for removal of a malignant melanoma. Which assessment data indicate the lesion is a malignant melanoma?
    1. The lesion is asymmetrical and has irregular borders.
    2. The lesion has a waxy appearance with pearl-like borders.
    3. The lesion has a thickened and scaly appearance.
    4. The lesion appeared as a thickened area after an injury.

33. The client has had a squamous cell carcinoma removed from the lip. Which discharge instructions should the nurse provide?
    1. Notify the HCP if a lesion that does not heal develops around the mouth.
    2. Squamous cell carcinoma tumors do not metastasize.
    3. Limit foods to liquid or soft consistency for one (1) month.
    4. Apply heat to the area for 20 minutes every four (4) hours.

34. Which client physiological outcome (goal) is appropriate for a client diagnosed with skin cancer who has had surgery to remove the lesion?
    1. The client will express feelings of fear.
    2. The client will ask questions about the diagnosis.
    3. The client will state a diminished level of pain.
    4. The client will demonstrate care of operative site.

35. The male client diagnosed with acquired immunodeficiency syndrome (AIDS) states that he has developed a purple–brown spot on his calf. Which action should the nurse do first?
    1. Refer the client to an HCP for a biopsy of the area.
    2. Assess the lesion for size, color, and symmetry.
    3. Discuss end-of-life decisions with the client.
    4. Report the sexually transmitted disease to the health department.

36. The nurse participating in a health fair is discussing malignant melanoma with a group of clients. Which information regarding the use of sunscreen is important to include?
    1. Sunscreen is only needed during the hottest hours of the day.
    2. Toddlers should not have sunscreen applied to their skin.
    3. Sunscreen does not help prevent skin cancer.
    4. The higher the number of the sunscreen, the more it blocks UV rays.

## Bacterial Skin Infection

37. The client comes to the emergency department complaining of pain in the left lower leg following a puncture wound from a nail in a board. The left lower leg is reddened with streaks, edematous, and hot to the touch, and the client has a temperature of 100.8°F. Which condition would the nurse suspect the client is experiencing?
    1. Cellulitis.
    2. Lyme disease.
    3. Impetigo.
    4. Deep vein thrombosis.

38. The client comes to the clinic complaining of sudden onset of high fever, chills, and a headache. The nurse assesses a patchy macular rash on the trunk and a circular type of rash that looks like an insect bite. Which question would be most appropriate for the nurse to ask during the interview?
    1. "Do you own dogs that stay in the yard?"
    2. "Have you been working in your garden lately?"
    3. "Have you been deer hunting in the last week?"
    4. "Do you use sunscreen when you are outside?"

39. The school nurse is discussing impetigo with the teachers in an elementary school. One of the teachers asks the nurse, "How can I prevent getting impetigo?" Which statement would be the most appropriate response?
    1. "Wash your hands after using the bathroom."
    2. "Do not touch any affected areas without gloves."
    3. "Apply a topical antibiotic to your hands."
    4. "Keep the child with impetigo isolated in the room."

40. The client is admitted to the medical floor diagnosed with cellulitis of the left arm. Which assessment data would warrant immediate intervention by the nurse?
    1. The client has bilaterally weak radial pulses.
    2. The client is able to move the left fingers.
    3. The client has a CRT less than 3 seconds.
    4. The client is unable to remove the wedding ring.

41. The nurse writes the client problem of "acute pain and itching secondary to bacterial skin lesions." Which intervention should be included in the care plan? Select all that apply.
    1. Keep humidity at less than 20%.
    2. Maintain a cool environment.
    3. Use a mild soap for sensitive skin.
    4. Keep lesions covered at all times.
    5. Apply skin lotion after bathing.

42. The nurse observes the unlicensed assistive personnel squeezing the "blackheads" on an elderly client. Which action should the nurse implement first?
    1. Notify the Unit Manager of witnessing this activity.
    2. Instruct the assistant to stop this behavior.
    3. Demonstrate the correct way to care for the skin.
    4. Complete an incident report regarding the action.

43. The client is diagnosed with acne vulgaris. Which psychosocial problem is priority?
    1. Impaired skin integrity.
    2. Ineffective grieving.
    3. Body-image disturbance.
    4. Knowledge deficit.

44. Which individual would most likely experience the skin disorder pseudofolliculitis barbae (shaving bumps)?
    1. A male African American soldier.
    2. A female Caucasian hairdresser.
    3. A male Asian food server.
    4. A female Hispanic schoolteacher.

45. The female client calls the clinic and tells the nurse that she has a really big "boil" in the perineal area that is causing a lot of pain. Which intervention should the nurse implement?
    1. Schedule an emergency appointment for the client.
    2. Instruct the client to apply warm, moist compresses to the area.
    3. Determine if someone can squeeze the boil.
    4. Explain that this will resolve on it own.

Integumentary

46. Which client would most likely be at risk for the development of a carbuncle?
    1. The young male who is just beginning to shave.
    2. The female with a fair complexion.
    3. The male who works out in the gym daily.
    4. The female diagnosed with diabetes mellitus.

47. The female teacher comes to the school nurse's office and shows the nurse a rash on her hands. The nurse tells the teacher she has probably contracted impetigo from one of the students. Which intervention should the nurse implement?
    1. Instruct the teacher to go to her HCP today.
    2. Tell the teacher to wash her hands with soap and water.
    3. Encourage the teacher to rub vitamin E oil on the lesions.
    4. Explain that the rash will go away in a few days.

48. The nurse is teaching a class on how to prevent Lyme disease. Which intervention should be included in the discussion?
    1. Instruct the clients to wear dark clothes when hunting.
    2. Use a sunscreen of at least SPF 30 when outside.
    3. Avoid dense undergrowth when in a wooded area.
    4. Do not use any type of insect repellant when deer hunting.

## Viral Skin Infection

49. The nurse is discussing the prevention of herpes simplex 2. Which intervention should the nurse discuss with the client?
    1. Encourage the client to get the chickenpox immunization.
    2. Do not engage in oral sex if you have a cold sore on the mouth.
    3. Wear nonsterile gloves when cleaning the genital area.
    4. Do not share any type of towel or washcloth with another person.

50. The client is complaining of burning, lancinating, stabbing pain that radiates around the left rib cage area. The nurse cannot find any type of skin abnormality. Which action should the nurse implement?
    1. Transfer the client to the ED for a cardiac workup.
    2. Inform the client that the nurse can't see anything.
    3. Administer a nonnarcotic analgesic to the client.
    4. Ask the client if he or she has ever had chickenpox.

51. The client is diagnosed with herpes simplex 2 and prescribed the antiviral medication valacyclovir (Valtrex). Which instructions should the nurse teach?
    1. This medication will prevent pregnancy and treat the virus.
    2. This medication must be tapered when discontinuing the medication.
    3. This medication will suppress symptoms but does not cure the disease.
    4. This medication may cause the client's urine to turn orange.

52. The nurse administered morphine sulfate, a narcotic analgesic, IVP 45 minutes ago to a client diagnosed with herpes zoster. On reassessment, the client complains the pain is at a "5" on a 1–10 scale. Which intervention should the nurse implement?
    1. Turn on soft music and shut the blinds.
    2. Apply warm, moist heat to the lesions.
    3. Notify the HCP for more pain medication.
    4. Encourage the client to ambulate with assistance.

53. The client is diagnosed with disseminated herpes zoster secondary to AIDS. Which interventions should the nurse implement? Select all that apply.
    1. Place in contact isolation.
    2. Administer a corticosteroid IVP.
    3. Assess the client's pain on a 1–10 scale.
    4. Request that the client not have any visitors.
    5. Ensure that only nurses who have had chickenpox care for this client.

54. Which statement by the client indicates that the client understands the teaching for the client diagnosed with chickenpox?
    1. "I should put rubbing alcohol on the lesions twice a day."
    2. "I should not scratch myself if at all possible. It might lead to scarring."
    3. "I can go to work when my lesions have all disappeared."
    4. "I need to take all my antibiotics no matter how I feel."

55. The client with viral skin lesions is experiencing pruritus. Which statement would be an appropriate long-term goal?
    1. The client will refrain from scratching the skin.
    2. The client will maintain intact skin integrity.
    3. The client will have relief from itching.
    4. The client will not develop a secondary bacterial infection.

56. The nurse is admitting an 88-year-old client diagnosed with a viral skin infection. Which nursing task could the nurse delegate to the unlicensed assistive personnel?
    1. Measure and document the client's skin lesions.
    2. Apply the antihistamine cream to the lesions.
    3. Set up the isolation equipment for the client.
    4. Determine if the client has prepared an advance directive.

57. The client is diagnosed with a viral infection and the HCP has prescribed an antiviral medication to be administered by weight. The client weighs 220 pounds and the order reads 10 mg per kilogram per day to be administered in equally divided doses every six (6) hours. How many milligrams will be administered in one dose?:

    _____

58. The 55-year-old client contracted chickenpox from his grandchild. The client had to be hospitalized because of the seriousness of the condition. Which complication is the client at risk for developing secondary to chickenpox?
    1. Deep vein thrombosis.
    2. Varicella pneumonia.
    3. Pericarditis.
    4. Scarring of the skin.

59. The nurse is assessing a young mother who came to the clinic complaining of sores on her skin. Which assessment data would support that the client has chickenpox?
    1. Crops of lesions that have pus and reddened base.
    2. Oval scaling lesions that occur on the legs and arms.
    3. Severe itching of the scalp with tiny eggs visible.
    4. Ringed red lesions on the face, neck, trunk, and extremities.

60. The long-term care nurse has received the A.M. shift report. Which client should the nurse assess first?
    1. The client who has not had a bowel movement today.
    2. The client who needs the indwelling catheter changed.
    3. The client with periorbital skin lesions.
    4. The client with a stage I pressure ulcer.

## Fungal/Parasitic Skin Infection

61. The school nurse is assessing a teacher who has pediculosis. Which statement by the teacher makes the nurse suspect that the teacher did not comply with the instructions that were discussed in the classroom with the children?
    1. I used the comb to remove all the nits.
    2. I washed my hair with Kwell shampoo.
    3. I removed all the sheets from my bed.
    4. I had to fix my daughter's hair with my brush.

62. The school nurse is discussing how to prevent tinea cruris to the football players. Which intervention should the nurse implement?
    1. Instruct the football players to wear tight, snug-fitting jock straps.
    2. Explain the importance of wearing white socks.
    3. Teach the football players to not share brushes or combs.
    4. Discuss the need to dry the groin area thoroughly after bathing.

63. The elderly client is admitted from the long-term care facility diagnosed with congestive heart failure. The client complains of severe itching on both hands and the nurse notes wavy, brown, threadlike lesions between the client fingers. Which comorbid condition would the nurse suspect the client of having based on these assessment data?
    1. Tinea capitis.
    2. Herpes simplex 2.
    3. Scabies.
    4. Psoriasis.

64. The HCP prescribed Kwell lotion to be applied to the entire body. Which instructions should the nurse teach the client concerning this medication?
    1. Leave the lotion on for two (2) hours after applying it to the body.
    2. Make sure that the skin is completely dry before applying the lotion.
    3. Repeat total body lotion application daily for at least one (1) week.
    4. Put the lotion in the bathwater and soak for at least 20 minutes.

65. The nurse in the long-term care facility must delegate a nursing task to unlicensed assistive personnel. Which nursing task would be most appropriate to delegate?
    1. Comb the nits out of the client's hair.
    2. Massage the reddened area on the hip.
    3. Scrape the burrows to remove the scabies mite.
    4. Apply antifungal lotion to the groin area.

66. The client has tinea pedis. Which intervention should the nurse teach to the client?
    1. Soak feet in a vinegar and water solution.
    2. Wear shoes without any type of socks.
    3. Alternate shoes on a monthly basis.
    4. Cut toenails straight across.

67. The client with thick, crusty, yellow toenails is diagnosed with tinea unguium (onychomycosis) and asks the clinic nurse what happens if he can't afford to take the medication the physician prescribed. The nurse's response will be based on which scientific rationale?
    1. The toes will become gangrenous and may have to be amputated.
    2. Over-the-counter antifungal creams can be substituted for the oral medication.
    3. The toenail plate will separate and the entire toenail may be destroyed.
    4. Take all the prescribed antibiotics or the infection may return.

68. There is an outbreak of scabies in a long-term care facility. Which instruction should the infection control nurse provide to all client care staff concerning the transmission of this parasitic infection?
    1. Use only hand-washing foam when caring for clients with scabies.
    2. Wear gloves when providing hands-on care for a client with scabies.
    3. Wash all linen and clothes in cold water and dry them outside in the sun.
    4. Instruct clients to use plastic eating utensils for meals.

69. The nurse in a dermatology clinic is taking the history of a client. Which questions should the dermatology nurse ask the client? Select all that apply.
    1. When did you first notice the skin problem?
    2. What cosmetics or skin products do you use?
    3. Have you experienced any loss of sensation?
    4. What is your current and previous occupation?
    5. Do you experience any itching, burning, or tingling?

70. The nurse is assessing the client diagnosed with scabies. Which assessment technique would be most appropriate?
    1. Gently palpate the affected area using sterile gloves.
    2. Apply vinegar to the affected area to identify the scabies.
    3. Use a magnifying glass and a penlight to visualize the skin.
    4. Obtain a Doppler to assess the movement of the mites.

71. The public health nurse is providing a class on skin disorders in the African American community. Which information should the nurse include in the presentation?
    1. People with dark skin suffer the same skin conditions as people with light skin.
    2. African American men are more likely to have skin cancer than women.
    3. Dark-skinned individuals are less likely to form keloids after any type of surgery.
    4. Buccal mucosa of dark-skinned individuals is usually a bluish-tinged color.

72. Which skin condition would most likely occur in the highlighted areas?

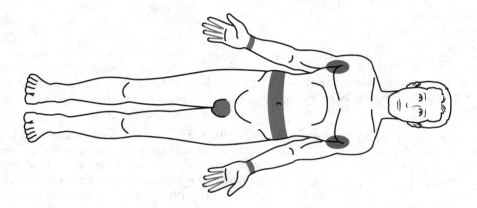

    1. Contact dermatitis.
    2. Herpes zoster.
    3. Seborrheic dermatitis.
    4. Scabies.

## Burns

1. 1. Sunburn is an example of this depth of burn; a superficial partial-thickness burn affects the epidermis and the skin is reddened and blanches with pressure.
   2. Deep partial-thickness burns are scalds and flash burns that injure the epidermis, upper dermis, and portions of the deeper dermis. This causes pain, blistered and mottled red skin, and edema.
   3. Full-thickness burns are caused by flame, electric current, or chemical burns and include the epidermis, entire dermis, and sometimes subcutaneous tissue and may also involve connective tissue, muscle, and bone.
   4. First-degree burn is another name for a superficial partial-thickness burn.

   **TEST-TAKING HINT: The adjectives in the stem are the most important words that assist the test taker when selecting a correct answer.**

2. 1. An 18-gauge catheter with lactated Ringer's infusion should be initiated to maintain a urine output of at least 30 mL per hour.
   2. Wounds should be covered with a clean, dry sheet.
   3. The client should be transferred with adequate pain relief, which requires intravenous morphine.
   4. **The client's legs should have pedal pulses and be warm to the touch, and the client must be able to move the toes.**

   **TEST-TAKING HINT: Note the adjectives "22-gauge," and "moist." If the test taker is unsure of the correct answer, then determine which system is affected and see if that will help determine the right answer. A client's extremities and a neurovascular assessment are similar; therefore the test taker should select this option.**

3. 1. After airway, the most urgent need is preventing irreversible shock by replacing fluids and electrolytes.
   2. This is important, but it is not priority over fluid volume balance, and this is not a collaborative intervention because the nurse can do this independently.
   3. Output must be monitored, but this is an independent intervention.
   4. An escharotomy, an incision that releases scar tissue that prevents the body from being able to expand, enables chest excursion in circum-

ferential chest burns. The client has not had time to develop eschar.

   **TEST-TAKING HINT: A collaborative intervention is an intervention that requires a HCP's order or working with another discipline. Therefore, options "2" and "3" should be eliminated immediately.**

4. 1. The client should be premedicated with an analgesic because this agent causes severe burning pain for up to 20 minutes after application.
   2. Silver nitrate solution is hypotonic and acts as a wick for sodium and potassium. Also, these electrolytes are WNLs and would not require immediate intervention.
   3. Sulfamylon is a strong carbonic anhydrase inhibitor that may reduce renal buffering and can cause metabolic acidosis. These ABGs indicate metabolic acidosis and therefore require immediate intervention.
   4. The client being able to perform ROM exercises does not warrant immediate intervention; this is a very good result.

   **TEST-TAKING HINT: "Warrants immediate intervention" means that the nurse must intervene independently or notify another health-care provider. The nurse must know how to interpret ABGs, and, even if the nurse is not familiar with the medication, metabolic acidosis requires intervention.**

5. 1. This is the explanation for an autograft.
   2. This is the description of a homograft.
   3. A xenograft or heterograft consists of skin taken from animals, usually porcine.
   4. This is "passing the buck"; the nurse can and should answer this question with factual information.

   **TEST-TAKING HINT: The test taker should eliminate options to help determine the correct answers. Option "1" can be eliminated because skin from self would be "auto," not "xeno." Option "4" should be eliminated because the nurse should answer the question and not pass the buck.**

6. 1. Although this is a potential problem, it is priority because the body's protective barrier, the skin, has been compromised and there is an impaired immune response.
   2. This psychosocial client problem is important, but in the ICU area the first priority is preventing infection so wound healing can occur.
   3. Burn wound edema, pain, and potential joint contractures can cause mobility deficits, but the

first priority is preventing infection so wound healing can occur.

4. Teaching is always important, but in the ICU the priority is the physiological integrity of the client.

**TEST-TAKING HINT:** The adjectives "intensive care" mean the client is critically ill; therefore a physiological problem is priority and options "2" and "4" can be eliminated. Although actual is usually higher priority than potential, in the case of a burn the risk for infection has to be priority.

7. 1. Addressing pain will not address impaired skin integrity.
2. **Daily cleaning reduces bacterial colonization.**
3. This intervention would be appropriate for a "risk for infection" nursing diagnosis.
4. Plants and flowers in water should be avoided because stagnant water is a source for bacterial growth.

**TEST-TAKING HINT:** The intervention addresses the etiology of the nursing diagnosis "open burn wounds," and the goal addresses the response "impaired skin integrity."

8. 1. Hand washing is the number-one intervention used to prevent infection, which is priority for the client with a burn.
2. **Aseptic techniques minimize risk of cross-contamination and spread of bacteria.**
3. **Aseptic techniques minimize risk of cross-contamination and spread of bacteria.**
4. Invasive lines and tubing should be changed daily.
5. **Antibiotics reduce bacteria.**

**TEST-TAKING HINT:** Alternative-type questions require the test taker to choose all options that apply. Infection is a priority for clients with burns.

9. 1. Severe pain would be expected in a client with these types of burns; therefore it would not warrant notifying the health-care provider.
2. A pulse oximeter reading greater than 93% is WNL. Therefore a 95% reading would not warrant notifying the health-care provider.
3. The client's vital signs show an elevated temperature, pulse, and respiration, along with a low blood pressure, but these vital signs would not be unusual for a client with severe burns.
4. **Fluid and electrolyte balance is the priority for a client with a severe burn. Fluid resuscitation must be maintained to keep a urine output of 30 mL/hour. Therefore a 25 mL/**

hour output would warrant immediate intervention.

**TEST-TAKING HINT:** The test taker must select an answer that is not expected for the client's disease or condition when being asked which data warrant immediate nursing intervention.

10. 1. The client needs sufficient nutrients for wound healing and increased metabolic requirements, and homemade nutritious foods are usually better than hospital food. This also allows the family to feel part of the client's recovery.
2. The client should be provided a high-calorie, high-protein diet along with vitamins.
3. The client should be weighed daily, and the goal is that the client loses no more than 5% of preburn weight.
4. The nurse would make a referral to a dietitian, not a social worker.

**TEST-TAKING HINT:** The nurse needs to be knowledgeable of different types of diets; this requires memorization.

11. 1. Ice should never be applied to a burn because this will worsen the tissue damage by causing vasoconstriction.
2. **Cool water gives immediate and striking relief from pain and limits local tissue edema and damage.**
3. Blisters should be maintained intact to prevent infection.
4. The client should be told to go to the ED, not the doctor's office, for burn care.

**TEST-TAKING HINT:** The test taker should select an answer that directly cares for the client's body. This eliminates "3" (blisters have not formed yet) and "4." Therefore the test taker has to decide between cool water and ice.

12. 1. The client should resume previous activities gradually and should not stay home; the client should go out and begin to live again.
2. The client should be honest with self, family, and friends about needs, hopes, and fears.
3. The client needs to know that it will take time to adjust to life after burns and that returning to work, family role, sexual intimacy, and body image will take time.
4. The client should feel free to discuss feelings with family, friends, and the therapist.

**TEST-TAKING HINT:** Even if the test taker is not familiar with the disease process, there are certain interventions that go with any chronic problem, such as getting back to normal life as soon as possible and being independent, but also getting help when needed and not expecting too much too soon.

## Pressure Ulcers

13. 1. The skin should be kept dry. The skin should be patted completely dry after each bath.
    2. Elderly people have decreased moisture in the skin. Applying lotion restores moisture.
    3. Clients should be turned at least every one (1) to two (2) hours to prevent pressure areas on the skin.
    4. All employees in any health-care facility are responsible for providing care within their scope of services.

    **TEST-TAKING HINT:** Option "2" has an absolute "any" in it. The test taker can eliminate this as an answer based on this. Option "4" has the absolute "only," so this option can be eliminated. Of the remaining options, option "3" can apply to all clients who are immobile.

14. 1. This can be an independent nursing problem or a collaborative one, but it does not relate to pressure ulcers.
    2. Altered nutrition is a collaborative problem involving the nurse, dietitian, and HCP. The client will need a diet high in protein and vitamins if there is a chance for the client to heal.
    3. Self-care deficit is an independent nursing problem.
    4. Altered coping is an independent problem and does not relate to skin integrity.

    **TEST-TAKING HINT:** The stem gives two (2) clues to the answer—"collaborative" and "pressure ulcers." Collaborative means that some other member of the health-care team must be involved and pressure ulcers are the client's problem. The correct answer must consider both of these variables.

15. 1. All the skin should be kept free of moisture. This is within the realm of nursing to provide this service. Clients with constant moisture on the skin are at high risk for impaired skin integrity.
    2. The clients who are able to reposition themselves would decrease the changes of developing pressure ulcers. This would not be a risk factor.
    3. Decreased elasticity occurs with aging, and it is not modifiable.
    4. Impaired cardiovascular perfusion of the skin in the periphery is not modifiable.

    **TEST-TAKING HINT:** The test taker must read the stem carefully. Which situation can the nurse modify with nursing care? The nurse cannot modify the changes that occur with aging or the sequelae that occur with disease processes.

16. 1. The pads will absorb moisture and will protect the bed but they also will keep the moisture next to the client's skin, which increases the risk of skin breakdown.
    2. The pads are made with plastic liners, which tend to contain heat next to the client's body, thereby increasing diaphoresis.
    3. The pads are a help to lift the client, but are not used to prevent workplace injuries. To prevent workplace injuries, the staff must practice good body mechanics.
    4. Lifting the client with a "lift" pad rather than pulling the client against the sheets helps to prevent skin damage from friction shearing.

    **TEST-TAKING HINT:** The stem asks for the rationale for using "lift" pads. Lifting a client involves repositioning the client. None of the other options mentions any kind of repositioning.

17. 1. The Braden and Norton scales are tools that identify clients at risk for skin problems. This client should be ranked on this scale, and appropriate measures should be initiated for controlling further damage to the skin.
    2. The Glasgow Coma Scale is a neurological coma scale used to determine the depth of neurological damage.
    3. A Babinski sign would not be attempted in a client who is paralyzed from the waist down. The nerve pathways are not working.
    4. A Brudzinski sign is used to assess for meningitis.

    **TEST-TAKING HINT:** The test taker must memorize the specific diagnostic tools used to assess clients.

18. 1. This describes a stage I pressure ulcer, which would be an improvement of the client's wound.
    2. This is a stage II pressure ulcer and is not a significant change in the wound.
    3. This implies that the skin has healed and is not at stage I.
    4. This is a stage III ulcer and is a worsening of the client's condition.

    **TEST-TAKING HINT:** The test taker could look at the description in the stem and then at the descriptions in the options. Only one (1) option appears to have a more involved skin condition.

19. 1. The head of a client eating in bed should be elevated. This is a correct action on the part of the unlicensed nursing assistant.
    2. It is important to turn bedfast clients every one (1) to two (2) hours and to encourage them, if they are able, to make minor readjustments to their position at least every 15 minutes. Allowing the client to lie in the same position for at least another 30 minutes before being turned should not be allowed.
    3. It is a courtesy to the oncoming staff to leave the rooms equipped to care for the clients.
    4. Thick-It frequently is added to the liquids of a client who has difficulty swallowing.

    **TEST-TAKING HINT:** This is an "except" question. All but one (1) option will be actions that are encouraged on the part of unlicensed assistive personnel. The test taker could jump to a conclusion that option "1" is correct if the test taker did not pay attention to the phrase "warrants immediate intervention."

20. 1. The client who is a quadriplegic cannot move his or her arms or legs. Quad means four (4) and none of the four (4) extremities move. This is expected for the client's problem.
    2. Weakness on one side of the body is expected in clients who have experienced a CVA (stroke).
    3. The client has a fever indicating an infection. Clients with pressure ulcers frequently develop infections in the wounds, which can lead to further complications.
    4. This is a psychological problem and should be addressed but not before assessing the infection.

    **TEST-TAKING HINT:** The test taker must decide if the situation is expected for the disease process or if it is life threatening. Physiologic problems come before psychological problems, according to Maslow.

21. 1. Using a pillow to suspend the heels of the bed when a client is supine prevents the development of pressure ulcers on the heels.
    2. Low air loss therapy beds are expensive and normally are provided only for clients who have stage III or stage IV impaired skin integrity. An egg-crate mattress may be applied to the bed for pressure relief, but many hospitals now have changed all of their regular mattresses for ones that provide the same pressure reduction surface as an egg-crate mattress.
    3. There is no indication that the client requires tube feeding.
    4. Physical therapists, not occupational therapists, work with the clients on strength train-

ing. Occupational therapists address activities of daily living deficits.

**TEST-TAKING HINT:** The test taker should not read into the question. The stem did not mention any swallowing problem, only a mobility problem. The correct answer must relate to the information provided in the stem.

22. 1. The question asks for therapeutic response. This response addresses a physiologic problem and does not address the client's concerns.
    2. This is restating and clarifying, both therapeutic responses.
    3. The client does not owe the nurse an explanation for the client's feelings. "Why" is not therapeutic.
    4. This does not address the client's feelings.

    **TEST-TAKING HINT:** When the stem asks the test taker for a therapeutic response, the correct answer must address the client's feelings.

23. 1. The client must be turned every one (1) to two (2) hours.
    2. Clients with pressure ulcers usually are debilitated and have a poor nutritional base for healing. An increase in protein and vitamins is needed in the diet to promote healing.
    3. Clients must sign consents if they are recognizable in the pictures. It is standard practice to document wounds by taking an instant imaging picture and placing the picture in the chart for reference by all concerned staff. In this instance a consent is not needed.
    4. A client with a stage IV pressure ulcer needs a higher level of pressure reduction than a normal hospital mattress can provide.
    5. The head of the bed can be in any position of comfort for the client, but the head should not be elevated at "all" times because the pressure applied to the lower body region.

    **TEST-TAKING HINT:** The test taker must notice time frames. Is three (3) to four (4) hours the correct time frame for turning a client with impaired skin integrity? Option "5" can be eliminated because of the word "all."

24. 1. A skin flap to graft an open wound is not a fecal diversion.
    2. This statement describes a debridement, not a fecal diversion.
    3. Hyperbaric chambers are used to increase oxygenation to nonhealing wounds, but surgery does not increase oxygenation.
    4. A fecal diversion is changing the normal exit of the stool from the body. A colostomy

is created to keep stool from contaminating the wounds and causing infection.

**TEST-TAKING HINT: The word "fecal" means "stool." Only one option mentions anything to do with the stool.**

## Skin Cancer

25. 1. The lower the number of sunscreen, the less protection. A sunscreen of SPF 15 is a minimum.
    2. Clients should avoid sunlight between 3 P.M. and 5 P.M. 0300–0500 refers to morning, the middle of the night.
    3. The American Cancer Society recommends a monthly skin check using mirrors to identify any suspicious skin lesion for early detection.
    4. Anything that prevents UV rays from reaching the skin helps to prevent skin cancer. Hats with a full brim are preferred to baseball caps, which leave the ears and back of the neck exposed.

    **TEST-TAKING HINT: The test taker must notice adjectives. In option "2" the use of 0300–0500 instead of 1500–1700, makes this option incorrect. In option "1" the number of the sunscreen makes this option wrong, and in option "4" the word "not" is an absolute word that could eliminate this option.**

26. 1. The nurse should complete an assessment of the lesion prior to notifying the HCP to check it.
    2. This is part of assessing the lesion and should be completed. The ABCDs of skin cancer detection include the following: 1) Asymmetry—Is the lesion balanced on both sides with an even surface? 2) Borders—Are the borders rounded and smooth or notched and indistinct? 3) Color—Is the color a uniform light brown or is it variegated and darker or reddish purple? 4) Diameter—A diameter exceeding 4–6 mm is considered suspicious.
    3. This may help as a comfort measure, but it is not the first and most important action.
    4. Instructing the client to also notify the HCP to assess the lesion should be done but does not have priority.

    **TEST-TAKING HINT: Assessment is the first step in the nursing process. The test taker should have a systematic decision-making model when determining a priority action.**

27. 1. This client has an unexpected situation occurring and should be assessed before any stable client.
    2. This client's surgery was three (3) hours ago and the client should be stable and allowed to rest.
    3. This client can be seen after assessing the client in option "1."
    4. This client could be escorted to the door by an unlicensed assistive personnel; the nurse before has prepared the client for discharge.

    **TEST-TAKING HINT: Physiological problems usually have priority over psychological ones, but none of the other clients have a life threatening or life-altering situation. The only unexpected situation is the client who is crying.**

28. 1. Darker-skinned individuals have a lower risk of developing skin cancer. It is living in the southwestern regions of the United States where sun exposure is the greatest that increases skin cancer risk.
    2. Hispanic clients have more melanin in the skin than Caucasian clients and moving from Mexico would have decreased the UV exposure.
    3. A family history of malignant melanoma increases the risk of developing malignant melanoma. Basal cell carcinoma is directly related to sun exposure and does not have an increased familial risk.
    4. Clients with very little melanin in the skin (fair-skinned) have an increased risk as a result of the UV damage to the underlying membranes. Damage to the underlying membranes never completely reverses itself; a lifetime of damage causes changes at the cellular level that can result in the development of cancer.

    **TEST-TAKING HINT: If the test taker noticed the similarities in the clients in options "1" and "2"—darker skin and living in an area with less sun exposure or moving from an area with greater sun exposure to an area with less—the test taker could eliminate these two (2) options. Based on skin color, the fair-skinned client would be most at risk.**

29. 1. The client should be taught to complete monthly skin checks to detect any future lesions.
    2. Basal cell lesions grow slowly and do not metastasize until the lesion has become very large. Prostheses are usually not needed.
    3. The area may need to have an antibiotic ointment, but sunscreen should not be applied until

after the operative area has healed and then only when the client is going to be in the sun.

4. On discharge, all clients should receive instructions in the care of surgical incisions.

**TEST-TAKING HINT: If the test taker did not know the specific information regarding this type of cancer surgery, then choosing an answer that is appropriate for all surgeries is a good option.**

30. 1. The diagnosis of cancer is concerning for clients; this is belittling the client's concerns and gives false reassurance.
2. This is the most commonly written therapeutic communication goal. This addresses the client's concerns.
3. The nurse is capable of discussing the client's concerns. Many clients feel more comfortable discussing fears with the nurse than with the HCP.
4. This should be done but does not directly address the client problem.

**TEST-TAKING HINT: The test taker must read the question carefully to decide what the question is asking. The answer must address the problem of fear.**

31. 1. The UAP can restock rooms.
2. These activities can be performed by a trained UAP.
3. This is part of assessing the client and cannot be delegated.
4. This is appropriate delegation.

**TEST-TAKING HINT: This is an "except question." The test taker must be careful to read the words in the stem of the question such as "not be delegated." All of the answers except one should be activities that the UAP can perform.**

32. 1. Malignant melanomas are the most deadly of the skin cancers. Asymmetry, irregular borders, variegated color, and rapid growth are characteristic of them.
2. A waxy appearance and pearl-like borders are characteristic of basal cell carcinoma.
3. A thickened and scaly appearance describes squamous cell carcinoma.
4. A thickened area after an injury describes a benign condition called a keloid.

**TEST-TAKING HINT: This is a knowledge-based question, but it does indicate the differences in the types of skin lesions. The test taker should concentrate on the differences when studying for an examination.**

33. 1. The client should be aware of symptoms that indicate development of another skin cancer. Squamous cell carcinoma can develop in areas of the skin and mucus membranes.
2. Of deaths from squamous cell carcinomas, 75% occur because of metastasize. Even basal cell carcinoma can metastasis but is usually so slow growing that surgical excision removes the cancer if the client does not delay treatment.
3. The surgery was on the lip, not in the mouth. Food can be of a regular consistency.
4. Applying heat to the area would increase circulation and edema, increasing the client's discomfort.

**TEST-TAKING HINT: Anatomical positioning, lip, could eliminate option "3." An HCP should be notified for any nonhealing wound.**

34. 1. This is a psychological goal.
2. This is a knowledge-deficit goal, not a physiological goal.
3. Pain is a physiological problem; this is an appropriate physiological goal.
4. This is a teaching goal, not a physiological goal.

**TEST-TAKING HINT: The test taker must read the question carefully to determine what the stem is asking. All of the goals are appropriate for the client with skin cancer, but only one is a physiological goal.**

35. 1. The client may need a biopsy, but the nurse should assess the area before deciding to refer the client.
2. This is the first step in deciding how to help the client. The nurse should assess the lesion to determine if the lesion could be a Kaposi's sarcoma tumor or a healing contusion.
3. This is important for all clients, even those without a chronic illness, but the question asks what should be done first. This is not the priority at this time.
4. AIDS is a reportable disease, but reporting is not the priority intervention.

**TEST-TAKING HINT: Assessment is the first step in the nursing process.**

36. 1. Sunscreen should be used whenever the client is going to be exposed to UV rays.
2. Infants younger than age six (6) months should not be placed in the sun or have sunscreen applied. This does not include the medical uses of a bili-light.
3. Sunscreen blocks absorption of UV rays, which, when allowed to penetrate the skin,

cause damage to the layers of the skin. This, in turn, causes cellular changes, which over time can develop into skin cancer.

4. Sunscreen products range in numerical value from 4 to 50; the higher the number of the sunscreen, the greater the UV protection.

TEST-TAKING HINT: Option "1" has the absolute word "only" and could be eliminated. "Toddler" is a key in this option. The test taker must decide if it is appropriate for a toddler to have sunscreen applied to the skin.

## Bacterial Skin Infection

37. 1. Cellulitis is a bacterial infection of the subcutaneous tissue usually associated with a break in the skin, and the nurse would suspect this with these signs/symptoms.
    2. Lyme disease is caused by the bite of a tick, resulting in a bull's eye–appearing lesion.
    3. Impetigo is characterized by large, fluid-filled blisters and is very contagious.
    4. Deep vein thrombosis signs/symptoms are a reddened, warm calf and pain on ambulation, but this condition is not caused by a nail puncture; it is caused by immobility.

TEST-TAKING HINT: If the test taker does not know the answer, look at the stem and identify that redness and fever are signs of inflammation; "itis" means inflammation and option "1" would be an appropriate selection.

38. 1. Dogs may have ticks, but these ticks do not carry Lyme disease, which is what these symptoms may represent.
    2. The client would most likely not be exposed to deer ticks while working in the garden.
    3. Deer ticks (*Ixodes dammini*) are responsible for the spread of Lyme disease, which is what this client is experiencing based on the signs/symptoms.
    4. Sunscreen is important, but it will not protect the client from any type of insect bites.

TEST-TAKING HINT: Option "4" could be eliminated as a possible answer if the test taker realized that the other three options all deal with some type of insect bite, which is stated in the stem of the question.

39. 1. Cleanliness and good hygiene prevent the spread of impetigo, but washing hands after going to the bathroom will not prevent the spread.
    2. Lesions are extremely contagious and should not be touched, except when wearing gloves.
    3. The topical antibiotic ointment is applied after

impetigo has developed. It will not help prevent impetigo. Usually the client with impetigo is given systemic antibiotics.

4. The child is kept at home until he or she has taken antibiotics for 48 hours; the child is not isolated in the room.

TEST-TAKING HINT: The test taker needs to think about what the options are saying. Option "4" can be eliminated because a child cannot be isolated in a room with many other children in the room. Washing hands after using the bathroom, option "1," is a general-hygiene tip encouraged for all individuals and is not specific to impetigo. Look at the word "prevent" in the stem; antibiotic ointment is only prescribed for bacterial infections, so option "3" should be ruled out as an answer.

40. 1. As long as the client has bilateral pulses, there is no need for the nurse to intervene.
    2. As long as the client is able to move the fingers, there is no need for the nurse to intervene.
    3. A CRT less than 3 seconds is normal and would not require immediate intervention.
    4. The client being unable to remove the wedding ring indicates that the arm is edematous and the ring must be removed immediately or it may cause impaired circulation to the left ring finger. This is a dangerous situation.

TEST-TAKING HINT: When the stem asks the test taker to identify data that warrant immediate intervention, the test taker must select the option that is abnormal for the disease process. All the options except "4" are normal neurovascular assessment data.

41. 1. Humidity should be kept high around 60% to prevent the skin from drying.
    2. Coolness deters itching.
    3. Mild soaps contain no detergents, dyes, or fragrances to cause an increase in itching.
    4. Lesions should be left open to air as much as possible; cloth rubbing the lesions is irritating.
    5. Effective hydration of the stratum corneum prevents compromise of the barrier layer of the skin.

TEST-TAKING HINT: "Select all that apply" questions require the test taker to make a determination for each option individually. Choosing one will not exclude another answer.

42. 1. The nurse is responsible for providing correct information to the assistants. This intervention would be appropriate if confronting the person has not altered the behavior.
    2. This action could result in the client developing a skin infection and should be

stopped immediately; therefore, stopping the behavior is the first intervention.

3. The nurse must be a role model for the assistant and demonstrate the correct way to care for the client's skin.

4. An incident report may need to be completed to document the situation, but it is not the first intervention.

**TEST-TAKING HINT:** When the question asks the test taker to select the first intervention, all four (4) options may be possible actions, but only one (1) should be done first. In this situation the behavior must be stopped prior to performing any other interventions.

43. 1. Impaired skin integrity is a physiological problem, not a psychosocial problem.

2. The nurse does not know if the client is grieving over the acne. Do not read more into the question than is available.

3. Acne occurs on the face and neck. This is the first impression that people get when looking at the client; therefore body-image disturbance is the priority.

4. Knowledge deficit is appropriate for this client, but it does not have priority over body image. Acne can be devastating to a client's self-image.

**TEST-TAKING HINT:** Remember to observe adjectives. "Psychosocial" is the key word to answering this question.

44. 1. This disease is a bacterial inflammatory reaction that occurs predominantly on the faces and necks of curly-haired men as a result of shaving. African American men who are in the military are allowed not to shave if this occurs. The sharp ingrowing hairs have a curved root that grows at a more acute angle and pierces the skin. The only treatment is to not shave.

2. This person will not get this disease.

3. This person will not get this disease.

4. This person will not get this disease.

**TEST-TAKING HINT:** If the test taker did not know the answer to this question, he or she could examine the root words and endings: "follicle" refers to "hair" and "itis" is an inflammation. The test taker should think about what type of hair each culture has and realize that an African American has a different type of hair than the other three options.

45. 1. A furuncle (boil) is not a life-threatening emergency, and an appointment is not needed for this client.

2. Warm, moist compresses increase vascularization and hasten the resolution of the furuncle.

3. With staphylococcal infections, such as a boil, it is important not to rupture the protective wall of induration that localizes the infection.

4. The client called the clinic to get help and this response does not help the client. A nurse can recommend heat, ice, elevation, or some type of independent treatment.

**TEST-TAKING HINT:** The test taker can always rule out options that don't address the client's needs, such as "4." Option "3" can also be ruled out: there are very few "nevers," but one is never squeeze or pop a boil or pimple.

46. 1. This client is not at increased risk for developing a carbuncle.

2. This client is not at increased risk for developing a carbuncle.

3. This client is not at increased risk for developing a carbuncle.

4. A carbuncle is an abscess of the skin and subcutaneous tissue and is an extension of a furuncle. These are more likely to occur in clients with underlying systemic diseases such as diabetes and hematologic malignances and in clients who are immunosuppressed.

**TEST-TAKING HINT:** If the test taker did not know what a carbuncle was, he or she could look at the options and note that only one has a disease process, which might be the best choice for the correct answer.

47. 1. Systemic antibiotics are the treatment of choice for impetigo. Therefore the teacher must go to the HCP to get the prescription today because impetigo is highly contagious.

2. Washing hands is always a good practice, but the teacher needs medication for this bacterial infection.

3. Vitamin E oil does help prevent scarring, but it will not treat this bacterial infection.

4. Impetigo is not a rash; it is raised, crusty lesions.

**TEST-TAKING HINT:** The test taker must know that impetigo is a bacterial infection requiring medical treatment. Vitamins do not treat skin infections. Washing with an antiseptic solution may help, but antibiotics are the treatment of choice.

48. 1. To help prevent deer tick bites, which spread Lyme disease, the individual should wear light-colored, tightly woven clothing with long pants and long-sleeved shirts. These allow the person to see the tick better.

2. Sunscreen will not help prevent the spread of Lyme disease.

Integumentary

3. Staying on paths and avoiding dense undergrowth will help the person keep away from tick-invested areas where the person is more likely to be bitten by a tick and perhaps subsequently develop Lyme disease.

4. Insect repellant should be used; there is special repellant, diethyltoluamide (DEET), used to help prevent Lyme disease.

**TEST-TAKING HINT: The test taker should be able to rule out sunscreen as an answer because the stem says "disease" and sunscreen cannot prevent an infectious disease. Not wearing insect repellant ("4") would not be appropriate for any teaching except teaching about infants.**

## Viral Skin Infection

49. 1. The virus that causes chickenpox is the herpes varicella virus, not the herpes simplex virus.
2. Herpes simplex 1 and 2 are caused by the same virus. Herpes simplex 1 refers to orolabial lesions and herpes simplex 2 refers to genital lesions, which can be transferred from one area to the other.
3. The question is asking which intervention the nurse should teach the client, and there is no reason for the client to have to wear nonsterile gloves for self-care. That is appropriate for the nursing personnel.
4. Herpes simplex is not transmitted via towels or cloths.

**TEST-TAKING HINT: In some instances the test taker simply must know about the disease process. Sexually transmitted diseases are common, and the nurse should know about how to prevent, discuss, and treat them.**

50. 1. The left rib cage area is not considered an area for revealing cardiac problems. The client with a cardiac problem would have chest pain radiating to the left arm, sweating, and nausea.
2. This negates the client's complaints and does not address the client's concerns. The nurse should always further assess when the client is in pain.
3. The nurse should not administer pain medication unless the cause of the pain is known. The client is complaining of severe pain, and Tylenol (a nonnarcotic) will not be effective.
4. The client's description of the pain suggests shingles. Shingles is caused by herpes zoster, which is the same virus as herpes varicella, which causes chickenpox. This virus is a retrovirus that never dies; it becomes dormant and lives in the body

along nerve pathways. During times of stress, it can erupt as herpes zoster, or shingles. The pain usually occurs prior to the eruption of the vesicles.

**TEST-TAKING HINT: If the test taker does not know the answer, then apply the nursing process. The "4" option is the only one (1) that involves assessment, which is the first part of the nursing process.**

51. 1. Valtrex is not a birth control medication.
2. Valtrex is usually prescribed for a set amount of time and does not need to be tapered.
3. Valtrex is an antiviral medication that suppresses the virus replication, but herpes is a retrovirus, which means it never dies as long as the host body is alive.
4. This medication does not cause the urine to turn orange.

**TEST-TAKING HINT: Medications are frequently advertised to the public; therefore, the nurse must know about medications that laypeople may be asking about.**

52. 1. Diversionary techniques, including music and television, are often used in conjunction with medication to manage pain. Shutting the blinds will help provide a calm, quiet atmosphere.
2. Warm, moist heat will exacerbate the pain from the lesions; cool compresses would help.
3. The client was medicated 45 minutes ago and would not be able to have more medication; therefore, there is no reason to notify the HCP.
4. Ambulating will not help decrease the client's pain and could aggravate it. In addition, the client has been given morphine, which causes drowsiness and could lead to a safety issue.

**TEST-TAKING HINT: The test taker could rule out "4" with no knowledge of the disease process because the nurse does not ambulate clients on morphine. The nurse often uses diversionary interventions when addressing pain issues.**

53. 1. The zoster lesions are contagious, so the client should be in contact isolation.
2. Corticosteroids decrease the inflammation, which helps with the healing process.
3. Assessment is always an appropriate intervention.
4. The client can have visitors as long as they do not have an infection that the client could get and the visitors comply with isolation protocol.
5. Herpes zoster is the same virus that causes chickenpox; therefore nurses who have not had chickenpox should not care for this client.

TEST-TAKING HINT: **This is an alternate-type question where the test taker must select all the interventions that are pertinent. If the test taker is aware that corticosteroid medications decrease inflammation, he or she should select "2" as a correct answer. Assessment ("3") is always an appropriate selection if the assessment data apply to the situation.**

54. 1. Rubbing alcohol will cause tremendous pain and will not help the lesions disappear.
    2. The lesions are very irritating and the client will want to scratch them. Clients with chickenpox should use calamine lotion, soak in oatmeal baths, and apply Benadryl topical cream or take oral Benadryl.
    3. The lesions are considered contagious until they are dry and crusted over, usually in five (5) to seven (7) days. The client does not have to wait until they have disappeared; this may take up to two (2) or three (3) weeks.
    4. Chickenpox is a virus and antibiotics are effective only with bacterial infections; antibiotics are not prescribed.

TEST-TAKING HINT: **The test taker may realize that options with absolutes such as "all" should not be selected as the right answer, but notice that this "all" is not used in the same manner as to mean "always."**

55. 1. This would be a short-term goal, but it is unrealistic to expect a client not to scratch when experiencing severe itching.
    2. The client currently has lesions; therefore the skin integrity is already compromised. The key word is "maintain."
    3. Relief of itching is a short-term goal for this client. For a long-term goal, the nurse needs to recognize the potential complications.
    4. A major complication of pruritus (itching) is the development of a bacterial skin infection, which is secondary to the client scratching and allowing bacteria from the dirty hands or nails to enter compromised tissue.

TEST-TAKING HINT: **The test taker must recognize what symptoms the client is experiencing. Lesions are open wounds; therefore "2" could be eliminated even if the test taker did not know what the word "pruritus" means. Furthermore, the test taker must look at adjectives; the question asks for long-term goals and the test taker should realize immediate behavior change (refrain from scratching) and pain relief are short-term goals.**

56. 1. The nurse cannot delegate assessment, which is what measuring the lesions is doing, and the nurse must document the assessment.

2. This is a medication and the nurse cannot delegate medication administration.
3. The nurse can delegate the setup of equipment to the assistant.
4. Determining if a client has an advance directive should not be delegated to the assistant because if the client has questions, the nurse must provide factual information.

TEST-TAKING HINT: **The nurse must know which nursing tasks can be delegated; assessment, teaching, evaluating, and medication administration cannot be delegated to unlicensed assistive personnel.**

57. 250 mg per dose. First, determine the client's weight in kilograms; there are 2.2 pounds per kilogram, so

    220 pounds ÷ 2.2 = 100 kilograms

Then, determine the total dosage to be given per day on the basis of the HCP order of 10 mg per kilogram per day

    100 × 10 = 1000 kilograms per day.

Then, determine how many doses in a day if a dose is to be given every six (6) hours.

    24 ÷ 6 = 4 doses.

Finally, determine how many milligrams per each dose to administer 1000 mg in 24 hours.

    1000 ÷ 4 = 250 mg per dose

TEST-TAKING HINT: **Math problems frequently require multiple steps. The test taker should replace each number as the conversion is made. The test taker must know conversion factors and how to use the drop-down calculator on the computer.**

58. 1. This is a complication of immobility, not specifically chickenpox.
    2. Herpes varicella is the causative agent for chickenpox, and pneumonia is a potential complication in adults.
    3. Pericarditis (inflammation of the sac surrounding the heart) is not a complication of chickenpox.
    4. Scarring of the skin is an expected sequelae of chickenpox, but it is not a complication.

TEST-TAKING HINT: **The question asks for a complication; therefore "4" could be ruled out because it is expected; if the test taker knows that chickenpox it caused by herpes varicella, then the most obvious answer is "2."**

59. 1. Chickenpox starts out with a macular rash. The lesions appear in crops first on the trunk and scalp, and then lesions move to the extremities. Then, they change to tear-

drop vesicles with an erythematous base and become pustular. Finally, they dry.

2. Oval scaling indicates fungal infections.

3. Severe itching of the scalp with tiny eggs visible supports the diagnosis of lice.

4. Ringed red lesions support the diagnosis of ringworm.

**TEST-TAKING HINT:** This is primarily a knowledge-based question. Either the test taker knows the signs and symptoms of different skin disorders or does not. One way to help identify the answer is to try to determine what condition each option describes. For example, "tiny eggs" should make the test taker think of a parasite (lice).

60. 1. This client would not be priority; elderly clients frequently think they need a daily movement.

2. A catheter change would not be priority.

3. Periorbital lesions may extend into the client's eyes, which is an ophthalmic emergency, especially if it is herpes zoster.

4. A stage I pressure ulcer requires changing the client's position, which can be delegated.

**TEST-TAKING HINT:** If the test taker knows medical terminology, then periorbital, "around the eye," would be priority.

## Fungal/Parasitic Skin Infection

61. 1. This statement indicates the teacher understands the teaching about the spread of lice (pediculosis).

2. Kwell shampoo or Rid are prescribed when lice are found in the hair.

3. All linens and pertinent clothing should be washed in hot water to help destroy the eggs.

4. Sharing brushes is one of the main ways that lice are spread. Therefore this indicates the teacher did not comply with the instructions.

**TEST-TAKING HINT:** This is an "except" question. Therefore, three (3) of the options will be a correct action for the problem and only one (1) option will be an incorrect action. Do not jump to conclusions after reading the first option. Always read all the options thoroughly.

62. 1. To prevent tinea cruris (jock itch) the football players should avoid wearing nylon underwear, tight-fitting clothing, and wet bathing suits.

2. This would be appropriate advice for tinea pedis (athlete's foot).

3. This would be appropriate advice to help prevent lice.

4. Tinea cruris (jock itch) results from a fun-

gal infection in warm, moist areas of the body. When such an infection occurs in the groin area, it is called tinea cruris.

**TEST-TAKING HINT:** All the options discuss prevention of something; therefore the test taker must know about disease processes. Test-Taking Hints do not substitute for studying and understanding the material. Remember that perfect test scores are few and far between.

63. 1. Tinea capitis is ringworm of the scalp, which does not support this client's signs/symptoms.

2. A herpes simplex 2 lesion is in the genital area.

3. Scabies is an infestation of the skin by the itch mite (*Sarcoptes scabiei*). The female burrows into the superficial layer of skin, and burrows are found between the fingers and on the wrist.

4. Psoriasis is a chronic noninfectious inflammatory disorder of the skin, which results in scales.

**TEST-TAKING HINT:** The nurse should be familiar with medical terminology, which can often help rule out incorrect options. "Capitus," for example, pertains to the head or scalp; therefore this could be eliminated as a possible answer.

64. 1. The lotion should be left on for at least 12–24 hours to be effective.

2. The application of Kwell lotion on wet skin can lead to increased absorption of the lotion, which increases the possibility of central nervous system abnormalities, including seizures.

3. One application may cure the infestation of lice or scabies, but another application may be needed in one (1) week; daily administration is contraindicated.

4. This medication must be applied to dry skin to prevent possible fatal complications.

**TEST-TAKING HINT:** The test taker should always be aware of adjectives; notice "two (2) hours," "20 minutes," and "daily." These are all adjectives that may help the test taker to choose the correct answer.

65. 1. The assistant could use a fine-toothed comb dipped in vinegar to remove any nits in the hair of the client with lice.

2. Reddened areas should not be massaged; that will lead to further damage.

3. Scraping the burrows is a diagnostic test and cannot be delegated to an assistant.

4. Assistants cannot administer medication.

**TEST-TAKING HINT:** The test taker must apply universal delegation rules. Nurses cannot delegate medication administration or diagnostic tests. Some states allow medication aides to administer routine medications to clients in long-term care facilities, but the stem does not identify this employee as a medication aide. Do not read into the question.

66. 1. Soaking the feet will help remove the crust, scales, and debris to reduce the inflammation in a client diagnosed with athlete's foot. Vinegar is mildly acidic, which helps remove crusts.
    2. White cotton socks should be recommended to help prevent athlete's foot. Colored socks have dyes that irritate the skin and cotton socks absorb moisture.
    3. Several pairs of shoes should be alternated so that shoes can be completely dry before wearing again.
    4. Cutting toenails straight across is correct, but it will not prevent or treat athlete's foot.

    **TEST-TAKING HINT:** There are basic interventions that are taught about foot care in general and trimming toenails is one of them. This could apply to many foot conditions. Wearing socks is always advisable because feet perspire. Not very many interventions are done on a monthly basis—usually daily or weekly—so option "3" can be eliminated.

67. 1. This sequela may occur with a client diagnosed with diabetes who develops a foot ulcer.
    2. Oral fungal agents must be taken for 12 weeks because the fungal infection is underneath the nail; topical medications would not reach the infection.
    3. This is a condition of ringworm of the toenail. The nurse must tell the client that the toenail will fall off if the client does not take the medication, and it might it fall off anyway.
    4. This is not a bacterial infection; therefore, oral antibiotics will not be administered. It is a fungal infection and antifungal medication will be administered.

    **TEST-TAKING HINT:** Gangrene is usually a circulation problem, not a toenail problem; therefore, "1" could be eliminated as a possible answer. Option "2" should be eliminated because nurses cannot prescribe or change physicians' orders. Of the two remaining options only "3" has the word toenail in it; therefore the test taker should select "3" as the correct answer.

68. 1. Foam or soap and water can be used to clean the hands.
    2. Because of the close living quarters, clients in long-term care facilities are at a high risk

for developing scabies. Clients may have poor hygiene as a result of limited physical ability and the nursing staff may transmit the parasite. Therefore, the nursing staff should wear gloves to provide a barrier to the mites.
3. Linens and clothing should be washed in hot water and dried in a hot dryer cycle because the mites can survive up to 36 hours in linens.
4. Plastic eating utensils will not help prevent the spread of scabies.

**TEST-TAKING HINT: If the test taker has no idea what the correct answer is, then eliminate "1" and "3" because of the words "only" and "all." There are very few absolutes in the health-care profession.**

69. 1. Dermatology is the study of the skin. Therefore asking about skin problems is appropriate.
    2. The nurse must differentiate between a dermatitis, which could result from a cosmetic or other skin product, and a skin infection.
    3. The skin is responsible for sensation so any loss would be significant.
    4. Many occupations, including those involved in working with chemicals, predispose a client to abnormal skin conditions.
    5. These are hallmark signs of skin abnormality.

    **TEST-TAKING HINT: In "select all that apply" questions each option stands or falls on its own. Do not try to second guess the item writer thinking that there is no way that all five (5) will be correct.**

70. 1. This technique will not help diagnose scabies.
    2. Vinegar will not help visualize and identify scabies.
    3. A magnifying glass and a penlight are held at an oblique angle to the skin while a search is made for small raised burrows, which indicate scabies.
    4. A Doppler is used to obtain faint pulses, but it will not help find a mite, which causes scabies.

    **TEST-TAKING HINT: The nurse must know about diagnostic equipment and a Doppler is commonly used in clients who have a nonpalpable pulse. Therefore, option "4" could be eliminated.**

71. 1. This is correct information.
    2. Dark-skinned people are less likely to have skin cancer.
    3. Dark-skinned people are more likely to have keloids (hypertrophied scar tissue) after surgery.

4. Bluish-tinged buccal mucosa in anyone indicates decreased oxygenation.

**TEST-TAKING HINT: The nurse should know that any blue color on the body is abnormal, thus ruling out option "4." Notice that options "2" and "3" have "more likely" and "less likely," which may encourage the test taker to rule out both answers and select "1."**

72. 1. Contact dermatitis usually occurs where cosmetics or perfume are applied or specific clothing items touch the skin.
    2. Herpes zoster in clients who are not immuno-

compromised occurs along nerve roots around the rib cage and back.

3. Seborrheic dermatitis occurs in the midline front and back of the body.
4. Scabies occurs around the waist, around the wrist, between the fingers, and in the axilla area.

**TEST-TAKING HINT: There may be questions that require the test taker to identify body parts when selecting the correct answer. The nurse must know about skin conditions to be able to answer the question.**

1. The nurse is conducting the interview of the client presenting to see the health-care provider with complaints of a rash and itching. Which information would be most important for the nurse to assess/teach?
   1. When did the rash appear and where did the appearance of the hirsutism first appear?
   2. Use the Wood's light in a darkened room to visualize the rash under the black light.
   3. Teach the client to clean the rash with cool alcohol water solution twice daily.
   4. What did the rash look like before and after the client's self-prescribed treatment?

2. The nurse is assessing the client diagnosed with psoriasis. Which data would support that diagnosis?
   1. Appearance of red, elevated plaques with silvery white scales.
   2. A burning, prickling row of vesicles located along the torso.
   3. Raised, flesh-colored papules with a rough surface area.
   4. An overgrowth of tissue with an excessive amount of collagen.

3. The nurse is preparing the plan of care for a client diagnosed with psoriasis. Which intervention should the nurse include in the plan of care?
   1. Apply a thin dusting with Mycostatin, an antifungal powder, over the area.
   2. Cover the area with an occlusive dressing after applying the steroid cream.
   3. Administer Acyclovir, an antiviral medication, to the affected areas six (6) times a day.
   4. Teach the client the risks and hazards of implanted radiation therapy.

4. The nurse has completed the teaching plan for the client diagnosed with psoriasis. What data indicate that further teaching is needed?
   1. The client will perform an inspection of the skin each day for redness with tenderness.
   2. The client will ingest psoralen, a photosensitizing agent, two (2) hours before treatment.
   3. The client will wear dark glasses all day and during ultraviolet light treatments.
   4. The client states coal-tar–derived ointments, shampoos, and lotions do not stain clothing.

5. The nurse is planning the care of a client diagnosed with psoriasis. Which client problem should be included in the plan?
   1. Anticipatory grieving.
   2. Altered body image.
   3. Potential for loss of extremity function.
   4. Fluid volume deficit.

6. The elderly client is complaining of intense pruritus and weeping blisters that started on the lower legs and have spread to the arms and abdomen. The health-care provider has diagnosed the client with an allergic reaction to poison ivy. The health-care provider prescribed prednisone by mouth. The nurse is preparing this client for discharge to home. Which intervention should the nurse include in the teaching about this medication?
   1. Come back to the office in one (1) week and then monthly for blood levels.
   2. Take the number of pills at the scheduled time on the information sheet.
   3. Take this medication on an empty stomach to increase the effectiveness.
   4. If any side effects occur, stop the medication abruptly and contact the HCP.

7. The nurse is teaching clients at a community center about skin diseases. Which information about pruritus should the nurse include? Select all that apply.
   1. Cool environments increase itching.
   2. Using soap increases itching.
   3. Use hot water to rinse off soap.
   4. Apply mild skin lotion for hydration.
   5. Blot gently but completely to dry the skin.

8. Which laboratory test should the nurse monitor that would identify an allergic reaction for the client diagnosed with contact dermatitis?
   1. IgA.
   2. IgD.
   3. IgE.
   4. IgG.

9. Which signs and symptoms should the nurse expect to find when assessing the client diagnosed with contact dermatitis?
   1. Erythema and oozing vesicles.
   2. Pustule and nodule form lesions.
   3. Varicosities and edema.
   4. Telangiectasia and flushing.

10. When caring for the client diagnosed with contact dermatitis, which collaborative intervention should the nurse implement?
    1. Encourage the use of support stockings.
    2. Administer a topical anti-inflammatory cream.
    3. Remove scales frequently by shampooing.
    4. Shampoo with lindane 1%, an antiparasitic, weekly.

11. The client returns to the clinic two (2) weeks after being diagnosed with an allergic reaction to poison oak. The client now has severe itching and a return of weeping vesicles that have spread from the legs to the arms. Which information should the nurse obtain to assist in preventive care for this client?
    1. Obtain a sample of the drainage for culture and sensitivities.
    2. Determine any allergic reactions to any medications taken recently.
    3. Inquire how the poison ivy/oak plants were destroyed.
    4. Assess for any temperature elevation since the last visit to the clinic.

12. The client is complaining of severe itching following a course of antibiotics. Which independent nursing action should the nurse implement?
    1. Refer to an allergy specialist to begin desensitization.
    2. Use a tar preparation gel after each shower or bath.
    3. Keep the covers tightly around the client at night.
    4. Take baths with an OTC colloidal oatmeal preparation.

13. The home health nurse is visiting with an elderly client. The client inquires about an area of skin that is rough with a greasy feel and multiple papules. Which information should the nurse provide the client?
    1. Contact the health-care provider immediately for an appointment.
    2. Tell the client that this is a normal aging change and that no action should be taken.
    3. Tell the client to discuss this with the HCP at the next appointment.
    4. Have the client buy a wart remover kit at the store.

14. The nurse is preparing the plan of care for a client diagnosed with Stevens–Johnson syndrome. Which interventions should the nurse include? Select all that apply.
    1. Monitor intake and output every eight (8) hours.
    2. Assess breath sounds and rate every four (4) hours.
    3. Assess vesicles, erosions, and crusts.
    4. Perform the whisper-test for auditory changes daily.
    5. Assess orientation to person, place, and time every shift.

15. Which expected outcome should the nurse include in the plan of care for the client diagnosed with seborrheic dermatitis?
    1. The client will have no further outbreaks.
    2. The client will be able to control the disorder.
    3. The client will shampoo three (3) times a week.
    4. The client will apply bacitracin twice daily.

16. The nurse working at the local health department is preparing the plan of care for a client diagnosed with leprosy (Hansen's disease). Which intervention should the nurse include?
    1. Prepare the client for admission to the hospital.
    2. Administer dapsone, a sulfone, for one (1) month only.
    3. Use skin moisturizing lotion to control the symptoms.
    4. Institute proper precautions since transmission is by direct contact over time.

17. The health department nurse is caring for the client who has leprosy, Hansen's disease. Which assessment data indicate the client is experiencing a complication of the disease?
    1. Elevated temperature at night.
    2. Brownish-black discoloration to the skin.
    3. Reduced skin sensation in the lesions.
    4. A high count of mycobacteria in the culture.

18. Which client problem should the nurse identify as a problem specific to the client diagnosed with leprosy (Hansen's disease)?
    1. Social isolation.
    2. Altered body image.
    3. Potential for infection.
    4. Alteration in comfort.

19. The nurse is teaching the client diagnosed with atopic dermatitis. Which information should the nurse include in the teaching?
    1. The need for meticulous skin care using hydrating lotions and minimal soap.
    2. Methods of treating secondary infection.
    3. Explain there are no adverse effects to using topical corticosteroids daily.
    4. Warning that inhaled allergens have been linked to exacerbations of the condition.

20. The nurse is working with clients in an aesthetic (plastic surgery) center. Which intervention should the nurse implement for clients undergoing a chemical peel?
    1. Teach the client to expect extreme swelling after the procedure.
    2. Apply the chemical mixture directly to skin after the face is cleansed.
    3. Administer general anesthesia to the client prior to the procedure.
    4. Explain that there will be no pain or discomfort during the procedure.

21. The nurse is preparing the client scheduled for a dermabrasion. Which information should the nurse include while teaching the client?
    1. Erythema will go away within 24 hours.
    2. Do not change the dressing until seen by the HCP.
    3. Stay out of extreme cold or heat situations.
    4. Avoid direct sunlight for three (3) days.

22. The nurse is caring for a client preoperative for facial reconstruction. Which information client problem should the nurse include in the plan of care?
    1. Loss of self-esteem.
    2. Alteration in comfort.
    3. Ineffective airway clearance.
    4. Impaired communication.

23. The nurse is caring for a client postoperative for facial reconstruction. Which intervention should the nurse implement to achieve an expected outcome of "a positive self-image"?
    1. Provide all activities of daily living.
    2. Allow client to voice fears and concerns.
    3. Monitor nutritional food and fluid intake.
    4. Monitor signs and symptoms of infection.

Integumentary

24. The nurse is caring for the client following reconstructive facial surgery. Which assessment data warrant immediate intervention?
    1. Generalized facial swelling.
    2. Blood clots on suture line.
    3. Blue pedicle flap.
    4. Hoarseness when the client speaks.

25. The nurse is caring for a male client diagnosed with a folliculitis. Which information should the nurse teach to prevent a reoccurrence?
    1. Do not shave the face.
    2. Rub on astringent aftershave lotion.
    3. Apply hot packs for 20 minutes before shaving.
    4. Use an antibacterial soap but do not lather it to shave.

26. The emergency department nurse is caring for a client admitted with extensive deep partial-thickness and full-thickness burns. Which interventions should the nurse implement? List in order of priority.
    1. Estimate the amount of burned area using the Rule of 9s.
    2. Insert two (2) 18-gauge catheters and begin fluid replacement.
    3. Apply sterile saline dressings to the burned areas.
    4. Determine the client's airway status.
    5. Administer morphine sulfate, a narcotic analgesic, IV.

1.
1. Hirsutism is an excessive amount of hair growth in unexpected areas. This is not associated with itching or a rash.
2. A Wood's light is used to examine certain infections. This would be used during the physical examination portion of the assessment.
3. Clients should not be cleaning a rash with alcohol or applying any treatment until the etiology is determined.
4. **It is important to assess the rash as it appeared. If the client treated the rash with an ointment or cream, its appearance may have changed. Many times the appearance has changed from first onset and from the treatment.**

2.
1. **Most clients with psoriasis have red raised plaques with silvery white scales.**
2. A burning, prickling row of vesicles located along the torso is the description of herpes zoster.
3. Raised, flesh-colored papules with a rough surface area is a description of a wart.
4. An overgrowth of tissue with excessive amount of collagen is the definition of keloids.

3.
1. Mycostatin is an antifungal medication and would not be useful to treat psoriasis.
2. **Covering the affected area with an occlusive dressing enhances the steroid's effectiveness. This intervention should be limited to 12 hours to reduce systemic and local side effects.**
3. Acyclovir is an antiviral medication and is used for viral diseases. It would not be used for psoriasis.
4. Implanted radiation is a treatment for some forms of cancer, but not for psoriasis. Radiation in the form of UV light therapy is sometimes used to treat psoriasis.

4.
1. The client needs to perform a complete inspection of skin to identify symptoms of generalized redness and tenderness. Treatments would be discontinued if they occur.
2. Psoralen, a photosensitizing agent, is administered two (2) hours before the ultraviolet light therapy to enhance the effects.
3. The client will wear dark glasses to protect the eyes during the treatments and for the remainder of the day. Prior to the treatment dark glasses are not needed.
4. **Coal tar comes in lotions, ointments, shampoos, and gels. They are used more in the hospital setting than in home settings because of the staining and mess associated with their use.**

5.
1. Psoriasis is not a terminal disease process. The client may have an altered coping problem.
2. **Altered body image is a problem that the nurse should assess in clients with psoriasis. Any chronic skin disease that affects appearance can cause psychosocial problems.**
3. Psoriasis does not cause disfigurement, but the scales may be on areas that are visible.
4. The condition of psoriasis does not affect fluid volume.

6.
1. Clients taking prednisone do not require laboratory testing for a therapeutic level.
2. **The client should take the medication exactly as instructed. The number of pills should be taken in a descending (tapering) manner.**
3. Prednisone by mouth can cause gastrointestinal bleeding. It should be taken with food or after eating.
4. Prednisone should not be stopped suddenly; it needs to be tapered off.

7.
1. A cool environment makes itching decrease, not increase.
2. **Soaps cause itching to increase. The client should avoid soap when experiencing pruritus.**
3. Tepid, cool water is better for the client who is itching.
4. **Mild lotion can help the skin stay hydrated.**
5. **The client should dry off completely after bathing and blot gently rather than rub vigorously.**

8.
1. IgA is a specific antibody/antigen reaction that occurs in anaphylactic transfusion reactions.
2. IgD is a protein that is activated in collagen disease.
3. **IgE is a protein responsible for allergic reactions.**
4. IgG is responsible for viruses, bacteria, and toxins.

9.
1. **Contact dermatitis presents with erythema and small oozing vesicles.**
2. Pustules and nodule formation indicate acne.
3. Statis dermatitis presents with varicosities and edema.
4. Clients diagnosed with rosacea present with telangiectasia and periodic flushing.

10.
1. Support stockings are used for stasis dermatitis, which is caused by impaired circulation.
2. **Topical corticosteroids are given to treat contact dermatitis, which comes from an**

allergic response to irritants. The irritant should be eliminated and topical anti-inflammatory creams should be used.

3. Seborrheic dermatitis is treated by frequent cleaning with medicated shampoos and soaps to remove the yellow scales.

4. Lindane 1% shampoo is used to treat lice. The client shampoos the hair and rinses after ten (10) minutes.

11. 1. Collecting a sample for culture would need an order from the health-care provider. This intervention would not be preventive care.

2. Allergic reactions to medications would not assist with prevention.

3. **Many people dispose of the poison oak plant in ways that spread the sap. Burning or pulling the plant without gloves can cause another allergic reaction. Pets can spread the allergen on fur. Tools should be cleaned prior to touching the skin.**

4. Clients do not have temperature elevation unless there is a secondary infection present.

12. 1. There is no indication for the need for the client to be desensitized to the medication. The client should inform health-care providers of any previous reactions to medications prior to taking any medication.

2. Tar solutions are used for psoriasis, not pruritus. Use of tar solutions would be a collaborative intervention, rather than an independent intervention.

3. Cool sleeping environments decrease itching. Warmth increases itching and should be avoided.

4. **Soothing baths, such as colloidal baths or emollient baths, are helpful in treating pruritus. Balneotherapy is a term used to refer to therapeutic baths.**

13. 1. An area that has a greasy rough feel and multiple papules does not require an immediate appointment with the HCP.

2. Seborrheic keratosis is a common occurrence in the elderly, but the skin lesion should be assessed by a health-care provider.

3. **The client should discuss any suspicious area with the health-care provider. This is not an emergency, but it should be assessed.**

4. An area that is wartlike in appearance that varies in color from flesh tones to black and has a greasy rough feel is probably a seborrheic keratosis. The home health nurse does not have the authority to diagnose as a health-care provider and therefore the nurse should not encourage the client to self-treat.

14. 1. The client with Stevens–Johnson syndrome must be assessed for fluid volume deficit (FVD), the need for fluid replacement, and renal failure. Intake and output monitors both.

2. **Breath sounds and respiratory status should be assessed because many clients develop respiratory failure and require mechanical ventilation.**

3. **The client with Stevens–Johnson syndrome has a combination of vesicles, erosions, and crusts at the same time. The skin should be assessed every eight (8) hours.**

4. Hearing is not affected by Stevens–Johnson syndrome, but blindness can be a complication; vision should be assessed for any changes.

5. Neurological status is not compromised.

15. 1. Seborrheic dermatitis is a chronic skin disorder that has remissions and exacerbations. To have an expected outcome for no further outbreaks would not be realistic.

2. **To control the disorder by following the medical protocols would be realistic and appropriate.**

3. The client needs to shampoo daily or a minimum of three (3) times each week for treatment. This is an intervention, not an outcome.

4. To apply bacitracin would treat a bacterial infection. This is an intervention, not a goal or expected outcome.

16. 1. Clients are treated on an outpatient basis by specialized clinics. In the United States, it is the health department's responsibility to care for these clients and ensure that the clients are taking their medications.

2. Dapsone, a sulfone, will be used to treat leprosy for several years up to the remainder of the client's life.

3. Moisturizing lotion will not treat the infectious process and therefore cannot control the symptoms.

4. **Contrary to popular thought, leprosy, although contagious, usually requires a prolonged exposure for the infection to spread to another person. Touching the lesions directly will increase the potential for infection.**

17. 1. The client does not usually have an elevated temperature.

2. A side effect of the medication Dapsone is a discoloration of the skin from pink to brownish black.

3. **The decrease in sensation of the lesions is the result of peripheral nerve damage.**

Integumentary

Leprosy is a peripheral nervous system disease.

4. A high mycobacterium count would be expected from the disease but would not be a side effect.

18. 1. The client diagnosed with leprosy (Hansen's disease) may feel ostracized because of the stigma of the disease. Historically, people have been isolated from society when diagnosed. Leprosy colonies were sites of treatment for those diagnosed. Today much of the public is unaware of the presence of the disease. Clients are treated on an outpatient basis by health departments.
2. Altered body image would be appropriate for any client with skin disorders.
3. Potential for infection is a problem for all skin disorders.
4. Clients with leprosy have a decreased sensation from peripheral nerve damage and have no discomfort.

19. 1. Skin care must be meticulous. Minimal soap and tepid water should be used when showering or bathing. Lotions that do not irritate should be used to keep the skin hydrated.
2. The client needs to know when to contact the health-care provider if signs and symptoms of secondary infection occur not treatment.
3. There are adverse effects of the topical use of corticosteroids.
4. There has been no link supported by research that inhaled allergens cause atopic dermatitis exacerbations (flare-ups).

20. 1. After the first six (6) to eight (8) hours, the client will have extreme edema that can cause the eyes to swell. This is expected.
2. The dermatologist will apply the chemical to begin the peeling procedure.
3. The client will be awake during the procedure, but an analgesic and a tranquilizer can be given for sedation. Only certified registered nurse anesthetists (CRNA) administer general anesthesia.
4. There is a sensation of burning during the application of the chemical and for several days after the procedure.

21. 1. Erythema can last from one (1) week to a month.
2. After 24 hours, the serum oozes from the dressing, and the client needs to apply a prescribed ointment to keep the area soft and flexible.
3. Extreme cold and heat, along with straining and lifting heavy objects, should be avoided.

4. Direct sunlight should be avoided for three (3) to six (6) months. Clients should be taught to wear a sunscreen.

22. 1. A loss of self-esteem can occur after a change in facial appearance through injury or disease. Age-related changes also cause a loss in self-esteem. This would be a nursing diagnosis that applies to the preoperative client.
2. Edema and pain would be appropriate postoperatively.
3. The airway has not been compromised preoperatively.
4. Communication may be a problem postoperatively but not prior to surgery.

23. 1. A client with a positive self-image would participate in as much self-care as possible and not allow someone else to do it.
2. The nurse allows the client to express fears and concerns to assist the client to have a positive self-image.
3. Monitoring the client's nutritional intake and fluid balance is important for healing, but this would not reflect a positive self-image.
4. Monitoring for complications such as infection is a responsibility of the nurse, but this would not alter a positive self-image.

24. 1. Generalized facial swelling is expected. Airway and breathing should be assessed frequently.
2. Blood clots may be present on suture lines and are expected.
3. A change in color of the pedicle flap (a procedure performed to supply blood to the operative area) can indicate that the blood supply to the site has been impaired. This needs to be assessed and reported to the surgeon.
4. Some hoarseness following intubation for general anesthesia is expected.

25. 1. Shaving is the cause of this condition, and refraining from shaving is the only cure. Special brushes are used. If the client must shave, he should use a depilatory cream or electric razor.
2. Aftershave will not prevent folliculitis.
3. Hot packs will not prevent folliculitis.
4. Antibacterial soap is too strong for use on the face. Shaving is the cause of folliculitis.

26. In order of priority: 4, 2, 3, 1, 5.
4. Airway is always the first priority for any process in which the airway might be compromised.
2. The nurse should start fluid resuscitation

Integumentary

as soon as possible before the client's blood pressure makes it more difficult to establish an IV route.

3. Covering the open burns will prevent further intrusion of bacteria.

1. Estimating the extent of the burned area should be done but does not have priority over airway, fluid replacement, and the prevention of infection.

5. Pain is priority but not over determining airway, fluid status, and prevention of infection.

*The secret of joy in work is contained in one word—excellence. To know how to do something well is to enjoy it.*—Pearl S. Buck

# 13

# Immune System Disorders

The immune system, which involves many tissues throughout the body, is subject to several inflammatory disorders. Some involve genetic predisposition, some result from infectious processes, and many are of uncertain etiology. This chapter includes questions on the most common immune disorders—multiple sclerosis, Guillain-Barré syndrome, rheumatoid arthritis, AIDS (acquired immunodeficiency syndrome), systemic lupus erythematosus, and allergies—and on other disorders affecting the body's immune system.

| KEYWORDS | ABBREVIATIONS |
| --- | --- |
| alopecia | Arterial Blood Gases (ABG) |
| arthralgia | Activities of Daily Living (ADL) |
| astringent | Acquired Immunodeficiency Syndrome (AIDS) |
| cogwheel rigidity | Apical Pulse (AP) |
| cutaneous | Blood Pressure (B/P) |
| demyelination | Electromyelogram (EMG) |
| diplopia | Erythrocyte Sedimentation Rate (ESR) |
| dysarthria | Guillain-Barré (GB) |
| dysmetria | Health-Care Provider (HCP) |
| eradicated | Human Immunodeficiency Virus (HIV) |
| erythema | Intramuscular (IM) |
| exacerbation | Intravenous (IV) |
| hirsutism | Intravenous Piggy Back (IVPB) |
| ocular | Intravenous Push (IVP) |
| plasmapheresis | Licensed Practical Nurse (LPN) |
| polymyositis | Magnetic Resonance Imaging (MRI) |
| pruritus | Myasthenia Gravis (MG) |
| Raynaud's phenomenon | Multiple Sclerosis (MS) |
| rhinitis | Nonsteroidal Anti-Inflammatory Drugs (NSAIDs) |
| scleroderma | Nothing By Mouth (NPO) |
| scotomas | Nurse Practitioner (NP) |
| spasticity | Osteoarthritis (OA) |
| wheal | Percutaneous Endoscopic Gastronomy (PEG) |
| | *Pneumocystis carinii* Pneumonia (PCP) |
| | Respiratory Rate (RR) |
| | Related To (R/T) |
| | Rule Out (R/O) |
| | Subcutaneous (SQ) |
| | Systemic Lupus Erythematosus (SLE) |
| | Ultraviolet (UV) |

## Multiple Sclerosis

1. The nurse is assessing a 48-year-old client diagnosed with multiple sclerosis. Which clinical manifestation assessed by the nurse would warrant immediate intervention?
   1. The client has scanning speech and diplopia.
   2. The client has dysarthria and scotomas.
   3. The client has muscle weakness and spasticity.
   4. The client has a congested cough and dyspnea.

2. The client newly diagnosed with multiple sclerosis (MS) states, "I don't understand how I got multiple sclerosis. Is it genetic?" The nurse's response would be based on which scientific rationale?
   1. Genetics may play a role in susceptibility to MS, but the disease may be caused by a virus.
   2. There is no evidence that suggests that there is any chromosomal involvement in developing MS.
   3. Multiple sclerosis is a caused by a genetically recessive gene, so both parents had to have the gene for the client to get MS.
   4. Multiple sclerosis is caused by an autosomal dominant gene on the Y chromosome, so only fathers can pass it on.

3. The 30-year-old female client is admitted with complaints of numbness, tingling, a crawling sensation affecting the extremities, and double vision. During the interview the client tells the nurse that she has been admitted twice before for the same complaints but nothing was found and the symptoms went away on their own. Which question would be important for the nurse to ask the client?
   1. "Have you experienced any difficulty with your menstrual cycle?"
   2. "Have you noticed a rash across the bridge of your nose?"
   3. "Do you get tired easily and sometimes have problems swallowing?"
   4. "Are you taking birth control pills to prevent conception?"

4. The nurse enters the room of a client diagnosed with acute exacerbation of multiple sclerosis and finds the client crying. Which statement would be the most therapeutic response for the nurse to make?
   1. "Why are you crying? The medication will help the disease."
   2. "You seem upset. I will sit down and we can talk for awhile."
   3. "Multiple sclerosis is a disease that has good times and bad times."
   4. "I will have the chaplain come and stay with you for a while."

5. The client diagnosed with multiple sclerosis is scheduled for a magnetic resonance imaging (MRI) scan of the head. Which information should the nurse teach the client about the test?
   1. The client will have wires attached to the scalp and lights will flash off and on.
   2. The machine will be loud and the client must not move the head during the test.
   3. The client will drink a contrast medium 30 minutes to one (1) hour before the test.
   4. The test will be repeated at intervals during a five (5)- to six (6)-hour period.

6. The 45-year-old client is diagnosed with primary progressive multiple sclerosis, and the nurse writes the nursing diagnosis "anticipatory grieving related to progressive loss." Which intervention should be implemented?
   1. Consult the physical therapist for assistive devices for mobility.
   2. Ask the dietitian to provide thickening on each tray.
   3. Teach the client self-catheterization and bowel management.
   4. Discuss the client's wishes regarding end-of-life care.

7. The home health nurse is assigned the following clients. Which client should be seen first?
   1. The 38-year-old male client diagnosed with multiple sclerosis who refused to have a gastrostomy feeding.
   2. The 22-year-old female client newly diagnosed with multiple sclerosis who is deciding whether her fiancé should be told before the wedding.
   3. The 40-year-old male client diagnosed with multiple sclerosis who called the office to tell the nurse that life is not worth living anymore.
   4. The 50-year-old female client diagnosed with relapsing remitting multiple sclerosis who needs a subcutaneous flu injection.

8. The nurse and a licensed practical nurse (LPN) are caring for a group of clients. Which nursing responsibility should not be assigned to the LPN?
   1. Administer a skeletal muscle relaxant to a client diagnosed with an exacerbation of multiple sclerosis.
   2. Discuss bowel regimen medications with the health-care provider for the client diagnosed with multiple sclerosis.
   3. Draw morning blood work on the client diagnosed with secondary progressive multiple sclerosis.
   4. Teach self-catheterization to the client diagnosed with multiple sclerosis.

9. The male client diagnosed with multiple sclerosis states he has been investigating alternative therapies to treat his disease. Which response would be most appropriate by the nurse?
   1. Encourage the therapy if it is not contraindicated by the medical regimen.
   2. Tell the client that only the health-care provider should discuss this with him.
   3. Ask how his significant other feels about this deviation from the medical regimen.
   4. Suggest that the client investigate an investigational therapy instead.

10. The client diagnosed with an acute exacerbation of multiple sclerosis is placed on high-dose intravenous injections of corticosteroid medication. Which nursing intervention should be implemented?
    1. Discuss discontinuing the proton pump inhibitor with the HCP.
    2. Hold the medication until after all cultures have been obtained.
    3. Monitor the client's serum blood glucose levels frequently.
    4. Provide supplemental dietary sodium with the client's meals.

11. The nurse writes the client problem of "altered sexual functioning" for a male client diagnosed with multiple sclerosis (MS). Which intervention should be implemented?
    1. Encourage the couple to explore alternative ways of maintaining intimacy.
    2. Make an appointment with a psychotherapist to counsel the couple.
    3. Explain that daily exercise will help increase libido and sexual arousal.
    4. Discuss the importance of keeping physically calm during sexual intercourse.

12. The nurse is admitting a client diagnosed with multiple sclerosis. Which clinical manifestation should the nurse assess? Select all that apply.
    1. Muscle flaccidity.
    2. Lethargy.
    3. Dysmetria.
    4. Fatigue.
    5. Dysphagia.

Immune

# Guillain-Barré Syndrome

13. Which assessment data would the nurse assess in the client diagnosed with Guillain-Barré syndrome?
    1. An exaggerated startle reflex and memory changes.
    2. Cogwheel rigidity and inability to initiate voluntary movement.
    3. Sudden severe unilateral facial pain and inability to chew.
    4. Progressive ascending paralysis of the lower extremities and numbness.

14. Which statement by the client supports the diagnosis of Guillain-Barré syndrome?
    1. "I just returned from a short trip to Japan."
    2. "I had a really bad cold just a few weeks ago."
    3. "I think one of the people I work with had this."
    4. "I have been taking some herbs for more than a year."

15. Which assessment intervention should the nurse implement specifically for the diagnosis of Guillain-Barré syndrome?
    1. Assess deep tendon reflexes.
    2. Complete a Glasgow Coma Scale.
    3. Check the Babinski reflex.
    4. Take the client's vital signs.

16. The health-care provider scheduled a lumbar puncture for a client admitted with rule out Guillain-Barré syndrome. Which pre-procedure intervention has priority?
    1. Keep the client NPO.
    2. Instruct the client to void.
    3. Place in the lithotomy position.
    4. Assess the client's pedal pulse.

17. Which priority client problem should be included in the care plan for the client diagnosed with Guillain-Barré syndrome?
    1. High risk for injury.
    2. Fear and anxiety.
    3. Altered nutrition.
    4. Ineffective breathing pattern.

18. The nurse caring for the client diagnosed with Guillain-Barré syndrome writes the client problem "impaired physical mobility." Which long-term goal should be written for this problem?
    1. The client will have no skin irritation.
    2. The client will have no muscle atrophy.
    3. The client will perform range-of-motion exercises.
    4. The client will turn every two (2) hours while awake.

19. The client diagnosed with Guillain-Barré syndrome is using a ventilator. Which action will help the client communicate with the nursing staff?
    1. Provide an erase slate board for the client to write on.
    2. Instruct the client to blink once for "no" and twice for "yes."
    3. Refer to a speech therapist to help with communication.
    4. Leave the call light within easy reach of the client.

20. The client diagnosed with Guillain-Barré syndrome asks the nurse, "Will I ever get back to normal? I am so tired of being sick." Which statement would be the best response by the nurse?
    1. "You should make a full recovery within a few months to a year."
    2. "Most clients with this syndrome have some type of residual disability."
    3. "That is something you should discuss with the health-care team."
    4. "The rehabilitation is short and you should be fully recovered within a month."

21. The client admitted with rule out Guillain-Barré syndrome has just had a lumbar puncture. Which intervention should the nurse implement post-procedure?
    1. Monitor the client for hypotension.
    2. Apply pressure to the puncture site.
    3. Test the client's cerebrospinal fluid.
    4. Increase the client's fluid intake.

22. The client diagnosed with Guillain-Barré syndrome is having difficulty breathing and is placed on a ventilator. Which situation would warrant immediate intervention by the nurse?
    1. The ventilator rate is set at 14 breaths per minute.
    2. A manual resuscitation bag is at the client's bedside.
    3. The client's pulse oximeter reading is 85%.
    4. The ABG results are pH 7.40, $PaO_2$ 88, $PaCO_2$ 35, and $HCO_3$ 24.

23. The client diagnosed with Guillain-Barré syndrome is on a ventilator. When the wife comes to visit for the first time she starts crying uncontrollably, and the client starts fighting the ventilator because his wife is upset. Which action should the nurse implement?
    1. Tell the wife she must stop crying.
    2. Escort the wife out of the room.
    3. Medicate the client immediately.
    4. Acknowledge the wife's fears.

24. The client diagnosed with Guillain-Barré syndrome is admitted to the rehabilitation unit after 23 days in the acute care hospital. Which interventions should the nurse implement? Select all that apply.
    1. Refer client to the physical therapist.
    2. Include the speech therapist in the team.
    3. Request a social worker consult.
    4. Implement a regimen to address pain control.
    5. Refer the client to the Guillain-Barré Syndrome Foundation.

## Myasthenia Gravis

25. Which ocular or facial signs/symptoms would the nurse expect to find when assessing the client diagnosed with myasthenia gravis?
    1. Weakness and fatigue.
    2. Ptosis and diplopia.
    3. Breathlessness and dyspnea.
    4. Weight loss and dehydration.

26. The client is being evaluated to rule out myasthenia gravis and being administered the Tensilon (edrophonium chloride) test. Which response to the test indicates the client has myasthenia gravis?
    1. The client has no apparent change in the assessment data.
    2. There is increased amplitude of electrical stimulation in the muscle.
    3. The circulating acetylcholine receptor antibodies are decreased.
    4. The client shows a marked improvement of muscle strength.

27. Which surgical procedure would the nurse anticipate the client with myasthenia gravis undergoing to help prevent the signs/symptoms of the disease process?
    1. There is no surgical option.
    2. A transsphenoidal hypophysectomy.
    3. A thymectomy.
    4. An adrenalectomy.

Immune

28. The client diagnosed with myasthenia gravis is being discharged home. Which intervention has priority when teaching the client's significant others?
    1. Discuss ways to help prevent choking episodes.
    2. Explain how to care for a client on a ventilator.
    3. Teach how to perform passive range-of-motion exercises.
    4. Demonstrate how to care for the client's feeding tube.

29. To which collaborative health-care team member should the nurse refer the client in the late stages of myasthenia gravis?
    1. Occupational therapist.
    2. Recreational therapist.
    3. Vocational therapist.
    4. Speech therapist.

30. The client with myasthenia gravis is undergoing plasmapheresis at the bedside. Which assessment data would warrant immediate intervention?
    1. The client's BP is 94/60 and AP is 112.
    2. A negative Chvostek's and Trousseau's sign.
    3. The serum potassium level is 3.5 mEq/L.
    4. Ecchymosis at the vascular site access.

31. Which statement by the female client diagnosed with myasthenia gravis indicates the client needs more discharge teaching?
    1. "I will not have any menstrual cycles because of this disease."
    2. "I should avoid people who have respiratory infections."
    3. "I should not take a hot bath or swim in cold water."
    4. "I will drink at least 2500 mL of water a day."

32. The client diagnosed with myasthenia gravis is admitted to the emergency department with a sudden exacerbation of motor weakness. Which assessment data indicate the client is experiencing a cholinergic crisis?
    1. The serum assay of circulating acetylcholine receptor antibodies is increased.
    2. The client's symptoms improve when administering a cholinesterase inhibitor.
    3. The client's blood pressure, pulse, and respirations improve after IV fluid.
    4. The Tensilon test does not show improvement in the client's muscle strength.

33. The client diagnosed with myasthenia gravis is admitted with an acute exacerbation. Which interventions should the nurse implement? Select all that apply.
    1. Assist the client to turn and cough every two (2) hours.
    2. Place the client in a high or semi-Fowler's position.
    3. Assess the client's pulse oximeter reading every shift.
    4. Plan meals to promote medication effectiveness.
    5. Monitor the client's serum anti-cholinesterase levels.

34. The significant other of a client diagnosed with myasthenia gravis is crying and shares with the nurse that they just don't know what to do. Which response would be the best action by the nurse?
    1. Discuss the Myasthenia Foundation with the significant other.
    2. Refer the client to a local myasthenia gravis support group.
    3. Ask the significant other if he or she would like to talk to a counselor.
    4. Sit down and allow the significant other to ventilate his or her feelings to the nurse.

35. The client with myasthenia gravis is prescribed the cholinesterase inhibitor, neostigmine (Prostigmin). Which data indicate the medication is effective?
    1. The client is able to feed self independently.
    2. The client is able to blink the eyes without tearing.
    3. The client denies any nausea or vomiting when eating.
    4. The client denies any pain when performing ROM exercises.

36. The client is diagnosed with myasthenia gravis. Which intervention should the nurse implement when administering the anti-cholinesterase pyridostigmine (Mestinon)?
    1. Administer the medication 30 minutes prior to meals.
    2. Instruct the client to take with eight (8) ounces of water.
    3. Explain the importance of sitting up for one (1) hour after taking medication.
    4. Assess the client's blood pressure prior to administering medication.

## Systemic Lupus Erythematosus

37. The 26-year-old female client is complaining of a low-grade fever, arthralgias, fatigue, and a facial rash. Which laboratory data would the nurse expect the HCP to order if SLE is suspected?
    1. Complete metabolic panel and liver function tests.
    2. Complete blood count and antinuclear antibody tests.
    3. Cholesterol and lipid profile tests.
    4. Blood urea nitrogen and glomerular filtration tests.

38. The client diagnosed with SLE is being discharged from the medical unit. Which discharge instructions would be important for the nurse to include? Select all that apply.
    1. Use a sunscreen of SPF 30 or greater when in the sunlight.
    2. Notify the HCP immediately when developing a low-grade fever.
    3. Some dyspnea is expected and does not need immediate attention.
    4. The hands and feet may change color if exposed to cold or heat.
    5. Explain that with continued therapy the client can be cured.

39. The nurse is developing a care plan for a client diagnosed with SLE. Which goal is priority for this client?
    1. Be able to maintain reproductive ability.
    2. Verbalize feelings of body-image changes.
    3. Have the body's organs remain functioning.
    4. No skin irritation or breakdown.

40. The nurse is admitting a client diagnosed with R/O SLE. Which assessment data observed by the nurse supports the diagnosis of SLE?
    1. Pericardial friction rub and crackles in the lungs.
    2. Muscle spasticity and bradykinesia.
    3. Hirsutism and clubbing of the fingers.
    4. Somnolence and weight gain.

41. The client diagnosed with an acute exacerbation of SLE is prescribed high-dose steroids. Which statement best explains the scientific rationale for using high-dose steroids in treating SLE?
    1. The steroids will increase the body's ability to fight the infection.
    2. The steroids will decrease the chance of the SLE spreading to other organs.
    3. The steroids will suppress tissue inflammation, thereby reducing damage to organs.
    4. The steroids will prevent scarring of skin tissues associated with SLE.

42. The nurse enters the room of a female client diagnosed with SLE and finds the client crying. Which statement would be the most therapeutic response?
    1. "I know you are upset, but stress makes the SLE worse."
    2. "Please explain to me why you are crying."
    3. "I'm sorry but I need to complete the shift assessment."
    4. "I see you are crying. We can talk if you would like."

43. The nurse is assessing a client with cutaneous lupus erythematosus. Which intervention should be implemented?
    1. Use astringent lotion on the face and skin.
    2. Inspect the skin weekly for open areas or rashes.
    3. Dry the skin thoroughly by patting.
    4. Apply anti-itch medication between the toes.

Immune

44. The nurse is caring for clients on a medical floor. Which client should be assessed first?
    1. The client diagnosed with SLE who is complaining of chest pain.
    2. The client diagnosed with multiple sclerosis who is complaining of pain at a "10."
    3. The client diagnosed with myasthenia gravis who has dysphagia.
    4. The client diagnosed with Guillain-Barré who can barely move his toes.

45. The nurse and a female unlicensed assistive personnel are caring for a group of clients on a medical floor. Which action by the assistant warrants immediate intervention by the nurse?
    1. The assistant washes her hands before and after performing vital signs on a client.
    2. The assistant dons sterile gloves prior to removing an indwelling catheter from a client.
    3. The assistant raises the head of the bed to a high Fowler's position for a client about to eat.
    4. The assistant uses a fresh plastic bag to get ice for a client's water pitcher.

46. The client recently diagnosed with SLE asks the nurse, "What is SLE and how did I get it?" Which statement best explains the scientific rationale for the nurse's response?
    1. SLE is thought to occur because the kidneys do not filter antibodies from the blood.
    2. SLE occurs after a viral illness as a result of damage to the endocrine system.
    3. There is no known identifiable reason for a client to develop SLE.
    4. This is an autoimmune disease that may have a genetic or hormonal component.

47. The client diagnosed with an acute exacerbation of SLE is being discharged with a prescription for an oral steroid that has the client taking smaller and smaller doses of the medication as each day progresses. Which statement is the scientific rationale for this type of medication dosing?
    1. Tapering the medication prevents the client from having withdrawal symptoms.
    2. So thyroid gland starts working because this medication stops it from working.
    3. Tapering the dose allows the adrenal glands to begin to produce cortisol again.
    4. This is the health-care provider's personal choice in prescribing the medication.

48. The nurse is discussing autoimmune diseases with a class of nursing students. Which signs and symptoms are shared by rheumatoid arthritis (RA) and systemic lupus erythematosus (SLE)?
    1. Nodules in the subcutaneous layer and bone deformity.
    2. Renal involvement and pleural effusions.
    3. Joint stiffness and pain.
    4. Raynaud's phenomenon and skin rash.

## Acquired Immunodeficiency Syndrome

49. The school nurse is preparing to teach a health class to 9th graders regarding sexually transmitted diseases. Which information regarding acquired immune deficiency syndrome (AIDS) should be included?
    1. Females taking birth control pills are protected from becoming infected with HIV.
    2. Protected sex is no longer an issue because there is a vaccine for the HIV virus.
    3. Adolescents with a normal immune system are not at risk for developing AIDS.
    4. Abstinence is the only guarantee of not becoming infected with sexually transmitted HIV.

50. The nurse is admitting a client diagnosed with protein calorie malnutrition secondary to AIDS. Which intervention would be the nurse's first action?
    1. Assess the client's body weight and ask what the client has been able to eat.
    2. Place in contact isolation and don a mask and gown before entering the room.
    3. Check the HCP's orders and determine what laboratory tests will be done.
    4. Teach the client about total parenteral nutrition and monitor the subclavian IV site.

51. The client diagnosed with AIDS is complaining of a sore mouth and tongue. When the nurse assesses the buccal mucosa, the nurse notes white, patchy lesions covering the hard and soft palates and the right inner cheek. Which interventions should the nurse implement?
    1. Teach the client to brush the teeth and patchy area with a soft-bristle toothbrush.
    2. Notify the HCP for an order for an antifungal swish-and-swallow medication.
    3. Have the client gargle with an antiseptic-based mouthwash several times a day.
    4. Determine what types of food the client has been eating for the last 24 hours.

52. Which type of isolation technique was designed to decrease the risk of transmission of recognized and unrecognized sources of infections?
    1. Contact Precautions.
    2. Airborne Precautions
    3. Droplet Precautions.
    4. Standard Precautions.

53. The nurse is describing the HIV virus infection to a client who has been told that he is HIV positive. Which information regarding the virus is important to teach?
    1. The HIV virus is a retrovirus, which means it never dies as long as it has a host to live in.
    2. The HIV virus can be eradicated from the host body with the correct medical regimen.
    3. It is difficult for the HIV virus to replicate in humans because it is a monkey virus.
    4. The HIV virus uses the client's own red blood cells to reproduce the virus in the body.

54. The client who has engaged in needle-sharing activities has developed a flulike infection. An HIV antibody test is negative. Which scientific rationale explains this finding?
    1. The client is fortunate to not have contracted HIV from an infected needle.
    2. The client must be repeatedly exposed to HIV before becoming infected.
    3. The client may be in the primary infection phase of an HIV infection.
    4. The antibody test is negative because the client has a different flu virus.

55. The nurse caring for a client who is HIV positive is stuck with the stylet used to start an IV. Which action should the nurse implement first?
    1. Flush the skin with water and try to get the area to bleed.
    2. Notify the charge nurse and complete an incident report.
    3. Report to the employee health nurse for prophylactic medication.
    4. Follow up with the infection control nurse to have lab work drawn.

56. The client on a medical floor is diagnosed with HIV encephalopathy. Which nursing problem is priority?
    1. Altered nutrition, less than body requirements.
    2. Anticipatory grieving.
    3. Knowledge deficit, procedures and prognosis.
    4. Risk for injury.

57. The client diagnosed with pneumocystis carinii pneumonia (PCP) is being admitted to the intensive care unit. Which HCP's order should the nurse implement first?
    1. Draw a serum for CD4 and complete blood count STAT.
    2. Give oxygen to the client, at four (4) L/minute.
    3. Administer trimethoprim sulfa, a sulfa antibiotic, IVPB.
    4. Obtain a sputum specimen for culture and sensitivity.

58. Which intervention is an important psychosocial consideration for the client diagnosed with AIDS?
    1. Perform a thorough head-to-toe assessment.
    2. Maintain the client's ideal body weight.
    3. Complete an advanced directive.
    4. Increase the client's activity tolerance.

Immune

59. The nurse on a medical floor is caring for clients diagnosed with AIDS. Which client should be seen first?
    1. The client who has flushed warm skin with tented turgor.
    2. The client who states that the staff ignores the call light.
    3. The client whose vital signs are T 99.9°F, P 101, R 26, and BP 110/68.
    4. The client who is unable to provide a sputum specimen.

60. The client diagnosed with AIDS is angry and yells at everyone entering the room and none of the staff members want to care for the client. Which intervention is the most appropriate for the nurse manager to use in resolving this situation?
    1. Assign a different nurse every shift to the client.
    2. Ask the HCP to tell the client not to yell at the staff.
    3. Call a team meeting and discuss options with the staff.
    4. Force one (1) staff member to care for the client a week at a time.

## Allergies and Allergic Reactions

61. The charge nurse observes the primary nurse interacting with a client. Which action by the primary nurse warrants immediate intervention by the charge nurse?
    1. The nurse explains that the IVP diuretic will make the client urinate.
    2. The nurse dons nonsterile gloves to remove the client's dressing.
    3. The nurse administers a medication without checking for allergies.
    4. The nurse asks the unlicensed assistive personnel for help moving a client up in bed.

62. The nurse in the emergency department is allergic to latex. Which action should the nurse implement regarding the use of nonsterile gloves?
    1. Use only sterile, nonlatex gloves for any procedure requiring gloves.
    2. Do not use gloves when starting an IV or performing a procedure.
    3. Keep a pair of nonsterile, nonlatex gloves in the pocket of the uniform.
    4. Wear white cotton gloves at all times to protect the hands.

63. The client diagnosed with a bee sting allergy is being discharged from the emergency department. Which discharge instruction should be taught to the client?
    1. Demonstrate how to use an EpiPen, an adrenergic agonist.
    2. Teach the client to never go outdoors in the spring and summer.
    3. Have the client buy diphenhydramine over the counter to use when stung.
    4. Discuss not wearing a Medic Alert bracelet when going outside.

64. The client comes to the emergency department complaining of dyspnea and wheezing after eating at a seafood restaurant. The client cannot speak and has a bluish color around the mouth. Which intervention should the nurse implement first?
    1. Initiate an IV with normal saline.
    2. Prepare to intubate the client.
    3. Administer oxygen at 100%.
    4. Ask the client about an iodine allergy.

65. The client in the HCP's office is complaining of allergic rhinitis. Which assessment question is important for the nurse to ask the client?
    1. "What time of year do the symptoms occur?"
    2. "Which over-the-counter medications have you tried?"
    3. "Do other members of your family have allergies to animals?"
    4. "Why do you think you have allergies?"

66. During which time of the year is allergic rhinitis least prevalent?
    1. Early spring.
    2. Early summer.
    3. Early fall.
    4. Early winter.

67. The client is highly allergic to insect venom and is prescribed venom immunotherapy. Which statement is the scientific rationale for this treatment?
    1. Immunotherapy can be effective in preventing anaphylaxis following a future sting.
    2. Immunotherapy will prevent all future insect stings from harming the client.
    3. This therapy will cure the client from having any allergic reactions in the future.
    4. This therapy is experimental and should not be undertaken by the client.

68. The client in the HCP's office has a red, raised rash covering the forearms, neck, and face and is experiencing extreme itching. The HCP diagnoses the rash as an allergic reaction to poison ivy. Which discharge instructions should the nurse teach?
    1. Tell the client never to scratch the rash.
    2. Instruct the client in administering IM Benadryl.
    3. Explain how to take a steroid dose pack.
    4. Have the client wear shirts with long sleeves and high necks.

69. The nurse is developing a care plan for a client diagnosed with allergic rhinitis. Which independent problem has priority?
    1. Ineffective breathing pattern.
    2. Knowledge deficit.
    3. Anaphylaxis.
    4. Ineffective coping.

70. The nurse on a medical unit has received the morning shift report. Which client should the nurse assess first?
    1. The client who has a 0730 sliding scale insulin order.
    2. The client who received an initial dose of IV antibiotic at 0645.
    3. The client who is having back pain at a "6" on a 1–10 scale.
    4. The client who has dysphagia and needs to be fed.

71. The nurse in the holding area of the operating room is assessing the client prior to surgery. Which information warrants immediate intervention by the nurse?
    1. The client is able to mark the correct site for the surgery.
    2. The client can only tell the nurse about the surgery in lay terms.
    3. The client is allergic to iodine and does not have an allergy bracelet.
    4. The client has signed a consent form for surgery and anesthesia.

72. The client in the emergency department begins to experience a severe anaphylactic reaction after an initial dose of IV penicillin, an antibiotic. Which interventions should the nurse implement? Select all that apply.
    1. Prepare to administer Solu-Medrol, a glucocorticoid, IV.
    2. Request and obtain a STAT chest x-ray.
    3. Initiate the emergency response team, Code Blue.
    4. Administer epinephrine, an adrenergic blocker SQ, then IV continuous.
    5. Assess for the client's pulse and respirations.

## Rheumatoid Arthritis

73. The client diagnosed with RA is receiving care through a nurse practitioner clinic. Which preventive care should the nurse include in the regularly scheduled clinic visits?
    1. Perform joint x-rays to determine progression of the disease.
    2. Send blood to the lab for an erythrocyte sedimentation rate (ESR).
    3. Recommend the flu and pneumonia vaccines.
    4. Assess the client for increasing joint involvement.

74. The client with RA has nontender movable nodules in subcutaneous tissue over the elbows and shoulders. Which statement is the best explanation for the nodules?
    1. The nodules indicate a rapidly progressive destruction of the affected tissue.
    2. The nodules are small amounts of synovial fluid that have become crystallized.
    3. The nodules are lymph nodes that have proliferated to try to fight the disease.
    4. The nodules present a favorable prognosis and mean the client is better.

75. The nurse is assessing a client diagnosed with RA. Which assessment findings warrant immediate intervention?
    1. The client complains of joint stiffness and the knees feel warm to the touch.
    2. The client has experienced one (1)-kg weight loss and is very tired.
    3. The client requires a heating pad applied to the hips and back to sleep.
    4. The client is crying, has a flat facial affect, and refuses to speak to the nurse.

76. The client diagnosed with RA who has been prescribed etanercept, a tumor necrosis factor alpha inhibitor, shows marked improvement. Which instruction regarding the use of this medication should the nurse teach?
    1. Explain that the medication loses its efficacy after a few months.
    2. Continue to have checkups and lab work while taking the medication.
    3. Have yearly magnetic resonance imaging to follow the progress.
    4. Discuss that the drug is taken for three (3) weeks and then stopped for a week.

77. The client diagnosed with RA has developed swan-neck fingers. Which referral would be most appropriate for the client?
    1. Physical therapy.
    2. Occupational therapy.
    3. Psychiatric counselor.
    4. Home health nurse.

78. The nurse is planning the care for a client diagnosed with RA. Which interventions should be implemented?
    1. Plan a strenuous exercise program.
    2. Order a mechanical soft diet.
    3. Maintain a keep-open IV.
    4. Obtain an order for a sedative.

79. The 20-year-old female client diagnosed with advanced unremitting RA is being admitted to receive a regimen of immunosuppressive medications. Which question should the nurse ask during the admission process regarding the medications?
    1. "Are you sexually active, and, if so, are you using birth control?"
    2. "Have you discussed taking these drugs with your parents?"
    3. "Which arm do you prefer to have an IV in for four (4) days?"
    4. "Have you signed an informed consent for investigational drugs?"

80. Which client problem is priority for a client diagnosed with RA?
    1. Activity intolerance.
    2. Fluid and electrolyte imbalance.
    3. Alteration in comfort.
    4. Excessive nutritional intake.

81. The nurse is caring for clients on a medical floor. Which client should the nurse assess first?
    1. The client diagnosed with RA who is complaining of pain at a "3" on a 1–10 scale.
    2. The client diagnosed with SLE who has a rash across the bridge of the nose.
    3. The client diagnosed with advanced RA who is receiving antineoplastic drugs IV.
    4. The client diagnosed with scleroderma who has hard, waxylike skin near the eyes.

82. The nurse and licensed practical nurse are caring for clients in a rheumatologist's office. Which task can the nurse assign to the licensed practical nurse?
    1. Administer methotrexate, an antineoplastic medication IV.
    2. Assess the lung sounds of a client with RA who is coughing.
    3. Demonstrate how to use clothing equipped with Velcro fasteners.
    4. Discuss methods of birth control that are compatible with treatment medications.

Immune

83. The client with early-stage RA is being discharged from the outpatient clinic. Which discharge instructions should the nurse teach regarding the use of nonsteroidal anti-inflammatory drugs (NSAIDs)?
    1. Take with an over-the-counter medication for the stomach.
    2. Drink a full glass of water with each pill.
    3. If a dose is missed, double the medication at the next dosing time.
    4. Avoid taking the NSAID on an empty stomach.

84. The nurse is preparing to administer morning medications. Which medication should the nurse administer first?
    1. The pain medication to a client diagnosed with RA.
    2. The diuretic medication to a client diagnosed with SLE.
    3. The steroid to a client diagnosed with polymyositis.
    4. The appetite stimulant to a client diagnosed with OA.

## Multiple Sclerosis

1. 1. These are clinical manifestations of multiple sclerosis and would be expected.
   2. These are expected clinical manifestations of multiple sclerosis.
   3. These are expected clinical manifestations of multiple sclerosis.
   4. Dysphagia is a common problem of clients diagnosed with multiple sclerosis and this places the client at risk for aspiration pneumonia. Some clients diagnosed with multiple sclerosis eventually become immobile and are at risk for pneumonia.

   **TEST-TAKING HINT: This question is asking the test taker to identify the assessment data that are unexpected for the disease process. Respiratory problems are high priority according to Maslow and often warrant immediate intervention.**

2. 1. The exact cause of MS is not known, but there is a theory that a slow virus is partially responsible. A failure of a part of the immune system may also be at fault. A genetic predisposition involving chromosomes 2, 3, 7, 11, 17, 19, and X may be involved.
   2. There is some evidence that there is a genetic component involved in developing MS.
   3. A specific gene has not been identified to know if the gene is recessive or dominant.
   4. The X chromosome, not the Y chromosome, may be involved.

   **TEST-TAKING HINT: Answer option "2" has the word "no" in it. Unless the test taker has absolute knowledge that this is true, then an absolute word such as "no," "never," " all," or "always" should rule out the option.**

3. 1. These are clinical manifestation of MS and can go undiagnosed for years because of the remitting relapsing nature of the disease. MS does not affect the menstrual cycle.
   2. A rash across the bridge of the nose would suggest systemic lupus erythematosus.
   3. These are clinical manifestation of MS and can go undiagnosed for years because of the remitting relapsing nature of the disease. Fatigue and difficulty swallowing are other symptoms of MS.
   4. Taking birth control medications should not produce these symptoms or the pattern of occurrence.

   **TEST-TAKING HINT: This stem is somewhat involved. The test taker must be sure to understand the important parts, which are client's age, complaints, and occurrence of complaints.**

This should cause the reader to think about what these have in common.

4. 1. "Why" is requesting an explanation, and the client does not owe the nurse an explanation.
   2. This is stating a fact and offering self. Both are therapeutic techniques for conversations.
   3. The client did not ask about the nature of MS. The client needs to be able to verbalize feelings.
   4. This is passing the buck. Therapeutic communication is an integral part of nursing.

   **TEST-TAKING HINT: The question is asking for a therapeutic response. Therapeutic responses address feelings.**

5. 1. This describes an evoked potential electroencephalogram (EEG).
   2. MRI scans require the client to lie still and not move the body; the client should be warned about the loud noise.
   3. The client does not drink any contrast medium. If contrast is used it will be given IVP or CT scan.
   4. The test is performed at one time.

   **TEST-TAKING HINT: The test taker must be knowledgeable about different tests and procedures and be able to teach about them to the client. There are no test-taking hints to help remember protocols for procedures and tests.**

6. 1. The problem is grieving R/T loss of functioning. Assistive devices will not prevent loss of functioning and do not address grieving.
   2. Thickening when used in liquids addresses the inability to swallow, not grieving.
   3. Self-catheterization and bowel training do not address grieving.
   4. The client should make personal choices about end-of-life issues while it is possible to do so. This client is progressing toward immobility and all the issues that attend this problem.

   **TEST-TAKING HINT: This is a psychological problem requiring a psychological answer. Options "1," "2," and "3" are physical interventions and therefore should be eliminated as correct answers.**

7. 1. This client could wait to be seen; a missed feeding is not life threatening.
   2. The nurse should see this client when the nurse can spend time with the client and make sure the client has all the information about MS the client needs to make this decision.
   3. The nurse should see this client first and determine if the client has a plan to carry

out the threat of suicide. This situation requires further assessment.

4. A flu injection is not priority.

**TEST-TAKING HINT: When the nurse is prioritizing, a systematic approach must be used. Safety is priority and a threat to a client's life is priority.**

8. 1. The licensed practical nurse (LPN) can administer a muscle relaxant.
   2. The licensed practical nurse can talk with a health-care provider about medication the LPN can give.
   3. The LPN can draw blood.
   4. When assigning tasks the nurse should not assign any task that includes teaching and evaluating the client's ability to perform self-care activities that require sterile technique.

**TEST-TAKING HINT: When deciding on assigning tasks the nurse must be aware of the capabilities of each classification of staff by licensure.**

9. 1. The nurse should listen without being judgmental about any alterative therapy the client is considering. Alternative therapies, such as massage and relaxation, are frequently beneficial and enhance the medical regimen.
   2. The nurse can discuss alternative therapy with the client.
   3. This is not addressing the client's concern of using alternative treatment.
   4. Investigational therapies are treatments that may have efficacy if proved by scientific methods. It is the health-care provider's responsibility to discuss these therapies with the client.

**TEST-TAKING HINT: Two options—"2" and "3"—don't address the issue. The answer must address the client's concern.**

10. 1. Steroid medications increase gastric acid; therefore a proton pump inhibitor would be an appropriate medication for the client.
    2. Cultures are ordered prior to administering antibiotics, not steroids.
    3. Steroids interfere with glucose metabolism by blocking the action of insulin; therefore the blood glucose levels should be monitored.
    4. Steroid medications cause the client to retain sodium; therefore a low-sodium diet should be encouraged.

**TEST-TAKING HINT: Steroid medications are some of the most common medications administered by nurses. They are also among the**

most dangerous; therefore the nurse must know about steroids, their actions, side effects, and adverse effects.

11. 1. This will assist the client and significant other to maintain a close relationship without putting undue pressure on the client.
    2. This is a real physical problem, not a psychological one.
    3. The problem is impotence, not libido.
    4. The problem is not psychosocial. It is a physical problem, and staying calm will not help.

**TEST-TAKING HINT: The nurse must differentiate physical and psychological problems.**

12. 1. Muscle flaccidity is a hallmark symptom of MS.
    2. Lethargy is the state of prolonged sleepiness or serious drowsiness and is not associated with MS.
    3. Dysmetria is the inability to control muscular action characterized by overestimating or underestimating range of movement.
    4. Fatigue is a symptom of MS.
    5. Dysphagia, or difficulty swallowing, is associated with MS.

**TEST-TAKING HINT: These questions are difficult because there are several correct answers. The test taker gets credit only if the entire question is answered correctly. The test taker should read each answer option carefully and rule it out as a potential correct answer before moving on to the next option.**

## Guillain-Barré Syndrome

13. 1. These signs/symptoms, along with sleep disturbances and nervousness, support the diagnosis of Creutzfeldt-Jakob disease.
    2. These signs/symptoms would support the diagnosis of Parkinson's disease.
    3. These are signs/symptoms of trigeminal neuralgia.
    4. Ascending paralysis is the classic symptom of Guillain-Barré syndrome.

**TEST-TAKING HINT: The test taker should try to remember at least one or two signs/symptoms of disease processes, and ascending paralysis is an unusual sign/symptom that is specific to this syndrome.**

14. 1. Visiting a foreign country is not a risk factor for contracting this syndrome.
    2. This syndrome is usually preceded by a respiratory or gastrointestinal infection one (1) to four (4) weeks prior to the onset of neurological deficits.

Immune

3. This syndrome is not a contagious or a communicable disease.

4. Taking herbs is not a risk factor for developing Guillain-Barré syndrome.

**TEST-TAKING HINT: There are some questions that require the test taker to be knowledgeable of the disease process. Herbs may aggravate a disease process, but as a rule they do not cause disease processes, so "4" can be eliminated.**

15. 1. Hyporeflexia of the lower extremities is the classic clinical manifestation of this syndrome. Therefore, assessing deep tendon reflexes is appropriate.

2. A Glasgow Coma Scale is used for clients with potential neurological deficits and used to monitor for increased intracranial pressure.

3. The Babinski reflex evaluates central nervous system neurological status, which is not affected with this syndrome.

4. Vital signs are a part of any admission assessment but are not a specific assessment intervention for this syndrome.

**TEST-TAKING HINT: Vital signs are general assessment skills and really do not help specifically diagnose a disease, except for blood pressure, which helps diagnose hypertension. The test taker should know that the Glasgow Coma Scale is for head or brain injuries.**

16. 1. The client does not need to be NPO prior to this procedure.

2. The client should void prior to this procedure to help prevent accidental puncture of the bladder during the procedure.

3. The lithotomy position has the client lying flat with legs in stirrups, such as when Pap smears are obtained.

4. The pedal pulses should be assessed post-procedure, not prior to the procedure.

**TEST-TAKING HINT: The adjective "pre-procedure" would help rule out "4" as a possible correct answer; it would be priority post-procedure. The test taker must know terminology that describes positioning such as lithotomy, side-lying, supine, Trendelenburg, or prone.**

17. 1. Safety is an important issue for the client, but this is not the priority client problem.

2. The client's psychological needs are important, but psychosocial problems are not priority over physiological problems.

3. Clients with this syndrome may have choking episodes and are at risk for inability to swallow as a result of the disease process, but this is not

the priority nursing problem because weight loss is not an expected complication of this syndrome.

4. Guillain-Barré syndrome has ascending paralysis that can cause respiratory failure. Therefore, breathing pattern is priority.

**TEST-TAKING HINT: Knowledge of the disease process would cause the test taker to select option "4," but applying Maslow's Hierarchy of Needs and choosing a client problem addressing airway is always a good option if the test taker is not sure of the correct answer.**

18. 1. This would be an appropriate long-term goal for the client problem "impaired skin integrity."

2. The client with Guillain-Barré syndrome will not be able to move the extremities; therefore, preventing muscle atrophy is an appropriate long-term goal.

3. The client will not be able to move the extremities. Therefore the nurse will have to do passive range-of-motion exercises; this is an intervention, not a goal.

4. This is a nursing intervention, not a goal, and the client should be turned while sleeping unless the client is on a special immobility bed.

**TEST-TAKING HINT: The adjective "long-term" should make the test taker eliminate option "4" because the words "two (2) hours" are in the goal. The word "perform" is an intervention, which is not a goal; therefore option "3" could be eliminated as the correct answer.**

19. 1. The ascending paralysis has reached his respiratory muscles; therefore the client will not be able to use his hands to write.

2. The client will not be able to use the arms as a result of the paralysis but can blink the eyes as long as the nurse asks simple yes or no questions.

3. A speech therapist will not be able to help the client communicate while the client is on the ventilator.

4. The ascending paralysis has reached the respiratory muscles; therefore the client will not be able to use the hands to push the call light.

**TEST-TAKING HINT: The test taker must realize that all the options except "3" are ways to communicate with a client on the ventilator. The test taker must think about what would make one more appropriate with the client with Guillain-Barré syndrome than the other two options. Options "1" and "4" both involve use of the hands, which might lead the test taker to eliminate these two options.**

20. 1. Clients with this syndrome usually have a full recovery, but it may take up to one (1) year.
    2. Only about 10% of clients are left with permanent residual disability.
    3. This is passing the buck. The nurse should answer the client's question honestly, which helps establish a trusting nurse–client relationship.
    4. This supports that the nurse does not understand the typical course for a client diagnosed with Guillain-Barré syndrome.

    **TEST-TAKING HINT:** The test taker could eliminate option "3" because this is passing the buck and is usually not the best action of a nurse. The nurse would need to be knowledgeable of the typical course of this syndrome to be able to answer this question.

21. 1. Very little cerebrospinal fluid is removed from the client. Therefore hypotension is not a potential complication of this procedure.
    2. A bandage is placed over the puncture site, and pressure does not need to be applied to the site.
    3. The laboratory staff, not the nurse, complete tests on the cerebrospinal fluid; the nurse could label the specimens and take them to the laboratory.
    4. Increased fluid intake will help prevent a post-procedure headache, which may occur after a lumbar puncture.

    **TEST-TAKING HINT:** The test taker could eliminate option "3" because nurses usually do not perform tests on bodily fluids at the bedside. A basic concept in many procedures is that if fluid is removed, it usually must be replaced, which might cause the test taker to select option "4."

22. 1. The rate of ventilation is usually 12 to 15 breaths per minute in adults who are on ventilators, so this would not require immediate intervention.
    2. A manual resuscitation bag (ambu) must be at the client's bedside in case the ventilator malfunctions; the nurse must bag the client.
    3. A pulse oximeter reading of less than 93% warrants immediate intervention; a 90% peripheral oxygen saturation indicates a $PaO_2$ of about 60 (normal 80–100). When the client is placed on the ventilator, this should cause the client's oxygen level to improve.
    4. These ABGs are within normal limits and do not warrant immediate intervention.

    **TEST-TAKING HINT:** The test taker must know specific norms for frequently performed tests for the client. Even if the test taker was not knowledgeable of the ventilator-based decisions based on norms, the test taker could ask, "Is a client with respiratory rate of 14 in respiratory failure or compromise?" Equipment at the bedside would probably not warrant immediate intervention.

23. 1. This action does not address the wife's fears, and telling her to stop crying will not help the situation.
    2. Making the wife leave the room will further upset the client and the client's wife.
    3. Medicating the client will not help the wife, but if the nurse can calm the wife, then it is hoped the client will calm down.
    4. It is scary to see your loved one with a tube down his mouth and all the machines around them. The nurse should help the wife by acknowledging her fears.

    **TEST-TAKING HINT:** The test taker should select the option that addresses the wife's needs first. By addressing the wife's needs the client will calm down. The test taker should not automatically select the option that medicates the client.

24. 1. The physical therapist is an important part of the rehabilitation team who addresses the client's muscle deterioration resulting from the disease process and immobility.
    2. There is no residual speech deficit from Guillain-Barré syndrome; therefore, this referral would not be appropriate.
    3. The social worker could help with financial concerns, job issues, and issues concerning the long rehabilitation time for this syndrome.
    4. Pain may or may not be an issue with this syndrome. Each client is different, but a plan needs to be established to address pain if it occurs.
    5. This is an excellent resource for the client and the family.

    **TEST-TAKING HINT:** The physical therapist and social worker are two members of the rehabilitation team who are always appropriate in long-term rehabilitation. Physical therapy addresses complications of immobility; social workers help the client get back home. Any resource referral is an appropriate intervention.

## Myasthenia Gravis

25. 1. These are musculoskeletal manifestations of myasthenia gravis.

2. These are ocular signs/symptoms of MG. Ptosis is drooping of the eyelid, and diplopia is unilateral or bilateral blurred vision.
3. These are respiratory manifestations of myasthenia gravis.
4. These are nutritional manifestations of myasthenia gravis.

**TEST-TAKING HINT: The keys to answering this question are the adjectives "ocular" or "facial." This information should make the test taker rule out options "1," "3," and "4" even if they don't know what ptosis or diplopia means.**

26. 1. No change in the client's muscles strength indicates that it is not MG.
2. There is reduced amplitude in an electromyelogram (EMG) in a client with MG.
3. The serum assay of circulating acetylcholine receptor antibodies is increased, not decreased, in MG, and this test is only 80% to 90% accurate in diagnosing MG.
4. Clients with MG show a significant improvement of muscle strength that lasts approximately five (5) minutes when Tensilon (edrophonium chloride) is injected.

**TEST-TAKING HINT: There are some questions that are knowledge-based questions. The test taker would need to know the test or that myasthenia gravis affects muscle strength to select option "4."**

27. 1. There is a surgical option available.
2. This surgery is performed in clients with pituitary tumors and is accomplished by going through the client's upper lip though the nasal passage.
3. In about 75% of clients with MG, the thymus gland (which is usually inactive after puberty) continues to produce antibodies that trigger an autoimmune response in MG. After a thymectomy, the production of autoantibodies is reduced or eliminated, and this may resolve the signs/symptoms of MG.
4. An adrenalectomy is the surgery for a client diagnosed with Cushing's disease, a disease in which there is an increased secretion of glucocorticoids and mineralocorticoids.

**TEST-TAKING HINT: This is a knowledge-based question, but the test taker may be able to eliminate options "2" and "4" if the test taker has a basic understanding of anatomy and physiology and knows that surgery involving the pituitary or adrenal glands would not help prevent signs and symptoms of a muscular disorder.**

28. 1. The client is at risk for choking; knowing specific measures to help the client helps decrease the client's, as well as the significant other's, anxiety and promotes confidence in managing potential complications.
2. Clients diagnosed with MG may end up on a ventilator at the end stage of the disease, but the client would not be cared for at home; this would be a very unusual situation.
3. The client should be encouraged to perform active range-of-motion exercises, but the most important intervention is treating choking episodes.
4. The client with MG doesn't necessarily have a feeding tube, and this information is not in the stem.

**TEST-TAKING HINT: The test taker should only consider the information in the stem of the question, which would cause the test taker to eliminate option "4." If the test taker could not decide between options "1" and "3" the test taker should apply Maslow's Hierarchy of Needs; airway is priority.**

29. 1. The occupational therapist assists the client with ADLs, but with MG the client has no problems with performing them if the client takes the medication correctly (30 minutes prior to performing ADLs).
2. A recreational therapist is usually in a psychiatric unit or rehabilitation unit.
3. A vocational therapist or counselor helps with the client finding a job that will accommodate the disease process; clients with MG are usually not able to work in the late stages.
4. Speech therapists address swallowing problems, and clients with MG are dysphagic and at risk for aspiration. The speech therapist can help match food consistency to the client's ability to swallow, which enhances client safety.

**TEST-TAKING HINT: The test taker must be aware of the responsibilities of the other health-care team members. Collaborative means working with another health-care team discipline.**

30. 1. Hypovolemia is a complication of plasmapheresis, especially during the procedure, when up to 15% of the blood volume is in the cell separator.
2. Positive signs would warrant intervention and indicate hypocalcemia, which is a complication of plasmapheresis.
3. This is a normal serum potassium level (3.5–5.5 mEq/L), which would not warrant

intervention, but the level should be monitored because plasmapheresis could cause hypokalemia.

4. Ecchymosis, bruising, would not warrant immediate intervention. Signs of infiltration or infection would warrant immediate intervention.

**TEST-TAKING HINT: If the test taker has no idea of the answer, then selecting signs of hypovolemia—hypotension and tachycardia—is an appropriate selection if the question asks which would warrant immediate intervention.**

31. 1. MG has no effect on the ovarian function and the uterus is an involuntary muscle, not a skeletal muscle, so the menstrual cycle is not affected.
    2. Infections can result in an exacerbation and extreme weakness.
    3. An extremely hot or cold environment may cause an exacerbation of MG.
    4. This will help the client mobilize and expectorate sputum.

**TEST-TAKING HINT: This question is an "except" question and is asking the test taker to select the option that is not appropriate for the client's disease process. Three (3) answers will be appropriate; sometimes if the test taker rethinks the question and asks, "Which statements indicate the client understands the teaching?" that will help identify the correct answer.**

32. 1. This is a diagnostic test that is done to diagnose MG.
    2. These assessment data would indicate the client is experiencing a myasthenic crisis, which is the result of undermedication, missed doses of medication, or the development of an infection.
    3. The vital signs do not indicate if the client is experiencing a cholinergic crisis.
    4. The injection of edrophonium chloride (Tensilon test) not only diagnoses MG but also helps to determine which type of crisis the client is experiencing. In a myasthenic crisis, the test is positive (the client's muscle strength improves), but in cholinergic crisis, the test is negative (there is no improvement in muscle strength), or the client will actually get worse and emergency equipment must be available.

**TEST-TAKING HINT: This question requires the test taker to be knowledgeable of the disease process, but this is an important concept that the test taker must understand about myasthenia gravis.**

33. 1. Position changes promote lung expansion, and coughing helps clear secretions from the tracheobronchial tree.
    2. This position expands the lungs and alleviates pressure from the diaphragm.
    3. The respiratory system and pulse oximeter reading should be assessed more frequently than every shift; it should be done every four (4) hours or more often.
    4. The medications should be administered 30 minutes before the meal to provide optimal muscle strength for swallowing and chewing.
    5. There is no serum level available for medications used to treat MG; the client's signs/symptoms are used to determine the effectiveness of this medication.

**TEST-TAKING HINT: An alternative-type question requests the test taker to select more than one option as the correct answer. The test taker must evaluate each option individually to determine if it is correct. The priority concerns for a client with MG are respiratory and eating.**

34. 1. This would be an appropriate action by the nurse, but it is not the best action.
    2. Support groups are helpful to the client's significant others, but in this situation, it is not the best action for the nurse.
    3. A counselor is an appropriate intervention, but it is not the best action.
    4. Directly addressing the significant other's feelings is the best action for the nurse in this situation. All the other options can be done, but the best action is to address the significant other's feelings.

**TEST-TAKING HINT: The test taker should select the option that directly addresses and helps the client or significant other. Remember if the word "best," "most important," or "first" is in the stem, then all four (4) options could be possible interventions, but only one is the highest priority.**

35. 1. This medication promotes muscle contraction, which improves muscle strength, which, in turn, would allow the client to perform ADLs without assistance.
    2. This medication does not affect secretions of the eye.
    3. This medication does not help with the digestion of food.
    4. This medication does not help with pain; clients with MG do not have muscle pain.

**TEST-TAKING HINT: The test taker must know about the disease process to be able to answer**

Immune

this question. Remember when answering pharmacology questions that the effectiveness of the medication is based on what sign/symptom the client is experiencing.

36. 1. This medication will increase muscle strength to help enhance swallowing and chewing during meals.
2. There is no need for the client to take this medication with eight (8) ounces of water.
3. The client does not have to sit up after taking this medication.
4. These assessment data would not cause the nurse to question administering this medication.

**TEST-TAKING HINT: There are very few medications that must be given specifically on time and this medication is one of them. The blood pressure is checked prior to administering antihypertensive medications.**

## Systemic Lupus Erythematosus

37. 1. SLE can affect any organ system, and these tests would be used to determine the possibility of the liver being involved but they are not used to diagnose SLE.
2. No single laboratory test diagnoses SLE, but the client usually presents with moderate to severe anemia, thrombocytopenia, leukopenia, and a positive antinuclear antibody.
3. Female clients with SLE develop atherosclerosis at an earlier age, but cholesterol and lipid profile tests are not used to diagnose the disease.
4. These tests may be done to determine SLE infiltration in the kidneys but not to diagnose the disease itself.

**TEST-TAKING HINT: A complete metabolic panel is ordered for many different diseases; cholesterol and lipid panels are usually ordered for atherosclerosis, and BUN and glomerular filtration tests are specific to the kidneys. These options could be ruled out because they are specific to other diseases or not specific enough.**

38. 1. Sunlight or UV light exposure has been shown to initiate an exacerbation of SLE, so the client should be taught to protect the skin when in the sun.
2. A fever may be the first indication of an exacerbation of SLE.
3. Dyspnea is not expected and could signal respiratory involvement.

4. Raynaud's phenomenon is a condition in which the digits of the hands and feet turn red, blue, or white in response to heat or cold and stress. It occurs with some immune inflammatory processes.
5. SLE is a chronic disease and there is no known cure.

**TEST-TAKING HINT: Dyspnea is an uncomfortable sensation of not being able to breathe. Usually clients are not told that this is normal regardless of the disease process.**

39. 1. SLE is frequently diagnosed in young women and reproduction is a concern for these clients, but it is not the most important goal.
2. The client's body image is important, but this is not the most important.
3. SLE can invade and destroy any body system or organ. Maintaining organ function is the primary goal of SLE treatment.
4. Measures are taken to prevent breakdown, but skin breakdown is not life threatening.

**TEST-TAKING HINT: When the question asks for "the most important" the test taker should determine if one of the options has information that could be life threatening or could result in a serious complication for the client.**

40. 1. SLE can affect any organ. It can cause pericarditis and myocardial ischemia as well as pneumonia or pleural effusions.
2. Muscle spasticity occurs in MS, and bradykinesia occurs in Parkinson's disease.
3. Hirsutism is an overgrowth of hair. Spotty areas of alopecia occur in SLE, and clubbing of the fingers occurs in chronic pulmonary or cardiac diseases.
4. Weight loss and fatigue are experienced by clients diagnosed with SLE.

**TEST-TAKING HINT: The nurse must know the signs and symptoms of disease processes.**

41. 1. Steroid medications mask the development of infections because steroids suppress the immune system's response.
2. SLE is not a cancer that metastasizes, or "spreads"; it does invade other organ systems, but steroids do not prevent this from happening.
3. The main function of steroid medications is to suppress the inflammatory response of the body.
4. Steroid medications can delay the healing process, theoretically making scarring worse.

**TEST-TAKING HINT: Steroids are a frequently administered medication drug class. The nurse must know the common actions, side**

effects, adverse effects, and how to administer the medications safely.

42. 1. Unless the nurse has SLE and has been through the exact same type of tissue involvement, then the nurse should not tell a client "I know." This does not address the client's feelings.
    2. The nurse should never ask the client "why." The client does not owe the nurse an explanation of his or her feelings.
    3. The nurse may need to perform an assessment, but this is not a therapeutic response.
    4. The nurse has stated a fact, "You are crying," and then offers self by saying "Would you like to talk?" This addresses the nonverbal cue, crying, and is a therapeutic response.

**TEST-TAKING HINT:** The question asks for a therapeutic response, which means a feeling must be addressed. Therapeutic responses do not ask "why," so the test taker could rule out option "2."

43. 1. Moisturizing lotions, not astringents, are applied. Astringent lotions have an alcohol base, which would be drying to the client's skin.
    2. The skin should be inspected daily for any breakdown or rashes.
    3. The skin should be washed with mild soap, rinsed, and patted dry. Rubbing can cause abrasions and skin breakdown.
    4. The stem does not tell the test taker that the client is itching, and SLE does not have itching as a symptom. Lotions are not usually applied between the toes because this would foster the development of a fungal infection between the toes.

**TEST-TAKING HINT:** If the test taker did not know what astringent meant, then the test taker should skip this option and continue looking for a correct answer. In option "2" the time frame of weekly makes this option wrong.

44. 1. Chest pain should be considered a priority regardless of the admitting diagnosis. Clients diagnosed with SLE can develop cardiac complications.
    2. Pain at a "10" is a priority but not above chest pain.
    3. Dysphagia is expected in clients diagnosed with MG.
    4. Clients diagnosed with GB have ascending muscle weakness or paralysis, which could eventually result in the client being placed on a ventilator, but the problem currently is in the distal extremities (the feet) and is not priority over chest pain.

**TEST-TAKING HINT:** When the test taker is deciding on which client has priority, a potentially life-threatening condition is always top priority.

45. 1. The assistant should wash the hands before and after client care.
    2. The assistant can remove an indwelling catheter with nonsterile gloves. This is a waste of expensive equipment. The nurse is responsible for teaching unlicensed personnel appropriate use of equipment and supplies and cost containment.
    3. Raising the head of the bed to a 90-degree angle (high Fowler's position) during meals helps to prevent aspiration.
    4. Using a clean plastic bag to access the ice machine indicates the assistant is aware of infection control procedures.

**TEST-TAKING HINTS:** This is really an "except" question—there will be three (3) answers with desired actions and only one (1) that needs to change.

46. 1. The kidneys filter wastes, not antibodies, from the blood.
    2. The problem is an overactive immune system, not a problem with the endocrine system. There is no research that supports a virus as an initiating factor.
    3. SLE is an autoimmune disease that is characterized by exacerbations and remission. There is empiric evidence that hormones are indicated in the development of the disease and some drugs can initiate the process.
    4. There is familial and hormonal evidence for the development SLE. SLE is an autoimmune disease process in which there is an exaggerated production of autoantibodies.

**TEST-TAKING HINT:** The test taker could eliminate options "1" and "2" " by referring to basic anatomy and physiology and the function of the kidneys and endocrine system.

47. 1. Steroids are not addicting.
    2. The adrenal gland, not the thyroid gland, produces the glucocorticoid cortisol.
    3. Tapering steroids is important because the adrenal gland stops producing cortisol, a glucocorticosteroid, when the exogenous administration of steroids exceeds what would normally be produced. The functions of cortisol in the body are to regulate glucose metabolism and maintain blood pressure.

Immune

4. Tapering the dose is standard medical practice, not a whim of the HCP.

**TEST-TAKING HINT: Basic knowledge of anatomy and physiology eliminates option "2." Tapering steroid medication is basic knowledge for the nurse administering a steroid.**

48. 1. Nodules and bony deformity are symptoms of RA but not of SLE.
    2. Organ involvement occurs in SLE but not RA.
    3. **Joint stiffness and pain are symptoms that occur in both diseases.**
    4. Raynaud's phenomenon and skin rashes are associated with SLE.

**TEST-TAKING HINT: There are a number of illnesses that have the same symptoms. The nurse must be aware of the symptoms that distinguish one illness from another.**

## Acquired Immunodeficiency Syndrome

49. 1. Birth control pills provide protection against unwanted pregnancy but they do not protect females from getting sexually transmitted diseases. In fact, because of the reduced chance of becoming pregnant, some women may find it easier to become involved with multiple partners, increasing the chance of contracting a sexually transmitted disease.
    2. There is no vaccine or cure for the HIV virus.
    3. Adolescents are among the fastest-growing population to be newly diagnosed with HIV and AIDS.
    4. **Abstinence is the only guarantee that the client will not contract a sexually transmitted disease, including AIDS. An individual who is HIV negative in a monogamous relationship with another individual who is HIV negative and committed to a monogamous relationship is the safest sexual relationship.**

**TEST-TAKING HINT: Answer option "1" is a form of an absolute, which could cause the test taker to eliminate this option. Option "4" is also an absolute—"only"—but it is a true statement. There are some absolutes in the health-care profession.**

50. 1. **The client has a malnutrition syndrome. The nurse would assess the body and what the client has been able to eat.**
    2. **Standard precautions are used for clients diagnosed with AIDS, the same as for every other client.**
    3. **The nurse should check the orders but not before assessing the client.**

4. The client will probably be placed on total parenteral nutrition and will need to be taught these things, but this is not the first action.

**TEST-TAKING HINT: Assessment is the first step in the nursing process. The nursing process is a good place to start when setting priorities for the nurse's actions.**

51. 1. This client probably has oral candidiasis, a fungal infection of the mouth and esophagus. Brushing the teeth and patchy areas will not remove the lesions and will cause considerable pain.
    2. **This most likely is a fungal infection known as oral candidiasis, commonly called thrush. An antifungal medication is needed to treat this condition.**
    3. Antiseptic-based mouthwashes usually contain alcohol, which would be painful for the client.
    4. The foods the client has eaten did not cause this condition.

**TEST-TAKING HINT: The client is complaining of a "sore mouth." The test taker must notice all the important information in the stem before attempting to choose an answer. How are brushing the area, an antiseptic mouthwash, or the foods that have been eaten going to alleviate the pain?**

52. 1. Contact precautions are a form of transmission-based precautions used when the infectious organism is known to be spread by contact with a substance.
    2. Airborne precautions are used for bacteria that are very small molecules that can be carried at some distance from the client on air currents. The bacterium that causes tuberculosis is an example of such bacteria. A special isolation mask is required to enter the client's negative air pressure room.
    3. Droplet precautions are used for organisms like those that cause the flu or some pneumonias. The organisms have a larger molecule and "drop" within three (3) to four (4) feet. A normal isolation mask is used with this client.
    4. **Standard precautions are used for all contact with blood and body secretions, except sweat.**

**TEST-TAKING HINT: Isolation procedures are basic nursing knowledge and the nurse must know, understand, and comply with all of the procedures.**

53. 1. Retroviruses never die; the virus may become dormant, only to be reactivated at a later time.
    2. Eradicated means to be completely cured or done away with. HIV cannot be eradicated.

3. The HIV virus originated in the green monkey, in whom it is not deadly. HIV in humans replicates readily using the CD4 cells as reservoirs.

4. The HIV virus uses the CD4 cell of the immune system as reservoirs to replicate itself.

**TEST-TAKING HINT:** If the test taker is not aware of the definition of a word, the individual monitoring the test may be able to define the word, but this is not possible on the RN-NCLEX examination. Of the answer options, option "1" has the most important information regarding prognosis and potential spread to noninfected individuals.

54. 1. The client may be in the primary infection stage when the body has not had time to develop antibodies to the HIV virus.

2. Repeated exposure to HIV increases the risk of infection, but it only takes one exposure to develop an infection.

3. The primary phase of infection ranges from being asymptomatic to severe flulike symptoms, but during this time, the test may be negative although the individual is infected with HIV.

4. The client may or may not have a different virus, but this is not the reason the test is negative.

**TEST-TAKING HINT:** Answer options "1" and "4" assume the client is negative for the HIV virus. Therefore these options should be eliminated as correct answers unless the test taker is completely sure that the statement is correct.

55. 1. The nurse should attempt to flush the skin and get the area to bleed. It is hoped that this will remove contaminated blood from the body prior to infecting the nurse.

2. The nurse should notify the charge nurse after flushing the area and trying to get it to bleed.

3. This should be done within four (4) hours of the exposure, not before trying to rid the body of the potential infection.

4. This is done at three (3) months and six (6) months after initial exposure.

**TEST-TAKING HINT:** In questions that ask the test taker to select the first action, all the options could be appropriate interventions, but the nurse must decide which has the most immediate need and the most benefit. Directly caring for the wound is of the most benefit.

56. 1. Altered nutrition may be a priority for a client with malnutrition, but HIV encephalopathy is a cognitive deficit.

2. The client might grieve if the client still has enough cognitive ability to understand the loss that is occurring, but this is not the most important consideration.

3. A client diagnosed with encephalopathy may not have the ability to understand instructions. The nurse would teach the significant other.

4. Safety is always an issue with a client with diminished mental capacity.

**TEST-TAKING HINTS:** The nurse must have a basis for deciding priority. Maslow's Hierarchy of Needs lists safety as a high priority.

57. 1. Serum blood work, although ordered STAT, does not have priority over oxygenation of the client.

2. Oxygen is a priority, especially with a client diagnosed with a respiratory illness.

3. It is extremely important to initiate IV antibiotic therapy to a client diagnosed with an infection as quickly as possible, but this does not have priority over oxygen.

4. Culture specimens should be obtained prior to initiating antibiotic therapy, but oxygen administration is still the first action.

**TEST-TAKING HINT:** Airway, breathing, and providing oxygen to the tissues is the top priority in any nursing situation. If the cells are not oxygenated, they die.

58. 1. Performing the head-to-toe assessment is a nursing consideration, not a client consideration. This is a physiological intervention, not a psychosocial one.

2. Maintaining body weight is physical.

3. Clients diagnosed with AIDS should be encouraged to discuss their end-of-life issue with the significant others and to put those wishes in writing. This is important for all clients, not just those diagnosed with AIDS.

4. Activity tolerance is a physical problem

**TEST-TAKING HINT:** All of the options except one (1) focus on the physical care of the client. The stem asked the test taker to consider a psychosocial need.

59. 1. Flushed warm skin with tented turgor indicates dehydration. The HCP should be notified immediately for fluid orders or other orders to correct the reason for the dehydration.

2. This is a concern but it can be taken care of after the client with the physical problem.

3. The temperature is slightly elevated and the pulse is one (1) beat higher than normal. This client could wait to be seen.

Immune

4. Many clients who have had sputum specimens ordered are unable to produce sputum, but it does not warrant immediate intervention.

**TEST-TAKING HINT: This is an "except" question that asks the test taker to identify abnormal data that indicate a life-threatening situation or a complication.**

60. 1. This does not provide continuity of care for the client. It does recognize the nurse's position, but it is not the best care for the client.
    2. The HCP should be asked to attend the care plan meeting to assist in deciding how to work with the client, but asking the HCP to "tell" the client to behave is not the best way to handle the situation. The client can always refuse to behave as requested.
    3. **The health-care team should meet to discuss ways to best help the client deal with the anger that is being expressed, and the staff should be consistent in working with the client.**
    4. Forcing a staff member to care for the client for a week could result in a buildup of animosity and make the situation worse.

**TEST-TAKING HINT: The test taker is being asked for the most appropriate method. Option "4" can be discarded because of the word "force." Option "3" gives the option for multiple individuals to work together toward an outcome.**

## Allergies and Allergic Reactions

61. 1. This is appropriate any time the nurse is administering a diuretic medication.
    2. A nurse uses nonsterile gloves to remove old dressings, then washes the hands and sets up the sterile field before donning sterile gloves to reapply the dressing.
    3. Checking for allergies is one (1) of the five (5) rights of medication. Is it the right drug? Even if the drug is the one that the HCP ordered, it is not the right drug if the client is allergic to it. The nurse should always assess a client's allergies prior to administering any medication.
    4. The nurse should ask for assistance in moving a client in bed to prevent on-the-job injuries.

**TEST-TAKING HINT: The stem asks the test taker to determine which is an incorrect action. This is an "except" question. Three (3) answers are actions the nurse should take. Explaining medications, using nonsterile gloves for removing a dressing, and asking for help in moving**

a client are all actions in which the test taker should not find fault.

62. 1. The nurse should use nonlatex gloves because of the latex allergy, but the gloves do not have to be sterile.
    2. The nurse must use gloves during procedures and starting an IV. Not using gloves is a violation of Office of Safety and Health Administration standards and places the nurse at risk for developing illnesses.
    3. **The nurse should be prepared to care for a client at all times and should not place himself or herself at risk because the facility does not keep nonlatex gloves available in the rooms. The nurse should carry the needed equipment (nonlatex gloves) with him or her.**
    4. White cotton gloves are made of cloth and would not provide the barrier against wet substances.

**TEST-TAKING HINT: The test taker must be aware of adjectives such as "sterile" in option "1." Basic concepts such as standard precautions should cause the test taker to eliminate option "2." Option "4" has the word "all" in it and could be eliminated as an answer because this is an absolute.**

63. 1. **Clients who are allergic to bee sting venom should be taught to keep an EpiPen with them at all times and how to use the device. This could save their life.**
    2. It is unrealistic to think that the client will never go outdoors, but the client should be taught to avoid exposure to bees whenever possible.
    3. Over-the-counter diphenhydramine, Benadryl, is a histamine 1 blocker, but it is oral and would not be useful in this situation.
    4. The client should wear a Medic Alert bracelet.

**TEST-TAKING HINT: Answer option "2" is an absolute and should be eliminated as a possible correct answer. Option "4" has the nurse telling the client not to wear a Medic Alert bracelet. The test taker must be aware of the descriptive adjectives in the stem and options.**

64. 1. This intervention should be implemented, but it is not the first action.
    2. This does address oxygenation and will take time to accomplish, so this intervention is not the first action.
    3. **The client is cyanotic with dyspnea and wheezing. The nurse should administer oxygen first.**
    4. The client may be allergic to iodine that is a

component of many shellfish, but the first need of the client is oxygenation.

**TEST-TAKING HINT: The test taker must apply some decision-making standard to determining what to do first. Maslow's Hierarchy of Needs ranks oxygen as first. Of the two (2) options that address oxygen, option "3" immediately attempts to provide oxygen to the client.**

65. 1. The symptoms are occurring at this time, so asking what time of the year the symptoms occur is not an appropriate question.
    2. There are many over-the-counter remedies available. Therefore the nurse should assess which medications the client has tried and what medications the client is currently taking.
    3. It was not in the stem that the client is allergic to animals. Many clients diagnosed with allergic rhinitis are allergic to seasonal environmental allergens such as pollen and mold.
    4. The client probably does not have any explanation for developing allergies.

**TEST-TAKING HINT: The test taker should not read into a question. Because animals were not mentioned in the stem, option "3" can be eliminated. Many over-the-counter medications and herbal remedies are available to clients and it is important for the nurse to determine what the client has been taking.**

66. 1. Tree pollen is abundant in early spring.
    2. Rose and grass pollen are prevalent in early summer.
    3. Ragweed and other pollen are prevalent in early fall.
    4. Early winter is the beginning of deciduous plants becoming dormant. Therefore, allergic rhinitis would be least prevalent during this time of year.

**TEST-TAKING HINT: The test taker could eliminate the three (3) options based on the growing plant season if the test taker realized that allergic rhinitis can be caused by environmental plant pollens and molds.**

67. 1. Immunotherapy does not cure the problem. However, if immunotherapy is done following a reaction, it provides passive immunity to the insect venom (similar to the way that RhoGAM prevents a mother who is Rh negative from building antibodies to the blood of a baby who is Rh positive). This is the purpose for immunotherapy in clients who are allergic.
    2. This is an untrue statement.

3. There is no cure for allergies to insect venom.
4. This therapy is standard procedure for clients who have severe allergies to insect venom.

**TEST-TAKING HINT: Answer options "2" and "3" contain forms of absolute adjectives such as "all" and "cure." Rarely is anything absolute in health care. The test taker should be absolutely sure of the correct answer before choosing any answer containing an absolute descriptive word or passage. The stem asks for the rationale and option "4" is giving advice, so it can be eliminated.**

68. 1. This is an unrealistic expectation for a client diagnosed with poison ivy. The pruritus is intense.
    2. The client should be instructed on how to use the EpiPen, not IM Benadryl.
    3. Clients with poison ivy are frequently prescribed a steroid dose pack. The dose pack has the steroid provided in descending doses to help prevent adrenal insufficiency.
    4. This may cause the client to be warm, which increases the likelihood of itching.

**TEST-TAKING HINT: Option "1" has the word "never," which is an absolute word and can be eliminated on this basis. Very few conditions require the nurse to teach the client to take intramuscular (IM) injections; therefore option "2" could be eliminated as a possible answer.**

69. 1. This can be an independent or collaborative nursing problem. It is an airway problem and has priority.
    2. Knowledge deficit is not a priority over the client with breathing problems.
    3. Anaphylaxis is a collaborative problem. The nurse will need to start IVs, administer medications, and possibly place the client on a ventilator if the client is to survive.
    4. Ineffective coping is a psychosocial problem; it does not have priority over breathing.

**TEST-TAKING HINT: The test taker must apply some problem-solving/decision-making standard. In this case Maslow's Hierarchy of Needs is a good option. Airway has priority.**

70. 1. This client should be seen but not before assessing for a possible anaphylactic reaction.
    2. This client has received an initial dose of antibiotic IV and should be assessed for tolerance to the medication within 30 minutes.
    3. Pain is a priority but not over a potential life-threatening emergency.
    4. This client can be seen last. A delayed meal is not life threatening.

Immune

**TEST-TAKING HINT: The test taker should determine which client has the most pressing need and rank the options in that order. Life-threatening situations have priority.**

71. 1. By the Joint Commission for Accreditation of Healthcare Organizations (JCAHO) standards, clients must mark any surgical site to make sure that the operation is not done on the incorrect site, such as the right arm instead of the left arm.
    2. The client should understand the surgery on his or her own terms.
    3. Iodine is the basic ingredient in Betadine, povidone iodine, which is a common skin prep used for surgeries. Therefore the nurse should notify the surgeon if the client has an allergy to iodine.
    4. The client should have a signed consent for the surgery and the anesthesia prior to surgery.

    **TEST-TAKING HINT: The options involve basic concepts for surgical preparation, and allergies must be identified on the client as well as in the client's chart.**

72. 1. Steroid medications decrease inflammation and therefore are one of the treatments for anaphylaxis.
    2. A STAT chest x-ray is not indicated at this time.
    3. A medical emergency team should be called because this client will be in respiratory and cardiac arrest very shortly.
    4. Because of its ability to activate a combination of alpha and beta receptors, epinephrine is the treatment of choice for anaphylactic shock.
    5. The first step in initiating CPR is to assess for a pulse and respirations.

    **TEST-TAKING HINT: This is an alternative type-question. If the test taker did not read the sentence "Select all that apply," the fact that there are five (5) not four (4) options should alert the test taker to go back and read the stem more closely. Each option must be decided on for itself. The test taker cannot eliminate one option based on the fact that another option is correct.**

## Rheumatoid Arthritis

73. 1. This would be done, but it will not prevent any disease from occurring.
    2. This will follow the progression of the disease of RA, but it is not preventive.
    3. RA is a disease with many immunologic abnormalities. The clients have increased

susceptibility to infectious disease, such as the flu or pneumonia, and therefore vaccines, which are preventive, should be recommended.
    4. Assessing the client does not address preventive care.

    **TEST-TAKING HINT: The stem requires the test taker to determine what action is preventive care for the client with RA. Only option "3" addresses preventive care.**

74. 1. The nodules may appear over bony prominences and resolve simultaneously. They appear in clients with the rheumatoid factor and are associated with rapidly progressive and destructive disease.
    2. There is a proliferation of the synovial membrane in RA, which leads to the formation of pannus and the destruction of cartilage and bone, but synovial fluid does not crystallize to form the nodules.
    3. The nodules are not lymph nodes. Lymph nodes may enlarge in the presence of disease, but they do not proliferate (multiply).
    4. The nodes indicate a progression of the disease, not an improving prognosis.

    **TEST-TAKING HINT: The test taker can rule out option "3" with knowledge of anatomy or physiology. Lymph nodes do not multiply; they do form chains throughout the body.**

75. 1. Joint stiffness and joints that are warm to the touch are expected in clients diagnosed with RA.
    2. Clients diagnosed with RA have bilateral and symmetrical stiffness, edema, tenderness, and temperature changes in the joints. Other symptoms include sensory changes, lymph node enlargement, weight loss, fatigue, and pain. A one (1)-kg weight loss and fatigue are expected.
    3. The use of heat is encouraged to provide comfort for a client diagnosed with RA.
    4. The client has the signs and symptoms of depression. The nurse should attempt to intervene with therapeutic conversation and discuss these findings with the HCP.

    **TEST-TAKING HINT: The test taker should not automatically assume that only physiological data require immediate intervention. There will be times when a psychological need will have priority. Because options "1," "2," and "3" are all expected in a client with RA, the psychological need warrants intervention by the nurse.**

76. 1. The drug does not lose efficacy, and clients are removed from the drug when the body cannot tolerate the side effects.

2. The drug requires close monitoring to prevent organ damage.
3. MRI scans are not used to determine the progress of RA.
4. There is no "off" period for the drug.

**TEST-TAKING HINT: If the test taker is not aware of the medication being discussed, option "2," the correct answer, is information that could be said of most medications.**

77. 1. Physical therapists work with gait training and muscle strengthening. Generally the physical therapist works on the lower half of the body.
2. **The occupational therapist assists the client in the use of the upper half of the body, fine motor skills, and activities of daily living. This is needed for the client with abnormal fingers.**
3. A counselor can help the client discuss feeling about body image, loss of function, and role changes, but the best referral is to the occupational therapist.
4. The client may need a home health nurse eventually, but first the client should be assisted to remain as functional as possible.

**TEST-TAKING HINT: The test taker must be aware of the role of all the health-care team members. The counselor can be ruled out as a possible correct answer because swan neck fingers are a physical problem.**

78. 1. The client diagnosed with RA is generally fatigued, and strenuous exercise would increase the fatigue, place increased pressure on the joints, and increase pain.
2. The client should be on a balanced diet that is high in protein, vitamins, and iron for tissue building and repair and should not require a mechanically altered diet.
3. There is no specific reason for the client to be ordered a keep-open IV; the client can swallow needed medications.
4. **Sleep deprivation resulting from pain is common in clients diagnosed with RA. A mild sedative can increase the client's ability to sleep, promote rest, and increase the client's tolerance of pain.**

**TEST-TAKING HINT: The test taker should be aware of adjectives that would lead to an option being eliminated—for example, the word "strenuous" in option "1."**

79. 1. **Immunosuppressive medications are considered class C drugs and should not be taken while pregnant. These drugs are teratogenic and carcinogenic and the client is only 20 years old.**

2. Any individual older than age 18 years old is considered an adult and does not need to discuss treatment with her parents unless she chooses to do so.
3. The medications can be administered on an outpatient basis, but if an inpatient has intravenous therapy, then IV sites are changed every 72 hours and there is no guarantee that an IV will last for four (4) days.
4. These are not investigational drugs and are standard therapy approved by the American College of Rheumatology and the Food and Drug Administration.

**TEST-TAKING HINT: The age of the client and the fact that the client is female could give the test taker an idea of the correct answer. This is a client in the childbearing years.**

80. 1. Activity intolerance is an appropriate client problem, but it is not priority over pain.
2. The client with RA does not experience fluid and electrolyte disturbance.
3. **The client diagnosed with RA has chronic pain; therefore alteration in comfort is a priority problem.**
4. Clients diagnosed with RA usually experience anorexia and weight loss, unless they are taking long-term steroids.

**TEST-TAKING HINT: The question is asking the priority problem, and pain is priority according to Maslow's Hierarchy of Needs.**

81. 1. The client in pain should receive medication as soon as possible to keep the pain from becoming worse, but the client is not at risk for a serious complication.
2. A butterfly rash across the bridge of the nose occurs in approximately 50% of the clients diagnosed with SLE.
3. **Antineoplastic drugs can be caustic to tissues; therefore the client's IV site should be assessed. The client should be assessed for any untoward reactions to the medications first.**
4. Scleroderma is a disease that is characterized by waxylike skin covering the entire body. This is expected for this client.

**TEST-TAKING HINT: Pain is a priority, but the test taker must determine if there is another client who could experience complications if not seen immediately.**

82. 1. Antineoplastic medications can be administered only by a registered nurse who has been trained in the administration and disposal of these medications.
2. Assessment cannot be assigned to a licensed practical nurse.

Immune

3. The licensed practical nurse (LPN) can demonstrate how to use adaptive clothing.

4. This is teaching that requires knowledge of medications and interactions and should not be assigned to an LPN.

**TEST-TAKING HINT: The nurse cannot assign assessment, evaluation, or teaching or any medication that requires specialized knowledge or skills to administer safely.**

83. 1. This is prescribing and the nurse is not licensed to do this unless the nurse has become a nurse practitioner.

2. NSAIDs do not require a specific amount of water to be effective, unlike bulk laxatives.

3. The medication should be taken in the usual dose when the client realizes that a dose has been missed.

4. NSAID medications decrease prostaglandin production in the stomach, resulting in less mucus production, which creates a risk for the development of ulcers. The client should take the NSAID with food.

**TEST-TAKING HINT: Knowledge of medication administration is a priority for every nurse. It is especially important for the nurse to be familiar with commonly used medications like NSAIDs, which can be purchased over the counter and may be taken by the client in addition to prescription medications.**

84. 1. Pain medication is important and should be given before the client's pain becomes worse.

2. Unless the client is in a crisis, such as pulmonary edema, this medication can wait.

3. Steroids do not have precedent over pain medication and should be administered with food.

4. Clients diagnosed with OA are usually overweight and do not require appetite stimulants. The nurse should question this medication before administering the medication.

**TEST-TAKING HINT: When determining priorities the test taker must employ some criteria to use as a guideline. According to Maslow, pain is a priority.**

1. The client is prescribed a prick epicutaneous test to determine the cause of hypersensitivity reactions. Which result indicates the client is hypersensitive to the allergen?
   1. The client complains of shortness of breath.
   2. The skin is dry, intact, and without redness.
   3. The pricked blood tests positive for allergens.
   4. A pruritic wheal and erythema occurs.

2. Which area of the body would the nurse assess to identify symptoms to support the early diagnosis of Guillain-Barré syndrome?

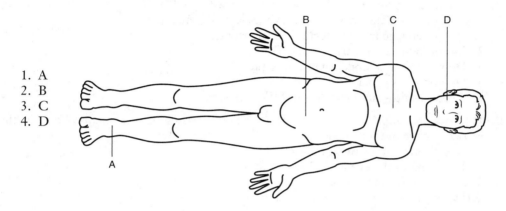

   1. A
   2. B
   3. C
   4. D

3. Which referral would be appropriate for a client with severe multiple allergies?
   1. Registered dietician.
   2. Occupational therapist.
   3. Recreational therapist.
   4. Social worker.

4. The client diagnosed with an anaphylactic reaction is admitted to the emergency room. Which assessment data indicate the client is not responding to the treatment?
   1. The client has a urinary output of 120 mL in two (2) hours.
   2. The client has an AP of 110 and a BP of 90/60.
   3. The client has clear breath sounds and an RR of 26.
   4. The client has hyperactive bowel sounds.

5. Which signs/symptoms would the nurse expect to assess in the client diagnosed with Sjögren's syndrome?
   1. Complaints of dry mouth and eyes.
   2. Complaints of peripheral joint pain.
   3. Complaints of muscle weakness.
   4. Complaints of severe itching.

6. Which intervention should the nurse implement for the client diagnosed with systemic sclerosis (scleroderma)?
   1. Instill artificial tears four (4) times a day.
   2. Apply moisturizers to the skin frequently.
   3. Instruct the client on how to apply braces.
   4. Encourage the client to decrease smoking.

7. Which diagnostic test would confirm the diagnosis of fibromyalgia?
   1. There is no diagnostic test to confirm fibromyalgia.
   2. A positive antinuclear antibody test.
   3. A magnetic resonance imaging (MRI) shows fibrosis.
   4. A negative erythrocyte sedimentation rate (ESR).

Immune

8. The primary nurse is administering medications to the assigned clients. Which client situation would require immediate intervention by the charge nurse?
   1. The client with congestive heart failure with an apical pulse of 64 who received 0.125 mg digoxin, a cardiac glycoside.
   2. The client with essential hypertension who received a beta blocker and has a blood pressure of 114/80.
   3. The client with myasthenia gravis who received the anticholinesterase medication 30 minutes late.
   4. The client with AIDS who received trimethoprim sulfamethoxazole, an antibiotic, and has a CD4 cell count of less than 200.

9. Which interventions should the nurse discuss with the female client who is positive for human immunodeficiency virus (HIV)? Select all that apply.
   1. Do not engage in unprotected sexual activity.
   2. Inform past sexual partners of HIV status.
   3. Do not donate blood, organs, or tissues.
   4. Do not get pregnant.
   5. Tell all health-care providers of HIV status.

10. Which sign/symptom would the nurse expect to assess in the client who is in the recovery stage of Guillain-Barré?
    1. Decreasing deep tendon reflexes.
    2. Drooping of the eyelids has resolved.
    3. A positive Babinski reflex.
    4. Descending increase in muscle strength.

11. The client is diagnosed with systemic lupus erythematosus (SLE). Which area of the body would the nurse expect to assess a butterfly rash?

    1. A
    2. B
    3. C
    4. D

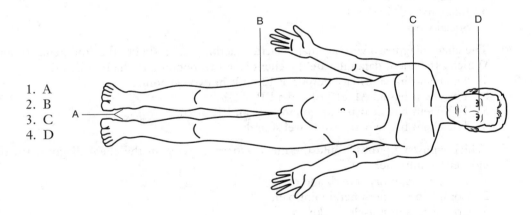

12. Which nursing intervention should the nurse include when teaching the client diagnosed with polymyositis?
    1. Explain the care of a percutaneous gastrostomy tube (PEG).
    2. Discuss the need to take corticosteroids every day.
    3. Instruct to wear long-sleeved shirts when exposed to sunlight.
    4. Teach the importance of strict hand washing.

13. The client recently diagnosed with rheumatoid arthritis is prescribed aspirin, a nonsteroidal anti-inflammatory medication. Which comment by the client would warrant immediate intervention by the nurse?
    1. "I always take the aspirin with food."
    2. "If I have dark stools, I will call my HCP."
    3. "Aspirin will not cure my arthritis."
    4. "I am having some ringing in my ears."

14. Which sign/symptom would make the nurse suspect the client has ankylosing spondylitis?
    1. Low back pain at night that is relieved by activity in the morning.
    2. Ascending paralysis of the lower extremities up to the spinal cord.
    3. A deep ache and stiffness in the hip joints radiating down the legs.
    4. Difficulty changing from lying to sitting position, especially at night.

15. The client diagnosed with multiple sclerosis is having trouble maintaining balance. Which intervention should the nurse discuss with the client?
    1. Discuss obtaining a motorized wheelchair for the client.
    2. Teach the client to stand with the feet slightly apart.
    3. Encourage the client to narrow his or her base of support.
    4. Explain the need to balance activity with rest.

16. The nurse is caring for the client diagnosed with acquired immune deficiency syndrome (AIDS) dementia. Which action by the unlicensed assistive personnel would require immediate intervention by the nurse?
    1. The assistant is helping the client to sit on the bedside chair.
    2. The assistant is wearing sterile gloves when bathing the client.
    3. The assistant is helping the client shave and brush the teeth.
    4. The assistant is providing a back massage to the client.

17. Which assessment data would make the nurse suspect that the client has chronic allergies?
    1. Jaundiced sclera and jaundiced palm of hands.
    2. Pale, boggy, edematous nasal mucosa.
    3. Lacy white plaques on the oral mucosa.
    4. Purple or blue patches on the face.

18. The client has had an anaphylactic reaction to insect venom, a bee sting. Which discharge instruction should the nurse discuss with the client?
    1. Take a corticosteroid dose pack when stung by a bee.
    2. Take antihistamines prior to outdoor activities.
    3. Use a cromolyn sodium (Intal) inhaler prophylactically.
    4. Carry a bee sting kit, especially when going outside.

19. The client with acquired immune deficiency syndrome (AIDS) dementia is referred to hospice. Which intervention has highest priority when caring for the client in the home?
    1. Assess the client's social support network.
    2. Identify the client's usual coping methods.
    3. Have consistent uninterrupted time with the client.
    4. Discuss and complete an advance directive.

20. The client with multiple sclerosis is prescribed the muscle relaxant baclofen (Lioresal). Which statement by the client indicates the client needs more teaching?
    1. "This medication may cause drowsiness so I need to be careful."
    2. "I should not drink any type of alcohol or take any antihistamines."
    3. "I will increase the fiber in my diet and increase fluid intake."
    4. "I stopped taking the medication because I can't afford it."

21. Which intervention has the highest priority when caring for a client diagnosed with rheumatoid arthritis?
    1. Encourage the client to ventilate feelings about the disease process.
    2. Discuss the effects of disease on the client's career and other life roles.
    3. Instruct the client to perform most important activities in the morning.
    4. Teach the client the proper use of hot and cold therapy to provide pain relief.

Immune

22. Which statement indicates that the female client with systemic lupus erythematosus (SLE) understands the discharge instructions?
    1. "I should wear sunscreen with at least a 5 SPF."
    2. "I am not going to any activities with large crowds."
    3. "I should not get pregnant because I have SLE."
    4. "I must avoid using hypoallergenic products."

23. Which is the highest priority nursing intervention for the client who is having an anaphylactic reaction?
    1. Administer parenteral epinephrine, an adrenergic agonist.
    2. Prepare for immediate endotracheal intubation.
    3. Provide a calm assurance when caring for the client.
    4. Establish and maintain a patent airway.

24. Which discharge instruction should the nurse implement for the client newly diagnosed with myasthenia gravis (MG)?
    1. Identify specific measures to help avoid fatigue and undue stress.
    2. Instruct the client to pad bony prominences, especially the sacral area.
    3. Discuss complementary therapies to help manage pain.
    4. Explain the possibility of having a splenectomy to help control the symptoms.

25. Which signs/symptoms would make the nurse suspect the most common opportunistic infection in the female client diagnosed with acquired immune deficiency syndrome (AIDS)?
    1. Fever, cough, and shortness of breath.
    2. Oral thrush, esophagitis, and vaginal candidiasis.
    3. Abdominal pain, diarrhea, and weight loss.
    4. Painless violet lesions on the face and tip of nose.

26. The client is experiencing an anaphylactic reaction to bee venom. Which interventions should the nurse implement? List in order of priority.
    1. Establish a patent airway.
    2. Administer epinephrine, an adrenergic agonist, IVP.
    3. Start an IV with 0.9% saline.
    4. Teach the client to carry an EpiPen when outside.
    5. Administer diphenhydramine (Benadryl), an antihistamine, IVP.

Immune

1.  1. This is a sign of an anaphylactic reaction to an allergen and will not happen during this test because of the small amount of allergen used.
    2. This would indicate a negative test and that the client is not sensitive to the allergen.
    3. The skin reaction, not the blood that is pricked, indicates a positive or negative test.
    4. During this test, a drop of diluted allergenic extract is placed on the skin and then punctured through the drop. A positive test causes a localized pruritic wheal and erythema, which occurs in five (5) to twenty (20) minutes.

2.  1. The presenting symptom of a client with Guillain-Barré syndrome is ascending paralysis that starts in the lower extremities.
    2. Abdominal symptoms would not be found early in the diagnosis.
    3. Chest symptoms would not be found early in the diagnosis.
    4. Head symptoms would not be found early in the diagnosis.

3.  1. A dietitian could help the client with any necessary dietary changes for food allergies and with ways to continue to meet nutritional needs.
    2. An occupational therapist addresses the client's ability to perform activities of daily living.
    3. A recreational therapist works in a psychiatric setting or rehabilitation setting and assists with the client's therapeutic recreational activities.
    4. A social worker addresses the client's financial needs.

4.  1. A urinary output of greater than 30 mL/hour is within normal limits and would indicate the client is responding to treatment.
    2. These vital signs indicate shock, which is a medical emergency and would require an immediate intervention.
    3. Clear breath sounds indicate response to treatment, and although the RR is increased, this could be the result of anxiety or fear.
    4. The client's bowel sounds would not be significant data to determine the client's response to treatment.

5.  1. Sjögren's syndrome is an autoimmune disorder that causes inflammation and dysfunction of exocrine glands throughout the body. Dry mouth and eyes are some of the signs/symptoms.
    2. Peripheral joint pain may be a symptom of rheumatoid arthritis.
    3. Muscle weakness is a symptom of a variety of disease processes and syndromes but not of Sjögren's syndrome.
    4. Severe itching is not a symptom of this syndrome.

6.  1. Artificial tears would be appropriate for a client diagnosed with Sjögren's syndrome.
    2. Nursing care addresses measures to maintain skin integrity and moisturizers help prevent dryness and cracking; once skin elasticity is lost, it cannot be regained.
    3. Braces are not prescribed for the client with scleroderma.
    4. The client should stop smoking, not just decrease smoking, because of the vasoconstrictive effect of nicotine and the respiratory effects of the disease.

7.  1. The diagnosis of fibromyalgia is based on the history and physical assessment. There is no laboratory or diagnostic test for fibromyalgia. However, tests may be performed to rule out other diagnoses.
    2. This test is not used to diagnose fibromyalgia.
    3. An MRI is not used to diagnose fibromyalgia.
    4. An ESR does not support the diagnosis of fibromyalgia.

8.  1. An apical heart rate of less than 60 would warrant intervention if the primary nurse gave the medication.
    2. A blood pressure of less than 90/60 would warrant intervention if the primary nurse gave the medication.
    3. These medications must be administered exactly on time so that increased strength can occur during activity such as eating or grooming. There are very few medications that must be administered exactly on time, but this is one of them.
    4. The client with AIDS receives prophylactic treatment for pneumocystis carinii pneumonia (PCP) when the CD4 count is less than 200–300.

9.  1. HIV is transmitted via sexual activity.
    2. HIV is transmitted via sexual activity, and the client may have been HIV positive for up to a year and not aware of it, so all past sexual partners should be informed of the HIV status.
    3. Blood donations are screened and excluded for this virus, as are organs/tissues from a client with HIV because the virus can be transmitted to clients receiving the organ or tissue.
    4. HIV can be transmitted to the fetus from the pregnant woman with HIV.

5. The client should tell the HCP, especially dentists, about the HIV status, but all health-care personnel should always follow Standard Precautions.

10. 1. This occurs in the acute stage of Guillain-Barré syndrome.
2. This would indicate that the client diagnosed with myasthenia gravis is getting better.
3. A positive Babinski reflex in an adult client is abnormal and indicates neurological deficits.
4. **The recovery stage may take from several months to two (2) years, and muscle strength and function return in a descending order.**

11. 1. The client diagnosed with SLE would not have a butterfly rash on the feet.
2. The client would not have a butterfly rash on the upper-thigh area.
3. The client would not have a butterfly rash on the chest area.
4. **The client with SLE often has a reddened area over both cheeks that is known as a butterfly rash; it is diagnostic of a client with SLE.**

12. 1. The client is at risk for aspiration as a result of muscle weakness, but modifications of dietary needs address this concern. The client does not require a PEG tube.
2. **Polymyositis is a systemic connective tissue disorder characterized by inflammation of connective tissues and muscle fibers and is treated with long-term corticosteroid therapy. Adrenal insufficiency may occur if the client quits taking the corticosteroid.**
3. Sunlight does not cause an exacerbation or irritation of polymyositis.
4. The client is not at risk for developing an infection, and an infection will not exacerbate the client's medical condition.

13. 1. Aspirin should be taken with food to prevent gastrointestinal upset.
2. Daily aspirin is used as an anticoagulant; therefore, abnormal bleeding should be reported to the HCP.
3. Aspirin is used to reduce the inflammatory process and manage the signs and symptoms, but it does not stop the disease process.
4. **Tinnitus, ringing in the ears, is a sign of aspirin toxicity and the client should be instructed to decrease the aspirin dosage or stop taking aspirin altogether. The client should be instructed to contact the health-care provider.**

14. 1. **Ankylosing spondylitis is a chronic inflammatory arthritis that primarily affects the spinal cord. The client complains of inter-**mittent bouts of low back pain with the pain worse at night, followed by morning stiffness that is relieved by activity.
2. This would make the nurse suspect Guillain-Barré syndrome.
3. A deep ache and stiffness may indicate osteoarthritis, which occurs in weight-bearing joints.
4. This is not a symptom of ankylosing spondylitis.

15. 1. Walkers or canes may be weighted to provide support and balance for the client; a wheelchair should be used as a last resort.
2. **Standing with the feet slightly apart widens the client's base of support and helps decrease balance problems.**
3. The client should widen his or her base of support by standing with the feet slightly apart. Narrowing the base of support would not help.
4. This intervention addresses fatigue, which does not cause balance problems.

16. 1. This action is appropriate and would not require any intervention by the nurse.
2. **The NA should wear nonsterile gloves, not sterile gloves. Wearing sterile gloves is not cost effective.**
3. The client has dementia, so helping the client with activities of daily living is appropriate to enable the client to maintain as much independence as possible.
4. This is an excellent intervention to help prevent skin breakdown; it is relaxing for the client and would not require intervention from the nurse.

17. 1. This may indicate a hemolytic reaction.
2. **Pale, boggy, edematous nasal mucosa indicates chronic allergies.**
3. This may indicate hemolysis or immune deficiency.
4. This may indicate Kaposi's sarcoma.

18. 1. Corticosteroids may be used in both systemic and topical forms for many types of hypersensitivity responses, but must be ordered by a health-care provider and are not automatically taken after a bee sting.
2. Antihistamines are the major class of drugs used to treat hypersensitivity responses, but they are not taken prophylactically. They are used when a reaction occurs.
3. This drug treats allergic rhinitis and asthma prophylactically. It does not help bee stings or insect bites.
4. **The kit usually includes a pre-filled syringe of epinephrine and an epinephrine nebulizer, which allows prompt self-treatment for any future exposures to insect venom or other potential allergen exposure.**

19. 1. This will help identify people who can help support the client, but it is not the highest priority.
    2. This will help the nurse identify methods that worked previously in stressful situations and may help the client deal with this disease.
    3. Developing a therapeutic relationship with the client is priority because the client probably has less than six (6) months to live. All the other interventions can be implemented, but establishing a therapeutic relationship will allow the nurse to discuss and implement additional interventions.
    4. An advance directive is important, but establishing a therapeutic relationship with the client is priority.

20. 1. Muscle relaxants have sedative effects, so appropriate safety measures should be taken.
    2. The client should avoid central nervous depressants because they can increase the sedative effects of the medication.
    3. This will help prevent constipation, which is a side effect of this medication.
    4. This medication must be tapered over one (1) to two (2) weeks when discontinuing because sudden withdrawal may cause seizures and paranoid ideation.

21. 1. Rheumatoid arthritis is a chronic illness and verbalization of feelings is helpful in dealing with disease processes, but it is not the highest priority intervention.
    2. This helps the client accept the disease process and body changes and helps the client to begin to identify strategies for coping with them, but it is not the highest priority intervention.
    3. Helping the client prioritize activities helps the client maintain independence as long as possible.
    4. Pain is priority over psychological problems and activity; remember Maslow's Hierarchy of Needs.

22. 1. A sunscreen with an SPF of at least 15 should be used by the client with SLE.
    2. The client with SLE is at risk for infections and should avoid large crowds.
    3. Pregnancy is not contraindicated in most women diagnosed with SLE.
    4. The client with SLE should use hypoallergenic products and should not use irritating soaps, shampoos, or chemicals.

23. 1. Epinephrine is the drug of choice for an anaphylactic reaction. It is a potent vasoconstrictor and bronchodilator that counteracts the effects of histamine, but this is not the priority intervention.
    2. This is an important intervention but it is not the priority intervention.
    3. Decreasing the client's anxiety is important, but it is not the priority intervention.
    4. Establishing a patent airway is priority because facial angioedema, bronchospasm, and laryngeal edema occur with an anaphylactic reaction. Inserting a nasopharyngeal or oropharyngeal airway would maintain an airway.

24. 1. The client must use measures to help prevent fatigue, which increases the depletion of acetylcholine and causes muscle weakness.
    2. The client with MG is not on strict bed rest and impaired skin integrity is not an expected complication of this disease process, especially in the early stages.
    3. Pain is not an expected complaint of clients diagnosed with MG.
    4. A thymectomy, not a splenectomy, may be recommended. Approximately 75% of clients with MG have dysplasia of the thymus gland.

25. 1. Pneumocystis carinii pneumonia (PCP) occurs in approximately 75% to 80% of clients diagnosed with AIDS. Signs/symptoms of it include fever, cough, and shortness of breath.
    2. This is an opportunistic infection, but it is not the most common infection.
    3. These are signs/symptoms of *Mycobacterium avium* complex (MAC), which affects up to 25% of client's with AIDS, but it is not the most common opportunistic infection.
    4. These are signs/symptoms of Kaposi's sarcoma, which is the most common cancer associated with AIDS; it is not an infectious disease.

26. In order of priority: 1, 3, 2, 5, 4.
    1. Airway is always the first priority for any process in which the airway might be compromised.
    3. The nurse should start an IV so that medications can be administered to treat the anaphylactic reaction.
    2. Epinephrine is the drug of choice for the treatment of anaphylaxis. The medication is administered every ten (10) to fifteen (15) minutes until the reaction has subsided. Epinephrine is given for its vasoconstrictive action.
    5. Benadryl, an antihistamine, is given to block histamine release, reducing capillary permeability.
    4. Teaching is important to prevent or treat further reactions, but this will be done after the crisis is over.

Immune

*The eye sees what the mind is prepared to comprehend.*—Henri Bergson

# Sensory Deficits

**14**

Some sensory deficits occur with normal aging, whereas others are the result of specific disease processes. Problems involving the senses—sight, hearing, smell, taste, touch—arise from many sources. Some are inflammatory, infectious, or both (otitis); some are the result of a specific disease process (cataract, glaucoma); and still others are the result of the normal aging process (decreased peripheral vision, decreased sense of smell). Many of these diseases/disorders can be treated with appropriate medical/surgical interventions. Still others can be addressed through safety precautions (smoke alarms) and assistive devices (hearing aids). The nurse must be familiar with how to assess the sensory system, identify specific problems, and help in the care of clients with these problems.

## KEYWORDS

Amsler grid
cataract
enucleation
glaucoma
intraocular
macular degeneration
Menière's disease
myopia
nephrotoxic
nystagmus
otitis
otorrhea
otoscope
ototoxic
perforation
presbycusis
ptosis
retrobulbar
Snellen chart
stapedectomy
tinnitus
tympanic membrane
vertigo

## ABBREVIATIONS

Health-Care Provider (HCP)
Intravenous (IV)
Laser-Assisted in situ Keratomileusis (LASIK)

## Eye Disorders

1. The client is diagnosed with glaucoma. Which symptom would the nurse expect the client to report?
   1. Halos around lights.
   2. Floating spots in the vision.
   3. A yellow haze around everything.
   4. A curtain coming across vision.

2. The client is scheduled for right-eye cataract removal surgery in five (5) days. Which preoperative instruction should be discussed with the client?
   1. Administer dilating drops to both eyes for 72 hours prior to surgery.
   2. Prior to surgery do not lift or push any objects heavier than 15 pounds.
   3. Make arrangements for being in the hospital for at least three (3) days.
   4. Avoid taking any type of medication that causes bleeding, such as aspirin.

3. The client is postoperative retinal detachment surgery, and gas tamponade was used to flatten the retina. Which intervention should the nurse implement first?
   1. Teach the signs of increased intraocular pressure.
   2. Position the client as prescribed by the surgeon.
   3. Assess the eye for signs/symptoms of complications.
   4. Explain the importance of follow-up visits.

4. The 65-year-old client is diagnosed with macular degeneration. Which statement by the nurse indicates the client needs more discharge teaching?
   1. "I should use magnification devices as much as possible."
   2. "I will look at my Amsler grid at least twice a week."
   3. "I am going to use low-watt light bulbs in my house."
   4. "I am going to contact a low-vision center to evaluate my home."

5. The nurse who is at a local park sees a young man on the ground and realizes he has fallen on a stick and it is lodged in his eye. Which action should the nurse implement at the scene?
   1. Carefully remove the stick from the eye.
   2. Stabilize the stick as best as possible.
   3. Flush the eye with water if available.
   4. Place the young man in a high-Fowler's position.

6. The employee health nurse is teaching a class on "Preventing Eye Injury." Which information should be discussed in the class?
   1. Read instructions thoroughly before using tools and chemicals.
   2. Wear some type of glasses when working around flying fragments.
   3. Always wear a protective helmet with eye shield around dust particles.
   4. Pay close attention to the surroundings so that eye injuries will be prevented.

7. The 65-year-old male client who is complaining of blurred vision reports that he thinks his glasses need to be cleaned all the time. He denies any type of pain in his eyes. Based on these signs/symptoms, which eye disorder would the nurse suspect the client has?
   1. Corneal dystrophy.
   2. Conjunctivitis.
   3. Diabetic retinopathy.
   4. Cataracts.

8. The nurse is administering eye drops to the client. Which guidelines should the nurse adhere to when instilling the drops into one eye? Select all that apply.
   1. Do not touch the tip of the medication container to the eye.
   2. Apply gently pressure on the outer canthus of the eye.
   3. Apply sterile gloves prior to instilling eye drops.
   4. Hold the lower lid down and instill drops into the conjunctiva.
   5. Gently pat the skin to absorb excess eye drops that run onto the cheek.

9. The client has had an enucleation of the left eye. Which intervention should the nurse implement?
   1. Discuss the need for special eyeglasses.
   2. Refer the client for an ocular prosthesis.
   3. Help the client obtain a seeing-eye dog.
   4. Teach the client how to instill eye drops.

10. The client diagnosed with glaucoma is prescribed a miotic cholinergic medication. Which data support that the medication has been effective?
    1. No redness or irritation of the eyes.
    2. A decrease in intraocular pressure.
    3. The pupil reacts briskly to light.
    4. The client denies any type of floaters.

11. The client is scheduled for laser-assisted in situ keratomileusis (LASIK) surgery for severe myopia. Which discharge teaching should the nurse discuss prior to the client's discharge from day surgery?
    1. Wear bilateral eye patches for three (3) days.
    2. Wear corrective lenses until the follow-up visit.
    3. Do not read any material for at least one (1) week.
    4. Teach the client how to instill corticosteroid ophthalmic drops.

12. The client is admitted to the emergency department after splashing chemicals into the eyes. Which intervention should the nurse implement first?
    1. Have the client move the eyes in all directions.
    2. Administer a broad-spectrum antibiotic.
    3. Irrigate the eyes with normal saline solution.
    4. Determine when the client had a tetanus shot.

## Ear Disorders

13. Which statement by the client would indicate that the client is experiencing some hearing loss?
    1. "I clean my ears every day after I take a shower."
    2. "I keep turning up the sound on my television."
    3. "My ears hurt, especially when I yawn."
    4. "I get dizzy when I get up from the chair."

14. Which factors increase the client's risk of developing hearing loss? Select all that apply.
    1. Perforation of the tympanic membrane.
    2. Chronic exposure to loud noises.
    3. Recurrent ear infections.
    4. Use of nephrotoxic medications.
    5. Multiple piercings in the auricle.

15. The client is diagnosed with acute otitis media. Which signs/symptoms support this medical diagnosis?
    1. Unilateral pain in the ear.
    2. Green, foul-smelling drainage.
    3. Sensation of congestion in the ear.
    4. Reports of hearing loss.

16. The client diagnosed with chronic otitis media is scheduled for a mastoidectomy. Which discharge teaching should the nurse discuss with the client?
    1. Instruct the client to blow the nose with the mouth closed.
    2. Explain that the client will never be able to hear from the ear.
    3. Instill ophthalmic drops in both ears and then insert a cotton ball.
    4. Do not allow water to enter the ear for six (6) weeks.

17. The client is diagnosed with Menière's disease. Which statement by the client supports that the client understands the medical management for this disease?
    1. "After intravenous antibiotic therapy, I will be cured."
    2. "I will have to use a hearing aid for the rest of my life."
    3. "I must adhere to a low-sodium diet, 2000 mg/day."
    4. "I should sleep with the head of my bed elevated."

18. The client reports to the nurse that there is a ringing in the ears. Which documentation would be most appropriate for the nurse to document in the client's chart?
    1. Complaints of vertigo.
    2. Complaints of otorrhea.
    3. Complaints of tinnitus.
    4. Complaints of presbycusis.

19. Which statement best describes the scientific rationale for the nurse to hold the otoscope in the right hand in a pencil-hold position when examining the client's ear?
    1. It is usually the most comfortable position to hold the otoscope.
    2. This allows the best visualization of the tympanic membrane.
    3. This prevents inserting the otoscope too far into the external ear.
    4. It ensures that the nurse will not cause pain when examining the ear.

20. The nurse is preparing to administer otic drops into an adult client's right ear. Which action should the nurse implement?
    1. Grasp the ear lobe and pull back and out when putting drops in the ear.
    2. Insert the eardrops without touching the outside of the ear.
    3. Instruct the client to close the mouth and blow prior to instilling drops.
    4. Pull the auricle down and back prior to instilling drops.

21. Which ototoxic medication should the nurse administer cautiously?
    1. An oral calcium-channel blocker.
    2. An intravenous aminoglycoside antibiotic.
    3. An intravenous glucocorticoid.
    4. An oral loop diuretic.

22. Which teaching instruction should the nurse discuss with students who are on the high school swim team when discussing how to prevent external otitis?
    1. Do not wear tight-fitting swim caps.
    2. Avoid using silicone earplugs while swimming.
    3. Use a drying agent in the ear after swimming.
    4. Insert a bulb syringe into each ear to remove excess water.

23. The client comes to the clinic and is diagnosed with otitis media. Which intervention should the clinic nurse include in the discharge teaching?
    1. Instruct the client not to take any over-the-counter pain medication.
    2. Encourage the client to apply cold packs to the affected ear.
    3. Tell the client to call the HCP if an abrupt relief of ear pain occurs.
    4. Wear a protective earplug in the affected ear.

24. The client is scheduled for ear surgery. Which statement indicates the client needs more preoperative teaching concerning the surgery?
    1. "If I have to sneeze or blow my nose, I will do it with my mouth open."
    2. "I may get dizzy after the surgery, so I must be careful when walking."
    3. "I will probably have some hearing loss after surgery, but hearing will return."
    4. "I can shampoo my hair the day after surgery as long as I am careful."

### Eye Disorders

1. 1. In glaucoma, the client is often unaware that he or she has the disease until the client experiences blurred vision, halos around lights, difficulty focusing, or loss of peripheral vision. Glaucoma is often called the "silent thief."
   2. Floating spots in the vision is a symptom of retinal detachment.
   3. A yellow haze around everything is a complaint of clients experiencing digoxin toxicity.
   4. The complaint of a curtain coming across vision is a symptom of retinal detachment.
   **TEST-TAKING HINT: The signs/symptoms of eye disorders are confusing for the nurse. The test taker must know which complaints will be made by the client with a specific eye disorder.**

2. 1. Dilating drops are administered every ten (10) minutes for four (4) doses one (1) hour prior to surgery, not for three (3) days prior to surgery.
   2. Lifting and pushing objects should be avoided after surgery, not prior to surgery.
   3. All types of cataract removal surgery are usually done in day surgery.
   4. To reduce retrobulbar hemorrhage, any anticoagulation therapy is withheld, including aspirin, nonsteroidal anti-inflammatory drugs (NSAIDs), and warfarin (Coumadin).
   **TEST-TAKING HINT: The test taker must notice the adjectives; these descriptors are important when selecting a correct answer. The test taker should notice "preoperative" and "prior to surgery."**

3. 1. This should be done, but it is not the first intervention the nurse should implement.
   2. The client will have to be specifically positioned to make the gas bubble float into the best position; some clients must lie face down or on their side for days, but it is not the first intervention.
   3. The nurse's priority must be assessment of complications, which include increased intraocular pressure, endophthalmitis, development of another retinal detachment, or loss of turgor in the eye.
   4. Follow-up visits are important, but it is not the first intervention the nurse should implement.
   **TEST-TAKING HINT: When the question asks which intervention should be implemented first, all four (4) answer options are possible interventions but only one (1) should be implemented first. Remember to apply the nursing process to help select the correct answer. Assessment is the first part of the nursing process.**

4. 1. Magnifying devices used with activities such as threading a needle will help the client's visual sight; therefore, this statement does not indicate the client needs more teaching.
   2. An Amsler grid is a tool to assess macular degeneration that often provides the earliest sign of a worsening of the condition. If the lines of the grid become distorted or faded, the client should call the ophthalmologist.
   3. Macular degeneration is the most common cause of visual loss in people older than age 60 years. Any intervention that can help increase vision should be included in the teaching such as bright lighting, not decreased lighting.
   4. Low-vision centers will send representatives to the client's home or work to make recommendations about improving lighting, thereby improving the client's vision and safety.
   **TEST-TAKING HINT: The test taker must be sure what the question is asking prior to looking at the answer options. This question is asking which statement indicates more teaching is needed. Therefore three (3) options will indicate that the client understands appropriate discharge teaching and only one (1) will indicate the client does not understand the teaching.**

5. 1. A foreign object should never be removed at the scene of the accident because this may cause more damage.
   2. The foreign object should be stabilized to prevent further movement that could cause more damage to the eye.
   3. Flushing with water may cause further movement of the foreign object and should be avoided.
   4. The person should be kept flat and not in a sitting position that may dislodge or cause movement of the foreign object.
   **TEST-TAKING HINT: In an emergency situation the first responder should first "do no harm." The test taker should examine each option and decide what will happen if this option is performed—will it help, harm, or stabilize the client? If the test taker determines that one (1) action may not help, then stabilization becomes the priority.**

6. 1. Instructions provide precautions that should be used and steps to take if eye injuries occur secondary to the use of tools or chemicals.
   2. The employee must wear safety glasses, not just any type of glasses and especially not regular prescription glasses.
   3. A protective helmet is usually used to help pre-

vent sports eye injuries, not work-related injuries.

4. Eye injuries will not be prevented by paying close attention to the surroundings. They are prevented by wearing protective glasses or eye shields.

**TEST-TAKING HINT: The test taker must make sure what the question is asking and must pay close attention to adjectives. An "employee health nurse" is in the workplace. If the test taker is going to select an option with a word such as "always," "never," or "only," he or she must be absolutely sure it is an intervention that is never questioned. In health care, there are very few absolutes.**

7. 1. Corneal dystrophy is an inherited eye disorder that occurs at about age 20 years and results in decreased vision and the development of blisters and is usually associated with primary open-angle glaucoma.

2. Conjunctivitis is an inflammation of the conjunctiva, which results in a scratching or burning sensation, itching, and photophobia.

3. Diabetic retinopathy results from deterioration of the small blood vessels that nourish the retina; it leads to blindness.

4. A cataract is a lens opacity or cloudiness, resulting in the signs/symptoms discussed in the stem.

**TEST-TAKING HINT: The test taker must know the signs/symptoms of eye disorders, especially those that commonly occur in the elderly. Option "2" could be ruled out because "itis" means inflammation and none of the signs/symptoms are inflammatory.**

8. 1. Touching the tip of the container to the eye could cause eye injury or an eye infection.

2. Gentle pressure should be applied on the inner canthus near the bridge of the nose for one (1) or two (2) minutes after instilling eye drops.

3. The nurse should wash hands prior to and after instilling medications; this is not a sterile procedure.

4. Medication should not be placed directly on the eye but in the lower part of the eye.

5. Eye drops are meant to go in the eye, not on the skin, so the nurse should use a clean tissue to remove excess medication.

**TEST-TAKING HINT: This is an alternate type question that requires the test taker to select all the options that are correct. Do not second guess the question. All five (5) can be selected or only one (1). Read each option, and if it is correct then select it.**

9. 1. Special eyeglasses are not needed for an enucleation.

2. An enucleation is the removal of the entire eye and part of the optic nerve. An ocular prosthesis will help maintain the shape of the eye after the enucleation.

3. The client had the left eye removed but is not blind because he or she still has the right eye.

4. The eyeball was totally removed and a pressure dressing is applied; therefore, there will be no need to instill eye drops.

**TEST-TAKING HINT: In some questions, the test taker must know the definition of the word (enucleation) to be able to apply it in a clinical situation.**

10. 1. Steroid medication is administered to decrease inflammation.

2. Both systemic and topical medications are used to decrease the intraocular pressure in the eye, which is what causes glaucoma.

3. Glaucoma does not affect the pupillary reaction.

4. Floaters are a complaint of clients with retinal detachment.

**TEST-TAKING HINT: To determine the effectiveness of a medication the nurse must know the signs/symptoms of the disease process. If the test taker knew glaucoma was the result of an increase in intraocular pressure, then the medication would be effective if there was a decrease in intraocular pressure.**

11. 1. The client does not have to wear eye patches after this surgery.

2. The purpose of this surgery is to ensure the client does not have to wear any type of corrective lens.

3. The client can read immediately after this surgery.

4. LASIK surgery is an effective, safe, predictable surgery that is performed in day surgery; there is minimal postoperative care, which includes instilling topical corticosteroid drops.

**TEST-TAKING HINT: Answer option "3" has the absolute word "any," so the test taker could eliminate it. LASIK is a corrective surgery, and if the problem is corrected, then corrective lenses should not be necessary.**

12. 1. Movement of the eye should be avoided until the client has received general anesthesia; therefore, this is not the first intervention that should be implemented.

2. Parenteral broad-spectrum antibiotics are initiated but not until the eyes are treated first.

3. Before any further evaluation or treatment,

the eyes must be thoroughly flushed with sterile normal saline solution.

4. Tetanus prophylaxis is recommended for full-thickness ocular wounds.

**TEST-TAKING HINT: If the test taker is not sure of the answer, the test taker should select the answer that directly addresses the client's condition. Options "1" and "3" directly affect the eyes, but when choosing between these two options, the test taker should ask, "How will moving the eyes help treat the eyes?" and then eliminate "1."**

## Ear Disorders

13. 1. Cleaning the ears daily does not indicate the client has a hearing loss.
    2. The need to turn up the volume on the television is an early sign of hearing impairment.
    3. Pain in the ears is not a clinical manifestation of hearing loss/impairment.
    4. This statement may indicate a balance problem secondary to an ear disorder, but it does not indicate a hearing loss.

**TEST-TAKING HINT: If the test taker has no idea of the answer, option "2" is the only answer that has anything to do with sound.**

14. 1. The tympanic membrane is the eardrum, and if it is punctured it may lead to hearing loss.
    2. Loud persistent noise, such as that from heavy machinery, engines, and artillery, over time has been found to cause noise-induced hearing loss.
    3. Multiple ear infections scar the tympanic membrane, which can lead to hearing loss.
    4. Nephrotoxic means harmful to the kidneys; ototoxic would be harmful to the ears.
    5. Multiple pierced earrings do not lead to hearing loss. The auricle (skin attached to the head) is composed mainly of cartilage, except for the fat and subcutaneous tissue in the earlobe.

**TEST-TAKING HINT: This alternate-type questions requires the test taker to select multiple correct answers. Many options can be eliminated as incorrect answers when the test taker knows medical terminology—"nephro" means kidney-related—and normal anatomy of the body—"auricle" means "skin attached to the head."**

15. 1. Otalgia, ear pain, is experienced by clients with otitis media.
    2. A green, foul-smelling drainage would support the diagnosis of external otitis, not of acute otitis media.

3. A sensation of congestion in the ear would support serous otitis media.
4. Hearing loss would support a diagnosis of chronic otitis media or serous otitis media.

**TEST-TAKING HINT: If the test taker was not sure of the answer, the adjective "acute" in the stem should cause the test taker to think "pain," which is included in option "1."**

16. 1. The client should blow the nose with the mouth open to prevent pressure in the Eustachian tube.
    2. There may be temporary deafness as a result of postoperative edema, but the hearing will return as the edema subsides.
    3. Ophthalmic drops would be used in the eyes, not the ears. Otic drops would be used for the ears.
    4. Water should be prevented from entering the external auditory canal because it may irritate the surgical incision and is a medium for bacterial growth.

**TEST-TAKING HINT: The test taker must be aware of adjectives. In option "3" the test taker should know that "ophthalmic" refers to the eye, which would cause the test taker to eliminate this as a possible answer.**

17. 1. Antibiotics will not cure this disease. Surgery is the only cure for Menière's disease, which may result in permanent deafness as a result of the labyrinth being removed in the surgery.
    2. Menière's disease does not lead to deafness unless surgery is performed that removes the labyrinth in attempts to eliminate the attacks of vertigo.
    3. Sodium regulates the balance of fluid within the body; therefore, a low-sodium diet is prescribed to help control the symptoms of Menière's disease.
    4. Sleeping with the head of the bed elevated will not affect Menière's disease.

**TEST-TAKING HINT: Sleeping with the HOB elevated is not a medical treatment; therefore "4" can be eliminated as a possible answer. The test taker must read the stem carefully.**

18. 1. Vertigo is an illusion of movement in which the client complains of dizziness.
    2. Otorrhea is drainage of the ear.
    3. Tinnitus is "ringing of the ears." It is a subjective perception of sound with internal origins.
    4. Presbycusis is progressive hearing loss associated with aging.

**TEST-TAKING HINTS: The test taker who is familiar with medical terminology can rule out options based on the understanding of medical terms.**

19. 1. This is not the rationale for holding the otoscope in this manner.
2. Holding the otoscope in this manner does not help visualize the membrane any better than does holding the otoscope in other ways.
3. Inserting the speculum of the otoscope into the external ear can cause ear trauma if not done correctly.
4. If the ear is inflamed, it may be impossible to prevent hurting the client on examination.

TEST-TAKING HINT: The scientific rationale is the critical-thinking component of nursing; the nurse must understand the "why" of nursing interventions.

20. 1. This is not the correct way to administer eardrops.
2. The nurse must straighten the ear canal; therefore the outside of the ear must be moved.
3. This will increase pressure in the ear and should not be done prior to administering eardrops.
4. This will straighten the ear canal so that the eardrops will enter the ear canal and drain toward the tympanic membrane (eardrum).

TEST-TAKING HINT: The test taker should notice that options "1" and "4" are opposite, which should clue the test taker into either eliminating both or deciding that one (1) of these two (2) is the correct answer. Either way the test taker now has a 50/50 chance of selecting the correct answer.

21. 1. Calcium channel blockers are not going to affect the client's hearing.
2. Aminoglycoside antibiotics are ototoxic. Overdosage of these medications can cause the client to go deaf, which is why peak and trough serum levels are drawn while the client is taking a medication of this type. These antibiotics are also very nephrotoxic.
3. Steroids cause many adverse effects, but damage to the ear is not one of them.
4. Administering an intravenous push loop diuretic too fast can cause auditory nerve damage, but an oral loop diuretic does not.

TEST-TAKING HINT: The test taker must be cautious of adjectives. The word "oral" in "4" would eliminate this option as a possible correct answer.

22. 1. Tight-fitting swim caps or wet suit hoods should be worn because they prevent water from entering the ear canal.
2. Silicone earplugs should be worn because they keep water from entering the ear canal without reducing hearing significantly.

3. A 2% acetic acid solution or 2% boric acid in ethyl alcohol is effective in drying the canal and restoring its normal acidic environment.
4. A bulb syringe with a Teflon catheter can be used to remove impacted debris from the ear, but it is not used to remove excess water.

TEST-TAKING HINT: If the test taker has no idea what the correct answer is, evaluate the answer options to see if two are similar. In this question both "1" and "2" say to not use ear protectors. Because there cannot be two correct answers, these two could be eliminated as possible correct answers.

23. 1. Mild analgesics such as aspirin or acetaminophen every four (4) hours as needed to relieve pain and fever are recommended; aspirin may help decrease inflammation of the ear.
2. Heat applied to the affected ear is recommended because heat dilates blood vessels, promoting the reabsorption of fluid and reducing edema.
3. Pain that subsides abruptly may indicate spontaneous perforation of the tympanic membrane within the middle ear and should be reported to the HCP.
4. Ear plugs should not be used in clients with otitis media, but cotton balls could be used to keep otic antibiotics in the ear canal.

TEST-TAKING HINT: The test taker must use basic principles when answering questions. Cold causes constriction and heat dilates. Except for aspirin not being given to children to prevent Reye syndrome, mild analgesics can be given for almost any discomfort.

24. 1. Leaving the mouth open when coughing or sneezing will minimize the pressure changes in the middle ear.
2. Surgery on the ear may disrupt the client's equilibrium, increasing the risk for falling.
3. Hearing loss secondary to postoperative edema is common after surgery, but the hearing will return after the edema subsides.
4. Shampooing, showering, and immersing the head in water are avoided to prevent contamination of the ear canal; therefore, this comment indicates the client does not understand the preoperative teaching.

TEST-TAKING HINT: This is an "except" question. The stem states "needs more teaching"; therefore three (3) of the distracters would reflect appropriate understanding of the teaching and only one (1) would indicate a misunderstanding of the teaching.

1. Which recommendation should the nurse suggest to an elderly client who lives alone when discussing normal developmental changes of the olfactory organs?
   1. Suggest installing multiple smoke alarms in the home.
   2. Recommend using a night light in the hallway and bathroom.
   3. Discuss keeping a high-humidity atmosphere in the bedroom.
   4. Encourage the client to smell food prior to eating it.

2. The elderly male client tells the nurse, "My wife says her cooking hasn't changed, but it is bland and tasteless." Which response by the nurse would be most appropriate?
   1. "Would you like me to talk to your wife about her cooking?"
   2. "Taste buds change with age, which may be why the food seems bland."
   3. "This happens because the medications sometimes cause a change in taste."
   4. "Why don't you barbecue food on a grill if you don't like your wife's cooking?"

3. The charge nurse is admitting a 90-year-old client to a long-term care facility. Which intervention should the nurse implement?
   1. Ensure the client's room temperature is cool.
   2. Talk louder to make sure the client hears clearly.
   3. Complete the admission as fast as possible.
   4. Provide extra orientation to the surroundings.

4. Which assessment technique would be indicated when assessing the client's cranial nerves for vibration?
   1. Move the big toe up and down and ask in which direction the vibration is felt.
   2. Place a tuning fork on the big toe and ask if the vibrations are felt.
   3. Tap the client's cheek with the finger and determine if vibrations are felt.
   4. Touch the arm with two sharp objects and ask if one (1) vibration or two (2) is felt.

5. Which intervention should the nurse include when conducting an in-service on caring for elderly clients that addresses normal developmental sensory changes?
   1. Ensure curtains are open when having the client read written material.
   2. Provide a variety of written material when discussing a procedure.
   3. Assist the client when getting out of the bed and sitting in the chair.
   4. Request a telephone for the hearing impaired for all elderly clients.

6. Which situation would make the nurse think the client has glaucoma?
   1. An automobile accident because the client not seeing the car in the next lane.
   2. The cake tasted funny because the client could not read the recipe.
   3. The client has been wearing mismatched clothes and socks.
   4. The client ran a stoplight and hit a pedestrian walking in the crosswalk.

7. The client with a retinal detachment has just undergone a gas tamponade repair. Which discharge instruction should the nurse include in the teaching?
   1. The client must lie flat with the face down.
   2. The head of the bed must be elevated 45 degrees.
   3. The client should wear sunglasses when outside.
   4. The client should avoid reading for three (3) weeks.

8. The nurse is conducting a Weber test on the client who is suspected of having conductive hearing loss in the left ear. Where should the nurse place the tuning fork when conducting this test?

   1. A
   2. B
   3. C
   4. D

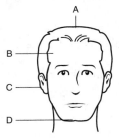

9. The student nurse asks the nurse, "Which type of hearing loss involves damage to the cochlea or vestibulocochlear nerve?" Which statement is the best response of the nurse?
   1. "It is called conductive hearing loss."
   2. "It is called a functional hearing loss."
   3. "It is called a mixed hearing loss."
   4. "It is called sensorineural hearing loss."

10. The client has undergone a bilateral stapedectomy. Which action by the client would warrant immediate intervention by the nurse?
    1. The client is ambulating without assistance.
    2. The client is blowing the nose with the mouth open.
    3. There is some slight serosanguineous drainage.
    4. The client reports hearing popping in the affected ear.

11. The female client tells the clinic nurse that she is going on a seven (7)-day cruise and is worried about getting motion sickness. Which information should the nurse discuss with the client?
    1. Make an appointment for the client to see the health-care provider.
    2. Recommend getting an over-the-counter scopolamine patch.
    3. Discourage the client from taking the trip because she is worried.
    4. Instruct the client to lie down and the motion sickness will go away.

12. The nurse writes the diagnosis "risk for trauma related to impaired balance" for the client diagnosed with vertigo. Which nursing intervention should be included in the plan of care?
    1. Provide information about vertigo and its treatment.
    2. Assess for level and type of diversional activity.
    3. Assess for visual acuity and proprioceptive deficits.
    4. Refer the client to a support group and counseling.

13. The nurse is assessing the client's cranial nerves. Which assessment data indicate that cranial nerve I is intact?
    1. The client can identify cold and hot on the face.
    2. The client does not have any tongue tremor.
    3. The client has no ptosis of the eyelids.
    4. The client is able to identify a peppermint smell.

14. The elderly client is complaining of abdominal discomfort. Which scientific rationale should the nurse remember when addressing an elderly client's perception of pain?
    1. Elderly clients react to pain the same way any other age group does.
    2. The elderly client usually requires more pain medication.
    3. Reaction to painful stimuli may be decreased with age.
    4. The elderly client should use the Wong scale to assess pain.

15. During a sensory assessment, which instruction should the nurse discuss with the client?
    1. Instruct the client to lie flat without a pillow during the assessment.
    2. Instruct the client to keep both eyes shut during the assessment.
    3. During the assessment the client must be in a treatment room.
    4. Keep the lights off during the client's sensory assessment.

16. Which signs/symptoms should the nurse expect to find when assessing the client with an acoustic neuroma?
    1. Incapacitating vertigo and otorrhea.
    2. Nystagmus and complaints of dizziness.
    3. Nausea and vomiting.
    4. Unilateral hearing loss and tinnitus.

17. Which assessment technique should the nurse use to assess the client's optic nerve?
    1. Have the client identify different smells.
    2. Have the client discriminate between sugar and salt.
    3. Have the client read the Snellen chart.
    4. Have the client say "ah" to assess the rise of the uvula.

18. Which referral would be most important for the client with permanent hearing loss?
    1. Aural rehabilitation.
    2. Speech therapist.
    3. Social worker.
    4. Vocational rehabilitation.

19. Which instruction should the nurse discuss with the female client with viral conjunctivitis?
    1. Contact the HCP if pain occurs.
    2. Do not share towels or linens.
    3. Apply warm compresses to the eyes.
    4. Apply makeup very lightly.

20. The client is two (2) hours postoperative right-ear mastoidectomy. Which assessment data should be reported to the health-care provider?
    1. Complaints of aural fullness.
    2. Hearing loss in the affected ear.
    3. No vertigo.
    4. Facial drooping.

21. Which behavior by the male client would make the nurse suspect the client has a hearing loss? Select all that apply.
    1. The client reports hearing voices in his head.
    2. The client becomes irritable very easily.
    3. The client has difficulty making decisions.
    4. The client's wife reports that he ignores her.
    5. The client does not dominate a conversation.

22. The client with cataracts who has had intraocular lens implants is being discharged from the day surgery department. Which discharge instructions should the nurse discuss with the client?
    1. Do not push or pull objects heavier than 50 pounds.
    2. Lie on the affected eye with two pillows at night.
    3. Wear glasses or metal eye shields at all times.
    4. Bend and stoop carefully for the rest of your life.

23. The nurse is assessing the client's sensory system. Which result would indicate an abnormal stereognosis test?
    1. The client is unable to identify which way the toe is being moved.
    2. The client cannot discriminate between sharp and dull objects.
    3. The toes contract and draw together when the sole of the foot is stroked.
    4. The client is unable to identify a key in the hand with both eyes closed.

24. Which statement by the daughter of an 80-year-old female client who lives alone would warrant immediate intervention by the nurse?
    1. "I put a night light in my mother's bedroom."
    2. "There are smoke alarms in every room."
    3. "I changed my mother's furniture around."
    4. "I got my mother large-print books."

25. The 72-year-old client tells the nurse that food does not taste good anymore and that he has lost a little weight. Which information should the nurse discuss with the client?
    1. Suggest using extra seasoning when cooking.
    2. Instruct the client to keep a seven (7)-day food diary.
    3. Refer the client to a dietitian immediately.
    4. Recommend eating three meals a day.

26. The male client diagnosed with Type 2 diabetes mellitus tells the nurse that he has begun to see yellow spots. Which interventions should the nurse implement? List in order of priority.
    1. Notify the health-care provider.
    2. Check the client's hemoglobin A1$_c$.
    3. Assess the client's vision using the Amsler grid.
    4. Teach the client about controlling blood glucose levels.
    5. Determine where the spots appear to be in the client's field of vision.

1. 1. The decreased sense of smell resulting from atrophy of olfactory organs is a safety hazard and clients may not be able to smell gas leaks or fire, so the nurse should recommend a carbon monoxide detector and a smoke alarm. This safety equipment is critical for the elderly.
   2. Night lights do not address the client's sense of smell.
   3. High humidity may help with breathing, but it does not help the sense of smell.
   4. The client's sense of smell is decreased; therefore, smelling food before eating is not an appropriate intervention.

2. 1. The nurse needs to discuss possible causes with the client and not talk to the wife.
   2. The acuity of the taste buds decreases with age, which could cause regular foods to seem bland and tasteless.
   3. Some medications may cause a metallic taste in the mouth, but medication would not cause foods to taste bland.
   4. Telling the client to cook if he doesn't like his wife's food is an argumentative and judgmental response.

3. 1. Because of altered temperature regulation, the client usually needs a warmer room temperature, not a cooler room temperature.
   2. The nurse should use a low-pitched, normal level, clear voice. Talking louder or shouting only makes it harder for the client to understand the nurse.
   3. The elderly client requires adequate time to receive and respond to stimuli, to learn, and to react; therefore the nurse should take time and not rush the admission.
   4. Sensory isolation resulting from visual and hearing loss can cause confusion, anxiety, disorientation, and misinterpretation of the new environment; therefore, the nurse should provide extra orientation.

4. 1. This assesses proprioception, or position sense; direction of the toe must be evaluated.
   2. Vibration is assessed by using a low-frequency tuning fork on a bony prominence and asking the client whether he or she feels the sensation and, if so, when the sensation ceases.
   3. Tapping the cheek assesses for tetany, not cranial nerve involvement.
   4. A two-point discrimination test evaluates integration of sensation, but it does not assess for vibration.

5. 1. Adequate lighting without a glare should be provided when having the client read written material; therefore, the curtains should be closed, not open.
   2. The nurse should provide material that is short, concise, and concrete, not a variety.
   3. Because fewer tactile cues are received from the bottom of the feet, the client may get confused as to body position and location. Safety is priority and assisting the client getting out of bed and sitting in a chair is appropriate.
   4. This is making a judgment. Not all elderly clients are hard of hearing, and telephones for the hearing impaired require special training for the user.

6. 1. Loss of peripheral vision as a result of glaucoma causes the client problems with seeing things on each side, resulting in a "blind spot." This problem can lead to the client having car accidents when switching lanes.
   2. This would be indicative of cataracts because clients with cataracts have blurred vision and cannot read clearly.
   3. This would be indicative of cataracts because there is a color shift to yellow–brown and there is reduced light transmission.
   4. This would be indicative of macular degeneration, in which the central vision is affected.

7. 1. If gas tamponade is used to flatten the retina, the client may have to be specially positioned to make the gas bubble float into the best position; clients must lie face down or on the side for days.
   2. The HOB should not be elevated after this surgery.
   3. There is no need for the client to wear sunglasses; this surgery does not cause photophobia.
   4. The client does not need to avoid reading.

8. 1. The tuning fork should be struck to produce vibrations and then placed midline between the ears on top of the head.
   2. The right temple area is not an appropriate place to assess for conductive hearing loss.
   3. The right occipital area is not the appropriate place to place the tuning fork; this is the area behind the ear where the Rinne test is performed.
   4. The chin area is not the appropriate area to put the tuning fork.

9. 1. Conductive hearing loss results from an external ear disorder, such as impacted cerumen, or a middle ear disorder, such as otitis media or otosclerosis.
   2. Functional (psychogenic) hearing loss is nonorganic and unrelated to detectable structural changes in the hearing mechanisms. It is usually a manifestation of an emotional disturbance.
   3. Mixed hearing loss involves both conductive loss and sensorineural loss. It results from dysfunction of air and bone conduction.
   4. **Sensorineural hearing loss is described in the stem of the question. It involves damage to the cochlea or vestibulocochlear nerve.**

10. 1. **Balance disturbance, or true vertigo, rarely occurs with other middle-ear surgical procedures, but it does occur for a short time after a stapedectomy. Safety is an important issue, and ambulating without assistance would require intervention by the nurse.**
    2. Pressure changes in the middle ear will be minimal if the client blows the nose with the mouth open instead of closed.
    3. Slightly bloody or serosanguineous drainage is normal after ear surgery.
    4. Popping and crackling in the operative ear is normal for about three (3) to five (5) weeks after surgery.

11. 1. This is not a condition that requires an appointment with the health-care provider.
    2. **Anticholinergic medications, such as scopolamine patches, can be recommended by the nurse; this is not prescribing. Motion sickness is a disturbance of equilibrium caused by constant motion.**
    3. Motion sickness can be controlled with medication and it may not even occur. Therefore, canceling the trip is not providing the client with appropriate information.
    4. This is providing the client with false information. Lying down may or may not help motion sickness. To be able to enjoy the cruise, the client needs medication.

12. 1. This would be appropriate for a diagnosis of "knowledge deficit."
    2. This would be appropriate for a diagnosis of "deficient diversional activity" related to environmental lack of activity.
    3. **Balance depends on visual, vestibular, and proprioceptive systems; therefore the nurse should assess these systems for signs/symptoms.**
    4. This would be appropriate for a diagnosis "ineffective coping."

13. 1. Being able to identify cold and hot on the face indicates an intact trigeminal nerve, cranial nerve V.
    2. Not having any tongue tremor indicates an intact hypoglossal nerve, cranial nerve XI.
    3. No ptosis of the eyelids indicates an intact oculomotor nerve (cranial nerve III), trochlear nerve (IV), and abducens nerve (VI). Tests also assess for ocular motion, conjugate movements, nystagmus, and papillary reflexes.
    4. **Cranial nerve I is the olfactory nerve, which involves the sense of smell. With the eyes closed the client must identify familiar smells to indicate an intact cranial nerve I.**

14. 1. This is an inaccurate statement.
    2. The elderly client usually requires less pain medication because of the effects of the normal aging process of the liver (metabolism) and renal (excretion) system.
    3. **Decreased reaction to painful stimuli is a normal developmental change; therefore, complaints of pain may be more serious than the client's perception might indicate and thus such complaints require careful evaluation.**
    4. The Wong scale is used to assess pain for the pediatric client, not the adult client.

15. 1. The client should be in the sitting position during a sensory assessment.
    2. **The eyes are closed so that tactile, superficial pain, vibration, and position sense (proprioception) can be assessed without the client seeing what the nurse is doing.**
    3. The sensory assessment can be conducted at the bedside; there is no reason to take the client to the treatment room.
    4. There is no reason the lights should be off during the sensory assessment; the client should close his or her eyes.

16. 1. Vertigo and otorrhea are not the signs/symptoms of an acoustic neuroma.
    2. Neither nystagmus, an involuntary rhythmic movement of the eyes, nor dizziness is a sign of an acoustic neuroma.
    3. Nausea and vomiting are not signs/symptoms of an acoustic neuroma.
    4. **An acoustic neuroma is a slow-growing, benign tumor of cranial nerve VII. It usually arises from the Schwann cells of the vestibular portion of the nerve and results in unilateral hearing loss and tinnitus, with or without vertigo.**

17. 1. This assesses cranial nerve I, the olfactory nerve.

2. This assesses cranial nerve IX, the glossopharyngeal nerve.

3. This assesses cranial nerve II, the optic nerve, along with visual field testing and ophthalmoscopic examination.

4. This assesses cranial nerve X, the vagus nerve.

18. 1. The purpose of aural rehabilitation is to maximize the communication skills of the client who is hearing impaired. It includes auditory training, speech reading, speech training, and the use of hearing aids and hearing guide dogs.

2. A speech therapist may be part of the aural rehabilitation team, but the most important referral is aural rehabilitation.

3. The client may or may not need financial assistance, but the most important referral is aural rehabilitation.

4. The client may or may not need assistance with employment because of hearing loss, but the most important referral is the aural rehabilitation.

19. 1. The client should be aware that eye pain (a sandy sensation and sensitivity to light) will occur with conjunctivitis.

2. Viral conjunctivitis is a highly contagious eye infection. It is easily spread from one person to another; therefore the client should not share personal items.

3. Cold compresses should be placed over the eyes for about ten (10) minutes four (4) to five (5) times a day to soothe the pain.

4. The client must not apply any makeup until the disease is over and should discard all old makeup to help prevent reinfection.

20. 1. Aural fullness or pressure after surgery is caused by residual blood or fluid in the middle ear. This is an expected occurrence after surgery, and the nurse should administer the prescribed analgesic.

2. Hearing in the operated ear may be reduced for several weeks because of edema, accumulation of blood and tissue fluid in the middle ear, and dressings or packing, so this would not be reported to the health-care provider.

3. Vertigo (dizziness) is uncommon after this surgery, but if it occurs the nurse should administer an antiemetic or antivertigo medication and does not need to report it to the health-care provider.

4. The facial nerve, which runs through the middle ear and mastoid, is at risk for injury during mastoid surgery; therefore, a facial paresis should be reported to the health-care provider.

21. 1. Voices in the head may indicate schizophrenia, but it is not a symptom of hearing loss.

2. Fatigue may be the result of straining to hear and a client may tire easily when listening to a conversation. Under these circumstances, the client may become irritable very easily.

3. Loss of self-confidence makes it increasingly difficult for a person who is hearing impaired to make a decision.

4. Often it is not the person with the hearing loss, but a significant other, that notices hearing loss; hearing loss is usually gradual.

5. Many clients who are hearing impaired tend to dominate the conversation because, as long as it is centered on the client, they can control it and are not as likely to be embarrassed by some mistake.

22. 1. The client should not lift, push, or pull objects heavier than 15 pounds; 50 pounds is excessive.

2. The client should avoid lying on the side of the affected eye at night.

3. The eyes must be protected by wearing glasses or metal eye shields at all times following surgery. Very few answer options with "all" will be correct, but if the option involves ensuring safety, it may be the correct option.

4. The client should avoid bending or stooping for an extended period—but not forever.

23. 1. This is an abnormal finding for testing proprioception, or position sense.

2. This is an abnormal finding for assessing superficial pain perception.

3. This is a normal Babinski reflex in an adult client.

4. Stereognosis is a test that evaluates higher cortical sensory ability. The client is instructed to close both eyes and identify a variety of objects (e.g., keys, coins) that are placed in one hand by the examiner.

24. 1. With normal aging comes decreased peripheral vision, constricted visual field, and tactile alterations. A night light addresses safety issues and would warrant praise, not intervention.

2. As a result of normal aging of the olfactory sense, the client may not smell fire, so smoke alarms address safety for the client and would warrant praise.

3. Decreased peripheral vision, constricted visual fields, and tactile alterations are associated with normal aging. The client needs a familiar arrangement of furniture for safety. Moving the furniture may cause the

client to trip or fall. The nurse should intervene in this situation.
4. As a result of normal aging, vision may become impaired, and the provision of large print books warrants praise.

25. 1. The acuity of taste buds decreases with age, which may cause a decreased appetite and subsequent weight loss. Extra seasoning may help the food taste better to the client.
2. This may be an appropriate intervention if excessive weight is lost or if seasoning the food does not increase appetite, but it is not necessary at this time.
3. The client does not need a dietary consult for food not tasting good. The nurse can address the client's concern.
4. This recommendation does not address the client's comment about food not tasting good.

26. In order of priority: 5, 3, 2, 1, 4
5. The nurse should question the client further to obtain information such as which eye is affected, how long the client been seeing the spots, and whether this ever occurred before.
3. The Amsler grid is helpful in determining losses occurring in the visual fields.
2. The hemoglobin $A1_3$ laboratory tests results indicate glucose control over the past two (2) to three (3) months. Diabetic retinopathy is directly related to poor blood glucose control.
1. The health-care provider should be notified to plan for laser surgery on the eye.
4. The client should be instructed about controlling blood glucose levels, but this can wait until the immediate situation is resolved or at least until measures to address the potential loss of eyesight have been taken.

# Emergency Nursing

# 15

Nurses in a medical-surgical unit may face emergency situations in the care of their clients. An important concept is shock. A client in shock needs immediate intervention. Other emergency situations occur because of outside factors—bioterrorism, disasters, physical abuse. Nurses must know what to do immediately, when to call a code, and what interventions are needed. In addition, because some emergency situations involve large numbers of people or people who pose a threat, there are specific public health and other governmental agencies that might need to be notified and whose rules must be followed in specific situations.

## KEYWORDS

corrosive
epistaxis
gastric lavage

## ABBREVIATIONS

Arterial Blood Gases (ABGs)
Automated External Defibrillator (AED)
Blood Pressure (BP)
Blood Urea Nitrogen (BUN)
Cardiopulmonary Resuscitation (CPR)
Emergency Department (ED)
Health-Care Provider (HCP)
Intravenous (IV)
Intravenous Piggy Back (IVPB)
Intravenous Push (IVP)
Licensed Practical Nurse (LPN)
Material Safety Data Sheet (MSDS)
Nasogastric Tube (NGT)
Nonsteroidal Anti-Inflammatory Drugs (NSAIDs)
Post-Traumatic Stress Disorder (PTSD)
Pulse (P)
Related To (R/T)
U.S. Environmental Protection Agency (EPA)

## Shock

1. The client diagnosed with hypovolemic shock has a BP of 100/60. Fifteen minutes later the B/P is 88/64. How much narrowing of the client's pulse pressure has occurred between the two readings? _____

2. The client is admitted into the emergency department with diaphoresis, pale, clammy skin, and BP of 120/80. Thirty minutes later the client's B/P is 90/70. Which intervention should the nurse implement first?
   1. Start an IV with an 18-gauge catheter.
   2. Administer dopamine intravenous infusion.
   3. Obtain arterial blood gases (ABGs).
   4. Insert an indwelling urinary catheter.

3. Which assessment data would warrant immediate intervention for the client diagnosed with septic shock?
   1. Vital signs T 100.4°F, P 104, R 26, and BP 102/60.
   2. A white blood cell count of 18,000 mm.
   3. A urinary output of 90 mL in the last four (4) hours.
   4. The client complains of being thirsty.

4. The client diagnosed with septicemia has the following health-care provider orders. Which order has the highest priority?
   1. Provide clear liquid diet.
   2. Initiate IV antibiotic therapy.
   3. Obtain a STAT chest x-ray.
   4. Perform hourly glucometer checks.

5. The client is diagnosed with neurogenic shock. Which signs/symptoms would the nurse assess in this client?
   1. Cool moist skin.
   2. Bradycardia.
   3. Wheezing.
   4. Decreased bowel sounds.

6. The nurse in the emergency department administered an intramuscular antibiotic in the left gluteal muscle to the client with pneumonia who is being discharged home. Which intervention should the nurse implement?
   1. Ask the client about drug allergies.
   2. Obtain a sterile sputum specimen.
   3. Have the client wait for 30 minutes.
   4. Place a warm washcloth on the client's left hip.

7. The nurse caring for a client with sepsis writes the client diagnosis of "alteration in comfort R/T chills and fever." Which intervention should be included in the plan of care?
   1. Ambulate the client in the hallway every shift.
   2. Monitor urinalysis, creatinine level, and BUN levels.
   3. Apply sequential compression devices to the lower extremities.
   4. Administer an antipyretic medication every four (4) hours PRN.

8. The nurse and an unlicensed assistive personnel member are caring for a group of clients on a medical floor. Which action by the assistant would warrant immediate intervention by the nurse?
   1. The assistant places a urine specimen in a biohazard bag in the hallway.
   2. The assistant uses the alcohol foam hand cleanser after removing gloves.
   3. The assistant puts soiled linen in a plastic bag in the client's room.
   4. The assistant obtains a disposable stethoscope for a client in an isolation room.

9. The elderly female client with vertebral fractures who has been self-medicating with ibuprofen, a nonsteroidal anti-inflammatory drug (NSAID), presents to the emergency department complaining of abdominal pain; is pale, clammy, and has a P 110 and a BP of 92/60. Which type of shock would the nurse suspect?
   1. Cardiogenic shock.
   2. Hypovolemic shock.
   3. Neurogenic shock.
   4. Septic shock.

10. The client has recently experienced a myocardial infarction. Which action by the nurse would help prevent cardiogenic shock?
    1. Monitor the client's telemetry.
    2. Turn the client every two (2) hours.
    3. Administer oxygen via nasal cannula.
    4. Place the client in the Trendelenburg position.

11. The client diagnosed with septicemia is receiving a broad-spectrum antibiotic. Which laboratory data require the nurse to notify the health-care provider?
    1. The client's potassium level is 3.8 mEq/L.
    2. The urine culture indicates high sensitivity to the antibiotic.
    3. The client's pulse oximeter reading is 94%.
    4. The culture and sensitivity is resistant to the client's antibiotic.

12. The client diagnosed with septic shock has hypotension, decreased urine output, and cool, pale skin. Which phase of septic shock is the client experiencing?
    1. The hypodynamic phase.
    2. The compensatory phase.
    3. The hyperdynamic phase.
    4. The progressive phase.

## Bioterrorism

13. The nurse in the emergency department has admitted five (5) clients in the last two (2) hours with complaints of fever and gastrointestinal distress. Which question would be most appropriate for the nurse to ask each client to determine if there is a bioterrorism threat?
    1. "Do you work or live near any large power lines?"
    2. "Where were you immediately before you got sick?"
    3. "Can you write down everything you ate today?"
    4. "What other health problems do you have?"

14. The health-care facility has been notified that an alleged inhalation anthrax exposure has occurred at the local post office. Which category of personal protective equipment (PPE) would the response team wear?
    1. Level A
    2. Level B
    3. Level C
    4. Level D

15. The nurse is teaching a class on bioterrorism and is discussing personal protective equipment (PPE). Which statement is the most important fact that must be shared with the participants?
    1. Health-care facilities should keep masks at entry doors.
    2. The respondent should be trained in the proper use of PPE.
    3. No single combination of PPE protects against all hazards.
    4. The EPA has divided PPE into four levels of protection.

16. The nurse is teaching a class on bioterrorism. What is the scientific rationale for designating a specific area for decontamination?
    1. Showers and privacy can be provided to the client in this area.
    2. This area isolates the clients who have been exposed to the agent.
    3. It provides a centralized area for stocking the needed supplies.
    4. It prevents secondary contamination to the health-care providers.

17. The triage nurse in a large trauma center has been notified of an explosion in a major chemical manufacturing plant. Which action should the nurse implement first when the clients arrive at the emergency department?
    1. Triage the clients and send them to the appropriate areas.
    2. Thoroughly wash the clients with soap and water and then rinse.
    3. Remove the clients' clothing and have them shower.
    4. Assume the clients have been decontaminated at the plant.

18. The nurse is teaching a class on biological warfare. Which information should the nurse include in the presentation?
    1. Contaminated water is the only source of transmission of biological agents.
    2. Vaccines are available and being prepared to counteract biological agents.
    3. Biological weapons are less of a threat than chemical agents.
    4. Biological weapons are easily obtained and result in significant mortality.

19. Which signs/symptoms would the nurse assess in the client who has been exposed to the anthrax bacillus via the skin?
    1. A scabby, clear fluid–filled vesicle.
    2. Edema, pruritus, and a 2-mm ulcerated vesicle.
    3. Irregular brownish-pink spots around the hairline.
    4. Tiny purple spots flush with the surface of the skin.

20. The client has expired secondary to smallpox. Which information about funeral arrangements is most important for the nurse to provide to the client's family?
    1. The client must be cremated.
    2. Suggest an open casket funeral.
    3. Bury the client within 24 hours.
    4. Notify the public health department.

21. A chemical exposure has just occurred at an airport. An off-duty nurse, knowledgeable about biochemical agents, is giving directions to the travelers. Which direction should the nurse provide to the travelers?
    1. Hold their breath as much as possible.
    2. Stand up to avoid heavy exposure.
    3. Lie down to stay under the exposure.
    4. Attempt to breathe through their clothing.

22. The nurse is caring for a client in the prodromal phase of radiation exposure. Which signs/symptoms would the nurse assess in the client?
    1. Anemia, leukopenia, and thrombocytopenia.
    2. Sudden fever, chills, and enlarged lymph nodes.
    3. Nausea, vomiting, and diarrhea.
    4. Flaccid paralysis, diplopia, and dysphagia.

23. Which cultural issues should the nurse consider when caring for clients during a bioterrorism attack?
    1. Language difficulties.
    2. Religious practices.
    3. Prayer times for the people.
    4. Rituals for handling the dead.
    5. Keeping the family in the designated area.

24. The off-duty nurse hears on the television of a bioterrorism act in the community. Which action should the nurse take first?
    1. Immediately report to the hospital emergency room.
    2. Call the American Red Cross to find out where to go.
    3. Pack a bag and prepare to stay at the hospital.
    4. Follow the nurse's hospital policy for responding.

## Codes

25. The nurse finds the client unresponsive on the floor of the bathroom. Which action should the nurse implement first?
    1. Check the client for breathing.
    2. Assess the carotid artery for a pulse.
    3. Shake the client and shout.
    4. Call a code via the bathroom call light.

26. Which behavior by the unlicensed assistive personnel who is performing cardiac compressions on an adult client during a code warrants immediate intervention by the nurse?
    1. Has one hand on the lower half of the sternum above the xiphoid process.
    2. Performs cardiac compressions and allows for rescue breathing.
    3. Depresses the sternum 0.5 to one (1) inch during compressions.
    4. Requests to be relieved from performing compressions because of exhaustion.

27. Which is the most important intervention for the nurse to implement when participating in a code?
    1. Elevate the arm after administering medication.
    2. Maintain sterile technique throughout the code.
    3. Treat the client's signs/symptoms; do not watch the monitor.
    4. Be sure to provide accurate documentation of what happened in the code.

28. The CPR instructor is explaining what an automated external defibrillator (AED) does to students in a CPR class. Which statement best describes an AED?
    1. It analyzes the rhythm and shocks the client in ventricular fibrillation.
    2. The client will be able to have synchronized cardioversion with the AED.
    3. It will keep the health-care provider informed of the client's oxygen level.
    4. The AED will perform cardiac compressions on the client.

29. The nurse is caring for clients on a medical floor. Which client is most likely to experience sudden cardiac death?
    1. The 84-year-old client exhibiting uncontrolled atrial fibrillation.
    2. The 60-year-old client exhibiting asymptomatic sinus bradycardia.
    3. The 53-year-old client exhibiting ventricular fibrillation.
    4. The 65-year-old client exhibiting supraventricular tachycardia.

30. Which health-care team member referral should be made when a code is being conducted on a client in a community hospital?
    1. The hospital chaplain.
    2. The social worker.
    3. The respiratory therapist.
    4. The director of nurses.

31. Which intervention is the most important for the nurse to implement when performing mouth-to-mouth resuscitation on a client who has pulseless ventricular fibrillation?
    1. Perform the jaw thrust maneuver to open the airway.
    2. Use the mouth to cover the client's mouth and nose.
    3. Insert an oral airway prior to performing mouth to mouth.
    4. Use a pocket mouth shield to cover client's mouth.

32. The nurse is teaching CPR to a class. Which statement best explains the definition of sudden cardiac death?
    1. Cardiac death occurs after being removed from a mechanical ventilator.
    2. Cardiac death is the time that the physician officially declares the client dead.
    3. Cardiac death occurs within one (1) hour of the onset of cardiovascular symptoms.
    4. The death is caused by myocardial ischemia resulting from coronary artery disease.

33. Which statement explains the scientific rationale for having emergency suction equipment available during resuscitation efforts?
    1. Gastric distention can occur as a result of ventilation.
    2. It is needed to assist when intubating the client.
    3. This equipment will ensure a patent airway.
    4. It keeps the vomitus away from the health-care provider.

34. Which equipment must be immediately brought to the client's bedside when a code is called for a client who has experienced a cardiac arrest?
    1. A ventilator.
    2. A crash cart.
    3. A gurney.
    4. Portable oxygen.

35. The nursing administrator responds to a code situation. When assessing the situation, which role must the administrator ensure is performed for legal purposes and continuity of care of the client?
    1. A person is ventilating with an ambu bag.
    2. A person is performing chest compressions correctly.
    3. A person is administering medications as ordered.
    4. A person is keeping an accurate record of the code.

36. The client in a code is now in ventricular bigeminy. The HCP orders a lidocaine drip at three (3) mg/min. The lidocaine comes prepackaged two (2) grams of lidocaine in 500 mL D5W. At what rate will the nurse set the infusion pump?_____

## Disasters/Triage

37. Which situation would warrant the nurse obtaining information from a material safety data sheet (MSDS)?
    1. The custodian spilled a chemical solvent in the hallway.
    2. A visitor slipped and fell on the floor that had just been mopped.
    3. A bottle of antineoplastic agent broke on the client's floor.
    4. The nurse was stuck with a contaminated needle in the client's room.

38. The triage nurse is working in the emergency department. Which client should be assessed first?
    1. The 10-year-old child whose dad thinks the child's leg is broken.
    2. The 45-year-old male who is diaphoretic and clutching his chest.
    3. The 58-year-old female complaining of a headache and seeing spots.
    4. The 25-year-old male who cut his hand with a hunting knife.

39. The nurse is teaching a class on disaster preparedness. Which are components of an Emergency Operations Plan (EOP)? Select all that apply.
    1. A plan for practice drills.
    2. A deactivation response.
    3. A plan for internal communication only.
    4. A pre-incident response.
    5. A security plan.

40. According to the North Atlantic Treaty Organization (NATO) triage system, which situation would be considered a level red (Priority 1)?
    1. Injuries are extensive and chances of survival are unlikely.
    2. Injuries are minor and treatment can be delayed hours to days.
    3. Injuries are significant but can wait hours without threat to life or limb.
    4. Injuries are life threatening but survivable with minimal interventions.

41. Which statement best describes the role of the medical-surgical nurse during a disaster?
    1. The nurse may be assigned to ride in the ambulance.
    2. The nurse may be assigned as a first assistant in the operating room.
    3. The nurse may be assigned to crowd control.
    4. The nurse may be assigned to the emergency department.

42. The nurse in a disaster is triaging the following clients. Which client would be triaged as an Expectant Category, Priority 4, and color black?
    1. The client with a sucking chest wound who is alert.
    2. The client with a head injury who is unresponsive.
    3. The client with an abdominal wound and stable vital signs.
    4. The client with a sprained ankle that may be fractured.

43. Which federal agency would be a resource for the nurse volunteering at the American Red Cross who is on a committee to prepare the community for any type of disaster?
    1. Joint Commission on Accreditation of Healthcare Organizations (JCAHO).
    2. Office of Emergency Management (OEM).
    3. Department of Health and Human Services (DHHS).
    4. Metro Medical Response Systems (MMRS).

44. Which situation would require the emergency department manager to schedule and conduct a Critical Incident Stress Management (CISM)?
    1. Caring for a two (2)-year-old child who died from severe physical abuse.
    2. Performing CPR on a middle-aged male executive who died.
    3. Participating in a 22-victim bus accident with no apparent fatalities.
    4. Being required to work 16 hours without taking a break.

45. During a disaster, a local news reporter comes to the emergency department requesting information about the victims. Which action would be most appropriate for the nurse to implement?
    1. Have security escort the reporter off the premises.
    2. Direct the reporter to the disaster command post.
    3. Tell the reporter that this is a violation of HIPAA.
    4. Request the reporter to stay out of the way.

46. The triage nurse has placed a disaster tag on the client. Which action would warrant immediate intervention by the nurse?
    1. The nurse documents the tag number in the disaster log.
    2. The unlicensed nursing assistant documents vital signs on the tag.
    3. The health-care provider removes the tag to examine the limb.
    4. The LPN securely attaches the tag to the client's foot.

47. The father of a child brought to the emergency department is yelling at the staff and obviously intoxicated. Which approach should the nurse take with the father?
    1. Talk to the father in a calm and low voice.
    2. Tell the father to wait in the waiting room.
    3. Notify the child's mother to come to the ED.
    4. Call the police department to come and arrest him.

48. A gang war has resulted in 12 young males being brought to the emergency department. Which action by the nurse is priority when a gang member points a gun at a rival gang member in the trauma room?
    1. Attempt to talk to the person who has the gun.
    2. Explain to the person that the police are coming.
    3. Stand between the client and the man with the gun.
    4. Get out of the line of fire and protect self.

## Poisoning

49. The parents of a toddler bring the child to the emergency department in a panic. The parents state the child had been playing in the kitchen and got into some cleaning agents and has swallowed an unknown quantity of the agents. Which health-care agency should the nurse contact at this time?
    1. Child Protective Services (CPS).
    2. The local police department.
    3. The Department of Health.
    4. The Poison Control Center.

50. Which is the primary goal of the ED nurse in caring for a client who has ingested poison?
    1. Remove or inactivate the poison before it is absorbed.
    2. Provide long-term supportive care to prevent organ damage.
    3. Administer an antidote to increase the effects of the poison.
    4. Implement treatment that prolongs the elimination of the poison.

51. The client has ingested a corrosive solution containing lye. Which intervention should the nurse implement?
    1. Administer syrup of ipecac to induce vomiting.
    2. Insert a nasogastric tube and connect to wall suction.
    3. Assess for airway compromise.
    4. Immediately administer water or milk.

52. The male client was found in a parked car with the motor running. The paramedics brought the client to the ED. In the ED the client complains of a headache, nausea, and dizziness and is not able to tell the ED nurse his name or address. On assessment the nurse notes the buccal mucosa is a cherry-red color. Which should the nurse implement first?
    1. Check the client's oxygenation level with a pulse oximeter.
    2. Apply oxygen via nasal cannula at 100%.
    3. Obtain a psychiatric consult to determine if this was a suicide attempt.
    4. Prepare the client for transfer to a facility with a hyperbaric chamber.

53. A gastric lavage has been ordered for a client who is comatose and who ingested a full bottle of acetaminophen, a nonnarcotic analgesic. Which should be included in the procedure? Select all that apply.
    1. Place the client on the left side with the head 15 degrees lower than the body.
    2. Insert a small bore feeding tube into the nare.
    3. Have standby suction available.
    4. Withdraw all stomach contents and then instill an irrigating solution.
    5. Send samples of the stomach contents to the lab for analysis.

54. A vat of chemicals spilled onto the client. Which action should the occupational health nurse implement first?
    1. Have the client stand under a shower while removing all clothes.
    2. Check the Material Safety Data Sheets for the antidote.
    3. Administer oxygen by nasal cannula.
    4. Collect a sample of the chemicals in the vat for analysis.

55. The client presents to the ED with acute vomiting after eating at a fast-food restaurant. There has not been any diarrhea. The nurse suspects botulism poisoning. Which nursing problem is the highest priority for this client?
    1. Fluid volume loss.
    2. Risk for respiratory paralysis.
    3. Abdominal pain.
    4. Anxiety.

56. The client has ingested the remaining amount of a bottle of analgesic medication. The medication comes 500 mg per capsule. Two (2) doses of two (2) capsules each have been used by another member of the family. The bottle originally had 250 capsules. How many mg of medication did the client take?_____

57. The nurse is providing first aid to a victim of a poisonous snakebite. Which should be the nurse's first action?
    1. Apply a tourniquet to the affected limb.
    2. Cut an X in across the bite and suck out the venom.
    3. Administer a corticosteroid medication.
    4. Have the client lie still and remove constrictive items.

58. The nurse is discharging a client diagnosed with accidental carbon monoxide poisoning. Which statement made by the client indicates the need for further teaching?
    1. "I should install carbon monoxide detectors in my home."
    2. "Having a natural bright-red color to my lips is good."
    3. "You cannot smell carbon monoxide, so it can be difficult to detect."
    4. "I should have my furnace checked for leaks before turning it on."

59. The nurse and unlicensed assistive personnel are caring for clients on a medical unit. Which nursing task cannot be delegated to the assistant?
    1. Obtaining the intake and output on a client diagnosed with food poisoning.
    2. Performing a dressing change on the client with a chemical burn.
    3. Assisting a client who overdosed on morphine to the bedside commode.
    4. Help a client with carbon monoxide poisoning turn, cough, and deep breathe.

60. The charge nurse is making assignments. Which client should be assigned to the most experienced nurse?
    1. The client diagnosed with a snakebite who is receiving antivenin.
    2. The client who swallowed a lye preparation and is being discharged.
    3. The client who is angry that the suicide attempt did not work.
    4. The client who required skin grafting after a chemical spill.

## Violence, Physical Abuse, and Neglect

61. The female client presents to the emergency department with facial lacerations and contusions. The spouse will not leave the room during the assessment interview. Which intervention should be the nurse's first action?
    1. Call the security guard to escort the spouse away.
    2. Discuss the injuries while the spouse is in the room.
    3. Tell the spouse that the police will want to talk to him.
    4. Escort the client to the bathroom for a urine specimen.

62. The elderly male client is admitted to the medical unit with a diagnosis of senile dementia. The client is 74 inches tall and weighs 54.5 kg. The client lives with his son and daughter-in-law, both of whom work outside the house. Which referral would be the most important for the nurse to implement?
    1. Adult Protective Services.
    2. Social worker.
    3. Medicare ombudsman.
    4. Dietitian.

63. The nurse working in a homeless shelter identifies an adolescent female that is sexually aggressive toward some of the males in the shelter. Which is the most common cause for this behavior?
    1. The client is acting in a learned behavior pattern to get attention.
    2. The client had to leave home because of promiscuous behavior.
    3. The client has a psychiatric disorder called nymphomania.
    4. The client is a prostitute and is trying to get customers.

64. The adolescent female comes to the school nurse of an intermediate school and tells the nurse she thinks she is pregnant. During the interview the client states that her father is the baby's father. Which should the nurse do first?
    1. Complete a rape kit.
    2. Notify Child Protective Services
    3. Call the parents to come to the school.
    4. Arrange for the client to go to a free clinic.

65. The nurse in an outpatient rehabilitation facility is working with convicted child abusers. Which characteristics would the nurse expect to observe in the abusers? Select all that apply.
    1. Calls the child a liar.
    2. Has a tendency toward violence.
    3. Exhibits a high self-esteem.
    4. Is unable to admit the need for help.
    5. Was spoiled as a child.

66. The nurse is teaching a class about rape prevention to a group of women at a community center. Which information is not a myth about rape?
    1. Women who are raped asked for it by dressing provocatively.
    2. If a woman says no, it is a come on and she really does not mean it.
    3. Rape is an attempt to exert power and control over the client.
    4. All victims of sexual assault are women; men can't be raped.

67. The nurse working in the emergency department is admitting a 34-year-old female client for one of multiple admissions for spousal abuse. The client has refused to leave her husband or to press charges against him. Which action should the nurse implement?
    1. Insist that the woman press charges this time.
    2. Treat the wounds and do nothing else.
    3. Tell the woman that her husband could kill her.
    4. Give the woman the number of a woman's shelter.

68. The 84-year-old female client is admitted with multiple burn marks on the torso and under the breasts along with contusions in various stages of healing. When questioned by the nurse the woman denies any problems have occurred. The woman lives with her son and does the housework. Which is the most probable reason the woman denies being abused?
    1. There has not been any abuse to report.
    2. The client is ashamed to admit being abused.
    3. The client has Alzheimer's disease and can't remember.
    4. The client has engaged in consensual sex.

69. Which is an appropriate interview question for the nurse to use with clients involved in abuse?
    1. "I know you are being abused. Can you tell me about it?"
    2. "How much does your spouse drink before he hits you?"
    3. "What did you do that caused your spouse to get mad?"
    4. "Do you have a plan if your partner becomes abusive?"

70. The client who was abused as a child is diagnosed with post-traumatic stress disorder (PTSD). Which intervention should the nurse implement when the client is resting?
    1. Call the client's name to awaken him or her, but don't touch the client.
    2. Touch the client gently to let him or her know you are in the room.
    3. Enter the room as quietly as possible to not disturb the client.
    4. Do not allow the client to be awakened at all when sleeping.

71. The emergency department nurse writes the problem of "ineffective coping" for a client who has been raped. Which intervention should the nurse implement?
    1. Encourage the client to take the "morning after" pill.
    2. Allow the client to admit guilt for causing the rape.
    3. Provide a list of rape crisis counselors.
    4. Discuss reporting the case to the police.

72. The nurse writes a nursing diagnosis of "risk for injury as a result of physical abuse by spouse" for a client. Which would be an appropriate goal for this client?
    1. The client will learn not to trust anyone.
    2. The client will admit the abuse is happening and get help.
    3. The client will discuss the nurse's suspicions with the spouse.
    4. The client will choose to stay with the spouse.

## Shock

1. **16 mm Hg pulse pressure.** The pulse pressure is the systolic B/P minus the diastolic B/P.

    100 − 60 = 40 mm Hg pulse pressure in first B/P reading

    88 − 64 = 24 mm Hg pulse pressure in second reading

    40 − 24 = 16 mm Hg pulse pressure narrowing.

    A narrowing or decreased pulse pressure is an earlier indicator of shock than a decrease in systolic blood pressure.

    **TEST-TAKING HINT: If the test taker is not aware of how to obtain a pulse pressure, the only numbers provided in the stem are systolic and diastolic blood pressures. The test taker should do something with the numbers.**

2. 1. There are many type of shock, but the one common intervention that should be done first in all types of shock is to establish an intravenous line with a large bore catheter. This client has signs and symptoms of shock, and the narrowing pulse pressure indicates the client is getting worse.
    2. This blood pressure would not require dopamine; fluid resuscitation is first.
    3. The client may need ABGs monitored, but this is not the first intervention.
    4. A Foley catheter may need to be inserted for accurate measurement of output, but it is not the first intervention.

    **TEST-TAKING HINT: This question asks for the first intervention, which means that all answer options may be appropriate interventions for the client, but only one should be implemented first.**

3. 1. These vital signs are expected in a client with septic shock.
    2. An elevated WBC count indicates an infection, which is the definition of sepsis.
    3. The client must have a urinary output of at least 30 mL/hr, so 90 mL in the last four (4) hours indicates impaired renal perfusion, which is a sign of worsening shock and warrants immediate intervention.
    4. The client being thirsty would not be an uncommon complaint for a client in septic shock.

    **TEST-TAKING HINT: The words "warrants immediate intervention" mean the nurse must do something, which frequently is notify the health-care provider. Any client in shock will have signs and symptoms requiring the nurse to intervene. In this question the test taker must determine priority and which data require immediate intervention.**

4. 1. The client's diet is not priority when transcribing orders.
    2. An IV antibiotic is the priority medication for the client with an infection, which is the definition of sepsis—a systemic bacterial infection of the blood. A new order for an IV antibiotic should be implemented within one (1) hour of receiving the order.
    3. Diagnostic tests are important but not priority over intervening in a potentially life-threatening situation such as septic shock.
    4. There is no indication that this client has diabetes in the stem of the question, and glucose levels are not associated with signs/symptoms of septicemia.

    **TEST-TAKING HINT: Remember if the test taker can rule out two answers—"1" and "4"—and cannot determine the right answer between "2" and "3," select the option that directly affects or treats the client, which would be the antibiotics. Diagnostic tests do not treat the client.**

5. 1. The client diagnosed with neurogenic shock will have dry, warm skin, rather than cool, moist skin as seen in hypovolemic shock.
    2. The client will have bradycardia instead of tachycardia, which is seen in other forms of shock.
    3. Wheezing would be associated with anaphylactic shock.
    4. Decreased bowel sounds occur in the hyperdynamic phase of septic shock.

    **TEST-TAKING HINT: The test taker should identify the body system that the question is addressing. In this case, the word "neuro" indicates that the question relates to the neurological system. With this information only, the test taker could possibly rule out "4," which refers to the gastrointestinal system, and "3," which refers to the respiratory system. Although bradycardia is in the cardiac system, the pulse rate is controlled by the brain.**

6. 1. It is too late to ask the client about drug allergies because the medication has already been administered.
    2. Obtaining a specimen after the antibiotic has been initiated will skew the culture and sensitivity results. It must be obtained before the antibiotic is started.
    3. Any time a nurse administers a medication for the first time, the client should be observed for a possible anaphylactic reaction, especially with antibiotics.
    4. The client is being discharged and the nurse can encourage the client to do this at home,

but it would not be appropriate to do in the emergency room

**TEST-TAKING HINT:** The test taker must be observant of information in the stem. The nurse has already administered the medication and checking for allergies after the fact will not affect the client's outcome. This is a violation of the five (5) rights; this medication cannot be the right medication if the client is allergic to it.

7. 1. Ambulating the client in the hall will not address the etiology of the client's chills and fever; in fact, this could increase the client's discomfort.
2. Monitoring these lab data does not address the etiology of the client's diagnosis.
3. Sequential compression devices help prevent deep vein thrombosis.
4. Antipyretic medication will help decrease the client's fever, which directly addresses the etiology of the client's nursing diagnosis.

**TEST-TAKING HINT:** The test taker must know that the problem "alteration in comfort" is addressed by the goal and the interventions address the etiology, which is "chills and fever."

8. 1. Specimens should be put into biohazard bags prior to leaving the client's room.
2. This is the appropriate way to clean hands and does not warrant intervention.
3. This is the appropriate way to dispose of soiled linens and does not warrant intervention.
4. Taking a stethoscope from a client who is in isolation to another room is a violation of infection-control principles.

**TEST-TAKING HINT:** This is an "except" question. The stem is asking which action warrants intervention; therefore the test taker must select the option that indicates inappropriate action by the unlicensed assistant.

9. 1. Cardiogenic shock occurs when the heart's ability to contract and pump blood is impaired and the supply of oxygen to the heart and tissues is inadequate, such as occurs in myocardial infarction or valvular damage.
2. This client's signs/symptoms would make the nurse suspect the client is losing blood, which leads to hypovolemic shock, which is the most common type of shock and is characterized by decreased intravascular volume. The client's taking of NSAID medications puts her at risk for hemorrhage because NSAIDs inhibit prostaglandin production in the stomach, which

increases the risk of developing ulcers, which can erode the stomach lining and lead to hemorrhaging.
3. In neurogenic shock, vasodilation occurs as a result of a loss of sympathetic tone. It can result from the depressant action of medication or lack of glucose.
4. Septic shock is a type of circulatory shock caused by widespread infection.

**TEST-TAKING HINT:** The test taker must look at the signs and symptoms and realize this client is in shock. Tachycardia and hypotension with clammy skin indicate shock. The additional information in the stem describes a particular medication, NSAID, which can cause stomach ulcers (abdominal pain).

10. 1. Monitoring the telemetry will not prevent cardiogenic shock. It might help identify changes in the hemodynamics of the heart, but it would not prevent anything from occurring.
2. Turning the client every two (2) hours will help prevent pressure ulcers, but it will do nothing to prevent cardiogenic shock.
3. Promoting adequate oxygenation of the heart muscle and decreasing the cardiac workload can prevent cardiogenic shock.
4. Placing the client's head below the heart will not prevent cardiogenic shock. This position can be used when a client is in hypovolemic shock.

**TEST-TAKING HINT:** If the test taker has no idea what the correct answer is, the test taker should apply Maslow's Hierarchy of Needs, which states oxygenation is most important. The nurse must know positions that the client may be put in during different disorders and diseases.

11. 1. This is a normal potassium level (3.5–5.5 mEq/L); therefore, the nurse would not need to notify the HCP.
2. A culture that shows high sensitivity to an antibiotic indicates this is exactly the antibiotic the client should be receiving.
3. A pulse oximeter reading of greater than 93% indicates the client is adequately oxygenated.
4. A sensitivity report that indicates a resistance to the antibiotic being given indicates the medication the client is receiving is not appropriate for the treatment of the infectious organism, and the HCP needs to be notified so that the antibiotic can be changed.

**TEST-TAKING HINT:** The key words in option "2" are "highly sensitive," and this would make the test taker think this is a good thing.

**In option "4" the word "resistant" would indicate something wrong with the antibiotic and would need intervention.**

12. 1. The hypodynamic phase is the last and irreversible phase of septic shock, characterized by low cardiac output with vasoconstriction. It reflects the body's effort to compensate for hypovolemia caused by the loss of intravascular volume through the capillaries.
    2. In the compensatory phase of shock, the heart rate, blood pressure, and respiratory rate are within normal limits, but the skin may be cold and clammy and urinary output may be decreased. However, this is the first phase of all types of shock and is not specific to septic shock.
    3. The hyperdynamic phase, the first phase of septic shock, is characterized by a high cardiac output with systemic vasodilation. The BP may remain within normal limits, but the heart rate increases to tachycardia and the client becomes febrile.
    4. The progressive phase is the second phase of all shocks. It occurs when the systolic BP decreases to less than 80–90 mm Hg, the heart rate increases to greater than 150 beats per minutes, and the skin becomes mottled.

**TEST-TAKING HINT: There are some questions that the test taker must know; they are called knowledge-based questions. The prefix "hypo" is in the stem with "hypodynamics" and matches the "hypo" of "hypotension," and decreased urine output, might help the test taker arrive at an answer.**

## Bioterrorism

13. 1. Power lines would not be a typical source of biological terrorism, which is what these symptoms represent.
    2. The nurse should take note of any unusual illness for the time of year or clusters of clients coming from a single geographical location who all exhibit signs/symptoms of possible biological terrorism.
    3. This might be appropriate for gastroenteritis secondary to food poisoning but is not the nurse's first thought to determine a biological threat. The nurse must determine if the clients have anything in common.
    4. This would be important information to obtain for all clients but is not pertinent to determine a biological threat.

**TEST-TAKING HINT: Answer option "4" is a question that the nurse would ask to all clients; therefore the test taker should eliminate it based on the specific question. Power lines are electrical and most bioterrorism threats involve chemical or biological threats, so option "1" can be eliminated.**

14. 1. Level A protection is worn when the highest level of respiratory, skin, eye, and mucous membrane protection is required. In this situation of possible inhalation of anthrax, such protection is required.
    2. Level B protection is similar to Level A protection, but it is used when a lesser level of skin and eye protection is needed.
    3. Level C protection requires an air-purified respirator (APR), which uses filters or absorbent materials to remove harmful substances.
    4. Level D is basically the work uniform.

**TEST-TAKING HINT: If the test taker was totally unaware of the correct answer, then the choice should be either "1" or "4" because these would be at either end of the spectrum. This gives the test taker a 50/50 chance of selecting the correct answer, instead of a 25% chance.**

15. 1. Masks are kept at designated areas, not at every entry door.
    2. This is a true statement, but it is not the most important information; in an emergency situation the respondent should use the equipment even if not trained.
    3. The health-care providers are not guaranteed absolute protection, even with all the training and protective equipment.
    4. This is a true statement, but it is not the most important statement.

**TEST-TAKING HINT: There are very few questions where the test taker should select an option with the word "all." Option "3" is stating that this is not an "always" situation. The test taker should not automatically assume that it is not a possible answer until understanding the context.**

16. 1. This is not a rationale; this is a statement of what is done at the area.
    2. This separates the clients until decontamination occurs, but the question is asking for the scientific rationale.
    3. This is false statement—the supplies should not be kept in the decontamination area.
    4. Avoiding cross contamination is a priority for personnel and equipment—the fewer number of people exposed, the safer the community and area.

**TEST-TAKING HINT: Options "1" and "2" are not rationales.**

17. 1. In most situations this is the first step, but with a potential chemical or biological exposure the first step must be the safety of the hospital; therefore the client must be decontaminated.
2. This is the second step in the decontamination process.
3. **This is the first step. Depending on the type of exposure, this step alone can remove a large portion of exposure.**
4. This assumption could cost many people in the hospital staff, as well as clients, their lives.

**TEST-TAKING HINT: If the test taker wants to select option "4" as the correct answer, be careful—assumptions are dangerous. The test taker may want to choose option "1" because it involves assessment, which is the first step of the nursing process, but the individual situation has to be evaluated. Bioterrorism violates many of the accepted rules.**

18. 1. Sources of biological agents include inhalation, insects, animals, and people.
2. The only known vaccine against a possible bioterrorism agent is the smallpox vaccine, which is not available in quantities sufficient to inoculate the public.
3. Because of the vast range of agents, biological weapons are more of a threat. A biological agent could be released in one city and affect people in other cities thousands of miles away.
4. **Because of the variety of agents, the means of transmission, and lethality of the agents, biological weapons, including anthrax, smallpox, and plague, are especially dangerous.**

**TEST-TAKING HINT: Answer option "1" should be eliminated because of the word "only." Even if the test taker has little knowledge of biological warfare, knowledge of the human body would suggest a wide range of ways biological agents could be transmitted.**

19. 1. Scabby, clear fluid–filled vesicles are characteristic of chickenpox.
2. **Exposure to anthrax bacilli via the skin results in skin lesions, which cause edema with pruritus and the formation of macules or papules that ulcerate, forming a one (1)- to (3)-mm vesicle. Then a painless eschar develops, which falls off in one (1) to two (2) weeks.**
3. Irregular brownish-pink spots around the hairline are characteristic of rubella.

4. Tiny purple spots flush with the skin surface are petechiae.

**TEST-TAKING HINT: This is a knowledge-based question. The test taker should try to determine which skin disease each answer option describes to rule out the incorrect answers.**

20. 1. **Cremation is recommended because the virus can stay alive in the scabs of the body for 13 years.**
2. An open casket might allow for the spread of the virus to the general public; therefore the nurse would not make this suggestion. The nurse should not tell the client's family how to make funeral arrangement for viewing.
3. Burying the body quickly would be the second best option for safety of the funeral home personnel and anyone who could come in contact with the body. The quicker the burial, the safer the situation (if the family refuses cremation).
4. The hospital, not the client's family, must notify the public health department.

**TEST-TAKING HINT: Option "4" could be eliminated because the test taker should know that the hospital staff, not family members, must make notifications to public health departments. The test taker should apply basic concepts when answering questions. Infection-control concepts would eliminate option "2" because an open casket would allow for spread of the virus.**

21. 1. The absence of breathing is death, and this is neither a viable option nor a sensible recommendation to terrified people.
2. **Standing up will avoid heavy exposure because the chemical will sink toward the floor or ground.**
3. Staying below the level of the smoke is the instruction for a fire.
4. Breathing through the clothing, which is probably contaminated with the chemical, will not provide protection from the chemical entering the lung.

**TEST-TAKING HINT: If the test taker does not know the answer, the test taker should realize that options "1" and "4" address breathing and options "2" and "3" address positioning and that one set of options should be eliminated, narrowing the choice to one (1) out of two (2) options. Therefore the test taker must choose between one of the sets when attempting to select the correct answer. Option "3" is pretty well known for fires, and holding one's breath, option "1," really doesn't make sense.**

22. 1. Anemia, leukopenia, and thrombocytopenia, signs of bone marrow depression, are signs/symptoms the client would experience in the latent phase of radiation exposure, which occurs from 72 hours to years after exposure. The client is usually asymptomatic in the prodromal phase of radiation exposure.
2. Sudden fever, chills, and enlarged lymph nodes are signs/symptoms of bubonic plague.
3. The prodromal phase (presenting symptoms) of radiation exposure occurs 48–72 hours after exposure and the signs/symptoms are nausea, vomiting, diarrhea, anorexia, and fatigue. Higher exposures of radiation signs/symptoms include fever, respiratory distress, and excitability.
4. These are signs/symptoms of inhalation botulism.

**TEST-TAKING HINT:** If the test taker knows the definition of "prodromal," which is an early sign of a developing condition or disease ("prodrom" is Greek for running before), then the option with vague and nonspecific signs/symptoms should be selected as the correct answer.

23. 1. Language difficulties can increase fear and frustration on the part of the client.
2. Some religions have specific practices related to medical treatments, hygiene, and diet and these should be honored if at all possible.
3. Prayers in time of grief and disaster are important to an individual and actually can have a calming affect on the situation.
4. Caring for the dead is as important as caring for the living based on religious beliefs.
5. For purposes of organization this may be needed, but it is not addressing cultural sensitivity and in some instances may violate cultural needs of the client and the family.

**TEST-TAKING HINT:** The stem asks the test taker to address cultural needs, and these are universal—in a bioterrorism attack or with an individual in the hospital. The test taker should select options addressing cultural needs. Dishonoring cultural needs can increase the client's anxiety and increase problems for the health-care team.

24. 1. Many hospital procedures mandate that off-duty nurses not report immediately so that relief can be provided for initial responders.
2. The nurse's first responsibility is to the facility of employment, not the community.
3. This is a good action to take when the nurse is notified of the next action. If, for example, the hospital is quarantined, the nurse may not report for days.

4. The nurse should follow the hospital's policy. Many times nurses will stay at home until decisions are made as to where the employees should report.

**TEST-TAKING HINT:** After looking at all the options the test taker should select the option that best assesses the entire situation, which would be following policy. There will be a tendency for mass hysteria to occur in the community, but following the terrorist attack on 9/11 all hospitals and communities are required by Homeland Security to have a disaster preparedness plan in place. The best action the nurse can take is follow the procedure and remain calm.

## Codes

25. 1. This is the third intervention based on the answer options available in this question.
2. This is the fourth intervention based on the options available in this question.
3. This is the first intervention the nurse should implement after finding the client unresponsive on the floor.
4. This is the second intervention based on the options available in this question.

**TEST-TAKING HINT:** Options "1," "2," and "3" are all assessment interventions, which is the first step in the nursing process. Of these three (3) possible options the test taker should select the intervention that is the easiest and fastest to determine if the client is alert, which is to shake and shout at the client.

26. 1. This hand position will help prevent positioning the hand over the xiphoid process, which can break the ribs and lacerate the liver during compressions.
2. This is the correct two-rescuer CPR; therefore no intervention is needed.
3. The sternum should be depressed 1.5 to 2 inches during compressions to ensure adequate circulation of blood to the body; therefore, the nurse needs to correct the assistant.
4. The assistant should request another health-care provider to perform compressions when exhausted.

**TEST-TAKING HINT:** The test taker must select which option is an incorrect procedure for cardiac compressions.

27. 1. This is an appropriate intervention, but it is not the most important.
2. Sterile technique should be maintained as much as possible, but the nurse can treat a live

body with an infection without using sterile technique, but the nurse cannot treat a dead body without an infection.

3. This is the most important intervention. The nurse should always treat the client based on the nurse's assessment and data from the monitors; an intervention should not be based on data from the monitors without the nurse's assessment.

4. Documentation is important but not priority over treating the client.

**TEST-TAKING HINT: The phrase "most important intervention" in the stem is the key to answering this question. All four (4) answer options are appropriate interventions for the question, but only one (1) is the most important. Remember to always select the option that directly affects the client, and this may mean not selecting an assessment intervention.**

28. 1. This is the correct statement explaining what an AED does when used in a code.
2. The Life Pack on the crash cart must be used to perform synchronized cardioversion.
3. This is the explanation for a pulse oximeter.
4. This is not the function of the AED.

**TEST-TAKING HINT: The test taker must know about equipment to be able to answer this question. The test taker may be able to eliminate options based on knowledge of what other equipment does.**

29. 1. Atrial fibrillation is not a life-threatening dysrhythmia; it is chronic.
2. Asymptomatic sinus bradycardia may be normal for the client, especially for athletes or long-distance runners.
3. Ventricular fibrillation is the most common dysrhythmia associated with sudden cardiac death; ventricular fibrillation is responsible for 65% to 85% of sudden cardiac deaths.
4. "Supraventricular" means "above the ventricle." The atrium is above the ventricle, and atrial dysrhythmias are not life threatening.

**TEST-TAKING HINT: The test taker should know that the left ventricle is responsible for pumping blood to the body (heart muscle and brain) and could eliminate options "1" and "4" as correct answers. The word "asymptomatic" should cause the test taker to eliminate "2" as the correct answer.**

30. 1. The chaplain should be called to help address the client's family or significant others. A small community hospital would not have a 24-hour on-duty pastoral service.

2. The social worker does not need to be notified of a code.
3. The respiratory therapist responds to the code automatically without a referral. The respiratory therapist is part of the code team and one (1) is on duty 24 hours a day, even in a small community hospital.
4. The director of nurses does not need to be notified of codes, but possibly the house supervisor should be notified.

**TEST-TAKING HINT: The test taker must know the role of the multidisciplinary health-care team and make appropriate referrals. The words "small community hospital" is an important phrase to help determine the correct answer.**

31. 1. A jaw thrust is used for a possible fractured neck. The nurse should use the head-tilt, chin-lift maneuver to open the airway.
2. The nurse should cover the client's mouth and nose with the nurse's mouth when giving mouth-to-mouth resuscitation to an infant but not when giving mouth-to-mouth resuscitation to an adult.
3. An oral airway is not mandatory to do effective breathing; therefore, it is not the most important intervention.
4. Nurses should protect themselves against possible communicable disease, such as HIV, hepatitis, or any types of sexually transmitted disease.

**TEST-TAKING HINT: Unless the stem provides an age for the client, the client is an adult client; therefore, the test taker could eliminate option "2" because it is for an infant.**

32. 1. This is not the definition of sudden cardiac death; this is sometimes known "as pulling the plug" on clients who are diagnosed as brain dead.
2. This is not the definition of sudden cardiac death.
3. Unexpected death occurring within one (1) hour of the onset of cardiovascular symptoms is the definition of sudden cardiac death.
4. This is not the definition of sudden cardiac death.

**TEST-TAKING HINT: If the test taker relates the word "sudden" with "unexpected," the best answer is option "3." The test taker must be aware of adjectives and adverbs.**

33. 1. Gastric distention occurs from overventilating clients. When compressions are performed, the pressure will cause vomiting that could be aspirated into the lungs.

2. The health-care provider does not require suctioning equipment to intubate.

3. Nothing ensures a patent airway, except a correctly inserted ET tube, and suction is needed to clear the airway.

4. Suction equipment is for the client's needs, not the health-care provider's needs.

**TEST-TAKING HINT: Answer option "4" could be eliminated because the equipment is for the client, not for the nurse or health-care providers. The word "ensures" is an absolute word, so the test taker should be cautious before selecting that option.**

34. 1. A ventilator is not kept on the medical-surgical floors and is not routinely brought to the bedside. The client is manually ventilated until arriving in the intensive care unit.

   2. **The crash cart is the mobile unit that has the defibrillator and all the medications and supplies needed to conduct a code.**

   3. The gurney, a stretcher, may be needed when the client is being transferred to another unit, but it is not an immediate need, and in some hospitals the client is transferred in the bed.

   4. Oxygen is available in the room and portable oxygen is on the crash cart, so it doesn't need to be brought separately.

**TEST-TAKING HINT: This is knowledge that the test taker must have. It is the primary piece of equipment and in most facilities there is a person assigned to bring the crash cart to the client's bedside.**

35. 1. This is providing immediate direct care to the client and is not performed for legal purposes.

   2. This is providing immediate direct care to the client and is not performed for legal purposes.

   3. This is providing immediate direct care to the client and is not performed for legal purposes. This is an occasion where someone else is allowed to document another nurse's medication administration.

   4. **The chart is a legal document and the code must be documented in the chart and provide information that may be needed in the intensive care unit.**

**TEST-TAKING HINT: Answer options "1," "2," and "3" have the nurse providing direct hands-on care. Option "4" is the only option that discusses documentation and should be selected as the correct answer because it is different.**

36. **45 mL/hr.** The test taker could remember the mnemonic, which is "For 1 mg, 2 mg, 3 mg, 4 mg is 15 mL, 30 mL, 45 mL, 60 mL." If the test taker has not memorized it, it is too late to figure it out in an emergency situation. But for math purposes:

First determine the number of mg in the 500 mL D5W.

$$2 \text{ gm} \times 1000 \text{ mg} = 2000 \text{ mg per } 500 \text{ mL}$$

Then determine how many milligrams per milliliters.

$$2000 \text{ mg} \div 500 \text{ mL} = 4 \text{ mg/mL}$$

Then find out how many milliliters must be infused per minute to give the ordered dose of 3 mg/min.

In algebraic terms: 4 mg : 1mL = 3 mg : x mL

Cross multiply and divide: x = 3/4

The number of milliliters to be infused in a minute is 3/4 mL.

The infusion pump is set at an hourly rate, so multiply 3/4 by 60 minutes

$$3/4 \times 60 = 45$$

The pump should be set at 45 mL per hour to infuse three (3) mg/min.

**TEST-TAKING HINT: The test taker must be familiar with basic nursing math and become comfortable with the equations the test taker uses to compute dosage calculations.**

## Disasters/Triage

37. 1. **The MSDS provides chemical information regarding specific agents, health information, and spill information for a variety of chemicals. It is required for every chemical that is found in the hospital.**

   2. This situation would require an occurrence or accident report.

   3. Any facility that administers antineoplastic agents (medications used to treat cancer) is required to have specific chemotherapy spill kits available and a policy and procedure that goes with them; in this situation the nurse already knows the chemical involved.

   4. This requires a hospital variance report and notifying the employee health or infection control nurse.

**TEST-TAKING HINT: If the test taker was not aware of MSDS, the name would tell the test taker to look for content in the answer option addressing materials; therefore options "2" and "4" could be eliminated as possible answers.**

38. 1. The child needs an x-ray to confirm the fracture, but the client is stable and does not have a life-threatening problem.

   2. **The triage nurse should see this client first because these are symptoms of a myocar-**

dial infarction, which is potentially life threatening.

3. These are symptoms of a migraine headache and are not life threatening.

4. A cut hand is priority, but not over a client having a myocardial infarction.

**TEST-TAKING HINT:** The test taker should evaluate each option on a scale of 1–10, with one (1) being the least critical client and ten (10) being life threatening. Option "2" would rate a ten (10).

39. 1. Practice drills allow for troubleshooting any issues before a real-life incident occurs.

2. A deactivation response is important so that resources are not overused, and the facility can then get back to daily activities and routine care.

3. Communication between the facility and external resources and an internal communication plan are critical.

4. A post-incident response is important to include a critique and debriefing for all parties involved; a pre-incident response is the plan itself. Be sure to read adjectives closely.

5. A coordinated security plan involving facility and community agencies is the key to controlling an otherwise chaotic situation.

**TEST-TAKING HINT:** The test taker must notice adjectives such as "only" in "3" and "pre" in "4." These words make these options incorrect. This question requires the test taker to select more than one option as the correct answer.

40. 1. That is a color black or priority 4 and is called expectant.

2. That is a color green or priority 3 and is called minimal.

3. That is a color yellow or priority 2 and is called delayed.

4. This is called the immediate category. Individuals in this group can progress rapidly to expectant if treatment is delayed.

**TEST-TAKING HINT:** This is basically a knowledge-based question, but often the color "red" would indicate a high priority.

41. 1. The nurse would not leave the hospital area; the nurse must wait for the casualties to come to the facility.

2. This is a position that requires knowledge of instruments and procedures that are not common to the medical-surgical floor.

3. The people in this area are usually chaplains or social workers, not direct client care personnel. In a disaster, direct care personnel cannot be spared for this duty.

4. New settings and atypical roles for nurses may be required during disasters; medical-surgical nurses can provide first aid and be required to work in unfamiliar settings.

**TEST-TAKING HINT:** The test taker should look at traditional nursing roles that require nursing expertise and eliminate crowd control or riding in an ambulance.

42. 1. This client would be an Immediate Category, Priority 1, and color red. If not treated STAT, a tension pneumothorax will occur.

2. This client has a very poor prognosis, and even with treatment, survival is unlikely.

3. This client would be a Delayed Category, Priority 2, and color yellow. This client would receive treatment after casualties requiring immediate treatment are treated.

4. This client would be a Minimal Category, Priority 3, and color green. This client can wait days for treatment.

**TEST-TAKING HINT:** If the test taker did not know the definition of the categories, looking at the words "black," which has a connotation of death, and the word "expectant" might lead the test taker to select the worst-case scenario.

43. 1. This organization mandates that all health-care facilities have an emergency operations plan, but it is a national agency, not a federal agency.

2. Most cities and all states have an OEM, which coordinates the disaster relief efforts at the state and local levels.

3. Federal resources include organizations such as DHHS and the Department of Justice. Each of these federal departments oversees hundreds of agencies, including the American Red Cross, that respond to disasters.

4. MMRS teams are local teams that are located in cities that are deemed to be possible terrorist targets.

**TEST-TAKING HINT:** The question asks for a federal agency. The word "metro" would mean "local"; therefore option "4" could be eliminated. All health-care providers should be aware of the role of JCAHO in the hospital and could eliminate "1."

44. 1. CISM is an approach to preventing and treating the emotional trauma that can affect emergency responders as a consequence of their job. Performing CPR and treating a young child affects the emergency personnel psychologically, and the death increases the traumatic experience.

2. Caring for this type of client is an expected part of the job. If the nurse finds this traumatic

enough to require a CISM, then the nurse should probably leave the emergency department.

3. This would require an intense time for triaging and caring for the victims, but without fatalities this should not be that traumatic for the staff.

4. This is a dangerous practice because medication errors and other mistakes may occur as a result of fatigue, but this is not a traumatic situation.

**TEST-TAKING HINT:** The test taker should examine the words "critical," "incident," and "stress." Each answer option should be examined to determine which would be the most traumatic. Needless deaths of innocent children are psychologically traumatic.

45. 1. The media has an obligation to report the news and can play a significant positive role in communication, but communication should come from only one source—the disaster command center.

2. Emergency operations plans will always have a designated disaster plan coordinator. All public information should be routed through this person.

3. Client confidentiality must be maintained, but the best action is for the nurse to help the reporter get to the appropriate area for information.

4. This would allow the reporter to stay in the emergency room, which is inappropriate.

**TEST-TAKING HINT:** The nurse should address the situation with the reporter and provide an access for the information. Options "1," "3," and "4" do not help the reporter get accurate information.

46. 1. This is the correct procedure when tagging a client and would not warrant intervention.

2. Vital signs should be documented on the tag. The tag takes the place of the client's chart, so this would not warrant intervention.

3. The tag should never be removed from the client until the disaster is over or the client is admitted and the tag becomes a part of the client's record. The HCP needs to be informed immediately of the action.

4. The tag can be attached to any part of the client's body.

**TEST-TAKING HINT:** This question is asking the test taker to identify an option that is incorrect for the situation. Sometimes asking which action is appropriate helps identify the correct answer.

47. 1. This will help diffuse the escalating situation and attempt to keep the father calm.

2. Sending the father to the waiting room does not help his behavior and could possibly make his behavior worse; loud and obnoxious behavior can become violent.

3. This will not help the current situation and could make it worse because the nurse doesn't know the home situation.

4. The nurse should notify hospital security before calling the police department.

**TEST-TAKING HINT:** The rule concerning dealing with anger is to directly address the client and diffuse the situation. There is only one option that addresses this rule, option "1."

48. 1. This puts the nurse in a dangerous position and might cause the death of the nurse.

2. This will escalate the situation.

3. This is a dangerous position for the nurse to put himself or herself in.

4. Self-protection is priority, and the nurse is not required to be injured in the line of duty.

**TEST-TAKING HINT:** Self-protection is a priority. There is no advantage to protecting others if the caregivers are also injured. The only option that protects the nurse is to get out of the line of fire.

## Poisoning

49. 1. CPS should be contacted only if the nurse suspects an intentional administration of the poison, but at this time determining which poison the child has swallowed and the antidote is the priority.

2. The local police department is only notified if the nurse suspects child abuse.

3. The Department of Health would not be notified.

4. The Poison Control Center can assist the nurse in identifying which chemical has been ingested by the child and the antidote.

**TEST-TAKING HINT:** The test taker should analyze each option to determine what information could be obtained. Then the test taker should put this information in order of priority. Even if the nurse suspects child abuse, the priority is to help the child immediately.

50. 1. The primary goal for the ED nurse is to stop the action of the poison and then maintain organ functioning.

2. ED nurses do no provide long-term care.

3. Antidotes are administered to neutralize the effects of poisons, not to increase the effects.
4. Treatment is implemented to hasten the elimination of the poison.

**TEST-TAKING HINT: The test taker should read each option carefully. ED nurse and "long-term care" don't match. Increasing the effects and prolonging the elimination of the poison would be damaging to the client.**

51. 1. Vomiting is never induced in clients who have ingested corrosive alkaline substances or petroleum distillates. More damage can occur to the esophagus and pharynx.
2. A gastric lavage may be done but not by inserting an NGT and attaching it to wall suction.
3. Airway edema or obstruction can occur as a result of the burning action of corrosive substances.
4. Water or milk may be administered to dilute the substance if the airway is not compromised.

**TEST-TAKING HINT: This is an emergency situation. If the test taker did not know the answer, Maslow's Hierarchy of Needs puts airway first.**

52. 1. These are signs and symptoms of carbon monoxide poisoning. Pulse oximetry is not a valid test because the hemoglobin is saturated with the carbon monoxide and a false high reading would be obtained.
2. These are signs and symptoms of carbon monoxide poisoning. Symptoms include skin color from a cherry red to cyanotic and pale, headache, muscular weakness, palpitations, dizziness, and confusion and can progress rapidly to coma and death. Oxygen should be administered 100% at hyperbaric or atmospheric pressures to reverse hypoxia and accelerate elimination of the carbon monoxide.
3. This may be done, but it is not the first action.
4. This may need to be done, but getting oxygen to the brain is first.

**TEST-TAKING HINT: Three (3) of the four (4) options concern oxygenation. The test taker must then decide which of the three (3) has a higher priority.**

53. 1. The client should be placed on the left side, which allows the gastric contents to pool in the stomach and decreases passage of fluid into the duodenum during lavage. After the placement of the orogastric tube, the head is lowered to facilitate removal of the gastric contents.

2. A large bore tube is placed through the mouth into the stomach of a client who is comatose and an endotracheal tube is inserted into the airway prior to beginning lavage to prevent aspiration.
3. Standby suction is an emergency measure to prevent aspiration in case the client vomits.
4. Removing all stomach contents before beginning the lavage helps to prevent over-distention of the stomach and aspiration.
5. Samples of the first two (2) lavage washings should be sent to the lab to be analyzed for chemical compounds.

**TEST-TAKING HINT: When deciding on the correct answers for an alternative-type-question, each option must be examined for its own merit. One good answer does not exclude another answer. In option "1" anatomical positioning can help the test taker determine if the position would be a good one. In option "2," the test taker must look at the adjective "small" and ask if this would facilitate or hinder irrigation of the stomach. Even if the test taker did not know what the circumstances are, option "3" could be a good action.**

54. 1. The skin should be immediately drenched with water from a hose or shower. A constant stream of water is applied. Time should not be lost by removing the clothes and then proceeding to rinsing with water. If the person has a dry powder form of white phosphorus or lye, it is brushed off and then the client is placed under the shower.
2. The first action is to remove the poison from the client's skin and prevent further damage.
3. If the client becomes dyspneic, the nurse would administer oxygen while waiting for the paramedics.
4. The vat should be labeled as to the chemical contents per Office of Safety and Health Administration (OSHA) regulations, but if not, then the nurse must determine which chemicals are in the vat so the HCP can treat the client appropriately.

**TEST-TAKING HINT: Usually oxygen is a priority, but in this scenario the client has dangerous chemicals on the skin. The stem did not tell the test taker that the respirations were a problem. It is important not to read into a question.**

55. 1. Fluid volume loss is a concern because of the potential for the client to go into hypovolemic shock, but this is not priority over airway.

2. Clients with botulism are at risk for respiratory paralysis, and this is the priority problem.

3. The client will be in pain and pain is a priority, but it does not come before airway and fluid volume.

4. The client may be anxious but a psychosocial problem usually can be ranked after a physiological one in priority.

**TEST-TAKING HINT: Maslow's Hierarchy of Needs lists airway as the highest priority.**

56. 123,000 mg of analgesic medication were consumed. The container originally contained 250 capsules. Two (2) doses of two (2) capsules each were removed.

$$2 \times 2 = 4.$$
$$250 \text{ capsules} - 4 \text{ capsules} = 246 \text{ capsules remaining.}$$

Each capsule contains 500 mg.

246 capsules $\times$ 500 mg = 123,000 mg of medication consumed.

**TEST-TAKING HINT: Do not overlook a step in the problem. On the NCLEX-RN be sure to check answers with the pull-down calculator.**

57. 1. Although this is seen as a first action in old television westerns, it is not a recommended action for clients who have been bitten by a snake. This action will cause further damage to the tissue by restricting blood flow to the tissue.

2. This is also an action that has been done in classic television programs and movies from the 1950s and 1960s, but this is not the current treatment for snakebite. If this is done the rescuer will suck the venom into the rescuer's mouth and possibly be poisoned.

3. Corticosteroid medications are contraindicated in the first six (6) to eight (8) hours after the bite because they might interfere with antibody production and hinder the action of the antivenin.

4. The client should lie down, all restrictive items such as rings should be removed, the wound should be cleansed and covered with a sterile dressing, the affected body part should be immobilized, and the client should be kept warm.

**TEST-TAKING HINT: The test taker should not jump to what is depicted in the mass media as the correct answer. Both options "1" and "2" have answers that have been portrayed in the media as the correct method of caring for snakebite. This should give the test taker a clue that if both cannot be right, then both are probably wrong.**

58. 1. Installing carbon monoxide detectors in the home would be a recommended safety measure.

2. The lips should be pink, not bright red or blue. This indicates a saturation of the hemoglobin with carbon monoxide. This client needs more instruction.

3. Because carbon monoxide is colorless and odorless it can be dangerous. It is detected with special detectors.

4. One of the major causes of accidental carbon monoxide poisoning is a faulty furnace.

**TEST-TAKING HINT: Three (3) options, "1," "3," and "4," are all about protecting the home and the client from inhaling carbon monoxide. If the test taker did not know the answer, a good option would be the option that is different.**

59. 1. Assistants can obtain intake and outputs, but evaluating the information is the nurse's responsibility.

2. This is a sterile dressing change and should not be delegated.

3. An assistant can assist clients to get up to the bedside commode as long as the assistant is knowledgeable about body mechanics.

4. The assistant can assist a client to turn and ask the client to cough and deep breathe.

**TEST-TAKING HINT: The task that requires knowledge of sterile procedures is the one the nurse should perform. Any task that requires specialized knowledge or nursing judgment cannot be delegated.**

60. 1. Before administering antivenin, the affected body part must be measured and remeasured every 15 minutes during a 4- to 6-hour procedure. The infusion is begun slowly and increased after 10 minutes. The affected part is measured every 30–60 minutes after the infusion and for 48 hours to detect symptoms of compartment syndrome (swelling, loss of pulse, increased pain, and paresthesias). Allergic reactions to the antivenin are not uncommon and are usually the result of a too-rapid infusion of the antivenin. The most experienced nurse should be assigned this client.

2. This client is beyond critical danger. This client is being discharged, so a less experienced nurse could care for this client.

3. This client has many needs, but anger is not a priority over a physiological need.

4. A less experienced nurse could care for this client.

**TEST-TAKING HINT: The test taker can rule out options "2" and "3" because of the discharge**

information and psychosocial versus physiological problem.

## Violence, Physical Abuse, and Neglect

61. 1. This action could cause the spouse to become violent. The security personnel should not attempt to remove the spouse unless the client wishes them to do so.
    2. Injuries resulting from spousal abuse should be discussed without the abuser present.
    3. This may or may not be true. The client will have to prosecute, and many times the abused client will not do so. The client may feel responsible for the abuse because she has been told that she is responsible and has such low self-esteem that she believes that it is true. She may decline to prosecute because she fears for her children's lives or for her own. There may be a financial hold the spouse has over the client. Battered woman syndrome has many facets.
    4. By escorting the client to a bathroom for any reason, the nurse can get the client to a safe area out of the hearing of the spouse. This is the most innocuous way to get the client alone.

    **TEST-TAKING HINT:** When dealing with a violent person, the nurse should use discretion to avoid the spouse erupting into violence directed against the nurse, client, or others in the emergency department.

62. 1. Adult protective services should be called only if it is determined that willful neglect or abuse of the client is occurring.
    2. The nurse should arrange for the social worker to see the client and family to determine if some arrangements could be made to provide for the client's safety and for the client to be provided with nutritious meals while the adult children are at work. A long-term care facility or adult day care may be needed.
    3. The Medicare ombudsman is a person who represents a Medicare client in a long-term care facility.
    4. The dietitian could see this client to determine eating preferences (74 inches = 6 foot 2 inches and 54.5 kg = 120 pounds), but the most appropriate is safety.

    **TEST-TAKING HINT:** The question asks for the test taker to determine a priority intervention. The client is diagnosed with senile dementia and is being left alone for hours of the day. Safety is priority.

63. 1. Research suggests that at least 67% of adolescents who are runaways or homeless have been abused in the home. This represents a learned behavior pattern that gets the female adolescent attention.
    2. One reason adolescents of both sexes run away from home is abuse in the home. Nothing in the stem indicates that the client was turned out of the home for any behavior.
    3. This has the nurse medically diagnosing the client.
    4. This is a judgmental statement.

    **TEST-TAKING HINT:** The test taker should not read into the question or choose an answer that has the nurse functioning outside of the nurse's role. Option "2" is assuming facts that are not in the stem, and option "3" is asking the nurse to make a medical diagnosis.

64. 1. The school nurse is not a Sexual Assault Nurse Examiner (SANE) nurse, and this child thinks she is pregnant, suggesting that the abuse has been occurring for a period of time or at least in some months past. The child should be taken for examination to a hospital.
    2. Child Protective Services should be notified to protect the child from further abuse and to initiate charges against the father. An intermediate school nurse would be caring for children in the 4th, 5th, 6th, or 7th grades, depending on the school district.
    3. This would bring the abuser to the school.
    4. Sending the child to a free clinic would not negate the nurse's responsibility to report suspected child abuse.

    **TEST-TAKING HINT:** All 50 states require the nurse to report suspected child abuse. Child Protective Services (CPS) is the advocate to notify. Nurses in a school clinic do not have the appropriate facilities to perform rape examinations. Option "4" does not address the abuse.

65. 1. Frequently child abusers will deny the child's reports of abuse and say that the child is a habitual liar.
    2. Child abusers believe that violence is an acceptable way to reduce tension. They tend to have a low tolerance for frustration and have poor impulse control.
    3. Child abusers have a tendency toward feelings of helplessness and hopelessness.
    4. Child abusers tend to blame the child for the abuse and not admit that the problem is their own.

5. The child abuser may have been abused as a child, but there is no evidence of the child abuser being spoiled as a child.

**TEST-TAKING HINT: This is an alternative-type question. The test taker should examine each option carefully to determine if it could be a correct answer. Option "3" could be eliminated because of the adjective "high" and "5" could be eliminated because of the adjective "spoiled."**

66. 1. This is a myth that has been believed by some people. Many individuals are raped ranging in age from infants to the 90s, male and female, heterosexuals and homosexuals. No one asks to be raped.
    2. If a person says they are not interested in any type of sexual activity it means no and anything else is forced and it is rape. No means no. It is considered rape if a prostitute says no.
    3. Rape is an act of violence motivated by the rapist's desiring to overpower and control the victim.
    4. Men and children can be victims of rape. Sexual arousal and orgasm do not imply consent; it may be a pathological response to stimulation.

**TEST-TAKING HINT: This is an "except" question, which means that three (3) of the options will contain correct information. In this question there are three (3) false statements about rape; this is a double-negative type of question.**

67. 1. The nurse can encourage the client to press charges but has no right to insist.
    2. The nurse should treat the wound and may find it frustrating that the client will not press charges, but the nurse is obligated to give the client information that will help the client to get to a safe place.
    3. The woman is more aware of this fact than the nurse.
    4. The nurse should help the client to devise a plan for safety by giving the client the number of a safe house or a woman's shelter.

**TEST-TAKING HINT: The test taker could eliminate option "3" based on common sense; the client lives in an abusive situation and would realize the abuser's potential more than the nurse. Option "2" could be eliminated by the phrase "do nothing else." Option "1" could be eliminated because of the principle of nurses empower their clients, not overpower them, which is what has been happening to the client already.**

68. 1. This client has signs of ongoing abuse: multiple burns and contusions in different stages of healing.
    2. Many times the elderly are ashamed to report abuse because they raised the abuser and feel responsible that their child became an abuser. The elder parent may feel financially dependent on the child or be afraid of being placed in a long-term care facility. Forty-seven states have Adult Protective Services (APS) created by the states to protect elder citizens.
    3. There is no evidence in the stem that the client is not mentally competent and there is evidence in the stem of physical abuse. This client is performing activities of daily living.
    4. Consensual sex does not involve the physical abuse noted in the assessment.

**TEST-TAKING HINT: The test taker could eliminate options "1," "3," and "4" by examining the stem and the physical abuse that is occurring and by the fact that the client is functioning by performing activities of daily living.**

69. 1. Unless the nurse is being personally abused in the same manner the client is being abused and has seen the abuse taking place, the nurse cannot "know" the client is being abused.
    2. Alcohol and drugs are implicated in the abuse of many clients, but not all abusers use alcohol or drugs.
    3. This is agreeing with the abuser that the client caused the abuse.
    4. This statement assesses the abused client's safety (or a plan for safety).

**TEST-TAKING HINT: Option "3" could be eliminated because it blames the victim. Option "1" can be eliminated because the nurse should not tell the client "I know" unless the nurse has proof or has been in the situation.**

70. 1. Clients diagnosed with PTSD are easily startled and can react violently if awakened from sleep by being touched.
    2. Touching the client can cause the client to become afraid, to believe himself or herself to be under attack, and to react violently. The nurse should not touch a sleeping client diagnosed with PTSD.
    3. If the client awakes with the nurse in the room, the client could become fearful and react to the fear.
    4. There may be times when the nurse must awaken the client to determine if the client is physically stable.

**TEST-TAKING HINT:** Option "4" can be eliminated because of the absolute statement "at all." Options "2" and "3" can be eliminated if the test taker would think of how it feels to be startled when perceiving another person around them when the test taker was not aware of the other person's presence.

71. 1. This plan for the client to take RU 486 or the morning-after pill prevents pregnancy from occurring, but it does not directly address coping skills.
    2. The client may talk about "what if I had not done," but the client is not guilty of causing the rape.
    3. The client should be provided the phone number of a rape crisis counseling center or counselor to help the client deal with the psychological feelings of being raped.
    4. This is a legal issue.

**TEST-TAKING HINT:** The test taker should read the stem "ineffective coping" and eliminate the physiologic problem in option "1" and the legal problem in option "4."

72. 1. The nurse should attempt to develop a relationship in which the client feels that he or she can trust the nurse (males are abused by significant others too).
    2. The first step in helping a client who has been abused is to get the client to admit that the abuse is happening.
    3. This could cause the abuse to escalate.
    4. This is what the nurse is trying to get the client to avoid.

**TEST-TAKING HINT:** Option "1" could be eliminated because it is the opposite of what the nurse tries to establish in a nurse–client relationship. Option "4" places the client in harm's way.

1. The nurse is working in the Emergency Department and receives a client diagnosed with multiple rib fractures. What specific data should the nurse include in the assessment of this client?
   1. Level of orientation to time and place.
   2. Current use and last dose of medication.
   3. Symmetrical movement of the chest.
   4. Time of last meal that the client ate.

2. The client is being treated in the Emergency Department for abdominal trauma. The nurse is preparing the plan of care for this client. Which intervention should the nurse include?
   1. Assess the returned fluid from the peritoneal lavage.
   2. Palpate the client for bilateral femoral pulses.
   3. Perform Leopold maneuvers every eight (8) hours.
   4. Collect information on the client's dietary history.

3. After gardening, the elderly client is brought into the Emergency Department complaining of cramps, headache, and weakness. The nurse applies the cardiac monitor and notes tachycardia. Which should the nurse include in the assessment?
   1. Determine if the client is experiencing any thirst.
   2. Administer D5W intravenously at 250 mL per hour.
   3. Maintain a cool environment to promote rest.
   4. Withhold the client's oral intake.

4. The nurse is working in the Emergency Department and is assigned a client who suffered a near-drowning. Which expected outcome should the nurse include in the plan of care for this client?
   1. Maintain cardiac function, including tachycardia.
   2. Promote a continued decrease in lung surfactant.
   3. Warm rapidly to minimize the effects of hypothermia.
   4. Keep the oxygen saturation level above 93%.

5. The nurse is assessing the client who suffered a near-drowning event. Which data would require immediate intervention?
   1. The onset of pink, frothy sputum.
   2. An oral temperature of 97°F.
   3. An alcohol level of 100 mg/dL.
   4. A heart rate of 100 beats/min.

6. A nurse is at the lake when a person experiences a near-drowning event. People at the scene remove the victim from the water. After breathing, which should the nurse assess first?
   1. Possibility of drug use.
   2. Spinal cord injury.
   3. Level of confusion.
   4. Amount of alcohol.

7. The nurse is preparing a discharge plan for the client admitted to the hospital with carbon monoxide poisoning. Which intervention should the nurse include in this plan?
   1. Report any black sputum or hypercapnia.
   2. Assess for suicidal thoughts or previous attempts.
   3. Keep annual physicals with the health-care provider.
   4. Notify the health-care provider of any stridor or dizziness.

8. The nurse is working the triage position in the ED. Which client should be treated first?
   1. A client who has multiple injuries from a motor-vehicle accident.
   2. A client complaining of epigastric pain and nausea after eating.
   3. An elderly client who fell and fractured the left femoral neck.
   4. The client suffering from a migraine headache and nausea.

9. The nurse is providing discharge teaching for the client with intermaxillary wiring after a fracture of the mandible. Which statement by the client would indicate to the nurse that teaching has been effective?
   1. Iced alcoholic drinks may be consumed by using a straw.
   2. Only one (1) food item should be consumed at one (1) time.
   3. Carbonated sodas should be limited to two (2) daily.
   4. Teeth can be brushed after tenderness and swelling subside.

10. The occupational health nurse is called to the scene of a traumatic amputation of a finger. Which intervention should the nurse implement prior to sending the client to the ED? Select all that apply.
    1. Rinse the finger with sterile normal saline.
    2. Place the finger in a sealed and watertight plastic bag.
    3. Place the finger into iced saline solution.
    4. Wrap the finger in saline-moistened gauze dressings.
    5. Replace the finger on the hand and wrap with gauze.

11. The nurse is teaching the client home care instructions for a reimplanted finger after a traumatic amputation. Which information should the nurse include?
    1. Perform range-of-motion exercises weekly.
    2. Smoking may be resumed if it does not causing nausea.
    3. Protect the finger and be careful not to reinjure the finger.
    4. An elevated temperature is the only reason to call the HCP.

12. The ED nurse is caring for a client diagnosed with frostbite of the feet. Which intervention should the nurse implement?
    1. Massage the feet vigorously.
    2. Soak the feet in warm water.
    3. Apply a heating pad to feet.
    4. Apply petroleum jelly to the feet.

13. A student reports to the school nurse with complaints of stinging and burning at the site of a wasp string. Which intervention should the nurse implement?
    1. Grasp the stinger and pull it out.
    2. Apply a warm, moist soak to the area.
    3. Cleanse the site with alcohol.
    4. Apply an ice pack to the site.

14. The ED nurse is caring for a client who has had a bee sting. Which intervention should the nurse implement?
    1. Instruct the client to wear a medical identification bracelet.
    2. Apply corticosteroid cream to the site to prevent anaphylaxis.
    3. Administer epinephrine 1:10,000 intravenously every three (3) minutes.
    4. Teach the client to avoid attracting insects by wearing bright colors.

15. The nurse working in the ED has a client with bladder trauma and a fractured pelvis occurring as a result of a motor-vehicle accident. Which should be included in this client's assessment?
    1. Monitor the serum creatine kinase level.
    2. Insert a suprapubic catheter.
    3. Note the amount and color of the urine.
    4. Listen for adventitious breath sounds.

16. The school nurse is caring for the child with a bleeding laceration. Which intervention should the nurse implement to prevent complications?
    1. Clean with saline solution.
    2. Apply a tight band bandage.
    3. Debride the edges bilaterally.
    4. Administer oral antibiotics to the child.

17. The nurse working in the ED receives a client involved in a motor-vehicle accident. The nurse notes a large hematoma on the right flank. Which intervention should the nurse implement first?
    1. Insert an indwelling urinary catheter.
    2. Take the vital signs every 15 minutes.
    3. Monitor the skin turgor every hour.
    4. Administer an aspirin, an analgesic.

18. Which expected outcome would be appropriate for the nurse to include in the plan of care for the client diagnosed with ureteral trauma from a gunshot injury?
    1. The client will have an absence of pain.
    2. The client will drink 2000 mL of water.
    3. The client will eat a high-protein diet.
    4. The client will maintain an output of 30 mL/hr.

19. Which nursing diagnosis would be appropriate for the client experiencing renal trauma?
    1. Infection of the renal tract.
    2. Ineffective tissue perfusion.
    3. Alteration in skin integrity.
    4. Alteration in temperature.

20. The nurse is conducting an interview with the client in the ED for a laceration. Which information is most important for the nurse to obtain?
    1. The date of the client's last tetanus injection.
    2. The name of the client's regular health-care provider.
    3. The dates of the client's hospital admissions.
    4. The person who provides spiritual support during stress.

21. The nurse working in an outpatient clinic is caring for a client who is experiencing an epistaxis. Which intervention should the nurse implement first?
    1. Teach the client to keep the nose clear by blowing forcefully.
    2. Hold the nose with thumb and finger for 15 minutes.
    3. Have the client sit with the head tilted back and hold a tissue.
    4. Administer silver nitrate, a cauterizing agent, with a packing applicator.

22. The client with a temperature of 94°F is being treated in the ED. Which intervention should the nurse implement that will directly elevate the client's temperature?
    1. Remove the client's clothing.
    2. Place a warm air blanket over the client.
    3. Have the client change into a hospital gown.
    4. Raise the temperature in the room.

23. The ED nurse is caring for the client who has taken an overdose of cocaine. Which intervention should the nurse delegate to the unlicensed assistive personnel?
    1. Evaluate the airway and breathing.
    2. Monitor the rate of intravenous fluids.
    3. Place the cardiac monitor on the client.
    4. Assess the vital signs every 15 minutes.

24. The client has been brought to the ED by ambulance following a motor-vehicle accident and has suffered a chest injury. Which intervention should the nurse implement first?
    1. Start a large bore intravenous access.
    2. Apply the cardiac monitor to the client.
    3. Assess the client's airway and breathing.
    4. Assess the cardiac rhythm on the monitor.

25. The ED nurse is completing the initial assessment on a client who becomes unresponsive. Which intervention should the nurse implement first?
    1. Assess the rate and site of the intravenous fluid.
    2. Administer an ampoule of sodium bicarbonate.
    3. Interpret the rhythm shown on the monitor.
    4. Prepare to cardiovert the client into sinus rhythm.

26. The nurse in an emergency department is caring for a female client with a greenstick fracture of the left forearm and multiple contusions on the face, arms, trunk, and legs. The significant other is in the treatment area with the client. Which nursing interventions should the nurse implement? List in order of priority.
    1. Determine if the client has a plan for safety.
    2. Assess the pulse, temperature, and capillary refill of the left wrist and hand.
    3. Ask the client is she feels safe in her own home.
    4. Request the significant other to wait in the waiting room during the examination.
    5. Notify the social worker to consult on the case.

1. 1. Orientation to person, place, and time should be assessed on all clients, but this information will not provide specific information about the chest trauma.
   2. Current use of all medication and the last doses should be assessed for all clients.
   3. **When a client suffers from multiple rib fractures, the client has an increased risk for flail chest. The nurse should assess the client for paradoxical chest wall movement and, if respiratory distress is present, for pallor and cyanosis.**
   4. The time of this last meal would be important if the client were to have surgery or intubation planned. A nutritional assessment should be performed on all clients.

2. 1. **A diagnostic peritoneal lavage is performed to assess the presence of blood, bile, and feces from internal bleeding induced by injury. If any of these are present, surgery should be considered to explore the extent of damage and repair of the injury.**
   2. Palpating the client's peripheral pulses would indicate blood flow to the extremities. Femoral pulses would not necessarily be assessed if all distal pulses are strong.
   3. Leopold maneuvers are performed on pregnant clients to assess the position of the fetus.
   4. Dietary history is information that should be assessed but not in an emergency situation. Assessments need to be efficient and direct to eliminate any time-wasting activities.

3. 1. Elderly clients lose the defense mechanism of increased thirst with dehydration. This would not accurately indicate fluid deficit.
   2. An intravenous fluid should be administered. The solution should correct fluid and electrolyte imbalances. D5W would not replace electrolytes lost, and 250 mL an hour could place the client at risk for heart failure if the body cannot adjust that rapidly to the fluid replacement.
   3. **The nurse should encourage the client to rest and should maintain a cool environment to assist the client to recover from heat exhaustion. The elderly are more susceptible to this condition.**
   4. If the client can tolerate oral fluids, the client should be encouraged to drink fluids that replace electrolytes lost in excessive sweating.

4. 1. An expected outcome would be a desired occurrence, not a common event. Tachycardia is a common manifestation of a near-drowning event but it is not desired. A combination of

physiologic changes, hypothermia, and hypoxia put the client at risk for life-threatening cardiac rhythms.
   2. Any near-drowning causes a decrease in alveolar surfactant, which results in alveolar collapse. A decrease in surfactant is not the desired outcome.
   3. The client needs to be rewarmed slowly to reduce the influx of metabolites. These metabolites, including lactic acid, would remain in the extremities.
   4. **The oxygen level needs to be maintained greater than 93%. The client needs as much support as necessary for this. Mechanical ventilation with peak end-expiratory pressure (PEEP) and high oxygen levels may be needed to achieve this goal.**

5. 1. **The onset of pinky, frothy sputum indicates that the client is experiencing pulmonary edema. This needs to be treated to prevent further decline in this client.**
   2. An oral temperature of 97°F is in the lower level of within normal limits.
   3. A blood alcohol of 100 mg/dL is an elevation but should not be considered priority over pulmonary edema. Treatments for elevations in toxicology levels can be considered after the client is stable.
   4. A heart rate of 100 beats/minute is tachycardia but not at a critical level. The nurse needs to follow the ABCs of treatment: A is for airway, B is for breathing, and C is for circulation. Pulmonary edema interferes with breathing.

6. 1. The use of drugs can alter the treatment and recovery of the near-drowning event. This is information that will be needed, but it is not priority at this time.
   2. An injury of the spinal cord should be considered and the spine should be assessed but after the client has been stabilized. The nurse would not complete an assessment of a potential spinal injury before assessing oxygenation status. If the client has sustained a spinal cord injury, then movement from the water by laypeople before stabilizing the injury may have caused irreparable damage to the spinal cord.
   3. **The nurse should assess the victim for hypoxia. Signs and symptoms of hypoxia include confusion or irritability and alterations in level of consciousness, such as lethargy.**
   4. The amount of alcohol ingestion will affect the treatment, but this is not a higher priority than oxygenation.

7. 1. The client diagnosed with carbon monoxide poisoning frequently has black sputum from inhaling soot, but this should resolve during the hospital stay. It should not return. Hypercapnia is a high level of $CO_2$. The nurse should be careful to use terms that the client will understand.

   2. The cause of the exposure to carbon monoxide needs to be explored. The environment needs to be corrected for the safety of the client prior to discharge. If exposure was a result of a suicide attempt, the client needs a psychiatric evaluation prior to being discharged. Interventions to prevent future attempts should be implemented.

   3. Keeping an annual physical would be an important health promotion activity, but this would not be an appropriate time for follow up for this client. This client should be seen by the health-care provider for any long-term complications.

   4. Stridor or dizziness would be present at the beginning of the hospitalization, not at discharge. If stridor occurs, the emergency medical system should be contacted. Treatment would be necessary to prevent arrest.

8. 1. Injuries from a motor-vehicle accident can be life threatening. This client should be assessed first to rule out respiratory difficulties and hemorrhage. Prioritizing nursing care is based on different criteria when in the Emergency Department. Triaging client treatment is based on rapid classification of the client's problem. The nurse assesses the client for the level of acuity of the presenting problem.

   2. Epigastric pain with nausea after eating sounds like gallbladder disease. Pain has high priority but not over breathing and hemorrhage.

   3. Elderly clients have special fluid and electrolyte issues after a fall. The cause of the fall may be cardiac, but the question does not indicate this. Based on this information, the client is not the highest priority.

   4. Migraine headaches are painful experiences, but they do not have a higher priority than breathing and hemorrhage.

9. 1. Alcoholic beverages should be avoided to prevent nausea and vomiting. The client should be taught where and how to cut wires if vomiting occurs.

   2. A combination of foods should be blended into a milkshake and consumed to maintain caloric intake and promote nutrition.

   3. Carbonated sodas can cause foam in the back of the throat and may induce vomiting.

   4. Hygiene is helpful in healing. The mouth should be rinsed and an irrigation device should be used frequently. Gentle brushing and rinsing the mouth after each meal and at bedtime can begin after swelling and tenderness subside.

10. 1. The amputated finger and all tissue should be rinsed with a sterile normal saline to remove dirt and sent to the Emergency Department with the client.

    2. Place the finger and all tissue in a water-sealed plastic bag to prevent loss and contamination.

    3. The finger or other tissue should not be placed on ice or in saline solution because this will cause severe damage to the tissue cells.

    4. The finger should be wrapped in gauze that has been moistened with sterile normal saline.

    5. The finger should not be replaced on the hand and wrapped with gauze in the field. The surgeon will determine if reattachment is possible.

11. 1. Exercises should be performed several times each day, not weekly.

    2. Smoking causes vasoconstriction, which will compromise the implanted finger's survival.

    3. The client should take extra care to prevent the finger from injury. The peripheral nerves that protect the finger can take months to regenerate.

    4. The client needs to report any signs of rejection of the finger, such as infection or impaired circulation, not just an elevated temperature.

12. 1. Massaging or rubbing tissue that has been frostbitten will cause further damage.

    2. Soaking feet in a warm bath of 107°F causes rapid continuous rewarming.

    3. Heating pads are not used to rewarm tissue that has frostbite. Heating pads can cause tissue damage from burns, especially in tissue with impaired sensation.

    4. Petroleum jelly would not affect the temperature of the tissue.

13. 1. The stinger should not be grasped because the wasp's venous sac may release more toxin. The stinger should be scraped in the opposite direction.

    2. Warmth increases the blood flow, which will increase the swelling.

    3. The site should be cleaned with soap and water, not alcohol.

    4. The nurse should apply an ice pack to the site. The cold will decrease the blood flow and sensation. The ice should be applied intermittently.

14. 1. Clients who have severe reactions to insect stings should wear identifying bracelets to provide information. If the client is unconscious, the bracelet can alert the health-care provider so that treatment can be started.
    2. Corticosteroid creams treat local reactions, not systemic ones.
    3. Epinephrine 1:10,000 is administered intravenously during a code situation or for a severe anaphylactic reaction to an allergen. This was not indicated in the stem.
    4. Bright-colored clothing attracts insects. Clients who that are allergic to insect stings should learn how to avoid them to decrease the risk. Flowery-smelling perfumes and lotions should also be avoided.

15. 1. A serum creatine kinase measures the enzyme from skeletal muscles, heart muscles, and the brain. With the trauma of the accident, the level would be elevated, but this monitoring would not assist with the diagnosis of the extent of bladder trauma.
    2. The nurse does not insert suprapubic catheters; this is done in surgery by the HCP.
    3. **The amount and color of urine would assist with diagnosing the extent of injury. Color would indicate the presence of blood. The amount would indicate whether the urine is contained throughout the pathway from bladder to urinary meatus.**
    4. Breath sounds should be assessed for a complete assessment, but they are not specific to this diagnosis.

16. 1. **The laceration should be cleaned well to prevent infection. A sterile saline solution or water should be used. A small amount of bleeding from the wound cleans the bacteria from the laceration.**
    2. Applying a "tight" bandage can impair circulation and cause tissue damage. Applying direct pressure until the bleeding stops is appropriate.
    3. Debridement is used to remove necrotic tissue, but this is a fresh injury.
    4. The nurse cannot prescribe antibiotics, and there may be no need for them.

17. 1. Inserting an indwelling catheter may cause further injury. Until the extent of injury is determined, prevention of further damage should have high priority.
    2. **Vital signs should be taken frequently to assess for covert bleeding. The hematoma in the flank area may indicate the presence of trauma to the kidney. Because of the large amount of blood flow through the kidney, hemorrhage is a high risk.**
    3. Assessing skin turgor would be important in determining the fluid balance, but it would not be higher priority than monitoring vital signs.
    4. The client may be in pain, but aspirin would not be administered when the client is at risk for bleeding. Aspirin interferes with the clotting of blood. This would result in further bleeding.

18. 1. An absence of pain would not be realistic for this client. Pain management is a goal for clients. At this time in the care of this client, it is not realistic to expect no pain.
    2. At this time, the client will remain NPO (nothing by mouth) for diagnostic tests and possible surgery.
    3. A high-protein diet will be appropriate later for healing.
    4. **A urine output of 30 mL/hour indicates the tissues are being adequately perfused and is an indicator of kidney functioning.**

19. 1. A potential for infection would be an appropriate nursing diagnosis, but there is no indication of infection from this question.
    2. **Bleeding results in an impairment of tissue perfusion. Because of the large amount of blood flow through the renal system, bleeding is a major problem.**
    3. Skin integrity is not necessarily an issue in trauma. There is no indication from the question that skin is not intact.
    4. An alteration in temperature is not a problem for this client unless infection occurs. That is not indicated at this time.

20. 1. **Any client who has not had a tetanus injection within five (5) years will need to receive an injection as prophylaxis.**
    2. The source of regular health care is obtained for all clients, but this client can be treated by the ED physician.
    3. This would be information collected on all clients, but it has no bearing on the current situation.
    4. The nurse should assess all clients for spiritual distress, but meeting this need during the short time that the client is in the Emergency Department is not the highest priority.

21. 1. Clients should be taught to avoid forcefully blowing the nose, straining, high altitudes, and nasal trauma.
    2. **Most nosebleeds will stop after applying pressure on the nose between thumb and index finger for 15 minutes.**
    3. The nurse should position the client head tilted forward. This position will prevent the client from swallowing the blood. The blood can be aspirated if the head is tilted back.

4. Most nosebleeds respond to pressure. If pressure for 15 minutes does not stop the bleeding, the health-care provider may need to use electrocautery or silver nitrate. This would be performed by the HCP, not the nurse.

22. 1. Removing clothing would cause further chilling.
2. **The warm air blanket blows warm air over the client and is an active warming method.**
3. Hospital gowns have openings that can cause the client to be colder.
4. Raising the temperature of the room will not actively raise the client's temperature.

23. 1. Evaluation of airway and breathing is assessment and cannot be delegated.
2. Monitoring the rate of intravenous fluid is a part of administering a medication. Medication administration cannot be delegated.
3. **Unlicensed assistive personnel who have been trained can attach the cardiac monitor to the clients.**
4. The act of taking vital signs can be delegated, but assessing vital signs cannot. Assessment requires nursing judgment.

24. 1. An intravenous access should be started with a large bore catheter as soon as possible to administer fluids and emergency medications if needed.
2. The client needs to be placed on the cardiac monitor before starting the intravenous access. Assessment has a higher priority than intervention. Airway and breathing have the highest priority.
3. Assessing the client's airway and respirations has the highest priority. Prioritizing care can be based on Maslow's Hierarchy of Needs or the American Heart Association's "A, B, Cs." Airway and respirations are first.
4. Assessing the cardiac rhythm is the "C" in the ABCs. This would follow assessing airway and breathing.

25. 1. Assessing the site and rate would not be the first intervention.
2. Sodium bicarbonate is not administered unless indicated by arterial blood gases.
3. **The rhythm on the monitor should be assessment. Many clients who become unresponsive have a lethal rhythm that requires defibrillation immediately.**
4. Cardioversion would not be useful. Defibrillation may be needed.

26. In order of priority: 4, 2, 3, 1, 5.
4. **This is done first before any action is taken to decrease suspicions on the part of the significant other. The nurse needs to ask the client questions regarding the injuries that may not get a truthful answer with the significant other in the room.**
2. **The nurse should assess the actual physical problems before assessing the potential abuse situation.**
3. **This is one of the first questions the nurse should ask to determine if abuse is occurring.**
1. **The nurse should determine if the client has a plan to escape the violence. The nurse should provide the client with hotline numbers for safe houses.**
5. **The nurse should refer the client to the social worker for further evaluation and referral needs.**

# Perioperative Care

# 16

Surgery is a serious experience for clients. Before the surgery, in preoperative care the nurse must prepare clients for the specific surgery, telling them what to expect during the procedure and afterward. During surgery, nurses help monitor the patient and maintain the proper condition of the operating room. The postoperative period is also important. The nurse must assess the client frequently during the immediate postoperative period, ensuring that the ABCs—airway, breathing, and circulation—are maintained. The client also must be assessed for any signs of complications, such as hemorrhage, evisceration, or infection. Because acute pain is associated with most surgeries, the nurse also must assess the level and type of pain and dispense pain-relieving medication as ordered by the health-care provider

## KEYWORDS

anesthesia
anesthesiologist
circulating nurse
evisceration
nurse anesthetist

## ABBREVIATIONS

Association of Operating Room Nurses (AORN)
Blood Pressure (BP)
Centers for Disease Control (CDC)
Electrocardiogram (ECG)
Health-Care Provider (HCP)
Intravenous (IV)
Medication Administration Record (MAR)
Nonsteroidal Anti-Inflammatory Drug (NSAID)
Nursing Assistant (NA)
Operating Room (OR)
Patient-Controlled Analgesia (PCA)
Post-Anesthesia Care Unit (PACU)
Related To (R/T)

## Preoperative

1. The nurse requests a client to sign the surgical consent form for an emergency appendectomy. Which statement by the client indicates that further teaching is needed?
   1. "I will be glad when this is over so that I can go home."
   2. "I will not be able to eat or drink anything prior to my surgery."
   3. "I need to practice relaxing by listening to my favorite music."
   4. "I will need to get up and walk as soon as possible."

2. The nurse in the holding area of the surgery department is interviewing a client who requests to keep his religious medal on during surgery. Which intervention should the nurse implement?
   1. Notify the surgeon about the client's request to wear the medal.
   2. Tape the medal to the client and allow the client to wear the medal.
   3. Request that the family member take the medal prior to surgery.
   4. Explain that taking the medal to surgery is against the policy.

3. The nurse must obtain surgical consent forms for the following clients who are scheduled for surgery. Which client would not be able to consent to surgery?
   1. The 65-year-old client who cannot read or write.
   2. The 30-year-old client who does not understand English.
   3. The 16-year-old client who has a fractured ankle.
   4. The 80-year-old client who is not oriented to the day.

4. When preparing a client for surgery, which intervention should the nurse implement first?
   1. Check the permit for the spouse's signature.
   2. Take and document intake and output.
   3. Administer the "on call" sedative.
   4. Complete the preoperative checklist.

5. When interviewing the surgical client in the holding area, which information should the nurse report to the health-care provider? Select all that apply.
   1. The client has loose, decayed teeth.
   2. The client is experiencing anxiety.
   3. The client smokes two packs of cigarettes a day.
   4. The client has had a chest x-ray that does not show infiltrates.
   5. The client reports using herbs.

6. Which nursing task can the nurse delegate to the unlicensed nursing assistant (NA)?
   1. Complete the preoperative checklist.
   2. Assess the client's preoperative vital signs.
   3. Teach the client about coughing and deep breathing.
   4. Assist the client to remove clothing and jewelry.

7. When completing the assessment for the client in the day surgery unit, the client states, "I am really afraid of having this surgery. I'm afraid of what they will find." Which statement would be the best therapeutic response by the nurse?
   1. "Don't worry about your surgery. It is safe."
   2. "Tell me why you're worried about your surgery."
   3. "Tell me about your fears of having this surgery."
   4. "I understand how you feel. Surgery is frightening."

8. The 68-year-old client scheduled for intestinal surgery does not have clear fecal contents after three tap water enemas. Which intervention should the nurse implement first?
   1. Notify the surgeon of the client's status.
   2. Continue giving enemas until clear.
   3. Increase the client's IV fluid rate.
   4. Obtain stat serum electrolytes.

9. The nurse is caring for a client scheduled for abdominal surgery. Which interventions should the nurse include in the plan of care? Select all that apply.
   1. Perform range-of-motion exercises.
   2. Discuss how to cough effectively.
   3. Explain how to perform deep-breathing exercises.
   4. Teach ways to manage postoperative pain.
   5. Discuss events that occur in the post-anesthesia care unit.

10. The client is scheduled for total hip replacement. Which behavior indicates to the nurse the need for further preoperative teaching?
    1. The client uses the diaphragm and abdominal muscles to inhale through the nose and exhale through the mouth.
    2. The client takes three slow, deep, breaths and coughs forcefully after inhaling for the third time.
    3. The client uses the incentive spirometer and inhales slowly and deeply so that the piston rises to the preset volume.
    4. The client gets out of bed by lifting straight upright from the waist and then swings both legs along the side of the bed.

11. While completing the preoperative assessment, the male client tells the nurse that he is allergic to codeine. Which intervention should the nurse implement first?
    1. Apply an allergy bracelet on the client's wrist.
    2. Label the client's allergies on the front of the chart.
    3. Ask the client what happens when he takes the drug.
    4. Document the allergy on the medication administration record.

12. Which laboratory result would require immediate intervention by the nurse for the client scheduled for surgery?
    1. Calcium 9.2 mg/dL.
    2. Bleeding time 2 minutes.
    3. Hemoglobin 15 gm/dL.
    4. Potassium 2.4 mEq/L.

## Intraoperative

13. Which activities are the circulating nurse's responsibilities in the operating room?
    1. Monitor the position of the client, prepare the surgical site, and ensure the client's safety.
    2. Give preoperative medication in the holding area and monitor the client's response to anesthesia.
    3. Prepare sutures; set up the sterile field; and count all needles, sponges, and instruments.
    4. Prepare the medications to be administered by the anesthesiologist and change the tubing for the anesthesia machine.

14. While working in the operating room the circulating nurse observes the surgical scrub technician remove a sponge from the edge of the sterile field with a clamp and place the sponge and clamp in a designated area. Which action should the nurse implement?
    1. Place the sponge back where it was.
    2. Tell the technician not to waste supplies.
    3. Do nothing because this is the correct procedure.
    4. Take the sponge out of the room immediately.

15. While the circulating nurse compares the final sponge count with that of the scrub nurse, a discrepancy in the count is found. Which action should the circulating nurse take first?
    1. Notify the client's surgeon.
    2. Complete an Occurrence Report.
    3. Contact the surgical manager.
    4. Re-count all sponges.

16. Which violation of surgical asepsis would require immediate intervention by the circulating nurse?
    1. Surgical supplies were cleaned and sterilized prior to the case.
    2. The circulating nurse is wearing a long-sleeved sterile gown.
    3. Masks covering the mouth and nose are being worn by the surgical team.
    4. The scrub nurse setting up the sterile field is wearing artificial nails.

17. The nurse identifies the nursing diagnosis "risk for injury related to positioning" for the client in the operating room. Which nursing action should the nurse implement?
    1. Avoid using the cautery unit that does not have a biomedical tag on it.
    2. Carefully pad the client's elbows before covering the client with a blanket.
    3. Apply a warming pad on the OR table before placing the client on the table.
    4. Check the chart for any prescription or over-the-counter medication use.

18. When positioning the intraoperative client for surgery, which client should the nurse consider at the highest rank for irreparable nerve damage?
    1. The 16-year-old client in the dorsal recumbent position having an appendectomy.
    2. The 68-year-old client in the Trendelenburg position having a cholecystectomy.
    3. The 45-year-old client in the reverse Trendelenburg position having a biopsy.
    4. The 22-year-old client in the lateral position having a nephrectomy.

19. Which situation demonstrates the circulating nurse acting as the client's advocate?
    1. Plays the client's favorite audio book during surgery.
    2. Keeps the family informed of the findings of the surgery.
    3. Keeps the operating room door closed at all times.
    4. Calls the client by the first name when the client is recovering.

20. Which statement would be an expected outcome when the circulating nurse evaluates the goal of the intraoperative client?
    1. The client has no injuries from the OR equipment.
    2. The client has no postoperative infection.
    3. The client has stable vital signs during surgery.
    4. The client recovers from anesthesia.

21. Which nursing intervention has the highest priority when preparing the client for a surgical procedure?
    1. Pad the client's elbows and knees.
    2. Apply soft restraint straps to the extremities.
    3. Prepare the client's incision site.
    4. Document the temperature of the room.

22. When making assignments for nurses working in the OR, which case would the manager assign to the new nurse?
    1. The client having open-heart surgery.
    2. The client having a biopsy of the breast.
    3. The client having laser eye surgery.
    4. The client having a laparoscopic knee repair.

23. While working in the operating room, the nurse notices that the client has tachycardia and hypotension. Which interventions should the nurse anticipate?
    1. Prepare ice packs and mix dantrolene sodium.
    2. Request the defibrillator to be brought into the OR.
    3. Draw a PTT and prepare a heparin drip.
    4. Obtain fingerstick blood glucose immediately.

24. When developing the plan of care for the surgical client having sedation, which intervention has highest priority for the nurse?
    1. Assess the client's respiratory status.
    2. Monitor the client's urinary output.
    3. Take a 12-lead ECG prior to injection.
    4. Attempt to keep the client focused.

## Postoperative

**25.** When receiving the client from the OR, which intervention should the PACU nurse implement first?
1. Assess the client's breath sounds.
2. Apply oxygen via nasal cannula.
3. Take the client's blood pressure.
4. Monitor the pulse oximeter reading.

**26.** Which assessment data indicate the postoperative client who had spinal anesthesia is suffering a complication of the anesthesia?
1. Loss of sensation on the lumbar (L5) dermatome.
2. Absence of the client's posterior tibial pulse.
3. The client has a respiratory rate of eight (8).
4. The blood pressure is within 20% of client's baseline.

**27.** After transferring the client from the PACU to the surgical unit, the client's vital signs are T 98°F, P 106, R 24, and BP 88/40. The client is awake and oriented times three (3). The client's skin is pale and damp. Which intervention should the nurse implement first?
1. Call the surgeon and report the vital signs.
2. Start an IV of D5RL with 20 mEq KCl at 125 mL/hour.
3. Elevate the feet and lower the head.
4. Monitor the vital signs every 15 minutes.

**28.** The nurse receives a report that the postoperative client received Narcan, an opioid antagonist, in PACU. Which client problem should the nurse add to the plan of care?
1. Alteration in comfort.
2. Risk for depressed respiratory pattern.
3. Potential for infection.
4. Fluid and electrolyte imbalance.

**29.** The 26-year-old male client in the PACU has a heart rate of 110, has a rising temperature, and complains of muscle stiffness. Which interventions should the nurse implement? Select all apply.
1. Give a back rub to the client to relieve stiffness.
2. Apply ice packs to axillary and groin areas.
3. Prepare a nice slush for the client to drink.
4. Prepare to administer Dantrolene, a smooth-muscle relaxant.
5. Reposition the client on a warming blanket.

**30.** Which data indicate the nursing care has been effective for the client who is one (1) day postoperative surgery?
1. Urine output was 160 mL in the past eight (8) hours.
2. Bowel sounds occur four (4) times per minute.
3. T 99.0°F, P 98, R 20, and BP 100/60.
4. Lungs are clear bilaterally in all lobes.

**31.** When working on the surgical floor, which task can the nurse delegate to the unlicensed nursing assistant (NA)?
1. Take vital signs every four (4) hours.
2. Check the Jackson-Pratt insertion site.
3. Hang the client's next IV bag.
4. Ensure that the client gets pain relief.

**32.** The charge nurse is making the shift assignments. Which postoperative client would be the most appropriate assignment to the graduate nurse?
1. The four (4)-year-old client who had a tonsillectomy and is swallowing frequently.
2. The 74-year-old client with a repair of the left hip who is unable to ambulate.
3. A 24-year-old client who had an uncomplicated appendectomy the previous day.
4. An 80-year-old client with small bowel obstruction and congestive heart failure.

33. Which statement would be an expected outcome for the postoperative client who had general anesthesia?
    1. The client will be able to sit in the chair for 30 minutes.
    2. The client will have a pulse oximetry reading of 97% on room air.
    3. The client will have a urine output of 30 mL per hour.
    4. The client will be able to distinguish sharp from dull sensations.

34. The postoperative client is transferred from the PACU to the surgical floor. Which action should the nurse implement first?
    1. Apply anti-embolism hose to the client.
    2. Attach the drain to 20 cm suction.
    3. Assess the client's vital signs.
    4. Listen to the report from the anesthesiologist.

35. Which client problem would be priority for client who is one (1) day postoperative?
    1. Potential for hemorrhaging.
    2. Potential for injury.
    3. Potential for fluid volume excess.
    4. Potential for infection.

36. The unlicensed nursing assistant reports the vital signs for a first-day postoperative client of T 100.8°F, P 80, R 24, and B/P 148/80. Which intervention would be most appropriate for the nurse to implement?
    1. Administer the antibiotic earlier than scheduled.
    2. Change the dressing over the wound.
    3. Help the client turn, cough, and deep breathe every two (2) hours.
    4. Encourage the client to ambulate in the hall.

## Acute Pain

37. The client is complaining of left shoulder pain. Which response would be best for the nurse to assess the pain?
    1. Request that the client describe the pain.
    2. Inquire if the pain is intense, throbbing, or stabbing.
    3. Ask if the client wants pain medication.
    4. Instruct the client to complete the pain questionnaire.

38. When preparing the plan of care for the client in acute pain as a result of surgery, the nurse should include which intervention?
    1. Administer pain medication as soon as the time frame allows.
    2. Use nonpharmacological methods to replace medications.
    3. Use cryotherapy after heat therapy because it works faster.
    4. Instruct family members to administer medication with the PCA.

39. Which situation is an example of the nurse fulfilling the role of client advocate?
    1. The nurse brings the client pain medication when it is due.
    2. The nurse collaborates with other disciplines during the care conference.
    3. The nurse contacts the health-care provider when pain relief is not obtained.
    4. The nurse teaches the client to ask for medication before the pain gets to a "5."

40. Which statement would be an expected outcome for a client experiencing acute pain?
    1. The client will have decreased use of medication.
    2. The client will participate in self-care activities.
    3. The client will use relaxation techniques.
    4. The client will repeat instructions about medications.

41. Which intervention has the highest priority when administering pain medication to a client experiencing acute pain?
    1. Monitor the client's vital signs.
    2. Verify the time of the last dose.
    3. Check for the client's allergies.
    4. Discuss the pain with the client.

42. Which intervention should the nurse delegate to the unlicensed nursing assistant when caring for the client experiencing acute pain?
    1. Take the pain medication to the room.
    2. Apply an ice pack to the site of pain.
    3. Check on the client 30 minutes after he or she takes the pain medication.
    4. Observe the patient's ability to use the PCA.

43. When administering an opioid narcotic, which interventions should the nurse implement to provide for client safety? Select all that apply.
    1. Compare the hospital number on the MAR to the client's bracelet.
    2. Have a witness verify the wasted portion of the narcotic.
    3. Assess the client's vital signs prior to administration.
    4. Determine if the client has any allergies to medications.
    5. Clarify all orders with the health-care provider.

44. Which intervention would be the best way for the nurse to assess a four (4)-year-old client for acute pain?
    1. Use words that a four (4)-year-old child can remember.
    2. Explain the 0–10 pain scale to the child's parent.
    3. Have the child point to the face that describes the pain.
    4. Administer the medication every four (4) hours.

45. Which nursing intervention would be priority for the client experiencing acute pain?
    1. Assess verbal and nonverbal behavior.
    2. Wait for the client to request pain medication.
    3. Bring the pain medication on a scheduled basis.
    4. Teach the client to use only imagery every hour for the pain.

46. While conducting an interview with a 75-year-old client admitted with acute pain, which question would have priority when assisting with pain management?
    1. "Have you ever had difficulty getting your pain controlled?"
    2. "What types of surgery have you had in the last 10 years?"
    3. "Have you ever been addicted to narcotics?"
    4. "Do you have a list of your prescription medications?"

47. At the end of the shift, the nurse clears the PCA and discovers that the client has used only a small amount of medication. Which intervention should the nurse implement?
    1. Determine why the client is not using the PCA.
    2. Document the amount and take no action.
    3. Chart that the client is not having pain.
    4. Contact the HCP and request oral medication.

48. Which client problem would be most appropriate for the client experiencing acute physical pain?
    1. Ineffective coping.
    2. Potential for injury.
    3. Alteration in comfort.
    4. Altered sensory input.

## Preoperative

1. 1. When recuperating from emergency surgery, the client will be in the hospital for a few days. This is not a day-surgery procedure. The client needs more teaching.
   2. Clients are NPO (nothing by mouth) prior to surgery to prevent aspiration during and after anesthesia.
   3. Listening to music and other relaxing techniques can be used to alleviate anxiety and pain.
   4. Clients are encouraged to get out of bed as soon as possible and progress until a return to daily activity is achieved.

   **TEST-TAKING HINTS: This question is asking the test taker to identify the answer option that is incorrect. Three (3) options will be appropriate statements that indicate the client understands the teaching.**

2. 1. The surgeon does not need to be notified of the client's request; this can be addressed by the nursing staff.
   2. **The medal should be taped and the client should be allowed to wear the medal because meeting spiritual needs is essential to this client's care.**
   3. The client should be allowed to bring the medal to surgery if the medal is taped to the client.
   4. Hospital policies should be established for the well-being of clients, and spiritual needs should be addressed.

   **TEST-TAKING HINT: Because answer options "3" and "4" both do not allow the client to wear the medal to surgery, these can be eliminated as possible answers because they are both saying the same thing.**

3. 1. The 65-year-old client who cannot read can mark an "X" on the form and is legally able to sign a surgical permit as long as the client understands the benefits, alternatives, and all potential complications of the surgery.
   2. The client who does not speak English can and should have information given and questions answered in the client's native language.
   3. A 16-year-old client is not legally able to give permission for surgery unless the adolescent is given an emancipated status by a judge. This information was not given in the stem.
   4. A client is able to give permission unless determined incompetent. Not knowing the day of the week is not significant.

   **TEST-TAKING HINT: Age in a stem or option gives the test taker a clue as to the correct**

answer. The nurse must be aware of legal issues when caring for the client.

4. 1. The client's signature, not the spouse's, should be on the surgical permit.
   2. This would be information that would be important if abnormal, but it is not the first intervention.
   3. "On call" sedations should be administered after the surgical checklist is completed.
   4. **Completing the preoperative checklist has the highest priority to ensure that all details are completed without omissions.**

   **TEST-TAKING HINT: A client should never be sedated until the permit has been verified and all legal issues are settled. The test taker should not read into a question by inserting facts that are not in the stem. For example, the test taker may think that option "1" could be a correct answer if the client is confused, but the stem does not include this information.**

5. 1. **Loose teeth or caries need to be reported to the health-care provider so he or she can make provisions to prevent breaking the teeth and causing the client to possibly aspirate pieces.**
   2. **The nurse should report any client who is extremely anxious.**
   3. **Smokers are at a higher risk for complications from anesthesia.**
   4. This is a normal finding and should not be reported.
   5. **Herbs—for example, St. John's wort, licorice, and ginkgo—have serious interactions with anesthesia and with bodily functions such as coagulation.**

   **TEST-TAKING HINT: This question is an alternate-type question that requires the test taker to select more than one (1) option as the correct answer. Safety is priority for a client undergoing surgery.**

6. 1. The nurse should complete this form because it requires analysis, which cannot be delegated to the NA.
   2. Nurses cannot delegate assessment.
   3. The nurse cannot delegate teaching to an NA.
   4. **The NA can remove clothing and jewelry.**

   **TEST-TAKING HINT: The nurse should consider the knowledge and training of the person receiving the assignments. The nurse should never delegate tasks that require assessment, teaching, or evaluation.**

7. 1. This statement is giving false reassurance.
   2. This statement is requesting an explanation.

3. This statement focuses on the emotion that the client identified and is therapeutic.
4. This statement belittles the client's fear, and no person understands how another person feels.

**TEST-TAKING HINT:** There are rules that the test taker should implement when answering these types of questions. The test taker should not select an option that asks the client "why," such as option "2," or an option that states, "I understand," such as option "4."

8. 1. The nurse should contact the surgeon because the client is at risk for fluid and electrolyte imbalance after three (3) enemas. Clients who are NPO, elderly clients, and pediatric clients are more likely to have these imbalances.
   2. Administering more enemas will put the client at further risk for fluid volume deficit and electrolyte imbalance.
   3. The IV may need to be increased, but the nurse would need an order for this intervention.
   4. The electrolyte status may need to be assessed, but the nurse would need an order for this intervention.

**TEST-TAKING HINT:** Very few questions will require the test taker to notify the health-care provider, but there will be some because the nurse must know when a potential complication may occur. The nurse cannot prescribe or order laboratory tests without a health-care provider's order.

9. 1. These exercises help prevent postoperative deep vein thrombosis.
   2. Coughing effectively aids in the removal of pooled secretions that can cause pneumonia.
   3. Deep-breathing exercises keep the alveoli inflated and prevent atelectasis.
   4. The client's postoperative pain should be kept within a tolerable range.
   5. These interventions help decrease the client's anxiety.

**TEST-TAKING HINT:** This is an alternate-type question that requires the test taker to select more than one (1) option as the correct answer. The nurse's priority after surgery is to prevent postoperative complications.

10. 1. This is the correct way to perform deep-breathing exercises; therefore, no further teaching is needed.
    2. This is the correct way to perform coughing exercises; therefore, no further teaching is needed.

3. This is the way to use a volume incentive spirometer; therefore, no further teaching is needed.
4. The correct way to get out of bed postoperatively is to roll onto the side, grasp the side rail to maneuver to the side, and then push up with one hand while swinging the legs over the side. The client needs further teaching.

**TEST-TAKING HINT:** This is an "except question." Therefore the test taker must select an option that shows that the client does not understand the teaching. Sometimes flipping the question and asking which behavior indicates the client understands the teaching will help in answering this type of question.

11. 1. This is an important step for the nurse to implement, but it is not the first intervention.
    2. This must be done, but it is not the first intervention.
    3. The nurse should first assess the events that occurred when the client took this medication because many clients think that a side effect, such as nausea, is an allergic reaction.
    4. This information must be put on the medication administration record (MAR), but it is not the first intervention.

**TEST-TAKING HINT:** The stem is asking the test taker to identify the first intervention. Therefore all four (4) options could be interventions that should be implemented, but assessment is the first part of the nursing process, so option "3" is the correct answer.

12. 1. Laboratory value is within normal limits.
    2. Laboratory value is within normal limits.
    3. Laboratory value is within normal limits.
    4. This potassium level is low and should be reported to the health-care provider because potassium is important for muscle function, including the cardiac muscle.

**TEST-TAKING HINT:** There are some items, such as normal laboratory values, that the test taker must memorize. Laboratory values may differ slightly between laboratories but the test taker must know them.

## Intraoperative

13. 1. The circulating nurse has many responsibilities in the OR, including coordinating the activities in the OR; keeping the OR clean; ensuring the safety of the client; and maintaining the humidity, lighting, and safety of the equipment.

2. This is the role of the nurse anesthetist or anesthesiologist.

3. This is the role of the scrub nurse or technologist.

4. If there is an anesthesia technologist, this would be his or her role or, or the nurse anesthetist and the anesthesiologist would assume that role.

**TEST-TAKING HINT: Options "2" and "4" discuss anesthesia and an anesthesiologist, which may lead the test taker to eliminate these as possible correct answers. Some questions are knowledge-based questions that require the test taker to know the information; this is an example of this type of question.**

14. 1. Items that are on the edge of the sterile field are considered contaminated and should be removed from the field.

2. The technician is not wasting supplies; the technician is following principles of asepsis.

3. The technician followed the correct procedure. Sponges are counted to maintain client safety, so all sponges must be kept together to repeat the count before the incision site is sutured. The sponge must be removed, not used, and placed in a designated area to be counted later.

4. Taking the contaminated sponge out of the room would cause a discrepancy in the sponge count.

**TEST-TAKING HINT: When answering this question the test taker must consider safety, which is always of the utmost importance when performing surgery on a client. Sponge count is a basic concept in operating room nursing theory.**

15. 1. When discrepancies occur in the count, it is usually a simple mistake that is discovered with a re-count. The surgeon will be notified if the count is wrong after a re-count.

2. If an error is found to have been made, an Occurrence Report will be completed, but it is not the first intervention.

3. This would be done if a correct count is not maintained, but it is not the first intervention.

4. A re-count of sponges may lead to the discovery of the cause of the presumed error. Usually it is just a miscount or a result of a sponge being placed in a location other than the sterile field, such as the floor or a lower shelf.

**TEST-TAKING HINT: When the test taker has no idea of the correct answer, the test taker should apply the nursing process and choose the option that addresses assessment because it is the first step in the nursing process.**

16. 1. These are appropriate activities in a surgery department; therefore, no intervention is required.

2. This is required to maintain surgical asepsis.

3. This follows the principle of surgical asepsis.

4. According to the Centers for Disease Control (CDC), the American Operating Room Nurses Association (AORN), and the Association of Professionals in Infection Control, artificial nails harbor microorganisms, which increase the risk for infection.

**TEST-TAKING HINT: The adjective "artificial" in option "4" and the word "violation" in the stem should cause the test taker to select option "4" as the correct answer if the test taker had no idea which distracter to select.**

17. 1. This would prevent an electrical injury, but the interventions must address positioning, which is the etiology of the nursing diagnosis.

2. Padding the elbows decreases pressure so that nerve damage and pressure ulcers are prevented. This addresses the etiology of the nursing diagnosis.

3. This would help to decrease hypothermia, but it does not address the etiology of the nursing diagnosis.

4. Checking the chart for medication use would help prevent interactions between anesthesia and routine medications, but it does not address the etiology of the nursing diagnosis.

**TEST-TAKING HINT: The test taker must be knowledgeable of nursing diagnosis and the nursing process. The assessment data support the response "risk for injury" and the interventions address the etiology "positioning."**

18. 1. The young client is not a high risk for nerve damage secondary to positioning.

2. The client's age, along with positioning with increased weight and pressure on the shoulders, puts this client at higher risk.

3. This client is sitting in an upright position, which would not put this client at risk for nerve damage.

4. A younger client would not be at a high risk for nerve damage when lying on the side.

**TEST-TAKING HINT: Clients who are at highest risk for nerve damage are clients who are elderly, obese, or emaciated and clients placed in positions that increase pressure on bony prominences.**

19. 1. The client is not awake during surgery so playing a favorite audio book would not be an example of client advocacy.

2. This would be a nice action to take, but it is not an example of client advocacy.

3. This would keep the client's dignity by maintaining privacy. With this action, the nurse is speaking for the client while they cannot speak as a result of anesthesia and is an example of client advocacy.

4. Clients should be referred to by their last name, rather than first, unless the client requests the staff to use his or her first name. This is not an example of client advocacy.

**TEST-TAKING HINT: The definition of a client advocate is a person designated to speak up for the client's rights when the client cannot.**

20. 1. This expected outcome addresses the safety of the client while in the OR.

2. This would be an expected outcome in the postoperative period.

3. The anesthesiologist or nurse anesthetist would monitor the client's vital signs during surgery.

4. This would be an expected outcome for the anesthesiologist or nurse anesthetist.

**TEST-TAKING HINT: The adjectives "intraoperative" and "circulating" are the key words to answering this question. Safety is priority in the operating room.**

21. 1. This intervention prevents nerve damage from positioning, but it is not a higher priority than preventing the client from falling off the OR table.

2. This action would prevent the client from falling off the table, which is the highest priority.

3. Preparing the incision site is not a higher priority than preventing the client from falling off the OR table.

4. The temperature of the room does not have a higher priority than safety.

**TEST-TAKING HINT: Client safety should always be a high priority. In order, the priorities would be preventing a fall, preventing nerve damage, preventing infection, and then documenting.**

22. 1. Open-heart surgery is complex, and the care of the client should be assigned to an experienced nurse with special training.

2. The case of a client having a biopsy of the breast would be a good case for an inexperienced nurse because it is simple.

3. Laser eye surgery requires that the nurse in the OR have additional training to operate the equipment.

4. Additional training to be in the OR would be required for this case because special care to prevent infection is needed in orthopedic cases.

**TEST-TAKING HINT: The test taker should select the option that requires the least amount of additional training because the nurse is new to the operating room. Technology required for specific surgeries requires additional training.**

23. 1. Unexplained tachycardia, hypotension, and elevated temperature are signs of malignant hyperthermia, which is treated with ice packs and Dantrolene sodium.

2. A defibrillator would be needed if the client were in ventricular tachycardia or ventricular fibrillation.

3. These interventions would not be appropriate for malignant hyperthermia.

4. These would be important if the client had diabetes, but it does not address malignant hyperthermia.

**TEST-TAKING HINT: The test taker could eliminate options based on basic concepts. Option "2" could be eliminated because the client is not coding. Option "3" would increase bleeding, which would not be appropriate for a client having surgery.**

24. 1. Assessing the respiratory rate, rhythm, and depth is the most important action.

2. The nurse needs to monitor all systems, but monitoring the urine output would not be priority over monitoring breathing.

3. Monitoring the client's ECG is appropriate, but it is not priority.

4. The client needs to be relaxed, not focused, but this is not priority over respiratory status.

**TEST-TAKING HINT: When the test taker must prioritize nursing care, assessment is usually first. Using Maslow's Hierarchy of Needs to prioritize, assessment of respiration is always first. All sedation agents can depress respirations.**

## Postoperative

25. 1. The airway should be assessed first. When caring for a client, the nurse should follow the ABCs: airway, breathing, and circulation.

2. After assessing the client's airway and breathing, the nurse can apply oxygen via a nasal cannula if it is necessary.

3. The blood pressure is taken automatically by the monitor, but this is not priority over airway.

4. The pulse oximeter is applied to the client's finger to obtain the peripheral oxygenation status, but the nurse should assess the client's breathing first.

**TEST-TAKING HINT: When the stem of the question asks the test taker to implement a nursing intervention first, the test taker should think of assessment and then apply Maslow's Hierarchy of Needs.**

26. 1. Loss of sensation in the L5 dermatome is expected from spinal anesthesia.
    2. Absence of a posterior tibial pulse is indicative of a block in the blood supply, but it is not a complication of anesthesia.
    3. If the effects of the spinal anesthesia move up rather than down the spinal cord, respirations can be depressed and even blocked.
    4. This is an expected outcome and does not indicate a complication.

**TEST-TAKING HINT: The test taker must know normal rates for vital signs, and a respiratory rate of eight (8) would be significantly low for any client and indicate a possible complication.**

27. 1. The surgeon should be notified, but this is not the first action; the client must be cared for.
    2. The postoperative client had lactated Ringer's infused during surgery. The rate should be increased during hemorrhage—which the vital signs indicate is occurring—but potassium should not be added.
    3. By lowering the head of the bed and raising the feet, the blood is shunted to the brain until volume-expanding fluids can be administered, which is the first intervention for a client who is hemorrhaging.
    4. When signs and symptoms of shock are observed, the nurse will monitor the vital signs more frequently than every 15 minutes.

**TEST-TAKING HINT: These are the signs of hypovolemic shock. The test taker should select the intervention that will directly affect the client's problem and can be implemented the fastest to ensure the client's safety.**

28. 1. Narcan does not cause pain for the client.
    2. A client with respiratory depression treated with Narcan can have another episode within 15 minutes after receiving the drug as a result of the short half-life of the medication.
    3. Infection would not be a concern immediately after surgery.
    4. Although the client may experience an imbalance in fluid or electrolytes, this problem would not be of concern as a result of the administration of Narcan.

**TEST-TAKING HINT: The test taker should be knowledgeable about medications commonly used in the postoperative period. If the test**

taker had no idea of the answer, selecting an option addressing the airway is an appropriate action.

29. 1. A back rub is a therapeutic intervention, but it is not appropriate for a life-threatening complication of surgery.
    2. Ice packs should be applied to the axillary and groin areas for a client experiencing malignant hyperthermia.
    3. The client would be NPO to prepare for intubation, but an ice slush would be used to irrigate the bladder and stomach per nasogastric tube.
    4. Dantrolene is the drug of choice for treatment.
    5. Cooling blankets, not a warming blanket, are used to decrease the fast-rising temperature.

**TEST-TAKING HINT: This is an alternate-type question that requires the test taker to select more than one (1) option as the correct answer. Malignant hyperthermia is a medical emergency that requires immediate treatment.**

30. 1. Adequate urine output should be 30 mL per hour or at least 240 mL in an eight (8)-hour period.
    2. These bowel sounds are sluggish; 5 to 30 times a minute is normal, which indicates ineffective nursing care.
    3. The client's temperature and pulse are slightly elevated and the BP is low, which does not indicate effective nursing care.
    4. Lung sounds that are clear bilaterally in all lobes indicate the client has adequate gas exchange, which prevents postoperative complications and indicates effective nursing care.

**TEST-TAKING HINT: If the test taker does not know the answer, then applying the testing rule that airway is priority would cause the test taker to select option "4" as the correct answer.**

31. 1. Taking the vital signs of the stable client may be delegated to the NA.
    2. Assessments cannot be delegated; "check" is a word that means to assess.
    3. IVs cannot be hung by the NA; this is considered administering a medication.
    4. Evaluating the client's pain relief is a responsibility of the RN.

**TEST-TAKING HINT: The test taker cannot delegate assessment, teaching, or evaluating care of the client.**

32. 1. This client appears stable, but pediatric clients can become unstable quickly and frequent

swallowing indicates bleeding; therefore, this would not be the best choice for an inexperienced nurse.

2. Because the client is unable to ambulate, the client requires further evaluation.

3. **A young client who had an appendectomy would require routine postoperative care and would be the most appropriate client to assign to the inexperienced nurse.**

4. An older client with a chronic disease would be a complicated case, requiring the care of a more experienced nurse.

**TEST-TAKING HINT: When questions ask for assignments for graduate nurses, the test taker should realize that clients whose condition can change quickly, such as pediatric clients or elderly clients who have a complicated condition, should be assigned with caution to the newly graduated nurse.**

33. 1. The postoperative client is expected out of bed as soon as possible, but this goal is not specific to having general anesthesia.

2. **The anesthesia machine takes over the function of the lungs during surgery so the expected outcome should directly reflect the client's respiratory status; the alveoli can collapse, causing atelectasis.**

3. Urine output should be 30 mL per hour, but the expected outcome is not specific to general anesthesia.

4. Sensation would be an outcome assessed after use of a spinal anesthesia or block, but it is not specific to general anesthesia.

**TEST-TAKING HINT: If the test taker has no idea what the answer is, the test taker should apply a test-taking rule such as apply the nursing process or Maslow's Hierarchy of Needs and select the option that addresses airway. This will not always result in the correct answer, but it is a rule that can be followed if the test taker has no idea of the correct answer.**

34. 1. Applying antiembolism hose may be appropriate, but it is not the first intervention.

2. Attaching a drain would be appropriate but not before assessing the client.

3. **Assessing the client's status after transfer from the PACU should be the nurse's first intervention.**

4. Receiving reports is not the nurse's first intervention.

**TEST-TAKING HINT: The test taker should apply the nursing process when answering questions that require identifying the first intervention. Assessment is the first step of the nursing process.**

35. 1. **All clients who undergo surgery are at risk for hemorrhaging, which is the priority problem.**

2. The client is at risk for injury, but the priority problem the first day postoperative is hemorrhaging.

3. A potential fluid imbalance would be for less fluid as a result of blood loss and decreased oral intake; it would not be for fluid volume excess.

4. Infection would be a potential problem but not priority over hemorrhaging on the first postoperative day.

**TEST-TAKING HINT: Remember to apply the ABCs of care: airway, breathing, and circulation. The test taker must apply testing rules when answering questions that require identifying priority problems.**

36. 1. Antibiotics need to be administered at the scheduled time.

2. This data would not support the need to change the dressing, and surgeons usually want to change the surgical dressing for the first time.

3. **Having the client turn, cough, and deep breathe is the best intervention for the nurse to implement because if a client has a fever within the first day, it is usually caused by a respiratory problem.**

4. The client is first-day postoperative and ambulating in the hall would not be appropriate.

**TEST-TAKING HINT: With clients who have undergone surgery, the priority problems are respiration and hemorrhaging. The test taker should select an option that addresses one of these two (2) areas.**

## Acute Pain

37. 1. **This request allows the client to use terms and descriptions so that the nurse can evaluate the pain and the effectiveness of the treatment.**

2. This is putting words in the client's mouth, which may need to be done if the client cannot describe the pain, but it would be best to let the client describe the pain in his or her own words.

3. The nurse must rule out complications that require medical intervention prior to medicating the client.

4. The client who is complaining of pain should not be asked to complete paperwork.

**TEST-TAKING HINT: The test taker should apply the nursing process when answering the question and select an option that addresses assess-**

ment, which would eliminate options "3" and "4" as possible correct answers.

38. 1. Pain medications should be administered at the frequency ordered by the HCP, not just when the client requests them, especially for acute pain.
  2. Nonpharmacological methods should never replace medications, but they should be used in combination to help keep the client comfortable.
  3. Cryotherapy (cold) is used immediately postoperative or post-injury. Heat applications are applied at a later time.
  4. Only clients should activate the PCA to prevent overdosing.

**TEST-TAKING HINT:** Option "4" should be eliminated because a basic concept is that the client should be the person in control of the pain, not a family member; pain is subjective.

39. 1. This exemplifies the role of provider of care, and it does not address client advocacy.
  2. This action is addressing the role of collaborator.
  3. When the nurse contacts the HCP about unrelieved pain, the nurse is speaking when the client cannot, which is the definition of a client advocate.
  4. This action is providing care to the client and does not address client advocacy.

**TEST-TAKING HINT:** One (1) of the most important roles of the nurse is to be a client advocate. The nurse must always identify problems and follow through to their resolution.

40. 1. A decrease in use of pain medication does not mean that the client's pain is managed; the client may be concerned about possible addiction to the pain medication.
  2. Clients experiencing acute pain will not be involved in self-care because of their reluctance to move, which increases the pain; therefore, participation indicates the client's pain is tolerable.
  3. Using relaxation techniques does not indicate the client's pain is under control.
  4. This would be an expected outcome of a knowledge-deficit problem.

**TEST-TAKING HINT:** The test taker must first determine what is the expected outcome, which should be "relief of pain," and then determine which option addresses the client's relief of pain.

41. 1. It is important to monitor vital signs, but it is not the priority intervention prior to administering the medication.

2. The nurse should verify the time that the last dose was administered to determine the time the next dose could be administered, but this is not the priority intervention.
  3. Prior to giving any medication, the nurse should assess any allergies, but it is not the priority intervention.
  4. The nurse should question the client to rule out complications and to determine which medication and amount would be most appropriate for the client. This is assessment.

**TEST-TAKING HINT:** When questions require a priority answer, the test taker should look for a option that addresses assessment, but remember there are many words that reflect assessment, such as "discuss," "determine," "monitor," or "obtain," to name a few.

42. 1. Medication administration cannot be delegated to an NA.
  2. This task does not require teaching, evaluating, or nursing judgment and therefore could be delegated.
  3. Assessment cannot be delegated to an NA.
  4. Evaluation of teaching cannot be delegated to an NA.

**TEST-TAKING HINT:** The terms "observe" and "check" are different from the term "evaluate," but reading the options, the tasks are clearly addressing the evaluation step of the nursing process. Evaluation cannot be delegated to the unlicensed nursing assistant.

43. 1. This procedure ensures client safety by preventing medication from being given to the wrong client.
  2. This is a legal requirement, not a safety issue.
  3. This intervention would prevent giving a narcotic to a client who is unstable or compromised.
  4. Determining allergies addresses client safety.
  5. It would not be realistic to recheck all orders.

**TEST-TAKING HINT:** This question specifically asks the test taker to identify interventions for safely administering medication to the client. Therefore options "2" and "4" could be eliminated because they do not address the client's safety. This is an alternate-type question that requires the test taker to select more than one (1) option as the correct answer.

44. 1. The nurse should use words that a four (4)-year-old child understands and remembers, but this is not the best way to assess pain.
  2. A child that age cannot use the 0–10 scale be-

cause lack of cognitive abilities and explaining it to the parents does not address the child's pain.

3. The face scale is the best way to assess pain for a four (4)-year-old child.

4. This does not assess the child's pain, and administering the pain medication every four (4) hours may compromise the child's safety.

**TEST-TAKING HINT: When age is listed, that is an indication that the question is asking for age-specific information. Consider developmental levels for that particular age.**

45. 1. Assessing verbal and nonverbal cues is the priority intervention because pain is subjective.

2. Some clients are hesitant to ask for medication or believe that it is a sign of weakness to ask.

3. There are times when pain medications are given on a routine basis, but it is not the best answer because assessment takes priority.

4. Alternative therapies, such as imagery, are used in combination with medications, but they never replace medications.

**TEST-TAKING HINT: Options such as "4" that have absolute words such as "only" usually can be eliminated as a correct answer. Remember to apply the nursing process, and the first step is assessment.**

46. 1. The answer to this request would indicate if the client has had a negative experience that may influence the client's pain management.

2. Previous surgeries would be pertinent information but not for pain management.

3. Before asking this question, the nurse should have specific information to suspect drug use.

4. Discussing the client's prescription medications is necessary, but asking for a list of medi-

cations will not address the client's pain management.

**TEST-TAKING HINT: Assessment, the first step of the nursing process, of pain perception is indicated when caring for a client with acute pain.**

47. 1. Assessing why the client is not using the medication is a priority and then, based on the client's response, a plan of care can be determined.

2. The fact that a client is not using pain medication warrants the nurse determining the cause so that appropriate action can be taken.

3. This may or may not be why the client is not using the PCA pump. The nurse must first determine why the client is not using pain medication.

4. This may or may not be indicated, but until the nurse determines why the client is not taking the medication, this action should not be implemented.

**TEST-TAKING HINT: Assessment is priority when caring for a client. It is the first step of the nursing process, and if the test taker is unsure of the correct answer, it is the best choice to select.**

48. 1. This is a psychosocial problem, which is not appropriate for an acute physiological problem.

2. A potential problem is not priority for a client in acute pain.

3. Alteration in comfort is addressing the client's acute physical pain.

4. Altered sensory input does not address the client's acute physical pain.

**TEST-TAKING HINT: The test taker should be familiar with NANDA's list of client problems and nursing diagnoses, which includes alteration in comfort for pain. Potential problems do not have priority over actual problems.**

1. Which client would the nurse identify as having the highest risk for developing postoperative complications?
   1. The 67-year-old client who is obese, has diabetes, and takes insulin.
   2. The 50-year-old client with arthritis taking nonsteroidal anti-inflammatory drugs.
   3. The 45-year-old client having abdominal surgery to remove the gallbladder.
   4. The 60-year-old client with anemia who smokes one (1) pack of cigarettes per day.

2. The nurse is completing the preoperative checklist on a client going to surgery. Which information should the nurse report to the surgeon?
   1. The client understands the purpose of the surgery.
   2. The client stopped taking aspirin three (3) weeks ago.
   3. The client uses the oral supplements licorice and garlic.
   4. The client has mild levels of preoperative anxiety.

3. Which statement explains the nurse's responsibility when obtaining a surgical permit for the client undergoing a surgical procedure?
   1. The nurse should provide detailed information about the procedure.
   2. The nurse should inform the client of any legal consultation needed.
   3. The nurse should write a list of the risks for postoperative complications.
   4. The nurse should ensure that the client is voluntarily giving consent.

4. Which client outcome would the nurse identify for the preoperative client?
   1. The client's abnormal laboratory data will be reported to the anesthesiologist.
   2. The nurse will develop a plan of care to prevent all postoperative complications.
   3. The client will demonstrate the use of a pillow to splint while deep breathing.
   4. The client will complete an advance directive before having the surgery.

5. Which client problem would be appropriate for the preoperative client preparing for an ankle repair?
   1. Alteration in skin integrity.
   2. Knowledge deficit of postoperative care.
   3. Alteration in gas exchange and pattern.
   4. Alteration in urinary elimination.

6. The nurse and unlicensed nursing assistant (NA) are caring for clients in a surgery holding area. Which nursing task could be delegated to the NA?
   1. Explain to the client how to cough and deep breathe.
   2. Discuss preoperative plans with the client and family.
   3. Determine the ability of the caregivers to provide postoperative care.
   4. Perform the skin preparation with povidone-iodine (Betadine).

7. Which action by the client would indicate that the preoperative teaching has been effective?
   1. The client demonstrates how to use the incentive spirometer device.
   2. The client demonstrates the use of the patient-controlled analgesia pump.
   3. The client names two (2) anesthesia agents that will be used.
   4. The client ambulates down the hall to the nurse's station each hour.

8. Which intervention has priority for the nurse in the surgical holding area?
   1. Verify the surgical checklist.
   2. Prepare the client's surgical site.
   3. Assist the client to the bathroom.
   4. Restrain the client on the surgery table.

9. The client in the surgical holding area tells the nurse "I am so scared. I have never had surgery before." Which statement would be the nurse's most appropriate response?
   1. "Why are you afraid of the surgery?"
   2. "This is the best hospital in the city."
   3. "Does having surgery make you afraid?"
   4. "There is no reason to be afraid."

10. The unlicensed nursing assistant (NA) can be overheard talking loudly to the scrub technologist discussing a problem that occurred during one (1) of the surgeries. Which intervention should the nurse implement?
    1. Close the curtains around the client's stretcher.
    2. Instruct the NA and scrub tech to stop the discussion.
    3. Tell the surgeon on the case what the nurse overheard.
    4. Inform the client that the discussion was not about their surgeon.

11. The nurse is completing the preoperative checklist. Which laboratory value should be reported to the surgeon immediately?
    1. Hemoglobin 13.1 g/dL.
    2. Glucose 90 mg/dL.
    3. White blood cells 6.0 mm ($10^3$).
    4. Potassium 3.2 mEq/L.

12. Which client problem would be appropriate for the client in the intraoperative phase of the surgery?
    1. Alteration in comfort.
    2. Disuse syndrome.
    3. Risk for injury.
    4. Altered gas exchange.

13. The client has been placed in the lithotomy position during surgery. Which nursing intervention should be implemented to decrease the risk of developing hypotension?
    1. Increase the intravenous fluids.
    2. Lower one leg at a time.
    3. Raise the foot of the stretcher.
    4. Administer epinephrine, a vasopressor.

14. The circulating nurse notices that a sponge is on the edge of the sterile field. Which action should the circulating nurse take?
    1. Don't include the sponge in the sponge count.
    2. Take the sponge off the field with forceps.
    3. Tell the surgical technologist about the sponge.
    4. Throw the sponge in the sterile trashcan.

15. The nurse notes a discrepancy in the needle count. What action should the nurse implement first?
    1. Inform the other members of the surgical team about the problem.
    2. Assume that the original count was wrong and change the record.
    3. Call the radiology department to perform a portable x-ray.
    4. Complete an occurrence report and notify the risk manager.

16. The client in the surgery holding area identifies the left arm as the correct surgical site, but the operative permits designate surgery to be performed on the right arm. Which interventions should the nurse implement? Select all that apply.
    1. Review the client's chart.
    2. Notify the surgeon.
    3. Immediately call a "time out."
    4. Change the surgical permit.
    5. Have the client mark the left arm.

17. The nurse has received a client from the post-anesthesia care unit. Which assessment data would warrant immediate intervention?
    1. The client's vital signs are T 97°F, P 108, R 24, and BP 80/40.
    2. The client is sleepy but opens the eyes to his name.
    3. The client is complaining of pain at a "5" on a 1–10 pain scale.
    4. There is 20 mL of urine in the drainage bag.

18. The client received naloxone (Narcan), an opioid antagonist, in the post-anesthesia care unit. Which nursing intervention should the nurse include in the care plan?
    1. Measure intake and output hourly.
    2. Administer sleep medications at night.
    3. Encourage the client to verbalize feelings.
    4. Monitor respirations every 15 to 30 minutes.

19. Which nursing task would be appropriate to delegate to the unlicensed nursing assistant (NA) on a postoperative unit?
    1. Change the dressing over the surgical site.
    2. Teach the client how to perform incentive spirometry.
    3. Empty and record the amount of drainage in the J-P drain.
    4. Auscultate the bowel sounds in all four (4) quadrants.

20. Which assessment data have priority when caring for clients in the post-anesthesia care unit?
    1. Breath sounds.
    2. Vital signs.
    3. IV fluid rate.
    4. Surgical site.

21. The male client in the postoperative day surgery unit complains of difficulty urinating. Which intervention should the nurse implement?
    1. Insert an indwelling catheter.
    2. Increase the intravenous fluid rate.
    3. Assist the client to stand to void.
    4. Encourage the client to increase fluids.

22. The postoperative client complains of hearing a "popping sound" and feeling "something opening" when ambulating in the room. Which intervention should the nurse implement first?
    1. Notify the surgeon that the client has had an evisceration.
    2. Contact the surgery department to prepare for emergency surgery.
    3. Assess the operative site and cover the site with a moistened dressing.
    4. Explain that this is a common feeling and tell the client to continue with activity.

23. The nurse received a report that the elderly postoperative client became confused during the previous shift. Which client problem would the nurse include in the plan of care?
    1. Altered gas exchange.
    2. Altered comfort level.
    3. Impaired circulation.
    4. Impaired skin integrity.

24. The client one (1) day postoperative develops an elevated temperature. Which intervention would have priority for the client?
    1. Encourage client to deep breathe and cough every hour.
    2. Encourage the client to drink 200 mL of water every shift.
    3. Monitor the client's wound for drainage every eight (8) hours.
    4. Assess the urine output for color and clarity every four (4) hours.

25. Which statement made by the client being discharged after abdominal surgery indicates that teaching has been effective?
    1. "I will take my temperature each week and report any elevation."
    2. "I will not need any pain medication when I go home."
    3. "I will take all of my antibiotics until they are gone."
    4. "I will not take a shower until my three (3)-month checkup."

26. The client diagnosed with appendicitis has undergone an appendectomy. At two (2) hours postoperative the nurse takes the vital signs and notes T 102.6°F, P 132, R 26, and BP 92/46. Which interventions should the nurse implement? List in order of priority.
    1. Increase the IV rate.
    2. Notify the health-care provider.
    3. Elevate the foot of the bed.
    4. Check the abdominal dressing.
    5. Determine if the IV antibiotics have been administered.

Perioperative

1. 1. This client has co-morbid conditions—advanced age, obesity, and diabetes—that put this client at a higher risk for postoperative complications.
   2. This client's risk factors of arthritis can make positioning in surgery and movement in the postoperative period more difficult, but this does not put the client at greater risk for postoperative complications. The NSAIDs can be held a few days prior to surgery to decrease the problems associated with NSAIDs.
   3. The client with abdominal surgery may have respiratory complications, but the client is not at as high risk as the older client with diabetes and obesity.
   4. The client's smoking increases the risk of pulmonary complications and increases the blood level of carboxyhemoglobin, but this client does not have the problems of delayed healing and age that the 67-year-old client with diabetes does.

2. 1. If the client does not understand the surgical procedure, the surgeon should be notified, not if the client understands.
   2. Aspirin should be stopped before surgery to help prevent bleeding.
   3. Licorice and garlic can interfere with coagulation; therefore the surgeon should be notified.
   4. Mild levels of anxiety and apprehension before surgery are normal.

3. 1. The nurse is not responsible for explaining details of surgery, and too much information can increase anxiety.
   2. The nurse is not responsible for informing the client of any need for legal representation.
   3. The surgeon is responsible for informing the client of the risks and hazards of the surgery.
   4. The nurse is responsible for ensuring that the client voluntarily signs the surgical consent form giving permission for the surgery without coercion.

4. 1. This would be an outcome for the health-care team, not the client.
   2. This would be an outcome for the nurse, not the client.
   3. This would be the expected outcome for the client during the preoperative phase. After the teaching has been completed, the client should be able to demonstrate how to splint with the pillow while deep breathing and coughing.
   4. This would not be an expected outcome for the preoperative client. All clients should be encouraged to complete an advance directive, but it is not required by law.

5. 1. This client problem would not be written until after the surgery.
   2. This would be an appropriate client problem for the preoperative client who is scheduled for ankle repair. Teaching is priority.
   3. This would not be a problem for a client scheduled for surgery.
   4. This would not be a problem for a client scheduled for surgery.

6. 1. Teaching cannot be delegated.
   2. Discussing the preoperative plans is part of the planning process and cannot be delegated.
   3. Evaluation cannot be delegated to the NA.
   4. Preparing the skin can be delegated to the NA.

7. 1. The teaching is effective if the client is able to demonstrate the use of the spirometer prior to surgery.
   2. The patient-controlled analgesia pump would not be available prior to surgery because the pumps are charged to the client on a daily basis and the client would not be able to demonstrate how to use it.
   3. Determining allergies to anesthesia medications is important prior to surgery, but the nurse would not teach the specific medication names.
   4. This would demonstrate increased mobility and would be encouraged after surgery, but it would not determine if teaching was effective.

8. 1. The surgical checklist is assessed when the client arrives in the surgery department holding area where clients wait for a short time before entering the operating room.
   2. Preparing the surgical site is completed in the surgery suite but not until the client and surgery have been verified.
   3. The client should have voided just prior to being transported to the surgery department.
   4. Securing the client onto the surgical table would be important in the operating room, not in the holding area.

9. 1. The nurse should never ask the client "why." The client does not owe the nurse an explanation.
   2. This response defends the hospital and does not address the client's feelings.
   3. This response is therapeutic and promotes communication of feelings.
   4. This statement is close-ended and will not encourage the continued discussion of "fear."

10. 1. Closing curtains will not keep loud conversations from being overheard.
    2. The NA and scrub tech are violating

HIPAA and should be told to stop the conversation immediately.

3. This is a nursing problem and the nurse should handle the situation. The surgeon is not in the chain of command of the NA or the scrub tech.

4. Telling the client that the situation does not involve their surgeon is involving the client even more in the overheard conversation.

11. 1. This hemoglobin is within normal limits and would not warrant immediate action.

2. This is a normal glucose level.

3. This white blood cell value is within normal range and would not be reported.

4. **This potassium level is low and would place the client at risk for cardiac complications.**

12. 1. This client problem would be appropriate for a postoperative client or, in some circumstances, a preoperative client, but not for a client in surgery.

2. This is a problem of long-term immobility and would not apply during surgery.

3. **This problem would be appropriate for the intraoperative phase. The circulating nurse would strap and carefully pad areas to prevent damage to tissues and nerves.**

4. The client is receiving oxygen or breathing by the ventilator. The client should not have an alteration in gas exchange.

13. 1. The anesthesiologist, not the nurse in the operating room, manages the intravenous fluids.

2. **The lithotomy position has both legs elevated and placed in stirrups. The legs should be lowered one leg at a time to prevent hypotension from the shift of the blood.**

3. Raising the foot of the bed would be a treatment of hypotension, but not hypotension resulting from the lithotomy position.

4. Epinephrine, a vasopressor, is used during codes to shunt blood from the periphery to the central circulation.

14. 1. All sponges must be included in the sponge count.

2. The circulating nurse, a person who is not sterile, should not alter the sterile field.

3. **The circulating nurse should inform the surgical technologist of any break in sterile technique or field.**

4. This action is below standards of the American Organization of Operating Room Nurses and violates the principles of sterility. The sponge is included in the count and will not be discarded until the end of the case, and all sponges have been accounted for.

15. 1. If the needle count does not correlate, the surgical technologist and the other surgical

team members should be informed. After repeating the count, a search for the missing needle should be conducted.

2. Assuming that the original count was wrong is illegal and dangerous for the client.

3. If the needle is not located, an x-ray will be done, but this is not the first intervention.

4. An Occurrence Report should be completed. If the missing needle is not located, an occurrence report should be completed and sent to the risk manager, but this it is not the first intervention.

16. 1. **When the client in the holding area states that the surgery site differs from the scheduled surgery, the nurse should identify the client and review the client's chart.**

2. **If there is a discrepancy, the nurse should notify the surgeon to explain the situation and resolve the issue.**

3. **In the current Joint Commission for Accreditation of Healthcare Organizations (JCAHO) surgical standards, a "time out" period is called and everything stops until the discrepancy is resolved.**

4. **The nurse should not change a permit. If an error is discovered, the nurse should correct the situation within legal and ethical guidelines.**

5. **Clients are encouraged to mark the correct side or site with indelible ink.**

17. 1. **These are symptoms of hypovolemic shock and require immediate intervention.**

2. This is a common response to anesthesia. Clients are sleepy until the anesthesia wears off.

3. Pain management is required, but this does not indicate a life-threatening complication.

4. Urine outputs should be monitored in the postoperative period, but indwelling catheter bags are emptied in the post-anesthesia care unit prior to transferring the client to the floor, so 20 mL would not warrant immediate intervention.

18. 1. Narcan does not alter the urinary elimination; therefore, this is not an appropriate intervention for this client.

2. Anesthesia may alter sleep patterns, but this nursing intervention does not take into account the need for Narcan to be administered to the client.

3. This nursing intervention does not address the use of Narcan.

4. **Narcan is given to reverse respiratory depression from opioid analgesic medications and has a short half-life. The client may experience a rebound respiratory depression in 15–20 minutes, so this nursing intervention of monitoring respirations every 15–30 minutes is appropriate.**

19. 1. The surgeon performs the first surgical dressing.
    2. Nurses cannot delegate teaching and assessment.
    3. **Emptying the drainage devices and recording the amounts on the bedside intake and output forms can be delegated.**
    4. Listening to bowel sounds is assessing and cannot be delegated.

20. 1. **The post-anesthesia care unit nurse should follow the ABCs format described by the American Heart Association. "A" is for airway, "B" is for breathing, and "C" is for circulation.**
    2. Vital signs would be done after assessing breathing.
    3. Intravenous fluids should be assessed after breathing and circulation have been assessed.
    4. The surgical site should be assessed after the intravenous fluid rate is assessed.

21. 1. This intervention is invasive, increases the client's risk for infection, requires an order from the HCP, and should be the last resort.
    2. The nurse would not increase the intravenous fluids unless the surgeon changes the order.
    3. **Helping the male client to stand can offer the assistance needed to void. The safety of the client should be ensured.**
    4. Drinking more fluids helps to increase urinary output but will not assist the client to empty the bladder.

22. 1. The nurse should assess the client before notifying the surgeon that the client felt or heard a "pop" and "something opening."
    2. The surgery department may or may not need to be notified. The incision should be assessed.
    3. **The nurse should assess the surgical site and, if the site has eviscerated, cover the opening with a sterile dressing that is moistened with sterile 0.9% saline. This will prevent the tissues from becoming dry and infected.**
    4. The nurse should not dismiss any complaint from a client without further assessment.

23. 1. **When a previously alert and oriented client becomes confused, the nurse should first consider hypoxia as the cause.**
    2. Confusion would not indicate a change in comfort level.
    3. Sudden confusion is usually not a circulation problem.
    4. Impaired skin integrity would not cause confusion.

24. 1. **When a postoperative client develops a fever within the first 24 hours, the cause is usually in the respiratory system. The client should increase deep breathing and coughing to assist the client to expand the lungs and decrease pulmonary complications.**
    2. Drinking fluid can bring down temperature, but 200 mL would not be a sufficient amount to accomplish this. Unless contraindicated, the client should drink from one (1) L to two (2) L per day.
    3. Wound infections may cause the fever later in the recovery but will usually not elevate within the first 24 hours after surgery.
    4. A urinary tract infection may occur later but would probably not be the cause of elevated temperature within 24 hours after surgery.

25. 1. The client should check the temperature twice a day.
    2. It not realistic to expect the client to experience no pain after surgery.
    3. **This statement about taking all the antibiotics ordered indicates that teaching is effective.**
    4. Clients may shower after surgery, but not taking a tub bath for three (3) months after surgery is too long a time.

26. In order of priority: 1, 3, 5, 4, 2.
    1. **The nurse should increase the IV rate to maintain the circulatory system function until further orders can be obtained.**
    3. **The foot of the bed should be elevated to help treat shock, the symptoms of which include elevated pulse and decreased blood pressure. Those signs and an elevated temperature indicate that an infection may be present and that the client could be developing septicemia.**
    5. **The nurse should administer any IV antibiotics that are ordered. A delay in administering IV antibiotics could cost the client his or her life. If the antibiotics have been given, then possibly the infection is resistant to the antibiotic. The nurse will need this information when reporting to the health-care provider.**
    4. **The dressing is two (2) hours old and would have been assessed when the client returned from PACU. This could provide some information, but it is not as important as the vital signs and antibiotic information.**
    2. **The health-care provider should be notified when the nurse has the needed information.**

# Cultural Nursing and Alternative Health Care

**17**

The use of alternative therapies to treat specific disorders and to promote health and well-being has increased in recent years. Many people use herbs, massage therapy, aromatherapy, rolfing, guided imagery, yoga, and numerous other techniques either alone or in addition to the techniques and drugs used by conventional medicine. The nurse should be aware of these practices and of the various health-related beliefs and traditions that people of different cultures have.

## KEYWORDS

ayurveda
curandero
mezuzah
nattuvidhyar
rolfing
tallis
Yom Kuppur

## ABBREVIATIONS

Acquired Immunodeficiency Syndrome (AIDS)
Activities of Daily Living (ADLs)
Blood Pressure (BP)
Complementary and Alternative Medicine (CAM)
Health-Care Provider (HCP)
International Normalized Ratio (INR)
National Center for Complementary and Alternative Medicine (NCCAM)
Nursing Assistant (NA)
Nonsteroidal Anti-Inflammatory Drug (NSAID)

1. The nurse is admitting the client to a medical unit. Which questions should the nurse specifically ask the client about the current use of medications? Select all that apply.
   1. "Have you used or do you currently use any type of herb?"
   2. "What over-the-counter medications do you take?"
   3. "Are you allergic to any medications or foods?"
   4. "When is the last time you took any medication?"
   5. "Do you take any prescription medications?"

2. The client who has had a cold for the last week is complaining of congestion and a stuffy nose. The client has been using medicated nasal spray several times a day. Which information should the nurse teach the client about frequent use of nasal spray?
   1. Nasal sprays are safe because they are available over the counter.
   2. Nasal sprays such as Afrin cause rebound congestion when used frequently.
   3. Nasal sprays have no adverse reactions, unlike over-the-counter oral decongestants.
   4. Nasal sprays must be alternated to help prevent developing a tolerance to the spray.

3. The client using contraceptive foam for birth control has not had her menses for the last two (2) months. Which intervention should the nurse implement first?
   1. Perform a vaginal examination.
   2. Check the urine for glucose and protein.
   3. Obtain vital signs to determine a baseline.
   4. Request a pregnancy test for this client.

4. The female client with a cold is prescribed warfarin (Coumadin), an anticoagulant, for chronic atrial fibrillation. The client calls the clinic and tells the nurse that she is bleeding and bruising more than normal. Which information indicates a need for further teaching?
   1. The client reports taking echinacea, an herb.
   2. The client had an INR drawn last month.
   3. The client uses acetaminophen, a nonopioid analgesic, for pain.
   4. The client reads labels on packaged foods.

5. Which intervention should the nurse implement when discussing health promotion activities for a client with a German heritage who leads a sedentary lifestyle?
   1. Refer the client to a support group for weight loss.
   2. Teach the client to never drink alcoholic beverages.
   3. Help the client to identify a routine exercise program.
   4. Assist the client to make a list of foods that must be avoided.

6. The elderly female client of Mexican heritage is upset and tells the nurse that the unlicensed nursing assistant (NA) complimented her grandchild's hair. Which intervention should the nurse implement?
   1. Ask the client why she is upset about the NA's saying the child's hair is pretty.
   2. Take no action because the unlicensed nursing assistant was being friendly.
   3. Notify the psychologist of the client's response to the NA's compliment.
   4. Explain to the NA about the cultural belief regarding the "evil eye."

7. The home health care nurse is visiting an elderly African American female client who is talking loudly. The client weighs 102 kg, is 5'4" tall, and has a BP of 154/98. The client lives with her daughter, son-in-law, and two grandchildren. Which intervention should the nursing implement?
   1. Maintain extended direct eye contact during the interview.
   2. Address what is assumed to be the client's anger because she is talking loudly.
   3. Discuss the client's care with the daughter and son-in-law.
   4. Discuss a weight-loss program for the client.

8. The home health nurse is making the initial visit to a 42-year-old male client with terminal cancer. The client is first-generation American-Vietnamese and lives with his parents, wife, and three children. Which behavior would best promote a therapeutic nurse–client relationship?
   1. Use questions that require "yes" and "no" answers when possible.
   2. Touch the client's head to assess warmth in case of a fever.
   3. Assume the client's smile means the client understands the teaching.
   4. Initially address conversation to the eldest family member.

9. When interviewing the client of Hindu heritage, which information should the nurse obtain to plan culturally sensitive care?
   1. Determine if the client has an advance directive.
   2. Assess the extent of the client's use of ayurveda.
   3. Request an interpreter to obtain the client's chief complaints.
   4. Inquire if the client has allergies to any foods or medications.

10. The unlicensed nursing assistant (NA) notices a strange amulet pinned to the client's gown and offers to remove it. The client does not want it removed. Which rationale should the nurse give the NA for allowing the client to continue to wear the amulet?
   1. The client is superstitious and may become distressed if it is removed.
   2. The amulet is a silly trinket that won't hurt the client in any way.
   3. The client brought the amulet because it gives the client emotional support.
   4. The amulet is worthless and no one would try to steal it if it stays on the gown.

11. After evaluating the meal tray of a Jewish client, the nurse notices that the client ate none of the meal. Which intervention should the nurse implement first?
   1. Request the client's family bring meals the client can eat.
   2. Contact the dietary department and request a kosher meal.
   3. Notify the local rabbi to request meals be provided for the client.
   4. Determine why the client is not eating any of the meal.

12. The client approaches the nurse about a weight-loss program. Which complementary therapy should the nurse suggest to assist the client's plan?
   1. Music therapy.
   2. Hypnotherapy.
   3. Hatha yoga.
   4. Alexander technique.

13. The nurse is incorporating complementary therapies in the routines of residents of a long-term care facility. Which information should the nurse consider when matching the clients with the therapy? Select all that apply.
   1. The client's preferences.
   2. The client's likes and dislikes.
   3. The benefits obtained from the therapy.
   4. The significant other's concerns.
   5. The client's ability to perform therapies.

14. Which form of complementary therapy should the nurse encourage as a relaxation technique for the anxious elderly client admitted for surgery?
   1. Meditation.
   2. Deep breathing.
   3. Rolfing.
   4. Scented candle.

15. The nurse is preparing the plan of care for the client diagnosed with migraine headaches. Which information regarding complementary therapies should the nurse include in this plan?
   1. Encourage the use of therapeutic touch.
   2. Purchase a textbook on autogenic therapy.
   3. Explain how to perform massage therapy.
   4. Discuss the need to avoid aromatic oils.

Cultural

16. The rehabilitation nurse is caring for an elderly client who had a surgical repair of a fractured hip. The client states that she misses her dog. Which intervention should the nurse implement?
    1. Put the television on a show with animal performers.
    2. Arrange for the family to bring the client's dog for a visit.
    3. Arrange for the client to have a visit from the pet therapy dog.
    4. Share that the client's feelings are completely understood by the nurse.

17. The nurse is caring for a client in the rehabilitation unit who is hearing impaired, is anxious, and who has elevated blood pressure. The client enjoys pet therapy but is allergic to dogs and cats. Which intervention should the nurse implement?
    1. Administer antihistamine medication prior to pet therapy.
    2. Spend extra time visiting at the client's bedside.
    3. Arrange for a volunteer to bring the client a radio.
    4. Provide a colorful fish in a small bowl for the client.

18. The nurse arranges for a dance movement therapist to lead a group session for clients with osteoarthritis. Which statement best describes the rationale for this intervention?
    1. Participants in dance movement form a unique bond while moving in unison.
    2. Dancing will help increase the amount of synovial fluid in the affected joints.
    3. Dance therapy helps decrease the client's pain in joints that are inflamed.
    4. Dancing causes the release of endorphins and helps the clients deal with pain.

19. The nurse is providing preoperative teaching about pain management techniques for the client having surgery. The client has a history of drug abuse. What should the nurse include in this client's plan of care?
    1. The nurse should know that these clients always require too much nursing care.
    2. The client should select two (2) alternate therapies to replace medications.
    3. The client should receive complementary therapies in addition to medications.
    4. The nurse should plan to administer a double dose of medication to this client.

20. Which intervention should the circulating nurse implement for the preoperative elderly client who is anxious and diaphoretic?
    1. Play soft, slow-beat music in the operating room.
    2. Encourage the client to take rapid, shallow breaths.
    3. Continue to talk to the client to promote relaxation.
    4. Open the door to the operating suite to increase the airflow.

21. The unlicensed nursing assistant (NA) is bathing a client who is comatose and the radio is playing current rock music. The client has tachycardia and elevated blood pressure. Which intervention should the nurse implement?
    1. No action by the nurse is indicated in this situation.
    2. Instruct the unlicensed NA to select baroque music.
    3. Administer medication to decrease the client's heart rate and blood pressure.
    4. Assist the NA to turn the client into the lateral position.

22. The nurse is caring for the surgical client who is experiencing pain at a "4" on a 1–10 pain scale and is receiving pain medication via patient-controlled analgesia (PCA). Which intervention should the nurse implement first to assist the client's pain management?
    1. Notify the health-care provider to increase the dosage of medication.
    2. Inform the client to relax and that the medication will relieve the pain soon.
    3. Assist the client to perform guided imagery to increase relaxation.
    4. Instruct the family member to continue to push the button for the medication.

23. Which expected outcome should be included in the plan of care for a postoperative client practicing guided imagery?
    1. The client will have a decreased white blood cell count.
    2. The client will report a decrease in pain using the pain scale.
    3. The client will have a urine output of 360 mL each shift.
    4. The client will have no drainage on the surgical dressing.

24. The nurse is teaching the client how to use guided imagery. Which information would indicate that the teaching has been effective?
    1. The client closes both eyes and makes a one-syllable sounding chant.
    2. The client rubs the right arm in firm stroking motions.
    3. The client selects meaningful music that has 50 beats per minute.
    4. The client visualizes a scene from a favorite place.

25. The client is complaining of nonspecific body aches, congestion, and coughing. The client's blood pressure is elevated. Which intervention should the nurse implement first?
    1. Instruct the client to decrease salt in the diet.
    2. Notify the HCP to request an antihypertensive medication.
    3. Determine if the client takes any over-the-counter medication.
    4. Discuss the long-term effects of atherosclerosis and hypertension.

Cultural

1. 1. The nurse should ask specifically about herbs because many clients do not consider them drugs and will not volunteer the information.
   2. The nurse should ask about the use of over-the-counter medications because many clients believe health-care providers are only concerned about prescribed medications.
   3. The nurse should assess the client for any previous reaction to medications.
   4. The nurse should be aware of when the last medication was taken to determine the effectiveness of the medication and to ensure that any further medication will not have an untoward effect.
   5. The health-care team must be aware of all prescriptions so the medications may be continued during hospitalization or discontinued if necessary.

   TEST-TAKING HINT: This is an example of an alternative-type question. There could be more than one (1) correct answer. The test taker should key into the descriptive words, such as "specifically," in the stem of the question.

2. 1. All medications have side effects, even the drugs that are available over the counter.
   2. Medicated nasal sprays, such as Afrin nasal spray, cause the arterioles to constrict, resulting in increased congestion after several days' use.
   3. Medicated nasal sprays, as well as oral decongestants, have adverse effects.
   4. Alternating several nasal sprays will not prevent the client from developing a tolerance to the sprays.

   TEST-TAKING HINT: If the client has no idea of the correct answer, answer option "2" has the word "decongestants" in the answer and the word "congestion" is in the stem of the question. This would be an appropriate option to select as the correct answer.

3. 1. A vaginal examination would be performed after the pregnancy test result was obtained.
   2. The first intervention is to determine if the client is pregnant.
   3. Baseline vital signs would be needed if the client were pregnant.
   4. The first intervention should be determining if the client is pregnant. The results of a pregnancy test will determine which interventions should be implemented next.

   TEST-TAKING HINT: The test taker must key in on the word "first," which indicates that one

(1) or all four (4) interventions are appropriate but only one (1) should be implemented first.

4. 1. Echinacea combines with warfarin (Coumadin) to increase bleeding time. It does not, however, alter the INR.
   2. Clients taking warfarin (Coumadin) should have their INR tested routinely.
   3. Clients taking anticoagulants should use acetaminophen (Tylenol) for pain, rather than aspirin or NSAIDs because these can cause bleeding.
   4. Prepared foods can interact with medications and medical treatments, but not many foods cause bleeding and bruising.

   TEST-TAKING HINT: Herbs often interfere with over-the-counter medications and prescription medications. Therefore this would be an appropriate choice for the correct answer if the test taker had no idea of the correct answer to this question.

5. 1. People with German heritage tend to be social, but nothing in the stem indicates the client is overweight.
   2. Unless contraindicated, a more realistic goal would be to restrict the number of alcoholic beverages to two (2) per day. Beer is a frequent beverage on many German tables.
   3. All clients would benefit from a routine daily exercise program, which promotes health, especially for those with a sedentary lifestyle.
   4. There is nothing in the stem that indicates the client has a specific disease process that warrants restricting foods.

   TEST-TAKING HINT: The adjective "sedentary" is the key to answering this question correctly. The test taker should not become distracted by excess verbiage in the stem. In option "2," the word "never" is an absolute term and makes this option incorrect.

6. 1. The nurse should not ask the client "why"; the client has a right to her feelings.
   2. An action should be implemented because the client is upset and the client's emotional state should be addressed.
   3. There is no reason for the nurse to refer the client to a psychologist.
   4. The NA should be informed about "the evil eye" so that the situation can be resolved. By complimenting the child, the grandmother might be afraid the child will become ill. The situation should be addressed, and the client may desire to perform a ritual to remove the "evil eye."

Cultural

**TEST-TAKING HINT:** The term "elderly" should inform the test taker that the question is age specific, and the word "Mexican" indicates that the question is probably addressing a cultural issue. In answer options "1" and "2" there is no action addressing the client's emotional state.

7. 1. The nurse should realize that maintaining direct eye contact with some African American clients can be interpreted as aggressive behavior.
   2. Loud expression of needs does not mean that the client is angry.
   3. The nurse should discuss the care with the client. Discussing her care with family members is a violation of HIPAA, and just because the client lives in their home does not mean they are the client's guardians.
   4. The nurse should discuss the importance of the management of ideal body weight because the client is overweight and hypertensive.

**TEST-TAKING HINT:** The test taker must realize that 102 kilograms is 240 pounds, which is overweight for a 5'4" woman. The test taker should not automatically select option "2" because the word "loudly" is in both the stem and the answer option. Speaking loudly could indicate a hearing impairment or her normal speech.

8. 1. Clients may use "yes" to answer questions to avoid conflict because of a desire to please the nurse.
   2. The head is considered sacred and should not be touched. If it is medically necessary to touch the head, the nurse should ask permission.
   3. The client may smile for various reasons. In the Vietnamese culture expression of emotions is viewed as a sign of weakness, and a stoic smile may be used to disguise negative emotions. The nurse should not interpret a smile as understanding.
   4. The nurse should talk to the eldest family member first. This is culturally acceptable behavior and will help establish a positive relationship with the client. However, addressing the conversation to the elder family member does not mean that the nurse discusses the client's health without the client's permission.

**TEST-TAKING HINT:** The question is asking for an intervention that will help establish a rapport with the client and cultural influences must be addressed, especially in the home. Answer option "1" is assuming the client has

decreased cognitive ability, which is information not provided in the stem.

9. 1. An advance directive would not be information that would help provide culturally sensitive nursing care.
   2. Ayurveda is the traditional health care of India and the nurse should determine if the client practices Ayurveda or uses a faith healer, nattuvidhyars. Many clients self-medicate with medications brought from India.
   3. An interpreter would not help the nurse provide culturally sensitive care but would help the nurse understand what the client is saying.
   4. Allergies to medications and environmental elements are assessed in the initial interviews of all clients and would not reflect cultural aspects of care.

**TEST-TAKING HINT:** This question is requesting specific information about the culture of the Hindu heritage. Answer options "1" and "4" are information that the nurse would require of any client and therefore could be eliminated because the stem is asking about culturally sensitive care.

10. 1. The nurse should not refer to the client's beliefs in a negative manner.
    2. This statement is belittling to the client's beliefs and would interfere with the nurse–client relationship.
    3. Good luck charms, such as amulets or medals, provide clients with emotional support. Folk remedies that are not harmful should be allowed while caring for the client.
    4. Personal belongings are usually sent home to prevent the loss of the items, but this statement would be false because the client values the amulet.

**TEST-TAKING HINT:** A basic concept in nursing is that the nurse should always try to support the client's cultural beliefs if they do not harm the client or interfere with the medical treatment.

11. 1. The nurse could request that the family bring meals, but this is not the first intervention.
    2. The nurse should notify the dietary department once it is determined why the client is not eating the meals provided.
    3. Many local Jewish communities will provide kosher meals for clients in the hospital if the dietary department is unable to provide them, but this is not the first intervention.
    4. The nurse should first assess and determine why the client is not eating. The not eating

could be because of the illness, medication, or cultural beliefs.

**TEST-TAKING HINT: Religious practices should be considered when clients are in the hospital. However, the nurse must first assess the situation to determine why the client is not eating. Remember, the first step of the nursing process is assessment.**

12. 1. Music therapy has been used in pain management and relaxation, but it is not used for weight loss.
    2. Hypnotherapy, or self-hypnosis, has been used successfully in weight-loss programs.
    3. There are several types of yoga that increase relaxation and promote health, but they do not assist with weight loss.
    4. The Alexander technique focuses on assisting clients become aware of movements and the relationship with health and performance, but it has not been used for weight loss.

**TEST-TAKING HINT: The test taker should be familiar with current treatments. Current treatment options being advertised for weight loss are hypnosis and self-hypnosis.**

13. 1. Selection of various therapies offers the client the ability to have some control over his or her care and may help maintain independence.
    2. Clients can select treatments that are pleasurable in addition to being effective.
    3. Many therapies decrease heart rate and blood pressure. Therefore the nurse should be knowledgeable so that referrals can be effective.
    4. The nurse should explain the benefits of the therapy to the significant other to alleviate concerns, but this would not be considered when the nurse is planning the therapy.
    5. Many therapies require movement or a specific cognitive ability to perform. If the client cannot perform the therapy, the client can become frustrated.

**TEST-TAKING HINT: This is an example of an alternative-type question. The test taker may have to select more than one (1) correct answer.**

14. 1. Meditation takes practice and the ability to focus. It is not the best way to help an elderly anxious client manage stress.
    2. Deep breathing begins to relax the muscles in the body, and this would be a method for an elderly client to learn and use to relax.
    3. Rolfing is a holistic method of structural integration. The client would not be able to per-

form this therapy independently because a therapist is needed to perform it.
    4. Scented candles would be unsafe in a hospital setting. Aromatherapy using essential oils can be used, but the client is admitted for surgery and any scent postoperatively can initiate nausea.

**TEST-TAKING HINT: The adjective "elderly" should cause the test taker to select the easiest and simplest way to help the client relax. The test taker must pay close attention to adjectives such as "elderly."**

15. 1. Therapeutic touch is used in the treatment of migraine headaches by some clients. The practitioner uses the hands to direct energy to correct imbalances that cause the migraine headache.
    2. Autogenic training is a method using mental relaxation to lead the body to healing. Because it may require several sessions by a certified trainer, the client would find it difficult to learn this technique from a book.
    3. Massage is the manual manipulation of the client's tissue, which affects the entire body and produces generalized relaxation and a feeling of well-being, but the client cannot perform massage therapy on himself or herself.
    4. Aromatherapy has been linked to the relief of the symptoms of migraine headaches by using certain essential oils such as rosemary, chamomile, and lavender..

**TEST-TAKING HINT: The test taker should be aware that the client will be unable to perform therapies on themselves. The test taker should be cautious when selecting an answer option that encourages the client to purchase a book explaining the therapy.**

16. 1. The nurse should not ignore the client's feelings of sadness and loneliness by turning on the television.
    2. The client is in a rehabilitation setting, which often allows pet visits. Therefore the nurse should investigate having the family bring the dog to the facility. This is being a client advocate.
    3. Pet therapy is being used to promote relaxation and a sense of well-being, but the client wants to see her own dog.
    4. The nurse should never claim to have a complete understanding of the client's feelings. This would belittle the client's feelings.

**TEST-TAKING HINT: The test taker must be aware of adjectives, and "rehabilitation" in the stem indicates the client is not in an acute care setting. Many rehabilitation units allow family pets to visit.**

17. 1. The nurse should not administer medication so that the client can visit with animals. The nurse cannot control all of the client's symptoms and this could present a danger to the client.
2. The nurse cannot realistically spend extra time visiting with the client when the nurse has many clients to care for and duties to complete.
3. Arranging for the volunteer to bring a radio for the client who is hearing impaired would not be helpful because it would need to be played loudly for the client to hear and that would interfere with other clients and staff.
4. **For clients who have allergies to pet dander, the nurse can provide fish therapy. Studies indicate that watching fish swim can decrease blood pressure and promote a calming effect.**

**TEST-TAKING HINT: The descriptive terms should guide the test taker to the correct answer. The test taker should eliminate "3" because of the words "hearing impaired" in the stem of the question.**

18. 1. **Dance movement therapy incorporates synchronized movement and creates an experience shared by all the participants which, in turn, contributes to the establishment of a bond between the participants. The sharing of emotions and experiences strengthens support-group relationships.**
2. Dance movements do not help increase the amount of synovial fluid in joints.
3. Dance movements don't help decrease pain; in fact, they may increase pain in some clients.
4. Endorphins are released by laughing, not dancing, and their release does not necessarily help with pain.

**TEST-TAKING HINT: The test taker should apply knowledge of anatomy and physiology to help answer this question. Synovial fluid does not increase for any reason; therefore, option "2" should be eliminated as a correct answer. Inflamed joints respond to cold or heat; therefore, option "3" should be eliminated as a correct answer.**

19. 1. The nurse is responsible for ensuring the client receives quality care regardless of the client's history or the amount of care required.
2. The client should be encouraged to use alternative therapies for pain management to supplement medication, not replace medication.
3. **The nurse should assist the client's pain management by using complementary therapies as well as medication, but never in place of pain medication.**

4. A double dose of medication requires an HCP's order, and, if administered, careful monitoring is required.

**TEST-TAKING HINT: The descriptive terms "preoperative teaching" can assist the test taker in eliminating options. Option "1" is judgmental and should be eliminated. Options "2" and "3" are opposites. Most of the time one (1) option is correct.**

20. 1. Studies show that music can calm the anxious client when the music has a slow beat. Faster beats or irregular rhythms tend to irritate elderly clients.
2. Taking deep breaths may help decrease anxiety. Rapid shallow breathing could cause the client to hyperventilate and lead to dizziness.
3. Talking makes some clients more anxious; a quiet environment would assist this client to relax.
4. The increased airflow could increase the risk for client infection and will not help the client's diaphoresis.

**TEST-TAKING HINT: The test taker should have basic concepts in operating room nursing, and often music is played to help decrease the anxiety of the client as well as the staff. Music can have a calming affect on people.**

21. 1. This situation indicates that the nurse should take some type of action. The client has an elevated heart rate and blood pressure.
2. **Baroque music has a slower pace and studies have shown that client's bodies attempt to synchronize with the beat and rhythm of the sounds in the room. The client's elevated vital signs could be a result of the rock music in the room.**
3. Medications should be used if other methods are not effective.
4. Changing the client's position should be done routinely and may decrease discomfort, but it will not affect the client's pulse and blood pressure.

**TEST-TAKING HINT: The test taker should recognize that words in the questions can aid in the selection of the correct answer. The description of "rock" music in the stem of the question and answer option "2" to change the music should assist in selecting the correct answer.**

22. 1. The pain and evaluation of the medication should be assessed prior to contacting the health-care provider.
2. Telling the client to relax does not help when the client is uncomfortable.
3. **Guided imagery can be used to increase**

relaxation and decrease the sensation of pain.

4. When clients are using a patient-controlled analgesia pump, family members should be discouraged from administering the medication for the client. The client can become over-sedated and develop respiratory depression.

**TEST-TAKING HINT:** If the test taker wants to select the answer option that says "notifies the health-care provider," the test taker must evaluate the other options to make sure another option does not include assessment data or an independent nursing intervention.

23. 1. Guided imagery is not used to prevent or treat infection; therefore assessing the white blood cell count would not be appropriate.
2. The postoperative client uses guided imagery to increase relaxation, which helps decrease the perception of pain.
3. This is a goal for a postoperative client, but it is not based on the use of guided imagery.
4. The expected outcome for the postoperative client would be to have a clean, dry dressing, but guided imagery would not affect the dressing.

**TEST-TAKING HINT:** The expected outcome must reflect the goal of guided imagery. Therefore the test taker must have knowledge of why guided imagery is used to be able to answer this question.

24. 1. This would be done during meditation.
2. Rubbing the arm in firm stroking motions is performing self-massage.

3. Music therapy is purposefully using music that has 50 to 60 beats per minute.
4. The client using guided imagery should use as many senses as possible to create an image of a scene that has meaning for the client.

**TEST-TAKING HINT:** Each answer option describes a type of complementary therapy. The test taker should pay attention to the word "imagery" and "visualize." To visualize is to use the imagination.

25. 1. Instructing on a low-salt diet may be needed, but assessment should be the first intervention implemented.
2. Antihypertensive medications may be needed, but assessment should be the first intervention implemented.
3. The nurse should first assess the client to determine if the client is taking any over-the-counter medication that may increase the blood pressure. Decongestants that contain ephedrine or pseudoephedrine elevate blood pressure and should be used with caution.
4. Teaching about the complications of hypertension would be important but not before assessing the client.

**TEST-TAKING HINT:** The test taker should use the nursing process when answering questions that ask the test taker to select the first intervention. Assessment is the first intervention of the nursing process.

Cultural

1. The client diagnosed with rheumatoid arthritis asks the nurse, "Is it all right for me to wear this copper bracelet to help cure my arthritis?" Which statement by the nurse would be most appropriate?
   1. "How do you know that the copper bracelet will help cure your arthritis?"
   2. "The bracelet will not cure your arthritis, but if it helps the pain, wear it."
   3. "You should talk to your health-care provider before wearing the copper bracelet."
   4. "I recommend not wearing the bracelet and taking your prescribed medications."

2. The client asks the nurse about using herbs and special teas to decrease blood pressure. Which question is most important for the nurse to consider before addressing the client's concerns?
   1. "How expensive is this treatment?"
   2. "Is this practice safe for the client?"
   3. "Do I have the knowledge to answer this question?"
   4. "Is this within the scope of the state's nursing practice act?"

3. The client is using acupuncture to help relieve severe back pain. Which client problem would the home health nurse identify in the plan of care?
   1. The likelihood of paralysis.
   2. The potential for infection.
   3. The possibility of contracting AIDS.
   4. No resolution of the pain.

4. The male Navajo client comes to the clinic complaining of chest pain and has a pouch filled with objects around his neck. Which statement best supports the nurse allowing the client to wear the pouch?
   1. This is a cultural practice shared by many Navajo clients, and the nurse should not remove it unless it interferes with the client's care.
   2. The client may get very upset and angry with the nurse if the pouch is removed and lose faith in the health-care system.
   3. The nurse should never ask any client to remove any type of cultural objects from the body.
   4. This is a preventive measure prescribed by the medicine man that wards off the evil of a witch.

5. The Mexican client requests a curandero to come to the hospital to visit. Which statement explains the role of the curandero in the Mexican culture?
   1. He is a person who treats muscle and joint problems using massage and manipulation.
   2. She is a person who uses herbs, teas, and roots to prevent or treat illnesses.
   3. She is a spiritualist who treats the person's condition that is caused by witchcraft.
   4. He is a person who receives his gift from God and treats traditional illnesses.

6. The home health nurse is visiting a Jewish client who has a small container on the doorpost of the house. Which term best describes this container?
   1. A tallis.
   2. A mezuzah.
   3. A synagogue.
   4. Yom Kippur.

7. The home health nurse is assessing a client diagnosed with congestive heart failure who has a slice of raw potato on a carbuncle on the abdomen. Which action should the nurse implement first?
   1. Explain that the client should not put raw potatoes on the boil.
   2. Ask the client to explain why there is a raw potato on the boil.
   3. Cleanse the wound and determine if there is an infection.
   4. Leave the raw potato on the boil and take no further action.

8. The female client is complaining of dyspepsia, insomnia, and upper-respiratory infection symptoms and has an elevated blood pressure. The client tells the nurse she recently moved to the area to care for an ill parent. Which statement best explains the client's clinical manifestations?
   1. The client has a psychosomatic illness.
   2. The client's immune system is altered by stress.
   3. The client's symptoms are cause by gastric reflux.
   4. The client has essential hypertension.

9. The nurse assessing an elderly client diagnosed with chronic obstructive pulmonary disease notes purple, round, nontender areas on the client's back. Which question should the nurse ask the client?
   1. "Have you had cupping performed?"
   2. "Do you always bruise this easily?"
   3. "Did someone living with you hurt you?"
   4. "What have you done to cause these?"

10. The nurse is preparing a teaching plan for a client diagnosed with chronic stress. Which information should the nurse include in the teaching care plan? Select all that apply.
    1. Discuss the relationship between stress and illness with the client.
    2. Define the terms "stress" and "relaxation" in words the client understands.
    3. Explain methods used to decrease stress that the nurse has used.
    4. Refer the client to a practitioner of traditional Chinese medicine.
    5. Provide Web site addresses for the client to investigate.

11. The nurse is assisting the client diagnosed with chronic pain to identify methods of complementary and alternative medicine (CAM). Which would indicate that an expected outcome was achieved?
    1. The client will spend 18 out of 24 hours in bed.
    2. The client will have an enhanced sensation of pain.
    3. The client will take his or her medication on a routine basis.
    4. The client will be able perform three (3) ADLs without pain.

12. The nurse and the unlicensed nursing assistant are performing post-mortem care on a client. Two (2) of the family members are seen laughing about a memory of the client. What explanation of this behavior would be best for the nurse to give the unlicensed nursing assistant?
    1. The two (2) family members probably did not love the client.
    2. The behavior is inappropriate for the situation and inexcusable.
    3. The family members are using laughter to cope with the pain.
    4. This behavior is demonstrated only by uneducated individuals.

13. The unlicensed nursing assistant asked the wound care nurse why a client has cabbage leaves on their wound. Which statement would be the best response by the nurse?
    1. "Cabbage leaves have antibacterial and anti-inflammatory properties."
    2. "Some people are ignorant and will believe or try anything to get better."
    3. "This is the placebo effect. If people believe something will work, it will."
    4. "The cabbage leaves will keep the wound moist and clean until it heals."

14. The nurse at the Family Planning Clinic is preparing a discussion for students attending a community college about contraception and methods to prevent pregnancy. Which information should the nurse include in the presentation?
    1. Condoms should be used to prevent sexually transmitted diseases.
    2. Sexually active females should have vaginal examinations yearly.
    3. Hormonal therapy can be used orally, subcutaneously, or topically.
    4. All methods of conception need prescriptions from the health-care provider.

15. The occupational health nurse is caring for the client with a superficial burn on the arm. The client states a preference to use holistic natural medication. Which medicinal plant should the nurse recommend to the client?
    1. Black cohosh.
    2. Fennel.
    3. Witch hazel.
    4. Aloe vera.

16. The client has been diagnosed with bronchitis. The client asks the nurse, "Can I use eucalyptus oil in steam and breathe it in deeply?" Which response by the nurse would be most appropriate?
    1. "I would not recommend using any type of folk medicine."
    2. "The steam and the oil may help open up your airway."
    3. "This type of treatment could interfere with your other medications."
    4. "Inhaled eucalyptus oil is not as affective as rubbing it on the chest."

17. The client with a deficiency of the immune system questions the nurse about the use of ginseng. Which information should the nurse teach the client?
    1. Take the ginseng daily to achieve a therapeutic level.
    2. Take ginseng with caffeine drinks to enhance its effects.
    3. Do not take ginseng continuously for more than two (2) months.
    4. There are no contraindications for any client taking ginseng.

18. The client with severe itching from an insect bite calls the clinic and asks the nurse, "What do I need to do for the itching?" Which intervention should the nurse implement for the client problem of alteration in comfort?
    1. Alternate Tylenol, an analgesic, with aspirin, an anti-platelet, every two (2) hours.
    2. Cover the area with Benadryl gel every six (6) hours as needed for itching.
    3. Wash the area with soap and hot water and cover with gauze pads.
    4. Apply 1% hydrocortisone cream, a steroid, every two (2) hours.

19. The client with anemia has been taking iron supplements. Which data would indicate to the nurse that treatment has been effective?
    1. The client is able to prepare a menu that is high in iron.
    2. The client is able to perform activities of daily living.
    3. The client has an increase in black tarry stools.
    4. The client has an increase in dystrophy of nails.

20. The nurse is teaching the elderly client about taking oral iron supplements. Which intervention should the nurse include in the teaching?
    1. Take the iron with an antacid to prevent a bleeding ulcer.
    2. If a dose is missed, take that dose with the next dose.
    3. The client should take the medication between meals.
    4. The client should recline for 30 minutes after dosage.

21. The nurse is teaching a 28-year-old client who was recently prescribed birth control pills. Which statement by the client indicates teaching has been effective?
    1. "I will use another birth control method if I have to take antibiotics."
    2. "If I miss a pill, I will take it at the end of the prescription."
    3. "I will use the contraceptive patch because it has fewer side effects."
    4. "If the contraceptive ring comes out, I will have to get a new one."

22. Which method of birth control would the nurse recommend for the homeless client who has had two (2) unplanned pregnancies?
    1. Prentif cavity-rim cervical caps.
    2. Subdermal levonorgestrel implants.
    3. Combination oral contraceptives.
    4. Depo-Provera injections intramuscularly.

23. Which information would be most important for the public health department nurse to obtain before giving the client condoms?
    1. Ask about the frequency of sexual activity.
    2. Find out the type of condom the client prefers.
    3. Determine if the client is allergic to latex.
    4. Discuss the client's sexual history.

24. The nurse and the unlicensed nursing assistant are caring for client who is anxious. Which task should the nurse delegate to the nursing assistant?
    1. Teach the client how to deep breathe.
    2. Give the client a backrub.
    3. Listen to the client's concerns.
    4. Instruct the client on how to perform guided imagery.

25. The nurse is teaching the client about relaxation techniques. Which interventions should be included in the teaching? Select all that apply.
    1. Instruct the client to contract and relax the muscles.
    2. Explain the importance of playing soothing music.
    3. Use all five (5) senses when using guided imagery.
    4. Discuss the need to eliminate all stress in the client's life.
    5. Insist the client write about his or her feelings in a journal.

26. The client is complaining of acute abdominal pain, and the next pain medication is not due for two (2) hours. Which interventions should the nurse implement? List in order of priority.
    1. Notify the health-care provider to increase pain medication
    2. Auscultate for bowel sounds and palpate the abdomen.
    3. Instruct the client to visualize a pleasant memory.
    4. Turn on the radio to soft, easy-listening music.
    5. Offer the client a therapeutic back massage.

Cultural

1.
1. This is challenging the client's question and will not help establish a therapeutic relationship with the client.
2. **The nurse should present facts and support the client's alternative health belief unless it hurts the client or makes the disease process worse.**
3. The nurse does not need to pass the buck to the HCP to answer this question.
4. Alternative medicine is often helpful to the client, and the nurse should support a client's beliefs as much as possible if it does not hurt the client.

2.
1. The nurse can be concerned about the cost of the herbs and teas, but it is not the most important question to consider.
2. The client's safety is priority, but if the nurse does not have the knowledge, then the nurse cannot answer the question.
3. **Teaching about herbs and alternative therapies is not a priority in nursing programs. Therefore, the nurse must determine if he or she has the knowledge to answer the client's question. The nurse should find a reputable resource before answering this question.**
4. The nurse must always practice within the scope of nursing, but providing correct and factual information is within the scope of the nurse's practice.

3.
1. Acupuncture does not usually cause paralysis because of the size of the needles/wires used.
2. **Acupuncture is a method of producing analgesia or altering the function of a system of the body by inserting fine, wire-thin needles into the skin at specific sites on the body. Infection does occur if a sterile procedure is not used when inserting the needles.**
3. AIDS is not a great concern because the health department regulates the centers that perform acupuncture and there is no sharing of the needles.
4. The pain not being resolved is a concern, but the potential for infection is priority.

4.
1. **Navajo people practice preventive medicine, and the nurse should support the client's culture if it does not interfere with the medical regimen.**
2. Most clients will not get upset and angry and lose faith if the nurse explains the importance of removing an object.
3. "Never" is an absolute word, and sometimes objects must be removed, such as when going to surgery.
4. This is the reason the object is worn, but it is not the best statement to explain why the nurse should not remove the pouch. Even if the nurse does not understand the reason for the object, the nurse should respect and honor the practice if possible.

5.
1. This is a Mexican folk practitioner known as a *sobadores*.
2. This is a Mexican folk practitioner known as a *Yerberos* or *Jerberos*.
3. This is a Mexican folk practitioner known as an *Espiritistas*.
4. **Curanderos receive their gift from God or serve an apprenticeship. Some even prescribe over-the-counter medications. They usually treat traditional illnesses not caused by witchcraft.**

6.
1. A tallis (or tallit) is a rectangular prayer shawl with fringes used during prayer.
2. **A mezuzah is a small container with scripture inside that is placed on the doorpost of the home; some wear the mezuzah as a necklace.**
3. A synagogue is a Jewish house of prayer; Jews may pray alone, or they may pray as a group.
4. Yom Kippur is a high holy day celebrated in September or early October. On Yom Kippur one fasts for a day to cleanse and purify oneself.

7.
1. The nurse should be sensitive to folk medicine, and if it does not hurt the client, the nurse should be respectful and honor the practice.
2. The nurse should not make the client explain his or her folk medicine beliefs.
3. **The nurse should first assess the carbuncle to determine if the raw potato is making the carbuncle worse; if it is not, the nurse should support the client's folk medicine.**
4. The nurse should assess the carbuncle before deciding not to take any further action.

8.
1. These are not typical signs and symptoms of a psychosomatic disorder.
2. **This would be the best explanation because the client has experienced major life changes, moving to another area and assuming the role of caregiver to a parent. Chronic unrelieved stress has been shown to decrease immunity, resulting in frequent upper-respiratory tract infections and increased blood pressure.**
3. Gastric reflux has been linked to asthma-type symptoms but not upper-respiratory infections.

Cultural

4. These signs/symptoms do not support the diagnosis of essential hypertension.

9. 1. Cupping is an alternative treatment modality in which heated cups are applied to the body. They produce round, red or purple circles that may remain for as long as one (1) week. It may be used for clients with respiratory difficulty.
   2. This response assumes that the areas are bruises resulting from injury or illness.
   3. This response assumes that the areas are bruises resulting from abuse, which could lead to false accusations and legal issues.
   4. This response sounds judgmental and blaming, and the nurse should avoid responses that damage the client–nurse relationship.

10. 1. The client should understand the relationship between stress and illness.
    2. For effective teaching, the nurse should use terms the client understands.
    3. Methods that the nurse has experienced personally or have observed to be successful with other clients can aid the client's selection.
    4. The nurse should not refer the client to alternative health-care providers. This is imposing the nurse's cultural beliefs onto the client.
    5. The nurse should provide a variety of referrals and resources to use to help reduce and control stressful situations.

11. 1. If the client spends more than three-fourths of the time in bed, then this would be a low quality of life and would not be the expected outcome.
    2. An expected outcome would be relief of pain or enhanced pain management. Enhanced sensation of pain would be unrelieved pain.
    3. CAM would not include medication, and taking medication is an intervention, not an expected outcome.
    4. A client performing activities of daily living (ADL) without pain represents an appropriate expected outcome.

12. 1. This behavior does not indicate lack of love; it is a coping mechanism.
    2. Family members' coping mechanisms should not be criticized by staff.
    3. Laughter during times of stress aids in coping with pain and increases relaxation.
    4. Laughter is used by many individuals as stress relief, regardless of educational levels.

13. 1. Cabbage leaves have been shown to have some antibacterial and anti-inflammatory

properties. Softened leaves are applied to wounds, ulcers, and arthritic joints.
   2. This response is belittling the client's beliefs and actions.
   3. Studies support the placebo effect, but this response does not answer the NA's question about the use of cabbage leaves.
   4. The leaves would not be the best way to keep the wound moist and clean.

14. 1. Condoms are helpful in preventing sexually transmitted diseases and in preventing pregnancy.
    2. Sexually active females do need vaginal examinations, but this statement does not address preventing pregnancy.
    3. Routes of hormonal therapy include birth control pills, creams, patches, and injections. All address ways to help prevent conception.
    4. All methods of birth control do not require a prescription. Condoms and contraceptive creams and ointments are sold over the counter.

15. 1. Black cohosh is used for gynecological disorders.
    2. Fennel is used as an expectorant or diuretic.
    3. Witch hazel has anti-inflammatory properties, but it is prepared with an alcohol base that would cause pain to the client when applying it to the burned area.
    4. Aloe vera has been used to promote wound healing. It has some antifungal properties and helps soothe the pain from the superficial burn.

16. 1. The nurse should support the use of folk and home remedies as long as they are not contraindicated by the medical treatment.
    2. Eucalyptus has been used by clients with congestion and as an expectorant; steam helps open the airway and liquefies secretions.
    3. This is an inhaled treatment that will provide the medication directly to the lungs and will limit systemic effects.
    4. The steam provides moisture to the lungs to liquefy secretions, and the efficacy of rubbing on the chest is provided by inhalation.

17. 1. Continuous, daily doses will not increase the effectiveness of the herb and could cause harm to the client.
    2. Ginseng is a stimulant; therefore additional stimulants, such as caffeine, should be avoided.
    3. Clients should take ginseng intermittently

for safety. Every two (2) months the client should omit the ginseng for two (2) or three (3) weeks.

4. There are contraindications to all medications. Ginseng elevates the blood pressure, so clients diagnosed with hypertension should avoid ginseng.

18. 1. Alternating Tylenol with aspirin is recommended for clients with fevers who do not respond to Tylenol alone.

2. **Benadryl gel can be applied to the area three (3) to four (4) times a day. The medication is absorbed topically. If the medication is applied more often, the client can develop systemic effects.**

3. Washing the area with soap and hot water will increase the itching.

4. Hydrocortisone cream is applied three (3) to four (4) times daily, not every two (2) hours.

19. 1. This outcome would be for a knowledge-deficit problem.

2. **Clients with anemia have decreased energy and are unable to complete activities of daily living. The ability to complete ADLs indicates that the treatment has been effective.**

3. Green–black stools are an expected side effect of taking iron supplements and can be confused with tarry stools that indicate blood in the stool.

4. Dystrophy of fingernails is an indication the treatment is ineffective.

20. 1. Antacids should be taken at least one (1) hour between doses of iron.

2. Clients should not double up on doses because that may lead to gastrointestinal upset.

3. **Food interferes with the absorption of oral supplements, but it is recommended that clients take iron between meals to minimize gastrointestinal upset and maximize iron absorption.**

4. The client needs to remain in an upright position for 30 minutes after taking oral iron supplements to reduce esophageal irritation or corrosion.

21. 1. **Antibiotics such as ampicillin and tetracycline increase the elimination of the oral contraceptive by killing the flora in the gastrointestinal tract. Clients should use another method of birth control while taking an antibiotic.**

2. The pills should be taken at the same time each day. If the client misses one (1), that pill should be taken as soon as the client remembers. If the

client misses taking the pill two (2) days in a row, then two (2) pills should be taken each day for the next two (2) days.

3. The transdermal patch has the same side effects as oral birth control pills. The advantage of the patch is that it does not have to be taken every day.

4. If the contraceptive ring comes out, it should be washed with warm water and replaced. One ring can be used for three (3) weeks.

22. 1. The Prentif cavity-rim cervical cap has a 40% failure rate for multiparous women.

2. Subdermal levonorgestrel implants are an effective method of birth control for up to five (5) years.

3. When taken as directed, oral contraceptives can be effective, but because this client has had two (2) unplanned pregnancies, compliance should be questioned.

4. **Depo-Provera is one of the most effective methods of birth control but lasts for only three (3) months; therefore, this should not be recommended for this client.**

23. 1. The frequency of sexual activity would indicate the number of condoms to be distributed, but it would not be the most important information.

2. The public health department provides free condoms and is not concerned with the client's style preference.

3. **The most effective condoms are made of latex, but they should not be used if the client is allergic to latex. The client should be instructed to ask their partner about latex allergies.**

4. Sexual history should be discussed only if the client has a STD because the public health department must notify all partners.

24. 1. Deep breathing would aid the client to relax, but teaching cannot be delegated.

2. **This relaxing intervention can be delegated to the unlicensed nursing assistant.**

3. Listening to why the client is anxious is part of assessment, which cannot be delegated.

4. Guided imagery is a method that assists clients to relax, but teaching it cannot be delegated.

25. 1. **Pogressive muscle relaxation is the systematic contracting and relaxing of muscles. It helps aid in relaxation when the client feels anxious.**

2. **Soothing music with the rate of 50 to 60 beats per minute can slow the client's heart rate and relax the client.**

3. Guided imagery is helpful to decrease anxiety. The more senses involved, the better the results of the guided imagery.
4. Stress is not always harmful, and the absence of all stress is death.
5. Journaling is useful for some individuals, but the nurse cannot insist or demand the client to do anything.

26. In order of priority: 2, 4, 1, 5, 3.
    2. Any pain not relieved with prescribed pain medication warrants assessment by the nurse to rule out any complications.
    4. Soft music is a method of distraction that can be implemented quickly and may have a calming effect on the client.
    1. The nurse should notify the HCP and discuss other possible medication regimens that can be provided for the client.
    5. According to the Gate Control theory of pain, flooding the brain with pleasurable sensations will block the transmission of pain.
    3. Clients in acute pain are not receptive to being taught; therefore, this intervention should be implemented as soon as the pain is tolerable and may be used by the client for future pain episodes.

Cultural

# End-of-Life Issues

**18**

End-of-life issues include some of the most sensitive issues a nurse must handle. Many times a nurse will need to confront his or her own feelings and fears about death to be able to help their clients. This chapter deals with advance directives, death and dying, chronic pain, ethical/legal issues, and organ/tissue transplants.

## ABBREVIATIONS

Advance Directive (AD)
American Nurses Association (ANA)
Apical Pulse (AP)
Blood Pressure (BP)
Blood Urea Nitrogen (BUN)
Cardiopulmonary Resuscitation (CPR)
Chronic Obstructive Pulmonary Disease (COPD)
Do Not Resuscitate (DNR)
Electroencephalogram (ECG)
Health-Care Provider (HCP)
Health Insurance Portability and Accountability Act (HIPAA)

Human Immunodeficiency Virus (HIV)
Human Leukocyte Antigen (HLA)
Intravenous (IV)
Intravenous Push (IVP)
Medication Administration Record (MAR)
Nonsteroidal Anti-Inflammatory Drug (NSAID)
Nursing Assistant (NA)
Pulse (P)
Respirations (R)
Transcutaneous Electrical Nerve Stimulation (TENS)

## Advance Directives

1. The client tells the nurse, "Every time I come in the hospital you hand me one of these advance directives (AD). Why should I fill one of these out?" Which statement by the nurse is most appropriate?
    1. "You must fill out this form because Medicare laws require it."
    2. "An AD lets you participate in decisions about your health care."
    3. "This paper will ensure that no one can override your decisions."
    4. "It is part of the hospital admission packet and I have to give it to you."

2. The nurse is presenting an in-service discussing do not resuscitate (DNR) orders and advance directives. Which statement should the nurse discuss with the class?
    1. Advance directives must be notarized by a notary public.
    2. The client must use an attorney to complete the advanced directive.
    3. Once the DNR is written it can used for every hospital admission.
    4. The health-care provider must write the DNR order in the client's chart.

3. In which client situation would the AD be consulted and used in decision-making?
    1. The client diagnosed with Guillain Barré who is on a ventilator.
    2. The client with a C-6 spinal cord injury in the rehabilitation unit.
    3. The client in end-stage renal disease who is in a comatose state.
    4. The client diagnosed with cancer who has Down syndrome.

4. The nurse is moving to another state that is part of the multistate licensure compact. Which information regarding ADs should the nurse be aware of when practicing nursing in other states?
    1. The laws regarding ADs are the same in all the states.
    2. Advance directives can be transferred from state to state.
    3. A significant other can sign a loved one's advanced directive.
    4. Advance directives are state regulated, not federally regulated.

5. Which client would be most likely to complete an advance directive?
    1. A 55-year-old Caucasian person who is a bank president.
    2. A 34-year-old Asian licensed vocational nurse.
    3. A 22-year-old Hispanic lawn care worker.
    4. A 65-year-old African American retired cook.

6. The client with an AD tells the nurse, "I have changed my mind about my AD. I really want everything possible done if I am near death since I have a grandchild." Which action should the nurse implement?
    1. Notify the health information systems department to talk to the client.
    2. Remove the AD from the client's chart and shred the document.
    3. Inform the client that they have the right to revoke their AD at any time.
    4. Explain that this document cannot be changed once it is signed.

7. The client has just signed an AD at the bedside. Which intervention should the nurse implement first?
    1. Notify the client's health-care provider about the AD.
    2. Instruct the client to discuss the AD with significant others.
    3. Place a copy of the advance directive in the client's chart.
    4. Give the original advance directive to the client.

8. The HCP has notified the family of a client in a persistent vegetative state on a ventilator of the need to "pull the plug." The client does not have an AD or a durable power of attorney for health care and the family does not want their loved one removed from the ventilator. Which action should the nurse implement?
    1. Refer the case to the hospital ethics committee.
    2. Tell the family they must do what the HCP orders.
    3. Follow the HCP's order and "pull the plug."
    4. Determine why the client did not complete an AD.

9. The client asks the nurse, "When will the Durable Power of Attorney for Health Care take effect?" On which scientific rationale would the nurse base the response?
   1. It goes into effect when the client needs someone to make financial decisions.
   2. It will be effective when the client is under general anesthesia during surgery.
   3. The client must say it is all right for it to become effective and enforced.
   4. It becomes valid only when the clients cannot make their own decisions.

10. The male client requested a DNR per the AD, and the HCP wrote the order. The client's death is imminent and the client's wife tells the nurse, "Help him please. Do something. I am not ready to let him go." Which action should the nurse take?
    1. Ask the wife if she would like to revoke her husband's AD.
    2. Leave the wife at the bedside and notify the hospital chaplain.
    3. Sit with the wife at the bedside and encourage her to say goodbye.
    4. Request the client to tell the wife he is ready to die, and don't do anything.

11. Which situation would cause the nurse to question the validity of an AD when caring for the elderly client?
    1. The client's child insists that the client make his or her own decisions.
    2. The nurse observes the wife making the husband sign the AD.
    3. A nurse encouraged the client to think about end-of-life decisions.
    4. A friend witnesses the client's signature on the AD form.

12. The nurse is aware that the Patient Self-Determination Act of 1991 requires the health-care facility to implement which action?
    1. Make available an AD on admission to the facility.
    2. Assist the client with legally completing a will.
    3. Provide ethically and morally competent care to the client.
    4. Discuss the importance of understanding consent forms.

## Death and Dying

13. The spouse of a client dying from lung cancer states, "I don't understand this death rattle. She has not had anything to drink in days. Where is the fluid coming from?" Which is the hospice care nurse's best response?
    1. "The body produces about two (2) teaspoons of fluid every minute on its own."
    2. "Are you sure that someone is not putting ice chips in her mouth?"
    3. "There is no reason for this, but it does happen from time to time."
    4. "I can administer a patch to her skin to dry up the secretions if you wish."

14. The nurse is discussing placing the client diagnosed with chronic obstructive pulmonary disease (COPD) in hospice care. Which prognosis must be determined to placed the client in hospice care?
    1. The client is doing well but could benefit from the added care by hospice.
    2. The client has a life expectancy of six (6) months or less.
    3. The client will live for about one (1) to two (2) more years.
    4. The client has about eight (8) weeks to live and needs pain control.

15. The client diagnosed with end-stage congestive heart failure and Type 2 diabetes is receiving hospice care. Which action by the nurse demonstrates an understanding of the client's condition?
    1. The nurse monitors the blood glucose four (4) times a day.
    2. The nurse keeps the client on a strict fluid restriction.
    3. The nurse limits the visitors the client can receive.
    4. The nurse brings the client a small piece of cake.

End of Life

16. The hospice care nurse is conducting a spiritual care assessment. Which statement is the scientific rationale for this intervention?
    1. The client will ask all of their spiritual questions and get answers.
    2. The nurse is able to explain to the client how death will affect the spirit.
    3. Spirituality provides a sense of meaning and purpose for many clients.
    4. The nurse is the expert when assisting the client with spiritual matters.

17. The nurse is caring for a dying client and the family. The male client is Muslim. Which intervention should the female nurse implement at the time of death?
    1. Allow the wife to stay in the room during post-mortem care.
    2. Call the client's minister to perform last rites when the client dies.
    3. Place incense around the bed, but do not allow anyone to light it.
    4. Do not touch the body, and have the male family members perform care.

18. The nurse writes a client problem of "spiritual distress" for the client who is dying. Which statement is an appropriate goal?
    1. The client will reconcile self and the higher power of his or her beliefs.
    2. The client will be able to express anger at the terminal diagnosis.
    3. The client will reconcile self to estranged member of the family.
    4. The client will have a dignified and pain-free death.

19. The hospice care nurse is planning the care of an elderly client diagnosed with end-stage renal disease. Which interventions should be included in the plan of care? Select all that apply.
    1. Discuss financial concerns.
    2. Assess any comorbid conditions.
    3. Monitor increased visual or auditory abilities.
    4. Note any spiritual distress.
    5. Encourage euphoria at the time of death.

20. The nurse is orienting to a hospice organization. Which statement does not indicate a right of the terminal client? The right to:
    1. Be treated with respect and dignity.
    2. Have particulars of the death withheld.
    3. Receive optimal and effective pain management.
    4. Receive holistic and compassionate care.

21. The client is on the ventilator and has been declared brain dead. The spouse refuses to allow the ventilator to be discontinued. Which collaborative action by the nurse is most appropriate?
    1. Discuss referral of the case to the ethics committee.
    2. Pull the plug when the spouse is not in the room.
    3. Ask the HCP to discuss the futile situation with the spouse.
    4. Inform the spouse that what is happening is cruel.

22. The client has been in a persistent vegetative state for several years. The family, who has decided to withhold tube feedings because there is no hope of recovery, asks the nurse, "Will the death be painful?" Which intervention should the nurse implement?
    1. Tell the family that the death will be painful but the HCP can order medications.
    2. Inform the family that dehydration provides a type of natural euphoria.
    3. Relate other cases where the clients have died in excruciating pain.
    4. Ask the family why they are concerned because they want the client to die anyway.

23. The family is dealing with the imminent death of the client. Which information is most important for the nurse to discuss when planning interventions for the grieving process?
    1. How angry are the family members about the death?
    2. Which family member will be making decisions?
    3. What previous coping skills have been used?
    4. What type of funeral service has been planned?

24. The client who is terminally ill called the significant others to the room and said good-bye, then dismissed them and now lies quietly and refuses to eat. The nurse understands that the client is in what stage of the grieving process?
    1. Denial.
    2. Anger.
    3. Bargaining.
    4. Acceptance.

## Chronic Pain

25. The nurse is assessing a client diagnosed with chronic pain. Which characteristics would the nurse observe?
    1. The client's blood pressure is elevated.
    2. The client has rapid shallow respirations.
    3. The client has facial grimacing.
    4. The client is lying quietly in bed.

26. The client had a mastectomy and lymph node dissection three (3) years ago and has experienced post-mastectomy pain (PMP) since. Which intervention should the nurse implement?
    1. Have the client see a psychologist because the pain is not real.
    2. Tell the client that the pain is the cancer coming back.
    3. Refer the client to a physical therapist to prevent a frozen shoulder.
    4. Discuss changing the client to a more potent narcotic medication.

27. The male client diagnosed with chronic pain since a construction accident that broke several vertebrae tells the nurse that he has been referred to a pain clinic and asks, "What good will it do? I will never be free of this pain." Which statement is the nurse's best response?
    1. "Are you afraid of the pain never going away?"
    2. "The pain clinic will give you medication to cure the pain."
    3. "Pain clinics work to help you achieve relief from pain."
    4. "I am not sure. You should discuss this with your HCP."

28. The client diagnosed with cancer is experiencing severe pain. Which regimen would the nurse teach the client about to control the pain?
    1. Nonsteroidal anti-inflammatory drugs (NSAIDs) around the clock with narcotics used for severe pain.
    2. Morphine sustained release, a narcotic, routinely with a liquid morphine preparation for breakthrough pain.
    3. Extra-Strength Tylenol, a nonnarcotic analgesic plus therapy to learn alternative methods of pain control.
    4. Demerol, an opioid narcotic, every six (6) hours orally with a suppository when the pain is not controlled.

29. The client is being discharged from the hospital for intractable pain secondary to cancer and is prescribed morphine, a narcotic. Which statement indicates the client understands the discharge instructions?
    1. "I will be sure to have my prescriptions filled before any holiday."
    2. "There should not be a problem having the prescriptions filled anytime."
    3. "If I run out of medications, I can call the HCP to phone in a prescription."
    4. "There are no side effects to morphine that I should be concerned about."

30. The client diagnosed with intractable pain is receiving an IV constant infusion of morphine, a narcotic opioid. The concentration is 50 mg of morphine in 250 mL of normal saline. The IV is infusing at ten (10) mL per hour. The client has required bolus administration of two (2) mg IVP × two (2) during the 12-hour shift. How much morphine has the client received during the shift?_____

31. The male client that has made himself a do not resuscitate (DNR) is in pain. The client's vital signs are P 88, R 8, and BP 108/70. Which intervention should be the nurse's priority action?
    1. Refuse to give the medication because it could kill the client.
    2. Administer the medication as ordered and assess for relief from pain.
    3. Wait until the client' respirations improve and then administer the medication.
    4. Notify the HCP that the client is unstable and pain medication is being held.

32. The charge nurse is making assignments on an oncology floor. Which client should be assigned to the most experienced nurse?
    1. The client diagnosed with leukemia who has a hemoglobin of 6.0 g/dL.
    2. The client diagnosed with lung cancer with a pulse oximeter reading of 89%.
    3. The client diagnosed with colon cancer who needs to irrigate the colostomy.
    4. The client diagnosed with Kaposi's sarcoma who is yelling at the staff.

33. The nurse and unlicensed nursing assistant are caring for a group of clients in a pain clinic. Which intervention would be inappropriate to delegate to the assistant?
    1. Assist to the bathroom the client diagnosed with intractable pain.
    2. Elevate the head of the bed for a client diagnosed with back pain.
    3. Perform passive range of motion for a client that is bedfast.
    4. Monitor the potassium levels on a client about to receive medication.

34. The client diagnosed with chronic back pain is being placed on a transcutaneous electric nerve stimulator (TENS) unit. Which information should the nurse teach?
    1. The TENS unit will deaden the nerve endings, and the client will not feel pain.
    2. The TENS unit could cause paralysis if the client gets the unit wet.
    3. The TENS unit stimulates the nerves in the area, blocking the pain sensation.
    4. The TENS unit should be left on for an hour, and then taken off for an hour.

35. The nurse is caring for clients on a medical floor. Which client should the nurse assess first after the shift report?
    1. The client with arterial blood gases of pH 7.36, $PaCO_2$ 40, $HCO_3$ 26, $PaO_2$ 90.
    2. The client with a T 99°F, P 101, R 28, and BP 120/80.
    3. The client complaining of pain at a "10" on a 1–10 scale but can't localize it.
    4. The client that is post-appendectomy with pain at a "3" on a 1–10 scale.

36. The female client in the oncology clinic tells the nurse that she has a great deal of pain but does not like to take pain medication. Which action should the nurse implement first?
    1. Tell the client that it is important for her to take her medication.
    2. Find out how the client has been dealing with the pain.
    3. Have the HCP tell the client to take the pain medications.
    4. Instruct the client not to worry—the pain will resolve itself.

## Ethical/Legal Issues

37. The nurse is teaching an in-service on legal issues in nursing. Which situation is an example of battery, an intentional tort?
    1. The nurse threatens the client to take a hypnotic medication.
    2. The nurse forcibly inserts a Foley catheter in a client who refused it.
    3. The nurse tells the client that a nasogastric tube insertion is not painful.
    4. The nurse gives confidential information over the telephone.

38. Which act protects the nurse against a malpractice claim when the nurse stops at a motor-vehicle accident and renders emergency care?
    1. The Health Insurance Portability and Accountability Act.
    2. The State Nurse Practice Act.
    3. The Emergency Rendering Aid Act.
    4. The Good Samaritan Act.

39. The family has requested that a client with terminal cancer not be told of the diagnosis. The client tells the nurse, "I think something is really wrong with me, but the doctor says everything is all right. Do you know if there is something wrong with me?" Which response by the nurse would support the ethical principle of veracity?
    1. "I think you should talk to your doctor about your concerns."
    2. "What makes you think that something is really wrong?"
    3. "Your family has requested that you not be told your diagnosis."
    4. "The doctor would never tell you incorrect information."

40. The nurse is obtaining the client's signature on a surgical permit form. The nurse determines that the client does not understand the surgical procedure and possible risks. Which action should the nurse take first?
    1. Notify the client's surgeon.
    2. Document the information in the chart.
    3. Contact the operating room staff.
    4. Explain the procedure to the client.

41. The client is in the psychiatric unit in a medical center. Which action by the psychiatric nurse is a violation of the client's legal and civil rights?
    1. The nurse tells the client that civilian clothes can be worn on the unit.
    2. The nurse allows the client to have family visits during visiting hours.
    3. The nurse delivers unopened mail and packages to the client.
    4. The nurse listens to the client talking on the telephone to a friend.

42. The client receiving dialysis for end-stage renal disease wants to quit dialysis and die. Which ethical principle supports the client's right to die?
    1. Autonomy.
    2. Self-determination.
    3. Beneficence.
    4. Justice.

43. Which document is the best professional source to provide direction for a nurse when addressing ethical issues and behavior?
    1. The Hippocratic Oath.
    2. The Nuremberg Code.
    3. Home Health Care Bill of Rights.
    4. ANA Code of Ethics.

44. Which element is not necessary to prove nursing malpractice?
    1. Breach of Duty.
    2. Identify the ethical issues.
    3. Injury to the client.
    4. Proximate cause.

45. The nurse is caring for a client who is confused and fell trying to get out of bed. There is no family at the client's bedside. Which action should the nurse implement first?
    1. Contact a family member to come and stay with the client.
    2. Administer a sedative medication to the client.
    3. Place the client in a chair with a sheet tied around them.
    4. Notify the health-care provider to obtain a restraint order.

46. Which entity mandates the registered nurse's behavior when practicing professional nursing?
    1. The Nurse Practice Act.
    2. Client's Bill of Rights.
    3. The United States legislature.
    4. American Nurses Association.

End of Life

47. The nurse must be knowledgeable of ethical principles. Which is an example of the ethical principle of justice?
    1. The nurse is administering a placebo, and the client asks if it will it help the pain.
    2. The nurse accepts a work assignment in an area in which he or she is not experienced.
    3. The nurse refuses to tell a family member that the client has a positive HIV test.
    4. The nurse provides an indigent client with safe and appropriate nursing care.

48. The nurse is discussing malpractice issues in an in-service class. Which situation is an example of malpractice?
    1. The nurse fails to report a neighbor who is abusing his two children.
    2. The nurse does not intervene in a client who has a BP of 80/50 and AP of 122.
    3. The nurse is suspected of taking narcotics that are prescribed for a client.
    4. The nurse falsifies vital signs in the client's medical records.

## Organ/Tissue Donation

49. The mother of a 20-year-old African American male client receiving dialysis asks the nurse, "My son has been on the transplant list longer than that white woman. Why did she get the kidney?" Which statement is the nurse's best response?
    1. "The woman was famous, and so more people will donate organs now."
    2. "I understand you are upset that your son is ill. Would you like to talk?"
    3. "No one knows who gets an organ. You just have to wait and pray."
    4. "The tissues must match, or the body will reject the kidney and it will be wasted."

50. The nurse is discussing the HCP's recommendation for removal of life support with the client's family. Which information concerning brain death should the nurse teach the family?
    1. Positive waves on the electroencephalogram (EEG) mean the brain is dead and any further treatment is futile.
    2. When putting cold water in the ear, if the client reacts by pulling away, that demonstrates brain death.
    3. Tests will be done to determine if any brain activity exists before the machines are turned off.
    4. Although the blood flow studies don't indicate activity, the client can still come out of the coma.

51. The client diagnosed with septicemia expired, and the family tells the nurse that the client is an organ donor. Which intervention should the nurse implement?
    1. Notify the organ and tissue organizations to make the retrieval.
    2. Explain that a systemic infection prevents the client from being a donor.
    3. Call and notify the health-care provider of the family's request.
    4. Take the body to the morgue until the organ bank makes a decision.

52. The client has received a kidney transplant. Which assessment would warrant immediate intervention by the nurse?
    1. Fever and decreased urine output.
    2. Decreased creatinine and BUN levels.
    3. Decreased serum potassium and calcium.
    4. Bradycardia and hypotension.

53. The client received a liver transplant and is preparing for discharge. Which discharge instruction should the nurse teach?
    1. The immune-suppressant drugs must be tapered off when discontinuing the drug.
    2. There may be slight foul-smelling drainage on the dressing for a few days.
    3. Notify the HCP immediately if a cough or fever develops.
    4. The skin will turn yellow from the anti-rejection drugs.

54. The pregnant client asks the nurse about banking the cord blood. Which information should the nurse teach the client?
    1. The procedure involves a lot of pain with a very poor result.
    2. The client must deliver at a large public hospital to do this.
    3. The client will be charged a yearly storage fee on the cells.
    4. The stem cells can be stored for about four (4) years before they ruin.

55. The nurse is caring for a client who received a kidney transplant from an unrelated cadaver donor. Which interventions should be included in the plan of care? Select all that apply.
    1. Collect a urine culture every other day.
    2. Prepare the client for dialysis three (3) times a week.
    3. Monitor urine osmolality studies.
    4. Monitor intake and output every shift.
    5. Check abdominal dressing every four (4) hours.

56. The client is three (3) hours post–heart transplant. Which data would support a complication of this procedure?
    1. The client has nausea after taking the oral anti-rejection medication.
    2. The client has difficulty coming off the heart-lung bypass machine.
    3. The client has saturated three (3) ABD dressing pads in one (1) hour.
    4. The client complains of pain at a six (6) on a one (1) to ten (10) scale.

57. The nurse and unlicensed nursing assistant are caring for clients on a postoperative transplant unit. Which task should the nurse delegate to the assistant?
    1. Assess the hourly outputs of the client who is postop kidney transplant.
    2. Raise the head of the bed for a client who is postop liver transplant.
    3. Monitor the serum blood studies of a client who has rejected an organ.
    4. Irrigate the nasogastric tube of the client who had a pancreas transplant.

58. The experienced medical-surgical nurse is being oriented to the transplant unit. Which client should the charge nurse assign to this nurse?
    1. The client who donated a kidney to a relative three (3) days ago and will be discharged in the morning.
    2. The client who had a liver transplant three days ago and was transferred from the intensive care unit two (2) hours ago.
    3. The client who received a corneal transplant four (4) hours ago and has developed a cough and is vomiting.
    4. The client who had a pancreas transplant and has a fever, chills, and a blood glucose monitor reading of 342.

59. The 6-year-old client diagnosed with cystic fibrosis (CF) needs a lung transplant. Which individual would be the best donor for the client?
    1. The 20-year-old brother who does not have cystic fibrosis.
    2. The 45-year-old father who carries the cystic fibrosis gene.
    3. The 18-year-old who died in a MVA who matches on four (4) points.
    4. The 5-year-old drowning victim who is a three (3)-point match.

60. Which tissue or organ can be repeatedly donated to clients needing a transplant?
    1. Skin.
    2. Bones.
    3. Kidneys.
    4. Bone marrow.

End of Life

# PRACTICE QUESTIONS ANSWERS AND RATIONALES

## Advance Directives

1. 1. Advance directives (AD) are not legally required. It is a standard of the Joint Commission on Accreditation of Healthcare Organizations (JCAHO), and any facility that accepts federal funds must ask and offer the AD.
   2. ADs allow the client to make personal health-care decisions about end-of-life issues, including cardiopulmonary resuscitation (CPR), ventilators, feeding tubes, and other issues concerning the client's death.
   3. This is not a legal document that stands up in a court of law; therefore the client should make sure all family members know the client's wishes.
   4. It is part of the hospital admission requirements, but it is not the reason why the client should complete an AD.

TEST-TAKING HINT: The test taker could eliminate answer option "1" because the nurse cannot make the client do anything. The client has a right to say no. Option "3" is an absolute, and unless the test taker knows for sure that this is correct information, the test taker should not select this option.

2. 1. This is not true; someone who is not family or directly involved in the client's care must witness the AD, but the document does not have to be notarized.
   2. This form can be filled out without the use of an attorney; copies of an AD can be obtained at hospitals or on-line from various sources.
   3. The DNR order must be written on each admission.
   4. The HCP writes the DNR order in the client's chart, and the client completes the AD.

TEST-TAKING HINT: Options "1" and "2" have other legal entities outside the health-care arena, which would make the test taker eliminate them.

3. 1. A client diagnosed with Guillain-Barré is mentally competent, and being on a ventilator does not indicate that the client has lost his or her decision-making capacity.
   2. A client in the rehabilitation unit would be alert, and spinal cord injuries do not cause the client to lose decision-making capacity.
   3. The client must have lost decision-making capacity as a result of a condition that is not reversible or must be in a condition that is specified under state law, such as a terminal, persistent vegetative state; irreversible coma; or as specified in the AD.

4. A client with Down syndrome may have some mental challenges, but unless the client has been declared legally incompetent in a court of law, the client can complete an AD.

TEST-TAKING HINT: If the test taker knows what an AD is, then the words "end-stage" and "comatose" would lead the test taker to select this as a correct answer. Remember that clients with congenital or genetic disorders are not incompetent, even if they are mentally challenged.

4. 1. Individual states are responsible for specific legal requirements for ADs.
   2. Moving from one state to another does not nullify or honor the AD; the nurse must be aware of the individual state's requirements.
   3. Only the individual can complete and sign an AD. The significant other may be asked to implement the AD.
   4. The state determines the definition of terms and requirements for an AD; individual states are responsible for specific legal requirements for ADs.

TEST-TAKING HINT: The test taker should know that the registered nurse must obtain a copy of the Nursing Practice Act of the state he or she is practicing in. The test taker should realize that every state has different regulations regarding ADs and other health-care issues. Option "4" is the only option that reflects this thought.

5. 1. ADs are more frequently completed by white, middle-to-upper class individuals.
   2. Many nurses do not have ADs, although they discuss them with clients daily.
   3. Culturally, Hispanics allow their family members to make decisions for them.
   4. Many cultures, including the African American culture, often distrust the health-care system and believe that necessary care will be withheld if an AD is completed.

TEST-TAKING HINT: If the test taker was not aware of the research, the test taker could examine the occupations and ask themselves, "Which client would want to direct their own care and make their own decisions?" Nurses may want this but many do not have ADs.

6. 1. This department has nothing to do with the AD.
   2. The most appropriate action would be for the nurse to have the client write on the AD that they are revoking the document; the nurse cannot shred legal documents from the client's chart.

3. The client must be informed that the AD can be rescinded or revoked at any time for any reason verbally, in writing, or by destroying his or her own AD. The nurse cannot destroy the client's AD, but the client can destroy his or her own.

4. This is incorrect answer because the client always has the right to change his or her mind.

**TEST-TAKING HINT: Option "4" can be eliminated by remembering that statements with absolutes should not be selected as correct answers unless the test taker knows for sure that the answer is correct. The client's chart is a legal document, and these papers cannot be shredded or altered by using white out or by erasing information.**

7. 1. The HCP should be made aware of the AD, but this is not the first intervention.

2. This is the most important intervention because the legality of the document is sometimes not honored if the family members disagree and demand other action. If the client's family is aware of the client's wishes, then the health-care team can support and honor the client's final wishes.

3. Copies of the AD should be placed in the chart and given to significant others, their attorney, and all health-care providers.

4. The original should be given to the client and a copy should be placed in the chart, but this is not the first intervention.

**TEST-TAKING HINT: This is a priority-setting question, and the test taker should read all the answer options and try to rank them in order of priority.**

8. 1. The ethics committee is composed of health-care workers and laypeople from the community to objectively review the situation and make a recommendation that is fair to both the client and health-care system. The family has the right to be present and discuss their feelings.

2. The nurse is legally obligated to be a client advocate.

3. This action could create a multitude of ramifications, including a lawsuit and possible criminal charges.

4. It really doesn't matter at this point why the client didn't complete an AD; the client cannot do it now.

**TEST-TAKING HINT: The test taker must be aware of the ethics committee and its role in helping resolve ethical dilemmas. Any answer option that has the word "why" should be evaluated closely before selecting it as the**

correct answer. Removing the endotracheal tube or turning off the ventilator ("pulling the plug") is a medical responsibility; therefore "3" could be eliminated as the correct answer.

9. 1. It is a Power of Attorney executed by a lawyer that allows a delegated other person to make financial decisions. That document has nothing to do with a Durable Power of Attorney for Health Care.

2. The client has not lost the capacity to make decisions; therefore a durable power of attorney cannot be used by the assigned person to make decisions.

3. The client must not be able to make his or her own decisions before this document can be used.

4. The client must have lost decision-making capacity as a result of a condition that is not reversible or must be in a condition that is specified under state law such as terminal, persistent vegetative state; irreversible coma; or as specified in the AD.

**TEST-TAKING HINT: The test taker should not confuse Power of Attorney and Durable Power of Attorney for Health Care. These are two separate, yet very important, documents with similar names.**

10. 1. Only the client can revoke the AD.

2. The wife should not be left alone, and the hospital chaplain may not be available for the client and his wife.

3. At the time of death, loved ones become scared and find it difficult to say goodbye. The nurse should support the client's decision and acknowledge the wife's psychological state. Research states that hearing is the last sense to go, and talking to the dying client is therapeutic for the client and the family.

4. The client is dying and should not be asked to exert himself for his wishes to be carried out.

**TEST-TAKING HINT: Logic would suggest that option "4" is not a viable answer. Leaving a grieving spouse would not be appropriate in any situation; therefore the test taker should eliminate option "2." Option "1" denies the client's autonomy and is not an ethical or legal choice.**

11. 1. This is appropriate for completing an AD and would not make the nurse question the validity of the AD.

2. This is coercion and is illegal when signing an AD. The AD must be signed by the client's own free will; an AD signed under duress may not be valid.

3. The nurse encouraging the client to think about ADs is an excellent intervention and would not make the AD invalid.

4. A friend can sign the AD as a witness; this would not cause the nurse to question its validity.

**TEST-TAKING HINT: This is an "except" question. The test taker could ask, "Which situation is valid for an AD?" Remember three answers are valid information for the AD and only one is not. Read all answer options and do not jump to conclusions.**

12. 1. The Patient Self-Determination Act of 1991 requires health-care facilities that receive Medicare or Medicaid funding to make ADs available to clients on admission into the facility.

2. This act is not concerned with completing a legal will.

3. Client care is not based on this act.

4. Consent forms are legal documents, which are not discussed in this act.

**TEST-TAKING HINT: The test taker should examine the words "self-determination" in the stem of the question, which match the words "advance" and "directive" in option "1." The words "legal," "ethical," and "moral" in options "2" and "3" apply to the nurse in the health-care setting, not the client.**

## Death and Dying

13. 1. The respiratory tract cells produce liquid as a defense mechanism against bacteria and other invaders. About nine (9) mL a minute are produced. The "death rattle" can be disturbing to family members, and the nurse should intervene but not with suctioning, which will increase secretions and the need to suction more.

2. This is a natural physical phenomenon and should be addressed.

3. There is an explanation.

4. The scopolamine patch applied to the skin helps to limit the secretions, but this does not answer the question.

**TEST-TAKING HINT: The test taker could eliminate "3" because it states there is no reason, "4" because it does not answer the question, and "2" because it is attempting to fix blame.**

14. 1. Hospice care does not assume care of a client with a prognosis of more than six (6) months and who is doing well.

2. The HCP must think that without life-prolonging treatment, the client has a life expectancy of six (6) months or less. The client may continue receiving hospice care if the client lives longer.

3. The client may live this long, but the HCP must think that the life expectancy is much shorter.

4. Hospice will attempt to manage symptoms of pain, nausea, and any other discomfort the client is experiencing, but the life expectancy is six (6) months.

**TEST-TAKING HINT: This is a knowledge-based question requiring an understanding of hospice.**

15. 1. This would be basic care, but it does not indicate the nurse is aware of the client's terminal prognosis.

2. This does not indicate an understanding of the client's terminal status.

3. The nurse should encourage visitors. There is not much time left for making memories, which will assist those left behind in dealing with the loss and allow the client time to say goodbye.

4. The client may have diabetes, but the client is also terminal, and allowing some food for pleasure is understanding of the client's life expectancy.

**TEST-TAKING HINT: This question requires the test taker to look not only at the disease processes but also at the descriptive words "end-stage" and "hospice" and ask, "What do these descriptors mean to the disease process?" Not limiting the client in small ways indicates the nurse is aware that the client has a limited time to live.**

16. 1. The nurse is not able to provide all spiritual answers to the client.

2. The nurse can explain physical aspects of death, but no one is able to tell the client with absolute knowledge what will happen to the soul or spirit at death. The beliefs of the client may differ greatly from those of the nurse.

3. Clients facing death may wish to find meaning and purpose in life through a higher power. This gives the clients hope, even if the life on earth will be temporary.

4. The nurse is not the expert but should be comfortable with his or her own beliefs to be able to allow the client to discuss personal beliefs and hopes. The experts would be chaplains and spiritual advisers from the client's faith.

**TEST-TAKING HINT: The test taker should recognize the nurse's expertise is not in the spiritual realm, although the nurse is frequently the one called on to perform the assessment and refer to the appropriate person.**

17. 1. No female is allowed to perform the post-mortem on a male Muslim client; this should be performed by a man.
2. Last rites are performed by a Catholic priest, not a Muslim minister.
3. Hindus use incense to pray, but Muslims do not.
4. Females, including the spouse, are not allowed to touch a male's body after death. The nurse should respect this and allow the male members of the family or mosque to perform post-mortem care.

**TEST-TAKING HINT: The question is requiring culturally sensitive knowledge. The test taker must be aware of the different beliefs of the clients being cared for.**

18. 1. The primary goal of spiritual care is to allow the client to be able to reconcile themselves with a higher being, maybe God. This goal is based on the belief that life comes from God, and to some degree for many people the process of living includes some separation from God. In the Western world, 95% of the people claim some belief in God.
2. This could be a goal for a diagnosis of anger, but it does not recognize the spiritual aspect of the client.
3. This would be a goal for altered family functioning.
4. This is the physiological goal for any client who is dying, but it is not a goal for spiritual distress.

**TEST-TAKING HINT: The identified problem is "spiritual distress," and the goal must have information that addresses the spiritual. This would eliminate option "4." Personal relationships with family members ("3") could also be eliminated.**

19. 1. The elderly are frequently on fixed incomes and financial concerns are important for the nurse to address. A social services referral may be needed.
2. The elderly may have many co-morbid conditions, which affect the type and amount of medications the client can tolerate and the client's quality of life.
3. Visual and auditory senses decrease with age; they do not increase.
4. The client may feel some spiritual distress at the terminal diagnosis. Even if the client possesses a strong faith, the unknown can be frightening.
5. A type of euphoria may accompany dehydration prior to death. This is a natural physiological occurrence that the nurse should

recognize, but it is not an intervention the nurse can implement.

**TEST-TAKING HINT: Three of the answer options can be answered on the basis of the descriptive word "elderly." Option "5" is not a nursing intervention.**

20. 1. The client has the right to be cared for with respect and dignity.
2. **The client has the right to discuss his or her feelings and direct his or her care. Withholding information would be lying to the client.**
3. The client has the right to the best care available and to have pain treated, regardless of the potential for hastening death.
4. All clients, even if they are not dying, have the right to holistic and compassionate care.

**TEST-TAKING HINT: This is an "except" question. All of the answer options except one have correct information. The test taker should read the stem carefully to recognize this type of question.**

21. 1. **The nurse should discuss using the ethics committee with the HCP to assist the family in making the decision to terminate life support. Many families feel that there may be a racial or financial reason the HCP wants to discontinue life support.**
2. This would be an illegal act on the part of the nurse and would destroy the nurse–client relationship with the family.
3. The stem already indicates the spouse is aware of the situation.
4. This is expressing a personal bias on the part of the nurse.

**TEST-TAKING HINT: The test taker could eliminate option "2" on the basis of legal and ethical issues. Option "3" is asking the HCP to do something that has already been done.**

22. 1. Death from dehydration occurs when the client is unable to take in fluid, but dehydration is not painful.
2. **Death from dehydration occurs when the client is unable to take in fluid. A natural euphoria occurs with dehydration. This is the body's way of allowing comfort at the time of death.**
3. This is needless.
4. Families who make this decision usually do so from a deep sense of love and commitment. It is an extremely difficult decision to make, and the nurse should not condemn the family decision.

**TEST-TAKING HINT: The test taker could examine options "3" and "4" and eliminate them on**

the basis of needless information or the nurse stepping outside of professional boundaries.

23. 1. The family may or may not be angry and this would need to be addressed, but it is not the most important.
    2. Who makes the decisions is not as important as discovering which coping skills the family uses when under stress.
    3. The nurse should assess previous coping skills used by the family and build on those to assist the family in dealing with their loss. Coping mechanisms are learned behaviors and should be supported if they are healthy behaviors. If the clients use unhealthy coping behaviors, then the nurse should attempt to guide the family to a counselor or support group.
    4. The type of funeral service may help the family to grieve, but it is not the most important intervention.

    **TEST-TAKING HINT:** The test taker must prioritize the interventions listed. All of the options could be addressed in "3."

24. 1. The client is not denying death; the client has said goodbye.
    2. Anger is the second stage of the grieving process, but this client appears to have accepted death.
    3. There is no evidence of bargaining in the client's actions.
    4. The client has accepted the imminent death and is withdrawing from the significant others.

    **TEST-TAKING HINT:** There are five (5) stages to Dr. Elisabeth Kübler-Ross's grieving process, and some authorities list several more, but this could only be withdrawal or acceptance.

## Chronic Pain

25. 1. Blood pressure elevates in acute pain. Chronic pain, by definition, lasts more than six (6) months, lasts far beyond the expected time for the pain to resolve, and may have an unclear onset. Changes in vital signs result from the fight-or-flight response by the body. The body cannot maintain this response and must adjust.
    2. Rapid shallow respirations might be attributed to acute pain if it was painful to breathe. The client with a chest injury or pain will splint the area and slow the respirations or attempt to breathe shallowly and rapidly.
    3. Facial grimacing will occur in acute pain and is an objective sign the nurse can identify. Clients with chronic pain may be laughing and still be

in pain. Remember that pain is whatever the client says it is and occurs whenever the client says it does.
    4. The client in chronic pain will have adapted to living with the pain, and lying quietly may be the best way for the client to limit the feeling of pain.

**TEST-TAKING HINT:** The test taker must be able to differentiate between acute and chronic pain. Answer options "1," "2," and "3" are objective symptoms of acute pain. If the test taker was aware of this, then choosing the only option left would be a good option.

26. 1. Pain is whatever the client says it is and occurs whenever the client says it does. The nurse should never deny the client's pain exists.
    2. This has been occurring for the past three (3) years and does not mean that the cancer has come back. Many clients will fear that the cancer has recurred and delay treatment; denial is a potent coping mechanism.
    3. PMP is characterized as a constriction accompanied by a burning sensation or prickling in the chest wall, axilla, or posterior arm resulting from movement of the arm. Because of this, the client limits movement of the arm and the shoulder becomes frozen.
    4. There are many problems associated with long-term narcotic use. Other strategies should be attempted prior to resigning the client to a lifetime of taking narcotic medications.

**TEST-TAKING HINT:** The test taker could eliminate distracter "1" because it violates all principles of pain management. Distracter "2" is not in the realm of the nurse's responsibility

27. 1. This is a therapeutic response and the client is requesting information.
    2. Pain clinics do not cure pain; they do help identify measures to relieve pain.
    3. Pain clinics use a variety of methods to help the client to achieve relief from pain. Some measures include guided imagery, transcutaneous electrical nerve stimulation (TENS) units, nerve block surgery or injections, or medications.
    4. This is not an appropriate answer, even if the nurse is not sure. The nurse should attempt to discover the information for the client and then give factual information.

**TEST-TAKING HINT:** The test taker should answer a question with factual information. If the stem asks for a therapeutic response, then the test taker should choose one that addresses feelings.

28. 1. NSAIDs around the clock are dangerous because of the potential for gastrointestinal ulceration. NSAIDS are not the drug of choice for cancer pain.
    2. Morphine is the drug of choice for cancer pain. There is no ceiling effect, it metabolizes without harmful byproducts, and is relatively inexpensive. A sustained-release formulation, such an MS Contin, is administered every six (6) to eight (8) hours, and a liquid fast-acting form is administered sublingually for any pain that is not controlled.
    3. Tylenol is not strong enough for this client's pain. The maximum adult dose within a 24-hour period is four (4) gm. Tylenol is toxic to the liver in higher amounts.
    4. Demerol, meperidine, metabolizes into normeperidine and is not cleared by the body rapidly. A buildup of normeperidine can cause the client to seize.

    TEST-TAKING HINT: **The test taker must be aware of medications and their uses.**

29. 1. Narcotic medications require handwritten prescription forms (Drug Enforcement Agency rules) that must be filled within a limited timeframe from the time the prescription is written. Many local pharmacies will not have the medication available or may not have it in the quantities needed. The client should anticipate the needs prior to any time when the HCP may not be available or the pharmacy may be closed.
    2. There can be several reasons that a legitimate prescription is not filled.
    3. Morphine needs a handwritten prescription on a triplicate form.
    4. All medications have side effects; most notably, narcotics slow peristalsis and cause constipation.

    TEST-TAKING HINT: **The test taker could eliminate both option "1" and "2" because they are opposites. Option "4" is untrue of all medications.**

30. 28 mg of morphine. First, determine how many milligrams of morphine are in each milliliter of saline.

    $$50 \div 250 \text{ mL} = 0.2 \text{ mg/mL}$$

    Then determine how many milliliters are given in a shift.

    $$10 \text{ mL per hour} \times 12 \text{ hour} = 120 \text{ mL infused}$$
    $$\text{shift} = 120 \text{ mL infused}$$

    If each milliliter contains 0.2 milligram of morphine, then

    $$0.2 \text{ mg} \times 120 \text{ mL} = 24 \text{ mg by constant infusion}$$

Then determine the amount given IVP:

$$2 \times 2 = 4 \text{ mg given IVP}$$

Finally add that bolus amount to the amount constantly infused:

$$24 + 4 = 28 \text{ mg}$$

TEST-TAKING HINT: **The nurse is responsible for being knowledgeable of all medications and the amount the client is receiving. The test taker can use the pull-down calculator on the RN-NCLEX exam or ask the examiner for scratch paper.**

31. 1. The client is in pain and has the right to have pain-control measures taken.
    2. The client is in pain. The American Nurse's Code of Ethics states that clients have the right to die as comfortably as possible even if the measures used to control the pain indirectly hasten the impending death. The Dying Client's Bill of Rights reiterates this position. The client should be allowed to die with dignity and with as much comfort as the nurse can provide.
    3. The client may be splinting to prevent the pain from being too severe. The client's respirations actually may improve when the nurse administers the pain medication.
    4. The HCP is aware that the client is unstable because the HCP must write the DNR order on the chart. There is no reason to withhold needed medication.

    TEST-TAKING HINT: **The position of administering medication that could hasten a client's death is a difficult one and requires the nurse to be aware of ethical position statements. Nurses never administer medications for the purpose of hastening death but sometimes must administer medications to provide what nurses do best, comfort.**

32. 1. This hemoglobin is low, but that would be expected for a client diagnosed with leukemia. A less experienced nurse could care for this client.
    2. This represents an arterial blood gas of less than 60%; this client should be assigned to the most experienced nurse.
    3. A client who needs to irrigate a colostomy could be assigned to a less experienced nurse.
    4. Psychological problems come second to physiological ones.

    TEST-TAKING HINT: **This is a priority question. The test taker should realize that option "1" is expected and may even be good for this client, that "3" is expected and not life threatening, and that "4," although not expected, is not life threatening. By doing this the test taker could** then look at what was determined for each option and realize that "2" needs the most experienced nurse.

33. 1. The assistant could perform this function.
2. The assistant could perform this function.
3. The assistant could perform this function.
4. The nurse should monitor any lab work needed to administer a medication safely.

**TEST-TAKING HINT:** The rules for delegation state that assessment, teaching, evaluating, or anything requiring nursing judgment cannot be delegated.

34. 1. The TENS unit does not deaden nerve endings; this would be accomplished through local anesthesia.
2. The unit could stop functioning if it got wet, but this would not cause paralysis.
3. The TENS unit works on the gate control theory of pain control and works by flooding the area with stimulation and blocking the pain impulses from reaching the brain.
4. The TENS unit should be applied and left in place unless the client is showering.

**TEST-TAKING HINT:** A unit that causes paralysis so easily would not be approved for use by the general population, so option "2" could be eliminated. The test taker would need to be aware of the gate control theory of pain control to eliminate the other options.

35. 1. These are normal arterial blood gases.
2. These temperature, pulse, and respiration rates are only slightly elevated, and the blood pressure is normal.
3. This is typical of clients with chronic pain. They cannot localize the pain and frequently describe the pain as always being there, as disturbing rest, and as demoralizing. This client should be seen, and appropriate pain-control measures should be taken.
4. This is considered mild pain and can be seen after the client in chronic pain.

**TEST-TAKING HINT:** Answer options "1" and "2" could be eliminated because the values are within normal limits or only slightly above normal. Option "4" could be eliminated because three (3) is less than ten (10) on the pain scale.

36. 1. This could be appropriate once the nurse assess the situation further.
2. The nurse should assess the situation fully. The client may be afraid of becoming addicted or may have been using alternative forms of treatment, such as music therapy,

distraction techniques, acupuncture, or guided imagery.
3. This is not appropriate. It is in the nurse's realm of responsibility to investigate the client's reasons for not wanting to take pain medication.
4. Chronic cancer pain does not resolve on its own.

**TEST-TAKING HINT:** Answer option "1" is advising without assessing. Assessment is the first step of the nursing process and should be implemented first in most situations unless a direct intervention treats the client in an emergency.

## Ethical/Legal Issues

37. 1. This is an example of assault that is a mental or physical threat without touching the client.
2. When a mentally competent adult is forced to have a treatment he or she has refused, battery occurs.
3. This is fraud, a willful and purposeful misrepresentation that could cause harm to a client.
4. This is called defamation, a divulgence of privileged information or communication. This is a violation of the Health Insurance Portability and Accountability Act (HIPAA).

**TEST-TAKING HINT:** If the test taker knows that battery is "bad" it may lead to selecting option "2," which has "forcibly" in the stem. The test taker could attempt to eliminate options based on knowledge. For example, breaking confidentiality is a violation of HIPPA; thus option "4" can be eliminated

38. 1. The Health Insurance Portability and Accountability Act (HIPAA) is a federal act that protects the client's privacy while receiving health care.
2. The state Nurse Practice Acts provides the laws that control the practice of nursing in each state.
3. There is no such law as this act.
4. The Good Samaritan Act protects healthcare practitioners against malpractice claims for care provided in emergency situations.

**TEST-TAKING HINT:** The test taker should be knowledgeable of the Good Samaritan Act and its implications in the nurse's professional career. The RN-NCLEX often asks questions on this Act.

39. 1. This response does not support veracity.
2. This response does not support veracity.

3. The principle of veracity is the duty to tell the truth. This response is telling the client the truth.
4. This response does not support veracity.

**TEST-TAKING HINT: The test taker must know certain ethical principles such as veracity, beneficence, nonmalfeasance, fidelity, autonomy, and justice, to name a few. Without knowing the definition of veracity the test taker would not be able to answer this question correctly.**

40. 1. The surgeon is responsible for explaining the surgical procedure to the client; therefore the nurse should first notify the surgeon.
2. This information should be documented on the chart, but it is not the first intervention.
3. The operating room staff may or may not need to be notified based on when or if the permit is being signed, but it is not the first intervention.
4. The nurse is not responsible for explaining the surgical procedure. The nurse is responsible for making sure the client understands and for obtaining the consent.

**TEST-TAKING HINT: The nurse is responsible for getting the permit signed and on the chart prior to going to surgery, but the nurse is not responsible for explaining the procedure to the client.**

41. 1. Wearing their own clothes, keeping personal items, and having a small amount of money are civil rights of clients in a psychiatric unit.
2. Seeing visitors is a civil right of the client.
3. Receiving and sending unopened mail is a civil right of the client; but any packages must be checked when the client is opening them to check for sharp items, weapons, or any type of medications.
4. This is a violation of the client's rights. The client has a right to have reasonable access to a telephone and the opportunity to have private conversations by telephone.

**TEST-TAKING HINT: The test taker must be aware of the client's legal and civil rights. The client in the psychiatric unit has the same rights as the client in the medical unit. Clients in a psychiatric hospital do not have to wear hospital gowns; they can wear their own clothes.**

42. 1. Autonomy implies that the client has the right to make choices and decisions about his or her own care even if it may result in death or is not in agreement with the health-care team.
2. Self-determination is not an ethical principle.

3. Beneficence is the duty to actively do good for clients.
4. Justice is the duty to treat all clients fairly.

**TEST-TAKING HINT: The test taker should be aware of ethical principles that mandate a nurse's behavior. Clients have rights, and autonomy is an important principle that the nurse must ensure every client has.**

43. 1. The Hippocratic Oath is the oath taken by medical doctors.
2. The Nuremberg Code identifies the need for voluntary informed consent when medical experiments are conducted on human beings. This source does not provide direction for the nurse addressing ethical issues.
3. This document informs clients and families receiving home health care of the ethical conduct they can expect from home care agencies and their employees when they are in the home. This source is not the best professional source for all nurses.
4. The American Nurse's Association (ANA) Code of Ethics outlines to society the values, concerns, and goals of the nursing profession. The code provides direction for ethical decisions and behavior by emphasizing the obligations and responsibilities that are entailed in the nurse–client relationship.

**TEST-TAKING HINT: The test taker must be aware of the word "best" to be able to answer this question. All four (4) answer options may or may not be potential answers, but the test taker must select the option that addresses all nurses. Option "3" should be eliminated as a possible answer because it only addresses home health care.**

44. 1. Breach of duty is one of the four (4) elements necessary to prove nursing malpractice. It is failure to perform according to the established standard of conduct.
2. This is one of the four (4) steps in ethical decision-making. It is not one (1) of the four (4) elements necessary to prove nursing malpractice.
3. Failure to meet the standard of care that results in an actual injury or damage to the client is required to prove nursing malpractice.
4. A connection must exist between conduct and the resulting injury to prove nursing malpractice.

**TEST-TAKING HINT: This is a knowledge-based question, but the test taker should realize that ethical issues and legal issues are two different concerns and that malpractice is a legal con-**

End of Life

cern. The test taker should also know the four (4) elements: 1) The nurse has a duty to the client. 2) The duty has been breached. The nurse failed to uphold a standard of care. 3) There is some harm to the client. 4) The breach of duty caused the harm.

45. 1. This action should be taken, but this is not the first action to keep the client safe.
2. This is a form of chemical restraint, and the nurse must have a health-care provider's order.
3. This is a form of restraint and is against the law unless the nurse has a health-care provider's order.
4. The nurse must notify the health-care provider before putting the client in restraints. Restraints are used in an emergency situation, for a limited time, and must be for the protection of the client.

**TEST-TAKING HINT:** The test taker must realize that when the stem asks which action is first, more than one option may be appropriate for the situation, but only one is implemented first. Restraining a client is considered battery and is against the law unless the client is a danger to self and there is a health-care providers order.

46. 1. Nurse Practice Acts provide the laws that control the practice of nursing in each state. All states have mandatory Nurse Practice Acts.
2. The Client's Bill of Rights, also known as "Your Rights as a Hospital Patient," is a document that explains the client's rights to participate in his or her own health care; it does not address the nurse's behavior.
3. Each state, not the United States Congress, is responsible for writing and implementing the state's Nurse Practice Act.
4. The American Nurses Association is a voluntary organization that provides standards of care and a code of ethics. It addresses issues in nursing, but it does not mandate the registered nurse's behavior.

**TEST-TAKING HINT:** This is a knowledge-based question that the test taker must know.

47. 1. This addresses the ethical principle of veracity. Should the nurse tell the client truthfully that a placebo will not help the pain?
2. This is an example of nonmalfeasance, the duty to prevent or avoid doing harm, whether intentional or unintentional. Is it harmful for a nurse to work in an area where they are not familiar?
3. This is an example of the ethical principle of fidelity, the duty to be faithful to commit-

ments. It involves keeping promises and information confidential and maintaining privacy.
4. Justice involves the duty to treat all clients fairly, without regard to age, socioeconomic status, or any other variables. Providing safe and appropriate nursing care to all clients is an example of justice.

**TEST-TAKING HINT:** The test taker must be knowledgeable of ethical principles; they are part of the RN-NCLEX blueprint. The word "justice" should make the test taker think about fairness, which might lead the test taker to select "4" as the correct answer. Do not automatically think, "I don't know the answer." Think about the words before selecting the correct answer.

48. 1. The law states that child abuse or suspected child abuse must be reported. The nurse is legally responsible to report child abuse or suspected child abuse. This is a legal issue, not malpractice.
2. Malpractice is a failure to meet the standards of care that result in harm or death of a client. Failing to heed warnings of shock is an example of malpractice.
3. Stealing narcotics is a legal situation, not a malpractice issue. The nurse could have his or her nursing license revoked for this illegal behavior.
4. Falsifying documents is against the law. It is not a malpractice issue.

**TEST-TAKING HINT:** The test taker must be knowledgeable of malpractice. Legal issues are dealt with by the laws of the state and government, and malpractice issues are dealt with in the state Nurse Practice Acts and in lawsuits in courts of law.

## Organ/Tissue Donation

49. 1. There is a feeling during times of stress that organs may be distributed unfairly. Tissue and organ banks use the United Network of Organ Sharing (UNOS) to be as fair as possible in the allocation of organs and tissues. Organs will be given to the best match for the organ in the community where the donor dies. If no match is found in that area, then the search for an HLA match will be expanded to other areas of the country. The recipient is chosen on the basis of HLA match, not fame or fortune.
2. The client is asking for information, which the nurse should provide.
3. There is a definite method of allocation of organs.

4. There are 27 known human leukocyte antigens (HLA). HLAs have become the principal histocompatibility system used to match donors and recipients. The greater the number of matches, the less likely the client will reject the organ. Different races have different HLAs.

**TEST-TAKING HINT: Answer option "2" can be eliminated because the client asked for information. Option "1" can be eliminated because the statement supports an unethical situation.**

50. 1. Positive brain waves on the EEG indicate brain activity, and the client is not brain dead.
   2. This is called the oculovestibular test. If the client reacts, then it indicates brain activity and the client is not brain dead.
   3. **The Uniform Determination of Brain Death Act states that brain death is determined by accepted medical standards that indicate irreversible loss of all brain function. Cerebral blood flow studies, EEG, and oculovestibular and oculocephalic tests may be done.**
   4. If the cerebral blood flow studies do not show acceptable blood flow to the brain, the client will not come out of the vegetative state.

**TEST-TAKING HINT: If the test taker examined all answer options and did not understand "1," "2," or "4," then simply reading "3" again would prove it to be the best choice because it simply states that the machine won't be turned off until brain death has been proved.**

51. 1. Many states require that tissue and organ banks are notified of all deaths, but the systemic infection eliminates this client from becoming a donor.
   2. **Septicemia is a systemic infection and will prevent the client from donating tissues or organs.**
   3. There is no reason to notify the HCP.
   4. If the client were to be an organ donor, then the client's body would remain in the intensive care unit on the ventilator and with IV medication support until the organ bank team arrives and takes the client to the operating room.

**TEST-TAKING HINT: Answer option "3" could be eliminated from consideration because the nurse should be able to handle this situation. Option "4" could be eliminated because the client would have to stay on life support if the organ bank was to retrieve viable organs.**

52. 1. Oliguria, fever, increasing edema, hypertension, and weight gain are signs of organ rejection.

2. A decrease in serum creatinine and BUN would indicate the transplanted kidney is functioning well.
3. Potassium and calcium are not monitored for rejection.
4. The client with a fever might have tachycardia. Hypertension is a sign of rejection.

**TEST-TAKING HINT: Answer option "2" could be eliminated because of the word "decreased." If the test taker was aware of the role the kidneys play in controlling blood pressure, then "4" could be eliminated. Decreased urine output in "1" would make the most sense to choose because the kidneys produce urine.**

53. 1. The client must take an immune-suppressant medication forever unless a rejection occurs, and then the client would die without another transplant.
   2. Foul-smelling drainage would indicate infection and is not expected. This would be an emergency situation.
   3. **Clients should be taught to notify the HCP immediately of any signs of an infection. The immune-suppressant drugs will mask the sign of an infection and superinfections can develop.**
   4. The skin turns yellow in liver failure; the anti-rejection drugs do not cause jaundice.

**TEST-TAKING HINT: Standard postoperative instructions include teaching the client to watch for any sign of an infection. Foul-smelling drainage is never normal.**

54. 1. There is no pain associated with storing cord blood. The blood is taken from the separated placenta at birth. Forty to 150 mL of stem cells can be retrieved from the umbilical vein.
   2. All hospitals that have an obstetrics department should be able to assist with the collection of stem cells. The client should notify the HCP to be prepared with the kit to obtain the specimens and to be able to send the stem cells to the Cord Blood Registry for processing and storage.
   3. There is an initial fee to process the stem cells and a yearly fee to maintain the stored stem cells until needed. Stem cells may be used by the infant in case of a devastating illness or can be donated at the discretion of the owner.
   4. There are stem cells that have been stored for more than 20 years.

**TEST-TAKING HINT: The test taker should recognize that pain could not be associated with tissue that is no longer a part of the body.**

End of Life

**55.** 1. Urine cultures are performed frequently because of the bacteriuria present in the early stages of transplantation.
2. A cadaver kidney may have undergone acute tubular necrosis and may not function for two (2) to three (3) weeks, during which time the client may experience anuria, oliguria, or polyuria and require dialysis.
3. Serum creatinine and BUN levels are monitored, but there is no need to monitor the urine osmolality.
4. Hourly outputs are monitored and compared with the intake of fluids.
5. The dressing is a flank dressing.

**TEST-TAKING HINT:** The test taker should notice timeframes. Any time a specific time reference is provided, the test taker must determine if the timeframe is the appropriate interval for performing the activity. In option "4," "every shift" is not appropriate.

**56.** 1. The client would be NPO at this time and would be receiving parenteral anti-rejection medications.
2. The client would have been taken off the heart-lung bypass machine in the operating room.
3. Saturating three (3) dressing pads in one (1) hour would indicate hemorrhage.
4. Pain is expected and is not a complication of the procedure.

**TEST-TAKING HINT:** The test taker should notice the timeframe provided in the stem—in this case, three (3) hours after surgery. This could eliminate "1" and "2."

**57.** 1. Assessment is always the nurse's responsibility and cannot be delegated. Hourly outputs are monitored to determine kidney function.
2. The assistant can perform this function. There is no nursing judgment required.
3. This requires nursing judgment and is outside the assistant's expertise.
4. Irrigating a nasogastric tube for a client who has undergone a pancreas transplant should be done by the nurse; this is a high-level nursing task.

**TEST-TAKING HINT:** When asked to choose a task that can be delegated, the test taker should determine which task requires the least amount of judgment and choose that option.

**58.** 1. This client is ready for discharge and is presumably stable. The client donated the kidney and still has one functioning kidney. An experienced medical–surgical nurse could care for this client.
2. This client must be observed closely for rejec-

tion of the organ and is newly transferred from the intensive care unit; therefore a more experienced nurse should care for this client.
3. This client has developed symptoms of a problem unrelated to the corneal transplant, but these symptoms will increase intracranial pressure, resulting in indirect pressure to the cornea. Therefore a more experienced nurse should care for this client.
4. This client is showing symptoms of organ rejection, which is a medical emergency and requires a more experienced nurse.

**TEST-TAKING HINT:** The test taker should choose the client with the least potential problems. The nurse is experienced as a medical–surgical nurse, but transplant recipients require more specialized knowledge.

**59.** 1. Living donors are able to donate some organs. The kidneys, liver, and lung may be donated, and the donor will still have functioning organs. An identical twin is the best possible match. However, in the situation in this question, the identical twin would also have CF because the genes would be identical. The next best chance for a compatible match comes from a sibling with both parents in common.
2. The father would have only half of the genetic makeup of the child.
3. There are at least 27 HLA types. A match is at least 7, and preferably 10 to 11 are required.
4. This is not an acceptable match; the client would reject the organ.

**TEST-TAKING HINT:** If the test taker did not know the rationale, then a choice between "1" and "2" would be the best option because of the direct familial relationships.

**60.** 1. Skin is taken from cadaver donors, so it is given once.
2. Bones are taken from cadaver donors, so it is given once.
3. A kidney can be donated while living or both can be donated as cadaver organs, but either way the donation is only once.
4. The human body reproduces bone marrow daily. There is a bone marrow registry for participants willing to undergo the procedure to donate to clients when a match is found.

**TEST-TAKING HINT:** The test taker could eliminate "3" because the stem asks for repeated times and the client cannot live without kidney function. The client would have to be placed on dialysis or he or she would die.

End of Life

1. The 38-year-old client was brought to the emergency department with CPR in progress and expires 15 minutes after arrival. Which intervention should the nurse implement for post-mortem care?
   1. Do not allow significant others to see the body.
   2. Do not remove any tubes from the body.
   3. Prepare the body for the funeral home.
   4. Send the client's clothing to the hospital laundry.

2. The primary nurse caring for the client who died is crying with the family at the bedside. Which action should the charge nurse implement?
   1. Request the primary nurse to come out in the hall.
   2. Refer the nurse to the employee assistance program.
   3. Allow the nurse and family this time to grieve.
   4. Ask the chaplain to relieve the nurse at the bedside.

3. The nurse is discussing advance directives with the client. The client asks the nurse, "Why is this so important to do?" Which statement would be the nurse's best response?
   1. "The federal government mandates this form must be completed by you."
   2. "This will make sure your family does what you want them to do."
   3. "Don't you think it is important to let everyone know your final wishes?"
   4. "Because of technology, there are many options for end-of-life care."

4. The client who is of the Jewish faith died during the night. The nurse notified the family, who does not want to come to the hospital. Which intervention should the nurse implement to address the family's behavior?
   1. Take no further action because this is an accepted cultural practice.
   2. Notify the hospital supervisor and report the situation immediately.
   3. Call the local synagogue and request the rabbi go to the family's home.
   4. Assume the family does not care about the client and follow hospital protocol.

5. The hospice nurse is making the final visit to the wife, whose husband died a little more than a year ago. The nurse realizes that the husband's clothes are still in the closet and chest of drawers. Which action should the nurse implement first?
   1. Discuss what the wife is going to do with the clothes.
   2. Refer the wife to a grief recovery support group.
   3. Do not take any action because this is normal grieving.
   4. Remove the clothes from the house and dispose of them.

6. The nurse is giving an in-service on end-of life-issues. Which activity should the nurse encourage the participants to perform?
   1. Discuss with another participant the death of a client.
   2. Review the hospital post-mortem care policy.
   3. Justify not putting the client in a shroud after dying.
   4. Write down his or her own beliefs about death and dying.

7. The 78-year-old Catholic client is in end-stage congestive heart failure and has a DNR order. The client has AP 50, RR 10, and BP 80/50, and Cheyne-Stokes respirations. Which action should the nurse implement?
   1. Bring the crash cart to the bedside.
   2. Apply oxygen via nasal cannula.
   3. Notify a priest for last rites.
   4. Turn the bed to face the sunset.

8. The Hispanic client who has terminal cancer is requesting a curandero to come to the bedside. Which intervention should the nurse implement?
   1. Tell the client it is against policy to allow faith healers.
   2. Assist with planning the visit from the curandero.
   3. Refer the client to the pastoral care department.
   4. Determine the reason the client needs the curandero.

End of Life

9. Which interventions should the nurse implement at the time of a client's death? Select all that apply.
   1. Allow gaps in the conversation at the client's bedside.
   2. Avoid giving the family advice about how to grieve.
   3. Tell the family the nurse understands their feelings.
   4. Explain that this is God's will to prevent further suffering.
   5. Allow the family time with the body in private.

10. The male client asks the nurse, "Should I designate my wife as durable power of attorney for health care?" Which statement would be the nurse's best response?
   1. "Yes, she should be because she is your next of kin."
   2. "Most people don't allow their spouse to do this."
   3. "Will your wife be able to support your wishes?"
   4. "Your children are probably the best ones for the job."

11. The client has been declared brain dead and is an organ donor. The nurse is preparing the wife of the client to enter the room to say goodbye. Which information is most important for the nurse to discuss with the wife?
   1. Inform the wife the client will still be on the ventilator.
   2. Instruct the wife to only stay a few minutes at the bedside.
   3. Tell the wife that it is all right to talk to the client.
   4. Allow another family member to go in with the wife.

12. Which client would the nurse exclude from being a potential organ/tissue donor?
   1. The 60-year-old female client with an inoperable primary brain tumor.
   2. The 45-year-old female client with a subarachnoid hemorrhage.
   3. The 22-year-old male client who has been in a motor-vehicle accident.
   4. The 36-year-male client recently released from prison.

13. The intensive care nurse is caring for a client who is an organ donor, and the organ donation team is in route to the hospital. Which statement would be an appropriate goal of treatment for the client?
   1. The urinary output is 20 mL/hr via a Foley catheter.
   2. The systolic blood pressure is greater than 90 mm Hg.
   3. The pulse oximeter reading remains between 88% and 90%.
   4. The telemetry shows the client in sinus tachycardia.

14. The nurse is teaching a class on ethical principles in nursing. Which statement supports the definition of beneficence?
   1. The duty to prevent or avoid doing harm.
   2. The duty to actively do good for clients.
   3. The duty to be faithful to commitments.
   4. The duty to tell the truth to the clients.

15. Which action by the unlicensed nursing assistant (NA) would warrant immediate intervention by the nurse?
   1. The NA is holding the phone to the ear of a client who is a quadriplegic.
   2. The NA refuses to discuss the client's condition with the visitor in the room.
   3. The NA put a vest restraint on an elderly client found wandering in the hall.
   4. The NA is assisting the client with arthritis to open up personal mail.

16. The nurse is teaching a class on chronic pain to new graduates. Which information is most important for the nurse to discuss?
   1. The nurse must believe the client's report of pain.
   2. Clients in chronic pain may not show objective signs.
   3. Alternate pain-control therapies are used for chronic pain.
   4. Referral to a pain clinic may be necessary.

17. The client with chronic low back pain is having trouble sleeping at night. Which nonpharmacological therapy should the nurse teach the client?
    1. Acupuncture.
    2. Massage therapy.
    3. Herbal remedies.
    4. Progressive relaxation techniques.

18. The client diagnosed with cancer is unable to attain pain relief despite receiving large amounts of narcotic medications. Which intervention should be included in the plan of care?
    1. Ask the HCP to increase the medication.
    2. Assess for any spiritual distress.
    3. Change the client's position every two (2) hours.
    4. Turn on the radio to soothing music.

19. The client diagnosed with chronic pain is laughing and joking with visitors. When the nurse asks the nurse to rate the pain on a one (1) to ten (10) scale the client rates the pain as ten (10). According to the pain scale, how would the nurse chart the client's pain?

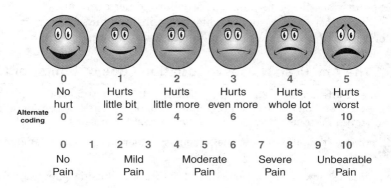

1. The client's pain is between a zero (0) and two (2) on the face scale.
2. The client's pain is a ten (10) on a one (1) to ten (10) pain scale.
3. The client is unable to accurately rate the pain on a scale.
4. The client's pain is moderate on the pain scale.

20. The client diagnosed with diabetes mellitus Type 2 wants to be an organ donor and asks the nurse, "Which organs can I donate?" Which statement is the nurse's best response?
    1. "That is wonderful you want to be an organ donor. Let's discuss this."
    2. "You can donate any organ in your body, except the pancreas."
    3. "You have to donate your body to science to be an organ donor."
    4. "You cannot donate any organs, but you can donate some tissues."

21. The client with multiple sclerosis who is becoming very debilitated tells the home health nurse that the Hemlock Society sent information on euthanasia. Which question should the nurse ask the client?
    1. "Why did you get in touch with the Hemlock Society?"
    2. "Did you know that this is an illegal organization?"
    3. "Who do you know that has committed suicide?"
    4. "What religious beliefs do you practice?"

22. Which intervention should the nurse implement to provide culturally sensitive health care to the European/American Caucasian elderly client who is terminal?
    1. Discuss health-care issues with the oldest male child.
    2. Determine if the client will be cremated or have an earth burial.
    3. Do not talk about death and dying in front of the client.
    4. Encourage the client's autonomy and answer questions truthfully.

End of Life

23. Which action by the primary nurse would require the unit manager to intervene?
    1. The nurse uses white out to correct a charting mistake.
    2. The nurse is shredding the worksheet at the end of the shift.
    3. The nurse circles an omitted medication time on the MAR.
    4. The nurse documents narcotic wastage with another nurse.

24. Which action should the nurse implement for the Chinese client's family that is requesting to light incense around the dying client?
    1. Suggest the family bring potpourri instead of incense.
    2. Tell the client that the door must be shut at all times.
    3. Inform the family the scent will make the client nauseated.
    4. Explain that the fire code does not allow any burning.

25. The nurse is caring for the client who has active tuberculosis of the lungs. The client does not have a DNR order. The client experiences a cardiac arrest, and there is no resuscitation mask at the bedside. The nurse waits for the crash cart before beginning resuscitation. According to the ANA Code of Ethics for Nurses (see below), which disciplinary action should be taken against the nurse?
    1. Report the action to the State Board of Nurse Examiners.
    2. The nurse should be terminated for failure to perform duties.
    3. No disciplinary action should be taken against the nurse.
    4. Refer the nurse to the American Nurses Association.

### TABLE 18-1 The American Nurses Association Code of Ethics for Nurses

The nurse, in all professional relationships, practices with compassion and respect for the inherent dignity, worth, and uniqueness of every individual, unrestricted by considerations of social or economic status, personal attributes, or nature of health problems.

The nurse's primary commitment is to the patient, whether an individual, family, group, or community.

The nurse promotes, advocates for, and strives to protect the health, safety, and rights of the patient.

The nurse is responsible and accountable for individual nursing practice and determines the appropriate delegation of tasks consistent with the nurse's obligation to provide optimum patient care.

The nurse owes the same duties to self as to others, including the responsibility to preserve integrity and safety, to maintain competence, and to continue personal and professional growth.

The nurse participates in establishing, maintaining, and improving health-care environments and conditions of employment conducive to the provision of quality health care and consistent with the values of the profession through individual and collective action.

The nurse anticipates the advancement of the profession through contributions in practice, education, administration, and knowledge development.

The nurse collaborates with other health-care professionals and the public in promoting community, national, and international efforts to meet health needs.

The profession of nursing is responsible for articulating nursing values, for maintaining the integrity of the profession and its practice, and for shaping social policy.

The American Nurses Association Code of Ethics for Nurses with interpretative statements. Copyright 2001, American Nurses Publishing, American Nurses Foundation/American Nurses Association, Washington, DC. Reprinted with permission.

26. The wife of a client in hospice being cared for at home calls the nurse to report that the client is restless and agitated. Which interventions should the nurse implement? List in order of priority.
    1. Request an order from the health-care provider for anti-anxiety medications.
    2. Call the medical equipment company and request oxygen for the client.
    3. Go to the home and assess the client and address the wife's concerns.
    4. Reassure and calm the wife over the telephone.
    5. Notify the chaplain about the client's change in status.

1. 1. There is no reason that the family members should not be able to see the client; this is important to allow the significant other closure.
   2. **This death should be reported to the medical examiner because the death occurred less than 24 hours after hospital admission and an autopsy may be required. Therefore, the nurse must leave all tubes in place; the medical examiner will remove the tubes.**
   3. This is a medical examiner case, and the nurse should not prepare the body by removing tubes or washing the body prior to taking the client to a funeral home.
   4. The client's clothing should be given to the family or to the police if foul play is suspected.

2. 1. The nurse is providing care for the family and should not have to leave the bedside.
   2. An employee assistance program is available at many facilities for counseling employees who are having psychosocial issues, but this nurse is being humane.
   3. **Crying was once considered unprofessional, but today it is recognized as simply an expression of empathy and caring.**
   4. The chaplain may come to the client's room and offer support but should not relieve the nurse who has developed a therapeutic nurse–client relationship with the client.

3. 1. Advance directives (AD) are not mandated by the federal government. The nurse must discuss this with the client, but the client does not have to complete it.
   2. ADs can be overridden by the family because the health-care provider is worried about being sued by family survivors.
   3. This response is not answering the client's question and it is argumentative.
   4. **Technology now allows for the body to maintain life functions indefinitely in some futile situations. ADs allow clients to make decisions that hopefully will be honored at the time of their death.**

4. 1. **Many of the Jewish faith do not believe in viewing or touching the dead body. The body is sent to the funeral home for burial within 24 hours, and a closed casket is preferred.**
   2. The hospital supervisor does not need to be notified that the family did not want to come to the hospital.
   3. The nurse needs to take care of the client, not the family, and should not call to request a rabbi to go visit the family.

   4. The nurse must be aware of cultural differences and not be judgmental.

5. 1. The nurse must first confront the wife about moving on through the grieving process. After one (1) year, the wife should be seriously thinking about what to do with her husband's belongings.
   2. This is an appropriate intervention, but the nurse must first talk directly to the client.
   3. The normal grieving process should take no more than two (2) years if it was an expected death, and because this client was receiving hospice care, it was expected.
   4. This will need to be done at some point, but it is not the nurse's responsibility. This action is crossing professional boundaries unless the wife asks the nurse to do this.

6. 1. This activity will not help the nurse address his or her own fear of death.
   2. This activity will not help the nurse address his or her own fear of death.
   3. This activity will not help the nurse address his or her own fear of death.
   4. **Many nurses are reluctant to discuss death openly with their clients because of their own anxieties about death. Therefore, coming face to face with the nurse's own mortality will address the fear of death.**

7. 1. The client has a DNR; therefore there is no need to bring the crash cart to the bedside.
   2. The client has a DNR and the nurse needs to help the client die peacefully.
   3. **The Catholic religion requires that last rites be performed immediately before or after death.**
   4. The client is Catholic, and there is no specific way for the bed to be placed.

8. 1. The hospital should not prevent the client from practicing his or her culture, and denying faith healers would be denying the client's spiritual guidance.
   2. **The nurse should support the client's culture as long as it is not contraindicated in the client's care. This client is terminal; therefore allowing the curandero, who is a folk healer and religious person in the Hispanic culture, would be appropriate.**
   3. There is no reason to refer this client to the pastoral care department; the nurse can assist the client.
   4. The nurse does not need to know why the client wants the curandero; the nurse should support the client's request without prejudice.

9. 1. The nurse needs to be sensitive to the family, and simply being present to support the family emotionally is important; the nurse does not have to talk.
   2. The nurse should avoid the impulse to give advice; each person grieves in his or her own way.
   3. The nurse should not tell the family that he or she understands; even if the test taker has lost a loved one, the test taker should never select an option that says the nurse understands another person's feelings.
   4. This is projecting the nurse's personal religious beliefs on the family and could cause more anger at God when the family needs to be able to draw on their own spiritual beliefs.
   5. **The family needs time for closure, and allowing the family to stay at the bedside is meeting the family's need to say goodbye.**

10. 1. The client can designate anyone he wishes to be the durable power of attorney.
    2. This is not true; many spouses are designated as the durable power of attorney for health care.
    3. **No matter who the client selects as the power of attorney, the most important aspect is to make sure the person, whether it be the wife, child, or friend, will honor the client's wishes no matter what happens.**
    4. The children must be at least 18 years old and willing to honor the client's wishes.

11. 1. **This is the most important action because when the wife walks in the room the client's chest will be rising and falling, the monitor will show a heartbeat, and the client will be warm. Many family members do not realize this and think the client is still alive but the brain is dead. The organs must be perfused until retrieved for organ donation.**
    2. The wife should be encouraged to stay a short time and leave the facility before the client is taken to the operating room, but it is not the most important intervention.
    3. It is all right for the wife to talk to the client, but because the client is brain dead and cannot hear her, it is not the most important intervention.
    4. It is all right for another family member to go into the room, but it is not the most important intervention.

12. 1. Primary brain tumors rarely metastasize outside the skull, and this client can be a donor; cancers other than primary brain tumors prevent organ/tissue donation.

2. This is an excellent potential donor because all other organs are probably healthy.
3. This is an excellent candidate because this is a young person with a traumatic death, not a chronic illness.
4. A male client who has been in prison is at risk for being HIV positive, which excludes him from being an organ/tissue donor.

13. 1. The urinary output should be at least 30 mL/hr.
    2. **The systolic blood pressure must be maintained at this rate to keep the client's organs perfused until removal.**
    3. The pulse oximeter should be greater than 93%.
    4. The client heart must be beating, but it can be normal sinus rhythm or even sinus bradycardia.

14. 1. This is the ethical principle of nonmalfeasance.
    2. **This is the ethical principle of beneficence.**
    3. This is the ethical principle of fidelity.
    4. This is the ethical principle of veracity.

15. 1. The client has a right to private phone conversations but because the client is a quadriplegic, holding the phone to the ear does not require immediate intervention.
    2. This is the appropriate action for the NA and should be praised.
    3. **Restraints are not allowed unless there is a health-care provider's order with documentation by the nurse that the client is a danger to himself or herself. The NA's putting the client in restraints warrants immediate intervention because it is battery.**
    4. The client has a right to send and receive mail, and the NA is just helping the client open the mail; therefore this does not require immediate intervention.

16. 1. **The most important information for a nurse caring for a client with acute or chronic pain is to believe the client. Pain is subjective, and the nurse should not be judgmental.**
    2. This is a true statement because the client's sympathetic nervous system cannot remain in a continual state of readiness. This results in no objective data to support the pain and a normal pulse and blood pressure.
    3. Transcutaneous electrical nerve stimulation (TENS), distraction, imagery, acupuncture, and acupressure are all alternate pain therapies that may be used for chronic pain, but it is not the most important information the new graduate should know.

4. Pain clinics treat clients with chronic pain, but it is not the most important information a new graduate should know.

17. 1. Acupuncture is an alternate therapy, but a nurse cannot teach it and the client cannot do this to themselves.
  2. A client cannot perform massage therapy on himself or herself.
  3. The nurse should not prescribe herbal remedies.
  4. **Progressive relaxation techniques involve visualizing a specific muscle group and mentally relaxing that muscle; this can be taught to the client, and it will allow the client to relax, which will foster sleep.**

18. 1. The client is already receiving large amounts of medication. The nurse should assess for other causes of pain.
  2. **Pain has many components, and spiritual distress or psychosocial needs will affect the client's perception of pain; remember, assessment is the first step of the nursing process.**
  3. Usually clients will naturally assume the most comfortable position, and forcing them to move may increase their pain.
  4. The client may or may not like this type of music, but it would not be the first intervention.

19. 1. The faces pain scale was devised to help children identify pain when they are unable to understand the concept of numbers. The nurse can use the pain scale when caring for adults who are unable to use the one (1) to (10) numerical scale. This client rated the pain at a ten (10).
  2. **Pain is whatever the client says it is and occurs whenever the client says it does. Pain is a wholly subjective symptom, and the nurse should not question the client's perception of pain. The client's pain is a ten (10).**
  3. The client did rate the pain on the pain scale. Laughing and talking with visitors may occur with excruciating chronic pain. The client in chronic pain must learn to adapt to pain and try to live as normal a life as possible.
  4. The client rated the pain at a ten (10).

20. 1. This is not answering the client's question.
  2. A client with Type 2 diabetes has organ damage as a result of the high glucose over time; therefore most organs are not usable.
  3. This is a false statement. The client does not

have to will his or her body to science to be a tissue/organ donor.
  4. **The client can donate corneas, skin, and some joints, but organ donation from clients with Type 2 diabetes mellitus usually is not allowed.**

21. 1. The nurse should not ask the client "why" he or she does something; this is judgmental.
  2. This answer option is giving erroneous information because it is not illegal; it is an organization that supports active euthanasia.
  3. This question is not relevant to the situation.
  4. **This question must be asked because Judeo-Christian belief supports the view that suicide is a violation of natural law and the laws of God. The tenets of the Hemlock Society are in direct opposition to Judeo-Christian beliefs. If the client is agnostic, then this organization may be helpful to the client.**

22. 1. Many Middle Eastern cultures practice this, but the Caucasian culture does not.
  2. Caucasians as a culture do not necessarily have a preference, but this does not affect culturally sensitive health care.
  3. Frequently Caucasians do not like to talk about death and dying, but this is an individual preference of the client and the nurse should allow the discussion.
  4. **The western Caucasian society values autonomy and truth telling in individual decision-making.**

23. 1. **The client's chart is a legal document, and if a mistake occurs, it should be corrected by marking one line through the entry in such a way that the entry can still be read in a court of law. Erasing, using white out, or obliterating the entry is illegal.**
  2. This is the correct method for disposing of any paper that has client information on it that is not a part of the client's permanent medical record.
  3. This is the correct method to indicate a medication was not administered to the client; the circle means that the person should go to the nurse's notes to read the reason why the medication was not administered.
  4. All narcotics not administered to the client must be verified when being wasted and documented.

24. 1. **The nurse must support the client's culture. Potpourri provides the scent without having the burning incense, which is against**

the fire code, and thus is a compromise that supports the client's culture.

2. Having the door shut does not matter; open flames are not allowed in any health-care facility.

3. This is not necessarily true, and if it is part of the culture beliefs about dying, then the nurse should medicate the client if he or she becomes nauseated.

4. This is a fact, but the nurse should attempt to compromise and support the client and family's cultural needs, especially at the time of death.

25. 1. There is no need to report this action to the state board; this is not malpractice.

2. This action does not warrant the nurse being terminated.

3. The Code states, "The nurse owes the same duty to self as to others including the responsibility to preserve integrity and safety." Therefore, if the nurse realizes that he or she could contract TB if unprotected

mouth-to-mouth resuscitation is performed, then not doing this action does not violate the code of ethics.

4. The ANA cannot discipline nurses; it is a voluntary nurse's organization.

26. In order of priority: 4, 3, 2, 1, 5.

4. The nurse should calm and reassure the wife over the telephone.

3. The nurse should then visit the client immediately to assess the change in condition.

2. Restlessness and agitation are symptoms of lack of oxygen. Therefore calling the medical equipment company to send oxygen would be the next intervention.

1. Terminal restlessness is difficult for the family to watch and client to experience, so anti-anxiety medications would be the next logical intervention.

5. Referral to the chaplain is needed because death may be imminent.

# Pharmacology

*Education makes a people easy to lead, but difficult to drive; easy to govern, but impossible to enslave.*—Lord Brougham

This chapter contains test-taking hints specific to pharmacology-related questions. Many of the general hints discussed in Chapter 1 and provided with the answer rationales in the other chapters are also helpful. Remember, however, that test-taking hints are useful for discriminating information and choosing among answer options, but they cannot substitute for knowledge. Nurses must be familiar with medications—their specific uses, modes of administration, side effects, possible adverse reactions, and ways to gauge their effectiveness in treating specific disorders/diseases.

## KEYWORDS

agranulocytosis
ataxia
doll's eye test
echinacea
mydriasis
tetany

## ABBREVIATIONS

Apical Pulse (AP)
As needed (PRN)
Beats Per Minute (BPM)
By mouth (PO)
Computed Tomography (CT)
Health-Care Provider (HCP)
Hour of Sleep (HS)
Intravenous Push (IVP)
Joint Commission for the Accreditation of Healthcare
  Organizations (JCAHO)
Licensed Practical Nurse (LPN)
Medication Administration Record (MAR)
Over-The-Counter (OTC)
Supraventricular Tachycardia (SVT)

## TEST-TAKING HINTS FOR PHARMACOLOGY QUESTIONS

The test taker must know medications and memorize specific facts about the different medications, including their uses, dosages, and side effects. This knowledge is part of administering medications safely. There are some specific tips to assist the test taker to learn about medications, and they will apply to the 101 questions in this chapter.

It is important to learn the different classifications of drugs—for example, diuretics, antibiotics, nonsteroidal anti-inflammatory drugs (NSAIDs). Learn the actions, uses, side effects, adverse effects, possible interactions, and method of administration (for example, oral, intravenous, intramuscular) of these drugs. Generally speaking, the various drugs in each classification will be similar in these factors.

Do not be too broad in the classifications. For example, do not combine all medications administered for hypertension in the same category. Angiotensin-converting enzyme (ACE) inhibitors, beta blockers, and calcium channel blockers, for example, are all used to treat hypertension, but they are different categories of medications, acting differently in the body and producing different effects. Diuretics and oral medications for diabetes mellitus fall into different specific classifications and must be learned by the specific classification. Each classification has its own effects on the body, side effects, and adverse effects, and each has steps the nurse must take before administering the medication.

When administering medications for a group of clients the test taker must realize that time is a realistic problem. The nurse will be unable to look up 50–60 medications and administer them all within the dosing timeframe, so it is imperative that the nurses learn the most common medications.

One tip for learning the medications is for the test taker to complete handmade drug cards. This is better than buying ready-made cards because in making the card, the test taker must involve more than one sense—reading, deciding which information to put on the card, and writing the pertinent information. Using more than one sense will assist the test taker to memorize the information.

## Drug Card

When the test taker is deciding which information is the most important to write on a drug card, there are five (5) questions that can be used as a guide.

1. **What is the scientific rationale for administering the medication?**
   The test taker should always ask "why" is this intervention being implemented.
   • What classification is the medication that the nurse is administering to the client?
   • Why is this client receiving this medication?
   • What action does the medication have in the body?

The answers to these questions provide the scientific rationale for administering the medication. It is also important to remember that many medications are in one classification but the client is receiving the medication for a different reason—for example, the anticonvulsant Depakote (Tegretol) is also administered as an anti-mania medication.

### EXAMPLE #1

Digoxin (Lanoxin) 0.25 mg po

• The classification of this medication is a cardiac glycoside.
• The medication is administered to clients with congestive heart failure or rapid atrial fibrillation.
• Cardiac glycosides increase the contractility of the heart and decrease the heart rate.

### EXAMPLE #2

Furosemide (Lasix) 40 mg IVP

• The classification of this medication is a loop diuretic.
• The medication is administered to clients with essential hypertension.
• This medication helps remove excess fluid from the body.
• Loop diuretics remove water from the kidneys along with potassium.

2. **When should the administration of a medication be questioned?**
   • When should the nurse question administering the medication?
   • Does the medication have a therapeutic serum level?
   • Which vital signs must be monitored?
   • Which physiological parameters should be monitored when the medication is being administered?

The answers to these questions will provide the nurse with information on which to base a decision on which medication orders should be questioned.

Pharmacology

## EXAMPLE #1

Digoxin (Lanoxin)

- Is the apical pulse less than 60 bpm?
- Is the digoxin level within the therapeutic range?
- Is the potassium level within normal range?

## EXAMPLE #2

Furosemide (Lasix)

- Is the potassium level within normal range?
- Does the client have signs/symptoms of dehydration?
- Is the client's blood pressure below 90/60?

3. **How can the nurse ensure the safety of the administration of medications?**
   - What interventions must be taught to the client to ensure the medication is administered safely in the hospital setting?
   - What interventions must be taught for taking the medication safely at home?

## EXAMPLE #1

Digoxin (Lanoxin)

- Explain to the client the importance of getting serum levels regularly.
- Teach the client to take radial pulse and to not take the medication if the pulse is less than 60.
- Tell the client to take the medication daily or as ordered and notify the HCP if not taking the medication.

## EXAMPLE #2

Furosemide (Lasix)

- Teach the client about orthostatic hypotension.
- Instruct the client to drink water to replace insensible fluid loss.
- Because the medication is intravenous push (IVP), how many minutes should the medication be pushed over; what primary IV is hanging; is it compatible with Lasix?

4. **What are the possible side effects and possible adverse reactions associated with a specific medication?**
   - What are the side effects? Side effects are not expected but are not unusual.
   - What are the possible adverse reactions associated with this medication?
   - Adverse reactions are any situations that would requiring notifying the health-care provider or discontinuing the medication.

## EXAMPLE #1

Digoxin (Lanoxin)

- Inform the client of the signs of toxicity, which are nausea, vomiting, anorexia, and yellow haze.

## EXAMPLE #2

Furosemide (Lasix)

- Side effects include dizziness and light-headedness.
- Adverse effects include hypokalemia and tinnitus (if Lasix is administered too quickly)

5. **How can the effectiveness of a medication be monitored?**

### EXAMPLE #1

Digoxin (Lanoxin)

- Have the signs/symptoms of congestive heart failure improved?
- Is the client able to breathe easier?
- How many pillows does the client have to sleep on when lying down?
- Is the client able to perform activities of daily living without shortness of breath?

### EXAMPLE #2

Furosemide (Lasix)

- Is the client's urinary output greater than the intake?
- Has the client lost any weight?
- Does the client have sacral or peripheral edema?
- Does the client have jugular vein distention?
- Is the client's blood pressure decreased?

## SAMPLE DRUG CARDS

### Front of Card:

**Classification of Drug:**          **Route:**

**Action of Drug:**

**Uses:**

**Nursing Implications (When would I question giving the medication?)**

**How will I monitor to see if it is working?**

### Back of Card:

**Side Effects:**

**Teaching Needs:**

**Drug Names:**

It is suggested that the test taker complete these cards from the pharmacology textbook and not your drug handbook because most test questions come from a pharmacology book.

## Front of Card: Digoxin

**Classification of Drug:** Cardiac Glycosides        **Route:** PO/IV

**Action:** Positive ionotropic action; increases force of ventricular contraction and thereby increases cardiac output; slows the heart, allowing for increased filling time.

**Uses:** Congestive heart failure and rapid atrial cardiac dysrhythmias

**Nursing Implications:** Check apical pulse for 1 full minute, hold if <60. Check digoxin level (0.5–2.0 normal; >2.0 is toxic). Check K+ level (3.5–5.5 MEq/L is normal). Hypokalemia is the most common cause of dysrhythmias in clients receiving digoxin. Monitor for S/S of CHF, crackles in lungs, I & O, edema. Question if the AP is <60 or abnormal lab values.

**IVP more than 5 minutes:** maintenance dose 0.125–0.25 mg q day

**Effective:** Breathing improves, activity tolerance improves, atrial rate decreases

## Back of Card: Digoxin

**Side Effects:** Toxic = yellow haze or nausea and vomiting, ventricular rate decreases. If a diuretic is given simultaneously, might increase the likelihood of hypokalemia.

**Teaching Needs:** To take pulse and hold digoxin if it is <60 and notify HCP.

K+ replacement: Eat food high in K+ or may need supplemental K+.

Report weight gain of 3 lbs or more.

**Drug names:** Digoxin (Generic)

Lanoxin

Lanoxicap

## Front of Card: Furosemide

**Classification of Drug:** Loop diuretic        **Route:** PO/IVP

**Actions:** Blocks reabsorption of sodium and chloride in the loop of Henle, which prevents the passive reabsorption of water and leads to diuresis.

**Uses:** CHF, fluid volume overload, pulmonary edema, HTN.

**Nursing Implications:** I & O, monitor K+ level, check skin turgor, monitor for leg cramps, provide K+-rich foods or supplements, give early in the day to prevent nocturia

If giving IVP: Give at prescribed rate (Lasix 20 mg/min), ototoxic if given faster.

**Effective:** Decrease in weight, output > intake, less edema, lung sounds clear.

## Back of Card: Furosemide

**Side Effects:** Hypokalemia, muscle cramps, hyponatremia, dehydration.

**Teaching Needs:** Take early in the day.

Eat foods high in K+.

**Drug Names:** Furosemide (Lasix)

Bumetanide (Bumex)

Torsemide (Demadex)

Ethacrynic acid (Edecrin)

Pharmacology

The test taker is encouraged to use the guidelines/test-taking hints given previously when taking the following medication test. The test is comprehensive for medications administered in a medical–surgical setting.

1. The client asks the clinic nurse if he should take 2000 mg of vitamin C a day to prevent getting a cold. On which scientific rationale should the nurse base the response?
   1. Vitamin C in this dosage will help cure the common cold.
   2. This vitamin must be taken with echinacea to be effective.
   3. This dose of vitamin C is not high enough to help prevent colds.
   4. Mega doses of vitamin C may cause crystals to form in the urine.

2. The client recently has had a myocardial infarction. Which medications should the nurse anticipate the health-care provider recommending to prevent another heart attack?
   1. Vitamin K and a nonsteroidal anti-inflammatory drug (NSAID).
   2. Vitamin E and a daily low-dose aspirin.
   3. Vitamin A and an anticoagulant.
   4. Vitamin B complex and an iron supplement.

3. The client diagnosed with essential hypertension calls the clinic and tells the nurse she needs something for the flu. Which information should the nurse tell the client?
   1. OTC medications for the flu should not be taken because of your hypertension.
   2. If OTC medications do not relieve symptoms within 3 days, contact the HCP.
   3. Tell the client to ask the pharmacist to recommend an OTC medication for the flu.
   4. Make an appointment for the client to receive the influenza vaccine.

4. Which laboratory test should the nurse monitor for the client receiving the intravenous steroid Solu-Medrol?
   1. Potassium level.
   2. Sputum culture and sensitivity.
   3. Glucose level.
   4. Arterial blood gases.

5. The client diagnosed with asthma is prescribed the mast cell inhibitor Cromolyn. Which statement by the client indicates the need for further teaching?
   1. "I will take two puffs of my inhaler before I exercise."
   2. "I will rinse my mouth with water after taking the medication."
   3. "After inhaling the medication, I will hold my breath for 10 seconds."
   4. "When I start to wheeze, I will use my inhaler immediately."

6. The client diagnosed with methicillin-resistant *Staphylococcus aureus* (MRSA) is receiving the aminoglycoside antibiotic vancomycin. A peak and trough level is ordered for the dose the nurse is administering. Which priority intervention should the nurse implement?
   1. Ask the client if he has had any diarrhea.
   2. Monitor the aminoglycoside peak level.
   3. Determine if the trough level has been drawn.
   4. Check the client's culture and sensitivity report.

7. The nurse is caring for an elderly client who is eight (8) hours postoperative hip replacement and is reporting incisional pain. Which intervention is priority for this client?
   1. Assist the client to sit in the bedside chair.
   2. Initiate pain medication at the lowest dose.
   3. Assess the client's pupil size and accommodation.
   4. Monitor the client's urinary output hourly.

8. The client is diagnosed with pernicious anemia. Which health-care provider order should the nurse anticipate in treating this condition?
   1. Subcutaneous iron dextran.
   2. Intramuscular vitamin $B_{12}$.
   3. Intravenous folic acid.
   4. Oral thiamine medication.

9. The client with Type 2 diabetes mellitus is prescribed glyburide (Micronase), a sulfonylurea. Which statement indicates the client understands the medication teaching?
   1. "I should carry some hard candy when I go walking."
   2. "I must take my insulin injection every morning."
   3. "There are no side effects that I need to worry about."
   4. "This medication will make my muscles absorb insulin."

10. The nursing assistant reports that the client's Glucometer reading is 380 mg/dL. The client is on regular sliding-scale insulin that reads:

| Glucometer Reading | Units of Insulin |
| --- | --- |
| <150 | 0 |
| 151–250 | 5 |
| 251–350 | 8 |
| 351–450 | 10 |
| 451+ | Notify the HCP |

How much insulin should the nurse administer to the client?_____

11. The nurse administers 18 units of Humulin N, an intermediate-acting insulin, at 1630. Which priority invention should the nurse implement?
   1. Monitor the client's hemoglobin $A1_c$.
   2. Make sure the client eats the evening meal.
   3. Check the ac blood Glucometer reading.
   4. Ensure that the client eats a snack.

12. The nurse is administering the following 1800 medications. Which medication should the nurse question before administering?
   1. The sliding-scale insulin to the client who has just been released to have the evening meal.
   2. The antibiotic to the client who is one (1) day postoperative exploratory abdominal surgery.
   3. Metformin (Glucophage), a biguanide, to the client having a CT scan in the morning.
   4. Protonix, a proton pump inhibitor, to the client diagnosed with peptic ulcer disease.

13. The nurse is administering the long-acting insulin glargine (Lantus) to the client at 2200. The nurse asks the charge nurse to check the dosage. Which action should the charge nurse implement?
   1. Ask the nurse why the insulin is being given late.
   2. Check the MAR with the dosage in the syringe.
   3. Instruct the nurse to complete a medication error form.
   4. Have the nurse notify the health-care provider.

14. The nurse is preparing to administer Synthroid, a thyroid hormone replacement, to the client diagnosed with hypothyroidism. Which assessment data would indicate the client is receiving too much medication?
   1. Bradypnea and weight gain.
   2. Lethargy and hypotension.
   3. Irritability and tachycardia.
   4. Normothermia and constipation.

15. The client is receiving a continuous intravenous infusion of heparin, an anticoagulant. Based on the most recent laboratory data:

| | |
|---|---|
| PT 13.2 | Control 12.1 |
| INR 1.3 | |
| PTT 72 | Control 39 |

Which action should the nurse implement?
1. Continue to monitor the infusion.
2. Prepare to administer protamine sulfate.
3. Have the lab reconfirm the results.
4. Assess the client for bleeding.

16. The elderly client is admitted to the emergency department from a long term care facility. The client has multiple ecchymotic areas on the body. The client is receiving digoxin, a cardiac glycoside; Lasix, a loop diuretic; warfarin, an anticoagulant; and Xanax, an anti-anxiety medication. Which order should the nurse request from the health-care provider?
1. A STAT serum potassium level.
2. An order to admit to the hospital for observation.
3. An order to administer Valium intravenous push.
4. A STAT International Normalized Ratio (INR).

17. The client with post-menopausal osteoporosis is prescribed the bisphosphonate alendronate (Fosamax). Which discharge instruction should the nurse discuss with the client?
1. The medication must be taken with the breakfast meal only.
2. Remain upright for at least 30 minutes after taking mediation.
3. The tablet should be chewed thoroughly before swallowing.
4. Stress the importance of having monthly hormone levels.

18. The nurse is administering AM medications. Which medication should the nurse administer first?
1. The daily digoxin to the client diagnosed with congestive heart failure.
2. The loop diuretic to the client with a serum potassium level of 3.1 mEq/L.
3. The mucosal barrier Carafate to the client diagnosed with peptic ulcer disease.
4. Solu-Medrol IVP to a client diagnosed with chronic lung disease.

19. The HCP ordered an angiotensin-converting enzyme (ACE) inhibitor for the client diagnosed with a myocardial infarction. Which statement best explains the rationale for administering this medication to this client?
1. It will help prevent the development of congestive heart failure.
2. This medication will help decrease the client's blood pressure.
3. ACE inhibitors increase the contractility of the heart muscle.
4. They will help decrease the development of atherosclerosis.

20. The client is receiving the angiotensin-converting enzyme (ACE) inhibitor enalapril (Zestril). When would the nurse question administering this medication?
1. The client is not receiving potassium supplements.
2. The client complains of a persistent irritating cough.
3. The blood pressure for two consecutive readings is 110/70.
4. The client's urinary output is 400 mL for the last eight (8) hours.

21. The nurse is preparing to administer the morning dose of digoxin, a cardiac glycoside, to a client diagnosed with congestive heart failure. Which data would indicate the medication is effective?
1. The apical heart rate is 72 beats per minute.
2. The client denies having any anorexia or nausea.
3. The client's blood pressure is 120/80 mm Hg.
4. The client's lungs sounds are clear bilaterally.

22. The client diagnosed with multiple sclerosis is receiving Lioresal (baclofen), a muscle relaxant. Which information should the nurse teach the client/family?
    1. The importance of tapering off medication when discontinuing medication.
    2. Baclofen may cause diarrhea, so the client should take anti-diarrheal medication.
    3. The client should not be allowed to drive alone while taking this medication.
    4. The need for follow-up visits to obtain a monthly white blood cell count.

23. The nursing is administering digoxin, a cardiac glycoside, to the client with congestive heart failure. Which interventions should the nurse implement? Select all that apply.
    1. Check the apical heart rate for one (1) full minute.
    2. Monitor the client's serum sodium level.
    3. Teach the client how to take his or her radial pulse.
    4. Evaluate the client's serum digoxin level.
    5. Assess the client for buffalo hump and moon face.

24. The client's vital signs are T 99.2°F, AP 59, R 20, and BP 108/72. Which medication would the nurse question administering?
    1. Theodur, a bronchodilator.
    2. Inderal, a beta blocker.
    3. Ampicillin, an antibiotic.
    4. Cardizem, a calcium channel blocker.

25. The client in end-stage renal disease is a Jehovah's Witness. The HCP orders erythropoietin (Epogen), a biologic response modifier, subcutaneously for anemia. Which action should the nurse take?
    1. Question this order because of the client's religion.
    2. Encourage the client to talk to his or her minister.
    3. Administer the medication subcutaneously as ordered.
    4. Obtain the informed consent prior to administering.

26. The elderly male client is admitted for acute severe diverticulitis. He has been taking Xanax, a benzodiazepine, for nervousness three (3) to four (4) times a day prn for six (6) years. Which intervention should the nurse implement first?
    1. Prepare to administer an intravenous anti-anxiety medication.
    2. Notify the HCP to obtain an order for the client's Xanax prn.
    3. Explain that Xanax causes addiction and he should quit taking it.
    4. Assess for signs/symptoms of medication withdrawal.

27. The nurse is administering an ophthalmic drop to the right eye. Which anatomical location would be correct when administering eye drops?
    1. A
    2. B
    3. C
    4. D

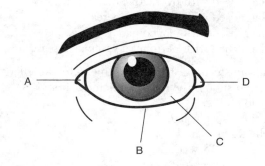

28. The nurse is administering the loop diuretic furosemide (Lasix) to the client diagnosed with essential hypertension. Which assessment data would warrant the nurse to question administering the medication?
    1. The client's potassium level is 4.2 mEq/L.
    2. The client's urinary output is greater than the intake.
    3. The client has tented skin turgor and dry mucous membranes.
    4. The client has lost two (2) pounds in the last 24 hours.

29. The client who has had a kidney transplant tells the nurse that he has been taking St. John's wort, an herb, for depression. Which action should the nurse take first?
    1. Praise the client for taking the initiative to treat the depression.
    2. Remain nonjudgmental about the client's alternative treatments.
    3. Refer the client to a psychologist for counseling for depression.
    4. Instruct the client to quit taking the medication immediately.

30. The nurse is administering an antacid to a client with gastroesophageal reflux disease. Which statement best describes the scientific rationale for administering this medication?
    1. This medication will suppress gastric-acid secretion.
    2. This medication will decrease the gastric pH.
    3. This medication will coat the stomach lining.
    4. This medication interferes with prostaglandin production.

31. The client is diagnosed with essential hypertension and is receiving a calcium channel blocker. Which assessment data would warrant the nurse holding the client's medication?
    1. The client's oral temperature is 102°F.
    2. The client complaints of a dry, nonproductive cough.
    3. The client's blood pressure reading is 106/76.
    4. The client complains of being dizzy when getting out of bed.

32. The client complains of leg cramps at night. Which medication should the nurse anticipate the HCP ordering to help relieve the leg cramps?
    1. Quinine, an antimalarial.
    2. Soma, a muscle relaxant.
    3. Ambien, a sedative-hypnotic.
    4. Darvon, an opioid analgesic.

33. The nurse is preparing to administer the initial dose of an antibiotic in the emergency department. Which interventions should the nurse implement? Select all that apply.
    1. Assess for drug allergies.
    2. Collect needed specimens for culture.
    3. Check the client's armband.
    4. Ask the client his or her birthday.
    5. Draw a peak and trough level.

34. For which client should the nurse question administering the muscarinic cholinergic agonist oxybutynin (Ditropan)?
    1. The client diagnosed with overactive bladder.
    2. The client diagnosed with Type 2 diabetes.
    3. The client diagnosed with glaucoma.
    4. The client diagnosed with peripheral vascular disease.

35. The nurse is administering a topical ointment to the client's rash on the right leg. Which intervention should the nurse implement first?
    1. Don nonsterile gloves.
    2. Cleanse the client's right leg.
    3. Check the client's armband.
    4. Wash the hands for 15 seconds.

36. The client is exhibiting multifocal premature ventricular contractions. Which antidysrhythmic medication should the nurse anticipate the HCP ordering for this dysrhythmia?
    1. Adenosine.
    2. Epinephrine.
    3. Atropine.
    4. Lidocaine.

37. The client in the intensive care department is receiving 2 mcg/kg/min of dopamine, an ionotropic vasopressor. Which intervention should the nurse include in the plan of care?
    1. Monitor the client's blood pressure every two (2) hours.
    2. Assess the client's peripheral pulses every shift.
    3. Use a urometer to assess hourly output.
    4. Ensure that the IV tubing is not exposed to the light.

38. The client is receiving thrombolytic therapy for a diagnosed myocardial infarction (MI). Which assessment data indicate the therapy is successful?
    1. The client's ST segment is becoming more depressed.
    2. The client is exhibiting reperfusion dysrhythmias.
    3. The client's cardiac isoenzyme CPK-MB is not elevated.
    4. The D-dimer is negative at two (2) hours post-MI.

39. The client with arthritis is self-medicating with aspirin, a nonsteroidal anti-inflammatory medication. Which complication should the nurse discuss with the client?
    1. Tinnitus.
    2. Diarrhea.
    3. Tetany.
    4. Paresthesia.

40. The client is receiving a loop diuretic for congestive heart failure. Which medication would the nurse expect the client to be receiving while taking this medication?
    1. A potassium supplement.
    2. A cardiac glycoside.
    3. An ACE inhibitor.
    4. A potassium cation.

41. The nurse is reviewing laboratory values for the woman diagnosed with cancer. Based on the laboratory report, which biologic response modifier would the nurse anticipate administering to the client?

| Laboratory Test | Client Values | Normal Values |
| --- | --- | --- |
| Red blood cells | 4.11 | M: 4.7–6.1 ($10^6$) |
|  |  | F: 4.2–5.4 ($10^6$) |
| Hemoglobin | 12.2 | M: 13.5–17.5 g/dL |
|  |  | F: 11.5–15.5 g/dL |
| Hematocrit | 37 | M: 40%–52% |
|  |  | F: 36%–48% |
| White blood cells | 2.0 | 4.5–11.0 ($10^3$) |
| Platelets | 160 | 140–400 ($10^3$) |

    1. Interferon.
    2. Neupogen.
    3. Neumega.
    4. Procrit.

42. The client admitted with pneumonia is taking Imuran, an immunosuppressive agent. Which question should the nurse ask the client regarding this medication?
    1. "Do you know this medication has to be tapered off when discontinued?"
    2. "Have you been exposed to viral hepatitis B or C recently?"
    3. "Why are you taking this medication, and how long have you taken it?"
    4. "Do you have a lot of allergies or sensitivities to different medications?"

43. The elderly client is in a long term care facility. If the client does not have a daily bowel movement in the morning, he requests a cathartic, bisacodyl (Dulcolax). Which action is most important for the nurse to take?
    1. Ensure the client gets a cathartic daily.
    2. Discuss the complications of a daily cathartic.
    3. Encourage the client to increase fiber in the diet.
    4. Refuse to administer the medication to the client.

44. The client received Narcan, a narcotic antagonist, following a colonoscopy. Which action by the nurse has the highest priority?
    1. Document the occurrence in the nurse's notes.
    2. Prepare to administer narcotic medication IV.
    3. Administer oxygen via nasal cannula.
    4. Assess the client every 15–30 minutes.

45. The client diagnosed with chronic obstructive pulmonary disease is being discharged and is prescribed the steroid prednisone. Which scientific rationale supports why the nurse instructs the client to taper off the medication?
    1. The pituitary gland must adjust to the decreasing dose.
    2. The beta cells of the pancreas have to start secreting insulin.
    3. This will allow the adrenal gland time to start to function.
    4. The thyroid gland will have to start producing cortisol.

46. The client is diagnosed with tuberculosis and prescribed rifampin and isoniazid (INH), both anti-tuberculosis medications. Which instruction is most important for the public health nurse to discuss with the client?
    1. The client will have to take the medications for 9–12 months.
    2. The client will have to stay in isolation as long as he or she is taking medications.
    3. Explain that the client cannot eat any type of pork products while taking the medication.
    4. The urine may turn turquoise in color, but this is an expected occurrence and harmless.

47. The employee health nurse is observing a student nurse administer a PPD tuberculin test to a new employee. Which behavior would warrant immediate intervention by the employee health nurse?
    1. The student nurse inserts the needle at a 45-degree angle.
    2. The student nurse cleansed the forearm with alcohol.
    3. The student nurse circles the injection site with ink.
    4. The student nurse instructs the employee to return in three (3) days.

48. The female diagnosed with herpes simplex 2 is prescribed valacyclovir (Valtrex), an antiviral. Which information should the nurse discuss with the client?
    1. Do not get pregnant while on this medication; it will harm the fetus.
    2. The medication does not prevent the transmission of the disease.
    3. There are no side effects when taking this medication by mouth.
    4. Get monthly liver function study tests.

49. The client diagnosed with coronary artery disease is prescribed an HMG-CoA reductase inhibitor to help reduce the cholesterol level. Which assessment data should be reported to the health-care provider?
    1. Complaints of flatulence.
    2. Weight loss of two (2) pounds.
    3. Complaints of muscle pain.
    4. No bowel movement for two (2) days.

50. The client with coronary artery disease is prescribed one baby aspirin a day. Which instructions should the nurse provide the client concerning this medication?
    1. Take medication on an empty stomach.
    2. Do not take Tylenol while taking this drug.
    3. If experiencing joint pain, notify the HCP.
    4. Notify the HCP if stools become dark and tarry.

51. The nurse is preparing to administer phenytoin (Dilantin), 100 mg intravenous push, to the client with a head injury who has an IV of D5W at 50 mL/hr. Which intervention should the nurse implement?
    1. Flush the IV tubing before and after with normal saline.
    2. Administer the medication if the Dilantin level is 22 mcg/mL.
    3. Push the Dilantin intravenous slowly over five (5) minutes.
    4. Expect the intravenous tubing to turn cloudy when infusing medication.

52. The client diagnosed with epilepsy is being discharged from the hospital with a prescription for phenytoin (Dilantin) by mouth. Which discharge instructions should the nurse discuss with the client?
    1. The client should purchase a self-monitoring Dilantin machine.
    2. The client should see the dentist at least every six (6) months.
    3. The client should never drive when taking this medication.
    4. The client should drink no more than one (1) glass of wine a day.

53. The female client with *Trichomonas vaginalis* is prescribed metronidazole (Flagyl), an anti-bacterial medication. Which statement indicates the client does not understand the discharge teaching?
    1. "I will not be able to drink any alcohol while taking this drug."
    2. "My boyfriend will need to take this same medication."
    3. "I cannot transmit the disease through oral sex."
    4. "I must make sure I take all the pills no matter how I feel."

54. The client diagnosed with angina must receive a two (2)-inch nitropaste application. Which interventions should the nurse implement? Select all that apply.
    1. Wear gloves when administering.
    2. Remove the old nitropaste paper.
    3. Apply the paper on a hairy spot.
    4. Put medication only on the legs.
    5. Report any headache to the HCP.

55. The nurse is hanging 1000 mL of IV fluids to run for eight (8) hours. The intravenous tubing is a microdrip. How many gtt/min should the IV rate be set? _____

56. The client with osteoarthritis is prescribed a nonsteroidal anti-inflammatory drug (NSAID). Which intervention should the nurse implement?
    1. Time the medication to be given with meals.
    2. Notify the HCP if abdominal striae develops.
    3. Do not administer if oral temperature is greater than 102°F.
    4. Monitor the liver function tests and renal studies.

57. The client in the intensive care department has a nasogastric tube for continuous feedings. The nurse is preparing to administer nifedipine (Procardia) XL via the N/G tube. Which procedure should the nurse follow?
    1. Crush the medication and dissolve it in water.
    2. Administer and flush the N/G tube with cranberry juice.
    3. Give the medication orally with pudding.
    4. Do not administer medication and notify the HCP.

58. The employee health nurse is discussing hepatitis B vaccines with new employees. Which statement best describes the proper administration of the hepatitis B vaccine?
    1. The vaccine must be administered once a year.
    2. Two (2) mL of vaccine should be given in each hip.
    3. The vaccine is given in three (3) doses over a six (6)-month time period.
    4. The vaccine is administered intradermally into the deltoid muscle.

Pharmacology

59. The nursing assistant reported an intake of 1000 mL and a urinary output of 1500 mL for a client who received a thiazide diuretic this morning. Which nursing task could the nurse delegate to the nursing assistant?
    1. Instruct the assistant to restrict the client's fluid intake.
    2. Request the assistant to insert a Foley catheter with an urimeter.
    3. Tell the assistant that urinary outputs are no longer needed.
    4. Ask the assistant to document fluids on the bedside I & O record.

60. The charge nurse is observing the new graduate administering a fentanyl (Duragesic) patch to a client diagnosed with cancer. Which action by the new graduate requires intervention by the charge nurse?
    1. The new graduate documents the date and time on the patch.
    2. The new graduate removes the patch 24 hours after it is placed on the client.
    3. The new graduate rotates the application site on the client's body.
    4. The new graduate checks the client's name band and date of birth.

61. The 68-year-old client is admitted to the emergency department with complaints of slurred speech, right-sided weakness, and ataxia. The emergency room physician ordered thrombolytic therapy for the client. Which action should the nurse implement first?
    1. Administer thrombolytic therapy via protocol.
    2. Send the client for a STAT CT of the head.
    3. Arrange for admission to the intensive care department.
    4. Check to determine if the client is cross-sensitive to the thrombolytic.

62. The client is admitted to the burn unit and prescribed pantoprazole (Protonix), a proton pump inhibitor (PPI). Which statement best supports the scientific rationale for administering this medication to a client with a severe burn?
    1. This medication will help prevent a stress ulcer.
    2. This medication will help prevent systemic infections.
    3. This medication will provide continuous vasoconstriction.
    4. This medication will stimulate new skin growth.

63. The nurse administered an IV broad-spectrum antibiotic scheduled every six (6) hours to the client with a systemic infection at 0800. At 1000 the culture and sensitivity prompted the HCP to change the IV antibiotic. When transcribing the new antibiotic order, when would the initial dose be administered?
    1. Schedule the dose for 1400.
    2. Schedule the dose for the next day.
    3. Check with the HCP to determine when to start.
    4. Administer the dose within one (1) hour of the order.

64. The client is receiving a continuous heparin drip, 20,000 units/500 mL D5W, at 23 gtt/min. How many units of heparin is the client receiving an hour?_____

65. The client with epilepsy is prescribed carbamazepine (Tegretol), an anticonvulsant. Which discharge instruction should the nurse include in the teaching?
    1. Wear SPF 15 sunscreen when outside.
    2. Obtain regular serum drug levels.
    3. Be sure to floss teeth daily.
    4. Instruct the client to take tub baths only.

66. The client diagnosed with bipolar disorder has been taking valproic acid (Depakote), an anticonvulsant, for four (4) months. Which assessment data would warrant the medication being discontinued?
    1. The client's eyes are yellow.
    2. The client has mood swings.
    3. The client's BP is 164/94.
    4. The client's serum level is 75 mcg/mL.

67. The client is complaining of nausea, and the nurse administers the antiemetic promethazine (Phenergan), IVP. Which intervention has priority for this client after administering this medication?
   1. Instruct the client to call the nurse before getting out of bed.
   2. Evaluate the effectiveness of the medication.
   3. Assess the client's abdomen and bowel sounds.
   4. Tell the client not to eat or drink for at least one (1) hour.

68. The client on bed rest is receiving enoxaparin (Lovenox), a low molecular weight heparin. Which anatomical site is recommended for administering this medication?
   1. The abdominal wall one (1) inch away from the umbilicus.
   2. The vastus lateralis with a 23-gauge needle.
   3. In the deltoid area subcutaneously.
   4. In the anterolateral abdomen.

69. The male client comes to the emergency department and reports he stepped on a rusty nail at home about two (2) hours ago. Which question would be most important for the nurse to ask during the admission assessment?
   1. "What have you used to clean the puncture site?"
   2. "Did you bring the nail with you so we can culture it?"
   3. "Do you remember when you had your last tetanus shot?"
   4. "Are you able to put any weight on your foot?"

70. The nurse is administering carbidopa/levodopa (Sinemet) to the client. Which assessment should the nurse perform to determine if the medication is effective?
   1. Assess the client's muscle strength.
   2. Assess for cogwheel movements.
   3. Assess the carbidopa serum level.
   4. Assess the client's blood pressure.

71. The client with coronary artery disease is prescribed atorvastatin (Lipitor) to help decrease the client's cholesterol level. Which intervention should the nurse discuss with the client concerning this medication?
   1. The client should eat a low-cholesterol, low-fat diet.
   2. The client should take this medication with each meal.
   3. The client should take this medication in the evening.
   4. The client should monitor daily cholesterol levels.

72. The client is in end-stage renal disease and is receiving sodium polystyrene sulfonate (Kayexalate) via an enema. Which data indicate the medication is effective?
   1. The client has 30 mL/hr urine output.
   2. The serum phosphorus level has decreased.
   3. The client is in normal sinus rhythm.
   4. The client's serum potassium level is 5.0 mEq/L.

73. The client has the following arterial blood gases: pH 7.19, $PaCO_2$ 33, $PaO_2$ 95, and $HCO_3$ 19. Which medication would the nurse prepare to administer based on the results?
   1. Intravenous sodium bicarbonate.
   2. Oxygen via nasal cannula.
   3. Epinephrine intravenous push.
   4. Magnesium hydroxide orally.

74. The client diagnosed with migraine headaches is prescribed propranolol (Inderal), a beta blocker, for prophylaxis. Which information should the nurse teach the client?
   1. Instruct to take medication at the first sign of headache.
   2. Teach the client to take his or her radial pulse for one (1) minute.
   3. Explain that this drug may make them thirsty and have a dry mouth.
   4. Discuss the need to increase artificial light in the home.

75. The client is experiencing supraventricular tachycardia (SVT). Which antidysrhythmic medication should the nurse prepare to administer?
    1. Atropine.
    2. Amiodarone.
    3. Adenosine.
    4. Dobutrex.

76. The client diagnosed with Parkinson's disease is taking levodopa (L-Dopa) and is experiencing an "on/off effect." Which action should the nurse take regarding this medication?
    1. Document the occurrence and take no action.
    2. Request that the HCP increase the dose of medication.
    3. Discuss the client's imminent death as a result of this complication.
    4. Explain that this is a desired effect of the medication.

77. The client in the emergency department is requiring sutures for a laceration on the left leg. Which information is most pertinent prior to suturing the wound?
    1. The client tells the nurse she has never had sutures.
    2. The spouse refuses to leave the room during suturing.
    3. The client shares that she is scared of needles.
    4. The client reports hives after having dental surgery.

78. The client diagnosed with diabetes insipidus is receiving vasopressin intranasally. Which assessment data indicate the medication is effective?
    1. The client reports being able to breathe through the nose.
    2. The client complains of being thirsty all the time.
    3. The client has a blood glucose of 99 mg/dL.
    4. The client is urinating every three (3) to four (4) hours.

79. The nurse is administering an otic drop to the 45-year-old client. Which procedure should the nurse implement when administering the drops?
    1. Place the drops when pulling the ear down and back.
    2. Place the drops when pulling the ear up and back.
    3. Place the drops in the lower conjunctival sac.
    4. Place the drops in the inner canthus and apply pressure.

80. The male client with a chronic urinary tract infection is prescribed trimethoprim sulfa (Bactrim). Which statement indicates the client needs more teaching?
    1. "I will drink six to eight glasses of water a day."
    2. "I am going to have to take this medication forever."
    3. "I can stop taking this medication if there is no more burning."
    4. "I may get diarrhea with this medication, but I can take Imodium."

81. The 54-year-old female client with severe menopausal symptoms is prescribed hormone replacement therapy (HRT). Which secondary health screening activity should the nurse recommend for HRT?
    1. A Pap smear every six (6) months.
    2. A yearly mammogram.
    3. A bone density test every three (3) months.
    4. A serum calcium level monthly.

82. The LPN is administering 0800 medications to clients on a medical floor. Which action by the LPN would warrant immediate intervention by the nurse?
    1. The LPN scores the medication to give the correct dose.
    2. The LPN checks the client's armband and birth date.
    3. The LPN administers sliding-scale insulin intramuscularly.
    4. The LPN is 30 minutes late hanging the IV antibiotic.

83. The client in end-stage renal disease is receiving aluminum hydroxide (Amphogel). Which assessment data indicate the medication is effective?
    1. The client denies complaints of indigestion.
    2. The client is not experiencing burning on urination.
    3. The client has had a normal, soft bowel movement.
    4. The client's phosphorus level has decreased.

84. The client diagnosed with diabetes mellitus Type 2 is scheduled for bowel resection in the morning. Which medication should the nurse question administering to the client?
    1. Ticlopidine (Ticlid), a platelet aggregate inhibitor.
    2. Ticarcillin (Timentin), an extended-spectrum antibiotic.
    3. Pioglitazone (Actos), a thiazolidinedione.
    4. Bisacodyl (Dulcolax), a cathartic laxative.

85. The client with Type 2 diabetes is diagnosed with gout and prescribed allopurinol (Zyloprim). Which instruction should the nurse discuss when teaching about this medication?
    1. The client will probably develop a red rash on the body.
    2. The client should drink two (2) to three (3) liters of water a day.
    3. The client should take this medication on an empty stomach.
    4. The client will need to increase oral diabetic medications.

86. The client is receiving atropine, an anticholinergic, to minimize the side effects of routine medications. Which intervention will help the client tolerate this medication?
    1. Teach the client about orthostatic hypotension.
    2. Instruct the client to eat a low-residue diet.
    3. Encourage the client to chew sugarless gum.
    4. Discuss the importance of daily isometric exercises.

87. The client is showing ventricular ectopy, and the HCP orders amiodarone (Cordarone) intravenously. Which interventions should the nurse implement? Select all that apply.
    1. Monitor telemetry continuously.
    2. Assess the client's respiratory status.
    3. Evaluate the client's liver function studies.
    4. Confirm the original order with another nurse.
    5. Prepare to defibrillate the client at 200 joules.

88. The HCP has ordered an intramuscular antibiotic. After reconstituting the medication the clinic nurse must administer 4.8 mL of the medication. Which action should the nurse implement first when administering this medication?
    1. Inform the HCP that this is too much medication.
    2. Administer the medication in the gluteal muscle.
    3. Discard the medication in the sharps container.
    4. Divide the medication and give 2.4 mL in each hip.

89. The client diagnosed with status asthmaticus is prescribed intravenous aminophylline, a bronchodilator. Which assessment data would warrant immediate intervention?
    1. The theophylline level is 12 mcg/mL.
    2. The client has expiratory wheezing.
    3. The client complains of muscle twitching.
    4. The client is refusing to eat the meal.

90. Which client would the nurse question when administering the osmotic diuretic mannitol (Osmotrol)?
    1. The client with 4+ pitting pedal edema.
    2. The client with decorticate posturing.
    3. The client with widening pulse pressure.
    4. The client with a positive doll's eye test.

Pharmacology

91. The male client is self-medicating with the H-2 antagonist cimetidine (Tagamet). Which complication can occur while taking this medication?
    1. Melena.
    2. Gynecomastia.
    3. Pyrosis.
    4. Eructation.

92. The client is complaining of low-back pain and is prescribed the muscle relaxant carisoprodol (Soma). Which teaching intervention has priority?
    1. Explain that this medication causes GI distress.
    2. Discuss the need to taper off this medication.
    3. Warn that this medication will cause drowsiness.
    4. Instruct the client to limit alcohol intake.

93. The client diagnosed with adult-onset asthma is being discharged. Which medication would the nurse expect the health-care provider to prescribe?
    1. A nonsteroidal anti-inflammatory medication.
    2. An antihistamine medication.
    3. An angiotensin-converting enzyme inhibitor.
    4. A proton pump inhibitor.

94. The client is complaining of incisional pain. Which intervention should the nurse implement first?
    1. Administer the pain medication STAT.
    2. Determine when the last pain medication was given.
    3. Assess the client's pulse and blood pressure.
    4. Teach the client distraction techniques to address pain.

95. The nurse is evaluating the client's home medications and notes the client with angina is taking an antidepressant. Which intervention should the nurse implement since the client is taking this medication?
    1. Ask the client if there is a plan for suicide.
    2. Assess the client's depression on a 1–10 scale.
    3. Explain that this medication cannot be taken because of the angina.
    4. Request a referral to the hospital psychologist.

96. The nurse is assessing the elderly client first thing in the morning. The client is confused and sleepy. Which intervention should the nurse implement first?
    1. Determine if the client received a sedative last night.
    2. Allow the client to continue to sleep and do not disturb.
    3. Encourage the client to ambulate in the room with assistance.
    4. Notify the health-care provider about the client's status.

97. The nurse is preparing to administer 37.5 mg of meperidine (Demerol) IM to a client who is having pain. The medication comes in a 50 mg/mL vial. Which action should the nurse implement?
    1. Notify the pharmacist to bring the correct vial.
    2. Have another nurse verify wastage of medication.
    3. Administer one (1) mL medication to the client.
    4. Request the HCP to increase the client's dose.

98. The client is to receive 3000 mg of medication daily in a divided dose every eight (8) hours. The medication comes 500 mg per tablet. How many tablets will the nurse administer at each dose?_____

99. The 38-year-old client with chronic asthma is prescribed a leukotriene receptor antagonist. Which is the scientific rationale for administering this medication?
    1. This medication is used prophylactically to control asthma.
    2. This medication will cure the client's chronic asthma.
    3. It will stabilize mast cell activities and reduce asthma attacks.
    4. It will cause the bronchioles to dilate and increase the airway.

100. The female nurse realizes that she did not administer a medication on time to the client diagnosed with a myocardial infarction. Which action should the nurse implement?
    1. Administer the medication and take no further action.
    2. Notify the director of nurses of the medication error.
    3. Complete a medication error report form.
    4. Report the error to the Peer Review Committee.

101. The nurse has received the morning report and has the following medications due or being requested. In which order should the nurse administer the medications? List in order of priority.
    1. Administer furosemide (Lasix), a loop diuretic, IVP daily to a client diagnosed with heart failure who is dyspneic on exertion.
    2. Administer morphine, a narcotic analgesic, IVP PRN to a client diagnosed with lower back pain who is complaining of pain at a "10" on an 1–10 scale.
    3. Administer neostigmine (Prostigmin), a cholinesterase inhibitor, po to a client diagnosed with myasthenia gravis.
    4. Administer lidocaine, an antidysrhythmic, IVP PRN to a client in normal sinus rhythm with multifocal premature ventricular contractions.
    5. Administer vancomycin, an aminoglycoside antibiotic, to a client diagnosed with a *Staphylococcus* infection who has a trough level of 14 mg/dL.

Pharmacology

1. 1. The normal recommended daily dose of vitamin C is 60–100 mg a day for healthy adults, but nothing cures the virus that causes the common cold.
   2. Echinacea is an herbal preparation thought to limit the severity of a cold and is sold in OTC preparations, but it does not have to be taken with vitamin C.
   3. This dose is already too high, and water-soluble vitamins in excess of the body's needs are excreted in the urine.
   4. **Mega doses can lead to crystals in the urine, and crystals can lead to the formation of renal calculi (stones) in the kidneys. Therefore, mega doses should not be taken because there is no therapeutic value.**

2. 1. Vitamin K helps prevent clotting, and NSAIDs are recommended for inflammatory disorders and to relieve mild to moderate pain.
   2. **Vitamin E is an antioxidant and is useful in the treatment and prevention of coronary artery disease, and aspirin is an antiplatelet that prevents platelet aggregation.**
   3. Vitamin A is required for healthy eyes, gums, and teeth and for fat metabolism. Anticoagulants are prescribed for clients with a high risk for clot formation.
   4. Vitamin B complex is used for healthy function of the nervous system, cell repair, and formation of red blood cells; iron supplements are recommended for clients with iron-deficiency anemia.

3. 1. **OTC decongestant medications used for the flu cause vasoconstriction of the blood vessels, which would increase the client's hypertension and therefore should be avoided. The client should let the flu run its course.**
   2. OTC medications should not be taken by the client with essential hypertension.
   3. The nurse should provide the information to the client about what medications to take and should not refer to the pharmacist.
   4. It is too late for the flu vaccine because the client is already ill with the flu.

4. 1. The potassium level is not affected by the administration of steroids.
   2. Culture and sensitivity reports should be monitored to determine if the proper antibiotic is being administered.
   3. **Steroids are excreted as glucocorticoids from the adrenal gland and are responsible** for insulin resistance by the cells, which may cause hyperglycemia.
   4. There is no reason why the nurse would question administering a steroid based on an ABG result.

5. 1. Cromolyn is used prophylactically to prevent exercise-induced asthma attacks. It is administered in routine daily doses to prevent asthma attacks.
   2. Rinsing the mouth will help prevent the growth of bacteria secondary to medication left in the mouth.
   3. Holding the breath for ten (10) seconds keeps the medication in the lungs.
   4. **This medication is used to stabilize the mast cells in the lung. During an asthma attack, the mast cells are already unstable; therefore this medication will not be effective in treating the acute asthma attack. This statement would require the nurse to reteach about the medication.**

6. 1. Diarrhea may indicate the client may have a superinfection, but it is not the priority intervention at this time because the antibiotic would still be administered.
   2. The peak level is not drawn until one (1) hour after the medication has been infused.
   3. **The trough level must be drawn prior to administering this dose; therefore, it is the priority intervention.**
   4. The culture and sensitivity (C&S) has already been done because it is known that the client has MRSA.

7. 1. At eight (8) hours postop the client should be on bed rest, and moving the client to a chair will not help the incisional pain and could cause hip dislocation.
   2. **Normal developmental changes in the organs of the elderly, especially the kidneys and liver, result in lower doses of pain medication needed to achieve therapeutic levels.**
   3. This is a neurological assessment, which is not pertinent to the extremity assessment.
   4. The urinary output would not affect the administration of pain medication.

8. 1. Iron dextran is administered for iron-deficiency anemia intravenously or intramuscularly, not subcutaneously.
   2. Vitamin $B_{12}$ is administered for pernicious anemia because there is insufficient intrin-

sic factor produced by the rugae in the stomach to be able to absorb and use vitamin $B_{12}$ from food sources.

3. Folic acid is administered orally or intravenously for folic acid deficiency, which is usually associated with chronic alcoholism.

4. Thiamine is administered intravenously in high doses to clients detoxifying from chronic alcoholism to prevent rebound nervous system dysfunction.

9. 1. **This medication stimulates the pancreas to secrete insulin. Therefore the client is at risk for developing hypoglycemic reactions, especially during exercise.**

2. The is an oral hypoglycemic medication.

3. There are side effects to every medication; this medication can cause hypoglycemia.

4. The medication stimulates the pancreas to produce more insulin, but it does not affect the muscles' absorption of glucose.

10. **10 units.** The nurse should administer the dosage for the appropriate parameters.

11. 1. This test monitors the client's average blood glucose level over the previous three (3) months.

2. The evening meal would prevent hypoglycemia for regular insulin administered at 1630.

3. The before-meal blood glucose level done at 1630 would not be affected by the insulin administered after that time.

4. **The intermediate-acting insulin peaks 6–8 hours after being administered; therefore, the nighttime snack (hs) will prevent late-night hypoglycemia.**

12. 1. The nurse would not question administering insulin to a client about to eat.

2. The client who is one (1) day postop would be receiving a prophylactic antibiotic.

3. **Glucophage must be held 24–48 hours prior to receiving contrast media (dye) because Glucophage, along with the contrast dye, can damage kidney function.**

4. The client with peptic ulcer disease would be ordered a proton pump inhibitor to help decrease gastric-acid production.

13. 1. This insulin is scheduled for bedtime.

2. **The charge nurse should double-check the dosage against the MAR to make sure the client is receiving the correct dose; this insulin does not peak and works for 24 hours.**

3. There is not a medication error at this time.

4. The HCP would only need to be notified if a serious medication error has occurred.

14. 1. These are sign/symptoms of hypothyroidism, which indicates not enough medication.

2. These indicate not enough medication is being administered.

3. **Irritability and tachycardia are signs/symptoms of hyperthyroidism, which indicates the client is receiving too much medication.**

4. Normothermia indicates a normal temperature, which does not indicate hypothyroidism or hyperthyroidism, and constipation is a sign of hypothyroidism.

15. 1. **The therapeutic heparin level is 1.5 to 2 times the control, which is 58–78; therefore, a PTT of 72 is within therapeutic range so the nurse should continue to monitor the infusion. PT/INR are used to monitor the oral anticoagulant warfarin (Coumadin).**

2. Protamine sulfate is the antidote for heparin toxicity, but the client is in therapeutic range.

3. There is no need for the laboratory to reconfirm the results.

4. The nurse would not need to assess for bleeding because the results are within the therapeutic range.

16. 1. A STAT potassium level would be needed for problems with digoxin or a diuretic, not for bleeding.

2. The nurse needs more information before requesting an admission into the hospital.

3. Valium IVP does not help bleeding.

4. **Ecchymotic areas are secondary to bleeding. The nurse should order an INR to rule out Coumadin toxicity.**

17. 1. The medication must be taken first thing in the morning before breakfast on an empty stomach; no food, juice, or coffee should be consumed for at least 30 minutes.

2. **Remaining in the upright position minimizes the risk of esophagitis; the drug should be taken with eight (8) ounces of water.**

3. The tablet should be swallowed, not chewed, and should not be allowed to dissolve until it is the stomach.

4. There is no monthly hormone level to determine the effectiveness of this medication; it is determined by a bone density test.

18. 1. A daily digoxin dose is not priority medication.

2. This potassium level is very low and the nurse should not administer the loop diuretic.

3. **The mucosal barrier must be administered on an empty stomach; therefore, it should be administered first.**

4. An IVP medication is not priority when administering a medication that must be given on an empty stomach.

19. 1. Attempting to prevent CHF is the rationale for administering ACE inhibitors to clients diagnosed with MIs. This medication is administered for a variety of medical diagnoses, such as heart failure and stroke, and to help prevent diabetic nephropathy.
    2. ACE inhibitors are prescribed to help decrease blood pressure, but the stem states the client has had an MI, not essential hypertension.
    3. Cardiac glycosides like digoxin, not ACE inhibitors, increase the contractility of the heart.
    4. Antilipidemics, not ACE inhibitors, help decrease the development of atherosclerosis.

20. 1. ACE inhibitors may increase potassium levels. The client should avoid potassium salt substitutes and supplements; therefore the nurse would not question the fact that the client is not receiving potassium supplements.
    2. An adverse effect of ACE inhibitors is the possibility of a persistent irritating cough, which might precipitate the HCP's changing the client's medication.
    3. This blood pressure indicates the medication is effective.
    4. A urinary output of 30 mL/hr indicates the kidneys are functioning properly.

21. 1. The apical heart rate is assessed prior to administering the dose, but it does not indicate that the medication is effective.
    2. Anorexia and nausea are signs of digoxin toxicity and do not indicate if the medication is effective.
    3. Digoxin has no effect on the client's blood pressure.
    4. Digoxin is administered for heart failure and dysrhythmias. Clear lung sounds indicate that the heart failure is being controlled by the medication.

22. 1. Abrupt discontinuation of baclofen is associated with hallucinations, paranoia, and seizures.
    2. This medication causes constipation and urinary retention.
    3. The client should not be allowed to drive at all when taking this medication because it causes drowsiness and the spasticity of MS makes driving dangerous for the client.
    4. WBC levels do not need to be monitored because the drug does not cause bone marrow suppression.

23. 1. If the apical heart rate is less than 60, the nurse should question administering this medication.
    2. The client's potassium level, not the sodium level, should be monitored.
    3. The client should be taught to monitor the radial pulse at home and not to take the medication if the pulse is less than 60 because this medication will further decrease the heart rate.
    4. The digoxin level should be between 0.8 and 2 ng/mL to be therapeutic.
    5. The client with digoxin toxicity would complain of anorexia, nausea, and yellow haze; buffalo hump and moon face would be assessed for the client taking prednisone, a glucocorticoid.

24. 1. The respiratory rate and pulse rate would not affect the administration of this medication.
    2. The apical heart rate (AP) of 59 would cause the nurse to question administering this medication because beta blockers decrease the sympathetic stimulation to the heart, thereby deceasing the heart rate.
    3. These vital signs would not warrant the nurse questioning administering an antibiotic.
    4. The blood pressure is higher than 90/60; therefore, the nurse would not question administering the calcium channel blocker.

25. 1. Epogen stimulates the client's own bone marrow to produce red blood cells; therefore this is not a violation of the client's religious beliefs about blood products.
    2. There is no reason for the client to have problems receiving this medication because of religious beliefs, so the client does not need to talk to the minister.
    3. This medication does not violate the Jehovah Witnesses' beliefs concerning receiving blood products; therefore the nurse should administer the medication via the correct route.
    4. This is not an invasive procedure or investigational medication and thus informed consent is not needed.

26. 1. Because the client is NPO as a result of the admitting diagnosis the client needs alternative anti-anxiety medication to prevent withdrawal symptoms, but this is not the first intervention.
    2. The client will be NPO as a result of the diverticulitis, and Xanax is administered orally; therefore another route of medication administration is needed, but this is not the first intervention.

3. This is correct information, but it is not the priority intervention.
4. **Xanax has a greater dependence problem than all the other benzodiazepines; therefore the nurse must assess for withdrawal symptoms first. Then the nurse can implement the other interventions. The client needs to be withdrawn slowly from the benzodiazepines, but assessment is priority.**

27. 1. This is the outer canthus and medications are not administered to this area.
2. **The correct placement of ophthalmic drops is to administer the medication in the lower conjunctival sac.**
3. This is the sclera and the correct placement of eye drops is in the lower conjunctival sac.
4. This is the inner canthus where pressure can be applied gently after instilling eye drops to help prevent the systemic absorption of ophthalmic medications.

28. 1. This potassium level is within normal limits; therefore the nurse would administer the medication.
2. This indicates that the medication is effective and the nurse should not question administering the medication.
3. **This indicates that the client is dehydrated and the nurse should discuss this with the HCP prior to administering another dose, which could increase the dehydration and could cause renal failure.**
4. This indicates the medication is effective. Daily weight changes reflect fluid gain and loss.

29. 1. The nurse should investigate any herbs a client is taking, especially if the client has a condition that requires long-term medication, such as anti-rejection medication.
2. The nurse should remain nonjudgmental but must intervene if the alternative treatment poses a risk to the client.
3. The client may need to be referred for psychological counseling, but it is not the first action the nurse should take.
4. **St. John's wort decreases the effects of many medications, including oral contraceptives, antiretrovirals, and transplant immunosuppressant drugs. Rejection of the client's kidney could occur if the client continues to use St. John's wort.**

30. 1. This is the rationale for H-2 antagonist and proton pump inhibitors.
2. **Antacids neutralize gastric acidity.**
3. This is the rationale for mucosal barrier agents.

4. Prostaglandin is responsible for production of gastric acid. Antacids do not interfere with prostaglandin production.

31. 1. The client's temperature would not affect the administration of this medication.
2. ACE inhibitors sometimes cause the client to develop a cough that requires discontinuing the medication, but this is a calcium channel blocker.
3. This blood pressure reading indicates the client's medication is effective.
4. **This indicates orthostatic hypotension, and the nurse should assess the client's BP before administering the medication.**

32. 1. **An unlabeled use for quinine is the prophylaxis and treatment of nocturnal leg cramps that are associated with arthritis, diabetes, varicose veins, and arteriosclerosis.**
2. A muscle relaxant is prescribed for muscle spasms, and leg cramps are not always the result of muscle spasms.
3. The question is addressing the relief of leg cramps, and sleeping pills will not help leg cramps.
4. The client does not need an opioid analgesic because it may cause addiction; this type of medication is given for acute pain for a short period. Prolonged use of Darvon compounds also predisposes the client to renal cell carcinoma.

33. 1. **The nurse should always assess for allergies, but especially when administering antibiotics, which are notorious for allergic reactions.**
2. **If specimens are not obtained for C&S prior to administering the first dose of antibiotic, the results will be skewed.**
3. **One (1) of the five (5) rights is to administer the medication to the "right client." Checking the armband on the client with the MAR and medication is a way to ensure this.**
4. **The 2005 JCAHO standards require two forms of identification prior to administering medications. The client's armband and medical record number provide one form of identifying information, and the client's birthday is the second form of identification in most health-care facilities. This is a nationwide emphasis to help prevent medication errors.**
5. The stem does not state it is an aminoglycoside antibiotic, and it is the initial dose, which

means there is no medication in the system even if it were an aminoglycoside antibiotic.

34. 1. This medication is prescribed for clients with an overactive bladder.
    2. There is no contraindication for a client with Type 2 diabetes receiving this medication.
    3. **These drugs cause mydriasis, which increases the intraocular pressure, which could lead to blindness. Glaucoma is caused by increased intraocular pressure.**
    4. There is no contraindication for a client with PVD receiving this medication.

35. 1. The nurse should use nonsterile gloves to apply ointment but should first wash his or her hands.
    2. The client's leg should be cleansed prior to administering a new application of ointment, but it is not the first intervention.
    3. The nurse should always check the client's armband, but it is not the first intervention when the nurse enters the room.
    4. **Hand washing is the first intervention that must be done when the nurse enters the client's room before any contact with the client; it is also the last intervention the nurse does after caring for the client and leaving the room.**

36. 1. Adenosine is ordered for supraventricular tachycardia.
    2. Epinephrine is administered during a code to vasoconstrict the periphery and shunt the blood to the central circulating system.
    3. Atropine is used for asystole or symptomatic sinus bradycardia.
    4. **Lidocaine is the drug of choice for ventricular irritability. It suppresses ventricular ectopy.**

37. 1. The blood pressure must be continuously monitored more often, at least every 10–15 minutes.
    2. The peripheral pulses should be monitored more frequently than every shift, but dopamine has no direct effect on the peripheral pulses.
    3. **The client's urine output should be monitored because low-dose dopamine is administered to maintain renal perfusion; higher doses can cause vasoconstriction of the renal arteries.**
    4. Dopamine is not inactivated when exposed to light.

38. 1. The ST segment that is becoming more depressed indicates a worsening of the oxygenation of the myocardial tissue.
    2. **Reperfusion dysrhythmias indicate that the ischemic heart tissue is receiving oxygen and is viable heart tissue.**

3. The CPK-MB elevates when there is necrotic heart tissue and does not indicate if thrombolytic therapy is successful.
    4. D-dimer is used to diagnose pulmonary embolus.

39. 1. **Tinnitus, ringing in the ears, is a sign of aspirin toxicity and needs to be reported to the HCP; the aspirin should be stopped immediately.**
    2. Diarrhea is a complication of many medications but not with aspirin.
    3. Tetany is muscle twitching secondary to hypocalcemia.
    4. Aspirin does not cause paresthesia, which is numbness or tingling.

40. 1. **Loop diuretics cause loss of potassium in the urine output; therefore the client should be receiving potassium supplements. Hypokalemia can lead to life-threatening cardiac dysrhythmias.**
    2. A cardiac glycoside, digoxin, is administered for congestive heart failure, but it is not necessary when administering a loop diuretic.
    3. An ACE inhibitor is not prescribed along with a loop diuretic. It t may be ordered for congestive heart failure.
    4. A potassium cation, Kayexalate, is ordered to remove potassium through the bowel for clients with hyperkalemia.

41. 1. Interferon is administered to treat hepatitis and some cancers, but it does not stimulate the bone marrow.
    2. **Neupogen is a granulocyte-stimulating factor that stimulates the bone marrow to produce white blood cells, which this client needs because the normal WBC is 4.-- 11.0($10^3$).**
    3. Neumega stimulates the production of platelets, but the client's platelet count of 160 is normal [100–400 mm ($10^3$)].
    4. Procrit stimulates the production of red blood cells and hemoglobin, but a hemoglobin of 12.2 is normal for a woman (11.5–15.5 g/dL).

42. 1. This medication must be taken for life because the client has to have had some type of transplant or severe rheumatoid arthritis for it to be prescribed.
    2. Exposure to hepatitis does not have anything to do with receiving this medication.
    3. **Imuran is not a drug of choice for treating pneumonia; therefore the nurse must find out why the client is taking it, either for a renal transplant or for severe rheumatoid arthritis.**
    4. Imuran does not affect the antigen–antibody reaction.

43. 1. A daily cathartic is a colonic stimulant, which results in dependency and a narrowing of the lumen of the colon, which increases constipation.
    2. **Although the client may think that a medication for bowel movements is necessary, the nurse should teach the client that this medication can cause serious complications, such as dependency and narrowing of the colon.**
    3. Fiber will help increase the roughage, which may help prevent constipation, but the most important action is to empower the client to make informed decisions about medications.
    4. The nurse should not refuse to administer the medication; the nurse should talk to the client and if needed the HCP before administering the medication.

44. 1. This should be documented in the client's nurse's notes because this is a PRN medication, but it is not the priority medication.
    2. The nurse would not administer another narcotic, which is what caused the need for Narcan in the first place.
    3. Oxygen will not help reverse respiratory depression secondary to a narcotic overdose.
    4. **Narcan is administered when the client has received too much of a narcotic. Narcan has a short half-life of about 30 minutes and the client will be at risk for respiratory depression for several hours; therefore the nurse should assess the client frequently.**

45. 1. The pituitary gland is not directly affected by the steroid and is not why the medication must be gradually tapered.
    2. Steroids do not affect the pancreas's production of insulin.
    3. **When the client is receiving exogenous steroids, the adrenal glands stop producing cortisol, and if the medication is not tapered, the client can have a severe hypotensive crisis, known as adrenal gland insufficiency or Addisonian crisis.**
    4. The adrenal gland, not the thyroid gland, produces cortisol.

46. 1. **This medication is taken up to one (1) year, and the public health department will pay for the medications and make sure the client complies because it is a public health risk.**
    2. The client is in isolation until three (3) consecutive early-morning sputum cultures are negative, which is usually in about two (2) to four (4) weeks.
    3. Pork products do not interact with these medications.

4. The client's urine and all body fluids may turn orange from the rifampin.

47. 1. **This medication should be administered intradermally with the needle barely inserted under the skin so that a wheal (bubble) forms after the injection.**
    2. Cleansing the forearm with an alcohol swab is standard procedure and would not warrant immediate intervention.
    3. Circling the site is an appropriate intervention so that when the skin test is read and no reaction is occurring, the nurse will be able document a negative skin test reading.
    4. The skin test is read in three (3) days to determine the results.

48. 1. This classification of medication is used to prevent transmission of this virus to the fetus during pregnancy; therefore it does not harm the fetus and the client can be pregnant while taking this medication.
    2. **Only condoms or abstinence will prevent transmission of the herpes virus.**
    3. There are side effects to every drug; this one causes headache, dizziness, nausea, and anorexia.
    4. This medication does not directly affect the liver, and liver function tests (LFTs) are not required monthly.

49. 1. Flatulence, "gas," is an expected side effect that is not life threatening and does not need to be reported to the HCP.
    2. A weight loss of two (2) pounds would not need to be reported to the HCP because this medication does not affect the client's weight.
    3. **Muscle pain may indicate arthralgias, myositis, or rhabdomyolysis, which are complications that would cause the HCP to discontinue the medication because its continued use may lead to liver failure.**
    4. Not having a bowel movement may be important to the client, but clients do not have to have daily bowel movements.

50. 1. Aspirin causes GI distress and should be taken with food.
    2. Tylenol is recommended for pain and can be safely taken with a daily baby aspirin.
    3. Aspirin does not cause joint pain; in fact, it may provide some relief because of its anti-inflammatory action, but when aspirin (ASA) is taken daily, it is an antiplatelet medication.
    4. **ASA is known to cause gastric upset that can lead to gastric bleeding, and dark, tarry stools may indicate upper gastrointestinal bleeding.**

Pharmacology

51. 1. Dilantin will crystallize in the tubing and is not compatible with any IV fluid, except normal saline. The IV tubing must be flushed before the medication is administered.
 2. The therapeutic Dilantin level is 10 to 20 mcg/mL; therefore, this is a toxic level.
 3. The medication is pushed at 50 mg per minute.
 4. If the tubing turns cloudy, it means it is not compatible, and the nurse must stop the IVP immediately and discontinue the IV.

52. 1. There is no machine for home use that monitors Dilantin levels. Levels are usually checked every six (6) months to a year by venipuncture and laboratory tests.
 2. Dilantin causes gingival hyperplasia, and mouth care and dental care are priority to help prevent rotting of the teeth.
 3. Some states allow seizure-free clients with epilepsy to drive, but some states don't. The word "never" in this distracter should eliminate it as a possible correct answer.
 4. Alcohol should be strictly prohibited when taking anticonvulsant medications.

53. 1. Alcohol creates a disulfiram reaction to the medication, which causes severe nausea, vomiting, and extreme hypertension.
 2. *Trichomonas vaginalis* is an asymptomatic sexually transmitted disease in males. If the male partner is not simultaneously treated, then he can reinfect the female.
 3. This sexually transmitted disease can be transmitted via oral routes.
 4. This is a concept that must be taught to all clients taking antibiotics: Take all the medications as prescribed.

54. 1. If the nurse does not wear the gloves, the nurse can absorb the medication and get a headache.
 2. The old nitropaste must be removed because it could cause an overdose of the medication.
 3. The paper should be applied to a clean, dry, hairless area.
 4. The medication can be placed on the chest, arms, back, or legs.
 5. A headache is a common side effect and should not be reported to HCP.

55. 125 gtt/min. A microdrip is 60 gtt/mL. The formula for this dosage problem is as follows:

$$\frac{1000 \text{ mL}}{480 \text{ min}} \times \frac{60}{480} = \frac{60,000}{480} = 125 \text{ gtt/mL}$$

56. 1. This medication is harsh on the lining of the stomach and should be taken with meals.
 2. Abdominal striae occur with steroids, not NSAIDs.
 3. The temperature does not affect the administration of this medication. NSAIDs would be prescribed for fever.
 4. The liver and kidneys are responsible for metabolizing and excreting all medications, but the tests are not routinely monitored for NSAIDs.

57. 1. The XL means the medication is extended release and cannot be crushed.
 2. Whole capsules or tablets cannot be administered through a feeding tube.
 3. The client has a feeding tube and is not able to swallow; therefore, the nurse should not administer the medications orally.
 4. Tablets that are enteric coated or extended release cannot be crushed and administered via the N/G tube. This would allow 24 hours worth of medication into the client's system at one time. The nurse should ask the HCP to change medication to a form that is not enteric coated and not extended release. Then it can be crushed and administered through the feeding tube.

58. 1. The vaccine is administered in a series of three (3) injections and is reported to be effective for life, but boosters may be given every five (5) years.
 2. This is the incorrect administration for hepatitis B vaccine.
 3. Hepatitis B is given in three (3) doses—initially, then at one (1) month, and then again at six (6) months.
 4. Hepatitis B vaccine is given intramuscularly in the deltoid muscle.

59. 1. An output greater than intake indicates the medication is effective, and there is no need to restrict the fluid intake.
 2. There is no reason to insert a Foley catheter in the client who is urinating without difficulties.
 3. As long as the client is receiving diuretics, the client should be on intake and output.
 4. The assistant can document the client's fluid intake and output numbers on the bedside record; this is one of the assistant's duties.

60. 1. This is a correct intervention when applying a patch; therefore the charge nurse would not have to intervene.

2. The fentanyl patch takes about 24 hours to develop full analgesic effect; the patch should be replaced every 72 hours.
3. The sites should be rotated to prevent irritation to the skin.
4. This is the correct way to administer all medications.

61. 1. The nurse should prepare to administer the medication, but it is not the first intervention.
2. **A CT scan must be done to rule out a hemorrhagic CVA because if it is a hemorrhagic stroke, thrombolytic therapy will increase bleeding in the head.**
3. The client receiving thrombolytic therapy will be in the ICU because the client needs constant surveillance during therapy. Heparin will be started, but this is not the first intervention.
4. The nurse should check to determine if the client is allergic to medications, but in this situation the client must have CT before any other action is taken. Cross sensitivity usually occurs with antibiotics, not thrombolytic therapy.

62. 1. **PPIs decrease gastric secretion and are prescribed for clients to prevent Curling's stress ulcer. PPIs are ordered for most clients in the intensive care department, not just clients with burns.**
2. PPIs do not treat infections; antibiotics treat infections.
3. PPIs do not cause continuous constriction. Dopamine might do this.
4. Positive nitrogen balance accomplished through nutritional interventions will help promote tissue regeneration.

63. 1. The new antibiotic must be started as soon as the medication arrives from the pharmacy.
2. Waiting until the next day could cause serious harm, with the client possibly going into septic shock.
3. The HCP does not determine when the medications are administered; this is a nursing intervention.
4. **A new IV antibiotic must be initiated as soon as possible, at least within one (1) hour. A broad-spectrum antibiotic is ordered until C&S results are determined. Then, an antibiotic that will specifically target the infectious organism must be started immediately.**

64. **920 units/hr.**
    20,000 U divided by 500 = 40 units/mL
    40 units/mL × 23 mL/hour = 920 units/hr.

65. 1. Tegretol is photosensitive, but the client must wear SPF of at least 30 to be protected.
2. **This medication has a therapeutic level that must be maintained to help prevent seizures. The therapeutic range is from 6 to 12 mcg/mL.**
3. Dilantin, another anticonvulsant, causes hyperplasia gingivitis, but carbamazepine does not.
4. The client with seizure disorder should only take showers because if a seizure occurs in the bathtub, the client could drown.

66. 1. **Yellow eyes would indicate the client is experiencing some type of hepatic toxicity, which would warrant the medication being discontinued immediately. During the first few months of treatment, the client is closely monitored for hepatic toxicity because deaths have occurred.**
2. The medication dose may be increased, but Depakote is administered to prevent the mood swings.
3. The BP is slightly elevated, but it is not related to the medication.
4. The therapeutic serum Depakote level is 50–100 mcg/mL; therefore the client is within therapeutic range.

67. 1. **Safety is priority when administering a phenothiazine because it causes sedative-like effects.**
2. Evaluation is not priority over safety.
3. The nurse should have assessed the client's GI system prior to administering the antiemetic, not after.
4. Withholding fluids/food is an appropriate intervention to help prevent emesis, but it is not priority over safety after administering this medication.

68. 1. This is the correct area to administer subcutaneous heparin, but not Lovenox.
2. This is in the client's anterior thigh, which may be used for insulin administration but not for Lovenox, and a 25-gauge 1/2-inch needle is used to administer Lovenox.
3. This is the upper arm area, which is used for subcutaneous insulin, but not Lovenox.
4. **Lovenox is administered in the "love handles," which is in the anterolateral abdomen; this helps prevent abdominal wall trauma.**

69. 1. This may be a question that the nurse asks, but it doesn't matter because the nurse will clean the site again.
2. The nail does not matter and it will not be cultured; it is assumed it is contaminated.

Pharmacology

3. The tetanus shot must be received every ten (10) years to prevent tetany, also known as "lock jaw."

4. Being able to walk on the foot is not a priority question. Determining the status of the tetanus shot is priority.

70. 1. Sinemet does not affect the client's muscle strength; it affects the smoothness of muscle movement.

2. Cogwheel motion (jerky, uneven movements) is a symptom of Parkinson's disease, and if the client is not experiencing these types of movements, then the medication is effective.

3. There is no such thing as a carbidopa therapeutic level. The client's signs/symptoms determine the effectiveness of the medication.

4. The client's blood pressure should be assessed to determine if the client is having hypotension, which is a side effect of the medication, but this does not determine the effectiveness of the medication.

71. 1. This diet is recommended for clients with coronary artery disease, but it is not an intervention specific for this medication.

2. This medication is taken once a day in the evening.

3. Atorvastatin (Lipitor) is taken at night to enhance the enzymes that metabolize cholesterol.

4. There is no machine to test daily cholesterol levels. The cholesterol level is checked every three (3) to six (6) months.

72. 1. The client in end-stage renal disease does not normally urinate, and urine output does not determine if this medication is effective.

2. Kayexalate does not affect phosphorus levels.

3. The client being in normal sinus rhythm is good, but it does not determine if the medication is effective.

4. Kayexalate is a cation and exchanges sodium ions for a potassium ions in the intestines, thereby lowering the serum potassium level. Therefore, a serum potassium level within normal limits would indicate the medication is effective. Normal potassium levels are 3.5–5.5 mEq/L.

73. 1. The ABG results indicate metabolic acidosis, and the treatment of choice is sodium bicarbonate.

2. Oxygen is the treatment of choice for respiratory acidosis.

3. Epinephrine is administered in a code situation.

4. This is milk of magnesia, which is an antacid/

laxative, but it is not the treatment for metabolic acidosis.

74. 1. Propranolol is taken prophylactically, which means the client should take the medication routinely whether they have a headache or not.

2. Beta blockers decrease the heart rate. If the radial pulse is less than 60 bpm, the client should hold the medication and notify the health-care provider.

3. This medication will mask tachycardia in clients with diabetes, an early symptom of hypoglycemia. Thirst and dry mouth are signs of hyperglycemia, but this client does not have diabetes.

4. Beta blockers do not affect the client's visual acuity; therefore a change in light is not necessary.

75. 1. Atropine is used in clients with asystole or symptomatic sinus bradycardia.

2. Amiodarone is a Class C medication used for ventricular dysfunction.

3. Adenosine is the drug of choice for clients in SVT.

4. Dobutrex is used for clients in cardiac heart failure.

76. 1. Loss of effect of the medication occurs near the end of a dosing interval and indicates that the plasma drug level has declined to subtherapeutic value. This is an expected occurrence with the medication and the chronic nature of the disease.

2. Increasing the dose increases the peripheral action of the drug on the heart and vessels. Because 75% of the drug never crosses the blood–brain barrier, the dose may not be increased.

3. This effect does not mean the client is dying. It means the medication is wearing off.

4. This is not the desired effect of the medication.

77. 1. This information really doesn't have bearing on the current situation.

2. The spouse can stay in the room if able to stay calm and not upset the client.

3. The nurse should address the client's fear, but it is not the most pertinent information.

4. A local anesthetic will be administered to numb the area prior to suturing. The same classification of drugs is used to numb the mouth before dental procedures, and this client may be allergic to the numbing medication.

78. 1. The medication is administered through the nose, but it has no effect on the client's ability to breathe.

2. Being thirsty all the time would indicate the medication is not effective.

3. Neither the medication nor the disease process has anything to do with the glucose level. A disease that affects glucose level is diabetes mellitus, not diabetes insipidus.

4. **Diabetes insipidus is characterized by the client not being able to concentrate urine and excreting large amounts of dilute urine. If the client is able to delay voiding for three (3) to four (4) hours, it indicates the medication is effective.**

79. 1. This is the correct procedure for instilling eardrops for children.

2. **"Otic" refers to the ear. Instilling eardrops in the adult must be done by pulling the ear up and back to straighten the eustachian tube.**

3. This is the correct procedure for placing ophthalmic drops in the eye.

4. Pressure is applied to the inner canthus to prevent eye medication from entering the systemic system.

80. 1. The client should increase fluid intake to help flush the bacteria through the kidneys and bladder.

2. The client has a chronic UTI, which will require antibiotics on a daily basis to keep the bacteria count under control.

3. **The key to answering this question is the word "chronic," which indicates a continuing problem; this statement would be appropriate for an acute UTI.**

4. Diarrhea is a sign of superinfection, which occurs when the antibiotic kills the good flora in the bowel. However, the client must keep taking the antibiotic and Imodium is an OTC anti-diarrheal.

81. 1. A Pap smear is usually done yearly and is used to detect cervical cancer; HRT does not increase the risk.

2. **The risk of developing breast cancer increases when the client is receiving HRT.**

3. A bone density test is used to detect osteoporosis, and HRT improves bone density.

4. Calcium levels are not effected by HRT.

82. 1. One (1) of the five (5) rights is the correct dose, and some medications must be divided prior to administering.

2. One (1) of the five (5) rights is the correct client, and this is making sure it is the correct client.

3. **One (1) of the five (5) rights is the correct route. Insulin cannot be administered**

intramuscularly. It must be administered subcutaneously or intravenously; therefore this action warrants immediate intervention.

4. One (1) of the five (5) rights is the right time, and the LPN has 30 minutes to one (1) hour to administer medications depending on hospital policy; therefore this would not require intervention by the nurse.

83. 1. This is an antacid, but it is not being administered to this client for that reason.

2. The client is in end-stage renal disease, but burning on urination is not a sign of ESRD; it is a sign of urinary tract infection.

3. A side effect of this medication is constipation, but having a normal bowel movement does not indicate the medication is effective.

4. **This medication decreases absorption of phosphates in the intestines, thereby decreasing serum phosphate levels. The normal phosphate level is 2.5–4.5 mg/dL.**

84. 1. **Any medication that will prolong bleeding, as a platelet aggregate inhibitor does, should not be administered to the client for at least two (2) to three (3) days prior to surgery.**

2. The nurse should not question administering an antibiotic before surgery, especially not before gastrointestinal surgery.

3. This is a medication for Type 2 diabetes and should be administered the day before the surgery.

4. The client will be receiving medications to evacuate the bowel.

85. 1. This rash indicates a sensitivity reaction, and the medication may need to be discontinued permanently or the dose should be decreased.

2. **Increased fluid intake minimizes the risk of renal calculi formation.**

3. To minimize gastric irritation, the medication should be taken with food or milk.

4. Allopurinol increases the effects of oral diabetic medications; therefore, the dose should be decreased.

86. 1. Atropine in this dosage will not cause orthostatic hypotension, but it will increase the pulse rate.

2. The client should increase the fiber in the diet because this medication may cause constipation.

3. **An expected side effect of anticholinergic medication is a dry mouth, and chewing gum will help relieve the dryness.**

4. Isometric exercises are muscle-building exer-

cises (weightlifting, pumping iron), which will not help the client tolerate this medication and should not be recommended for any client.

87. 1. Telemetry should be monitored during therapy to ensure the client does not develop worsening of dysrhythmias.
2. The client taking amiodarone is at risk for pulmonary toxicity and developing adult respiratory distress syndrome (ARDS); therefore, the nurse should monitor the client's respiratory status.
3. When the client is receiving medications intravenously, monitoring the liver and renal function is appropriate; this drug causes hepatomegaly.
4. Intravenous vasoactive medications are inherently dangerous; fatalities have occurred from amiodarone, so the nurse confirming the order with another nurse is appropriate.
5. The nurse should never defibrillate a client who has a heartbeat, and nothing in the stem states the client is in ventricular fibrillation.

88. 1. This medication amount is too much and must be divided into two injections to be given safely, but the nurse can do this independently and does not need to notify the HCP.
2. The nurse should not administer 4.8 mL in one (1) injection. No more than three (3) mL should be administered in an intramuscular injection.
3. There is no reason for the nurse to discard this medication. Divide the medication and give two (2) injections.
4. The nurse should never administer more than three (3) mL in an intramuscular injection because a larger amount could cause damage to the muscle. The nurse should divide the dose and administer two (2) injections.

89. 1. The client's drug level is between the therapeutic level of 10–20 mcg/mL.
2. Expiratory wheezing would be expected in the client with status asthmaticus and therefore would not warrant intervention.
3. Muscle twitching indicates the client is receiving too much medication and may experience a seizure.
4. The client is having trouble breathing, and eating requires energy. Therefore the client may not want to eat a meal or the client may not like the hospital food, which would not warrant immediate intervention.

90. 1. The client with pitting pedal edema is in fluid volume overload, which should make the nurse question administering an osmo-

tic diuretic because this medication will pull more fluid from the tissues into the circulatory system, causing further fluid volume overload.
2. An osmotic diuretic is administered for increased intracranial pressure; therefore a client who is exhibiting decorticate posturing would need this medication.
3. A widening pulse pressure indicates increased intracranial pressures; therefore the client needs the osmotic diuretic.
4. The doll's eye test indicates increased intracranial pressure, which is why the HCP would prescribe the osmotic diuretic.

91. 1. Melena is black, tarry stool, which should not occur from taking this medication.
2. Gynecomastia, breast development in men, is a complication of this medication.
3. Pyrosis, or heartburn, is why the client would be taking this medication.
4. Eructation, belching, is not a complication of this medication.

92. 1. Muscle relaxants do not cause GI distress.
2. Muscle relaxants, with the exception of baclofen, do not need to be tapered off.
3. Initially muscle relaxants cause drowsiness, so safety is an important issue.
4. As a safety precaution the client should avoid drinking alcohol while taking muscle relaxants.

93. 1. The client may be given a steroid, such as prednisone, but not an NSAID.
2. An antihistamine is prescribed to decrease symptoms of a cold or the flu, but it is not prescribed for asthma.
3. An ACE inhibitor prevents deterioration of heart muscle and kidneys, but it is not a drug of choice for the respiratory system.
4. Because 80% to 90% of adult-onset asthma is caused by gastroesophageal reflux disease, a proton pump inhibitor would be prescribed to decrease acid reflux into the esophagus and subsequent aspiration.

94. 1. The pain medication should be administered as soon as possible but not before assessing for complications that might be causing pain.
2. The nurse must not administer the medication too close to the last dose, but this is not the first intervention the nurse would implement.
3. The first step of the nursing process is to assess and the nurse must determine if this is routine postop pain the client should have or if this is a complication that requires immediate intervention. Decreased blood pressure and increased pulse indicates hemorrhaging.

Pharmacology

4. Teaching distraction techniques is an appropriate intervention, but the nurse should medicate the client.

95. 1. Just because a client is taking an antidepressant does not mean he or she is suicidal.
2. **The nurse should determine if the client is in a depressed state or if the medication is effective, so the nurse should ask the client to rate the depression on the 1–10 scale, 1 being no depression and 10 being the most depressed.**
3. Antidepressants must be tapered off because of rebound depression.
4. The client taking an antidepressant medication does not automatically need a referral to a psychologist.

96. 1. **Many times, especially with elderly clients, sedatives extend the desired effects longer than expected; therefore the nurse should check to see if the client received any sleeping medication.**
2. The nurse should assess why the client is sleepy and then allow the client to sleep if the sleepiness is a result of receiving a sedative the previous night.
3. If an elderly client is confused and drowsy, the client should not be allowed to ambulate, even if assistance is being provided, because of safety issues.
4. The nurse must determine if this is an expected occurrence or a decrease in neurologic function before notifying the health-care provider.

97. 1. Medication does not always come in the exact amount of the HCP's order.
2. **Because this is a narcotic, the nurse preparing the medication must have someone to verify and document the wastage of 12.5 mg of the Demerol.**
3. This would be a medication error because the order is for 37.5 mg, not 50 mg.
4. This would not be an appropriate intervention. The nurse can safely and accurately administer the prescribed dose to the client. If the pain is not controlled with the amount, then the HCP could be notified.

98. **2 tablets.** The nurse needs to determine how many doses are to be given in 1 day (24 hours) if doses are to be eight (8) hours apart.

$$24 \div 8 = 3 \text{ doses}$$

If 3000 mg are to be given in 3 doses, then determine how much is given in each dose:

$$3000 \div 3 = 1000 \text{ mg per dose}$$

If the medication comes in 500 mg tablets, then to give 1000 mg, the nurse must give:

$$1000 \div 500 = 2 \text{ tablets}$$

99. 1. **This medication decreases inflammation by stabilizing the leukotrienes in the lung that initiate an asthma attack.**
2. Children may outgrow asthma attacks, whereas adult asthmatics can control their disease, but there is no cure for asthma at this time.
3. This is the scientific rationale for mast cell inhibitors.
4. This is the scientific rationale for bronchodilators.

100. 1. Although many nurses will do this, the correct and ethical action is to take responsibility for the error and just be thankful the client did not have a problem.
2. There is a chain of command to report medication errors, which includes the charge nurse and the health-care provider, not the director of nurses.
3. **The ethical and correct action is to report and document the medication error; remember to always assess the client.**
4. The Peer Review Committee would not be involved in one medication error unless the client died or a life-threatening complication occurred or if the nurse has a pattern of behavior with multiple medication errors.

101. In order of priority: 4, 3, 2, 1, 5
4. **Although the lidocaine is a PRN order, this client is exhibiting a life-threatening dysrhythmia, multifocal PVCs.**
3. **The client diagnosed with myasthenia gravis must have this medication as close to the specific time as possible. This medication allows skeletal muscle to function; if this medication is delayed, the client may experience respiratory distress.**
2. **Pain is a priority and should be attended to after administering medications to clients in life-threatening situations.**
1. **This client is symptomatic, and the loop diuretic should relieve some of the symptoms of dyspnea.**
5. **Intravenous antibiotics are priority, but this client has received several doses of the medication or there would not be a trough level, so this client's medication could wait until the other medications have been administered.**

# Comprehensive Final Examination

20

This book is designed to assist the test taker to recognize elements of test construction and to be able to think critically to arrive at the correct answer. Many hints have appeared in the previous chapters. Some are general hints that apply to preparing for class and subsequently to taking examinations (Chapter 1), some are specific tips for the different types of questions about disorders/diseases of the different body systems (Chapters 2–18), and some are specific to pharmacology (Chapter 19). The test taker should now apply these hints, use all the knowledge gained in class and study, and take the comprehensive examination.

1. The 44-year-old female client calls the clinic and tells the nurse that while performing breast self examination (BSE) she felt a lump. Which question should the nurse ask the client?
   1. "Are you taking birth control pills?"
   2. "Do you eat a lot of chocolate?"
   3. "When was your last period?"
   4. "Are you sexually active?"

2. Which problem is priority for the 24-year-old client diagnosed with endometriosis who is admitted to the gynecological unit?
   1. Hemorrhage.
   2. Pain.
   3. Constipation.
   4. Dyspareunia.

3. The 28-year-old client diagnosed with testicular cancer is scheduled for a unilateral orchiectomy. Which intervention should have priority in the client's plan of care?
   1. Encourage the client to bank his sperm.
   2. Discuss completing an advance directive.
   3. Explain follow-up chemotherapy and radiation.
   4. Allow the client to express his or her feelings regarding having cancer.

4. The nurse is teaching a class on sexually transmitted diseases to high school sophomores. Which information should be included in the discussion?
   1. Oral sex decreases the chance of transmitting a sexual disease.
   2. Sexual activity during menses decreases transmission of diseases.
   3. Frequent sexual activity is necessary to transmit a sexual disease.
   4. Unprotected sex puts the individual at risk for many diseases.

5. The nurse has taught Kegel exercises to the client who is para 5, gravida 5. Which information would indicate the exercises have been effective?
   1. The client reports no SOB when walking up stairs.
   2. The client has no complaints of stress incontinence.
   3. The client denies being pregnant at this time.
   4. The client has lost 10 lbs in the last two (2) months.

6. Which diagnostic procedure would the nurse anticipate being ordered for the 27-year-old female client who is reporting irregular menses and complaining of lower left abdominal pain during menses?
   1. Pelvic sonogram.
   2. Complete blood count (CBC).
   3. Kidney, ureter, bladder (KUB) x-ray.
   4. Computed tomography (CT) of abdomen.

7. The client is diagnosed with Stage IV prostate cancer and is receiving chemotherapy. Which lab value would the nurse assess prior to administering the chemotherapy?
   1. Prostate-specific antigen (PSA).
   2. Serum calcium level.
   3. Complete blood count (CBC).
   4. Alpha fetoprotein (AFP).

8. Which client would the charge nurse of the day surgery unit assign to a new graduate nurse in orientation?
   1. The client who had an arthroscopy with an AP of 110 and BP of 94/60.
   2. The client with open reduction of the ankle who is confused.
   3. The client with a total hip replacement who is being transferred to the ICU.
   4. The client diagnosed with low back pain who has had a myelogram.

9. The client in the long term care facility has severe osteoarthritis. Which nursing task should the nurse delegate to the unlicensed nursing assistant (NA)?
   1. Feed the client the breakfast meal.
   2. Give the client Maalox, an antacid.
   3. Monitor the client's INR results.
   4. Assist the client to the shower room.

10. The primary nurse is applying antiembolism hose to the client who had a total hip replacement. Which situation would warrant immediate intervention by the charge nurse?
    1. Two fingers can be placed under the top of the band.
    2. The peripheral capillary refill time is <3 seconds.
    3. There are wrinkles in the hose behind the knees.
    4. The primary nurse does not place a hose on the foot that has a venous ulcer.

11. The 54-year-old female client is diagnosed with osteoporosis. Which interventions should the nurse discuss with the client? Select all that apply.
    1. Instruct the client to swim 30 minutes every day.
    2. Encourage drinking milk with added vitamin D.
    3. Refer the client to a smoking-cessation group.
    4. Recommend that the client not go outside.
    5. Teach about safety and fall precautions.

12. The 33-year-old client had a traumatic amputation of the right forearm as a result of a work-related injury. Which referral by the rehabilitation nurse would be most appropriate?
    1. Physical therapist.
    2. Occupational therapist.
    3. Worker's compensation.
    4. State rehabilitation commission.

13. The client has a fractured right tibia. Which assessment data would warrant immediate intervention?
    1. The client complains of right calf pain.
    2. The nurse cannot palpate the radial pulse.
    3. The client's right foot is cold to touch.
    4. The nurse notes ecchymosis on the right leg.

14. The nurse writes the problem "high risk for complications" for the client with a right total hip replacement who is being discharged from the hospital. Which problem would have the highest priority?
    1. Self-care deficit.
    2. Impaired skin integrity.
    3. Abnormal bleeding.
    4. Prosthetic infection.

15. The client has sustained severe burns on both the anterior right and left leg and the anterior chest and abdomen. According to the rule of nines, what percentage of the body has been burned?

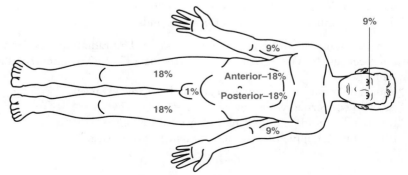

16. The nurse is planning the care for the client with multiple stage IV pressure ulcers. Which complication could result from these pressure ulcers?
    1. Wasting syndrome.
    2. Osteomyelitis.
    3. Renal calculi.
    4. Cellulitis.

17. The client comes to the clinic complaining of itching on the left wrist. The nurse notes an erythematous area along with pruritic vesicles around the left wrist. Which condition would the nurse suspect?
    1. Contact dermatitis.
    2. Herpes simplex 1.
    3. Impetigo.
    4. Seborrheic dermatitis.

18. Which diagnostic test would the nurse expect to be ordered for the client who has a nevus that is purple and brown with irregular borders?
    1. Bone scan.
    2. Skin biopsy.
    3. Carcinogenic embryonic antigen (CEA).
    4. Sonogram.

19. The client is admitted to the neurointensive care unit following a motor-vehicle accident resulting in a closed head injury. Which goal would be an appropriate short-term goal for the client?
    1. The client will maintain optimal level of functioning.
    2. The client will not develop extremity contractures.
    3. The client's intracranial pressure will not be >15 mm Hg.
    4. The client will be able to verbalize feelings of anger.

20. The 25-year-old client who has a C-6 spinal cord injury is crying and asks the nurse, "Why did I have to survive? I wish I was dead." Which statement would be the nurse's best response?
    1. "Don't talk like that. At least you are alive and able to talk."
    2. "God must have something planned for your life. Pray about it."
    3. "You survived because the people at the accident saved your life."
    4. "This must be difficult to cope with. Would you like to talk?"

21. The client is newly diagnosed with epilepsy. Which statement indicates that the client does not understand the discharge teaching?
    1. "I can drive as soon as I see my HCP for my follow-up visit."
    2. "I should get at least eight (8) hours of sleep at night."
    3. "I should take my medication every day even if I am sick."
    4. "I will take showers instead of taking tub baths."

22. The nurse observes the unlicensed nursing assistant (NA) taking vital signs on an unconscious client. Which action by the NA would warrant intervention by the nurse?
    1. The NA uses a vital sign machine to check the BP.
    2. The NA takes the client's temperature orally.
    3. The NA verifies the blood pressure manually.
    4. The NA counts the respirations for 30 seconds.

23. The client diagnosed with a brain tumor who has had radiation treatment and developed alopecia asks, "When will my hair grow back?" Which statement should be the nurse's response?
    1. "Your hair should start growing back within three (3) weeks."
    2. "Are you concerned your hair will not grow back?"
    3. "It may take months, if your hair grows back at all."
    4. "It may take a couple of years for the hair to grow back."

24. Which assessment data indicate the treatment for the client diagnosed with bacterial meningitis is effective?
    1. There is a positive Brudzinski's and photophobia.
    2. The client tolerates meals without nausea.
    3. There is a positive Kernig's sign and an elevated temperature.
    4. The client is able to flex the neck without pain.

25. The client is being evaluated to rule out Parkinson's disease. Which diagnostic test confirms this diagnosis?
    1. A positive magnetic resonance imaging (MRI) scan.
    2. A biopsy of the substantia nigra.
    3. A stereotactic pallidotomy.
    4. There is no test that confirms this diagnosis.

26. The client diagnosed with a transient ischemic attack (TIA) is being discharged from the hospital. Which medication would the nurse expect the HCP to prescribe?
    1. The oral anticoagulant warfarin (Coumadin).
    2. The antiplatelet medication, a baby aspirin.
    3. The beta blocker propranolol (Inderal).
    4. The anticonvulsant valproic acid (Depakote).

27. The nurse has just received the shift assessment. Which client should the nurse assess first?
    1. The client with encephalitis who has myalgia.
    2. The client who is complaining of chest pain.
    3. The client who refuses to eat hospital food.
    4. The client who is scheduled to go to the whirlpool.

28. Which client should the charge nurse on the substance abuse unit assign to the licensed practical nurse (LPN)?
    1. The client with chronic alcoholism who has been on the unit three (3) days.
    2. The client who is complaining of palpitations and has a history of cocaine abuse.
    3. The client diagnosed with amphetamine abuse who tried to commit suicide.
    4. The client diagnosed with cannabinoid abuse who is threatening to leave against medical advice (AMA).

29. The telemetry nurse is monitoring the following clients. Which client should the telemetry nurse instruct the primary nurse to assess first?
    1. The client who has occasional premature ventricular contractions (PVCs).
    2. The client post-cardiac surgery who has three (3) unifocal PVCs in a minute.
    3. The client with a myocardial infarction who had two (2) multifocal PVCs.
    4. The client diagnosed with atrial fibrillation who has an AP of 116 and no P wave.

30. The nurse is teaching the clients in a cardiac rehabilitation unit. Which dietary information should the nurse discuss with the clients?
    1. No more than 30% of daily food intake should be fats.
    2. Eighty percent of calories should come from carbohydrates.
    3. Red meat should comprise at least 50% of daily intake.
    4. Monosaturated fat in the daily diet should be increased.

31. The client diagnosed with end-stage congestive heart failure is being cared for by the home health nurse. Which interventions should the nurse teach the caregiver?
    1. Report any time the client starts having difficulty breathing.
    2. Notify the HCP if the client gains more than 5 lbs in a week.
    3. Teach how to take the client's apical pulse for one (1) full minute.
    4. Encourage the client to participate in 30 minutes of exercise a day.

32. The client is diagnosed with aortic stenosis. Which assessment data would indicate a complication is occurring?
    1. Barrel chest and clubbing of the fingers.
    2. Intermittent claudication and rest pain.
    3. Pink, frothy sputum and dyspnea on exertion.
    4. Bilateral wheezing and friction rub.

33. The client who has just received a permanent pacemaker is admitted to the telemetry floor. The nurse writes the problem "knowledge deficit." Which interventions should be included in the plan of care? Select all that apply.
    1. Take tub baths instead of showers the rest of their life.
    2. Do not hold electrical devices near the pacemaker.
    3. Carry the pacemaker identification card at all times.
    4. Count the radial pulse one (1) full minute every morning.
    5. Notify the HCP if the pulse is 12 beats slower than the preset rate.

34. Which question should the nurse ask the client who is being admitted to rule out infective endocarditis?
    1. "Do you have a history of a heart attack?"
    2. "Have you had a cardiac valve replacement?"
    3. "Is there a family history of rheumatic heart disease?"
    4. "Do you take nonsteroidal anti-inflammatory medications?"

35. The client diagnosed with arterial occlusive disease is prescribed an antiplatelet medication, clopidogrel (Plavix). Which assessment indicates the medication is effective?
    1. The client's pedal pulse is bounding.
    2. The client's blood pressure has decreased.
    3. The client does not exhibit signs of a stroke.
    4. The client has decreased pain when ambulating.

36. The client diagnosed with atherosclerosis has coronary artery disease. The client experiences sudden chest pain when walking to the nurse's station. Which action should the nurse implement first?
    1. Administer sublingual nitroglycerin.
    2. Apply oxygen via nasal cannula.
    3. Obtain a STAT electrocardiogram.
    4. Have the client sit in a chair.

37. The nurse and the unlicensed nursing assistant (NA) are caring for clients on a medical floor. Which nursing task could be delegated to the NA?
    1. Retake the BP on a client who received a STAT nitroglycerin sublingual.
    2. Notify the health-care provider of the client's elevated blood pressure.
    3. Obtain and document the routine vital signs on all the clients on the floor.
    4. Call the laboratory technician and discuss a hemolyzed blood specimen.

38. The client with venous insufficiency tells the nurse, "The doctor just told me about my disease and walked out of the room. What am I supposed to do?" Which statement would be the nurse's best response?
    1. "I will have your HCP come back and discuss this with you."
    2. "When you are watching TV you should elevate your legs."
    3. "You will probably need to have surgery within a few months."
    4. "This will go away after you lose about 20 pounds and start walking."

39. The client is admitted with rule out leukemia. Which assessment data support the diagnosis of leukemia?
    1. Cervical lymph node enlargement.
    2. An asymmetrical dark purple nevus.
    3. Petechiae covering the trunk and legs.
    4. Brownish-purple nodules on the face.

40. The client diagnosed with non-Hodgkin's lymphoma tells the nurse, "I am so tired. I just wish I could die." Which stage of the grieving process would this statement represent?
    1. Anger.
    2. Denial.
    3. Bargaining.
    4. Acceptance.

41. The nurse writes the goal "the client will list three (3) food sources of vitamin $B_{12}$" for the client diagnosed with pernicious anemia. Which foods listed by the client indicate the goal has been met?
    1. Brown rice, dried fruits, and oatmeal.
    2. Beef, chicken, and pork.
    3. Broccoli, asparagus, and kidney beans.
    4. Liver, cheese, and eggs.

42. The client diagnosed with stomach cancer has developed disseminated intravascular coagulopathy (DIC). Which collaborative intervention would the nurse expect to implement?
    1. Prepare to administer intravenous heparin.
    2. Assess for frank hemorrhage from venipuncture sites.
    3. Monitor for decreased level of consciousness.
    4. Prepare to administer total parenteral nutrition.

43. The nurse is administering 250 mL of packed red blood cells with 50 mL of preservative. The client has no jugular vein distention and has clear breath sounds. After the first 15 minutes, at what rate should the nurse set the IV infusion pump?_____

44. The 24-year-old African American female client tells the nurse that she has a brother with sickle cell disease. She is engaged to be married and is concerned about giving this disease to her future children. Which information is most important to provide to the client?
    1. Tell the client that she won't pass this on if she has never had symptoms.
    2. Encourage the client to discuss this concern with her fiancé.
    3. Recommend that she and her fiancé see a genetic counselor.
    4. Discuss the possibility of adopting children after she gets married.

45. The nurse is at home preparing for the 7 A.M. to 7 P.M. shift and has the flu with a temperature of 100.4°F. Which action should the nurse take?
    1. Notify the hospital that the nurse will not be coming into work.
    2. Go to work and wear an isolation mask when caring for the clients.
    3. Request an alterative assignment that does not involve direct client care.
    4. Take over-the-counter cold medication and report to work on time.

46. The client is being admitted into the hospital with a diagnosis of pneumonia. Which HCP order would the nurse implement first?
    1. Initiate intravenous antibiotics.
    2. Collect a sputum specimen for culture.
    3. Obtain a clean voided midstream urinalysis.
    4. Request a chest x-ray to confirm the diagnosis.

47. Which medical client problem should the nurse include in the plan of care for a client diagnosed with cardiomyopathy?
    1. Heart failure.
    2. Activity intolerance.
    3. Powerlessness.
    4. Anticipatory grieving.

48. The client comes to the emergency department complaining of pain in the right fore-arm. The nurse notes a large area of redness and edema over the forearm, and the client has an elevated temperature. Which condition would the nurse suspect?
    1. Cellulitis.
    2. Intravenous drug abuse.
    3. Raynaud's syndrome.
    4. Thromboangiitis obliterans.

49. The client is performing breast self examination (BSE) by the American Cancer soci-ety's recommended steps and has completed palpating the breast. Which is the next step in the BSE process?
    1. Stand before the mirror and examine the breast.
    2. Lean forward and look for dimpling or retractions.
    3. Examine the breast using a circular motion.
    4. Pinch the nipple to see if any fluid can be expressed.

50. Which assessment information is the most critical indicator of a neurological deficit?
    1. Changes in pupil size.
    2. Level of consciousness.
    3. A decrease in motor function.
    4. Numbness of the extremities.

51. The nurse is initiating a blood transfusion. Which interventions should the nurse implement? Select all that apply.
    1. Assess the client's lung fields.
    2. Have the client sign a consent form.
    3. Start an IV with a 22-gauge IV catheter.
    4. Hang 250 mL of D5W at a keep open rate.
    5. Check the chart for the HCP's order.

52. When the nurse is assessing the client with psoriasis, what data would support this diagnosis?
    1. Appearance of red, elevated plaques with silvery white scales.
    2. A burning, prickling row of vesicles located along the torso.
    3. Raised, flesh-colored papules with a rough surface area.
    4. An overgrowth of tissue with an excessive amount of collagen.

53. Which comment by the client diagnosed with rule out Guillain-Barré (GB) syndrome would be most significant when completing the admission interview?
    1. "I had a bad case of gastroenteritis a few weeks ago."
    2. "I never use sunblock and I use a tanning bed often."
    3. "I started smoking cigarettes about 20 years ago."
    4. "I was out of the United States for the last 2 months."

54. Which laboratory result would warrant immediate intervention by the nurse for the female client diagnosed with systemic lupus erythematosus (SLE)?
    1. A hemoglobin and hematocrit of 13 g/dL and 40%.
    2. A erythrocyte sedimentation rate of 9 mm/hr.
    3. A serum albumin level of 4.5 g/dL.
    4. A white blood cell count of 15,000 mm.

55. The client diagnosed with gastroesophageal reflux disease (GERD) has undergone surgery for a hiatal hernia repair. The client has a nasogastric tube in place. Intravenous fluid replacement is to be at 125 mL per hour plus the amount of drainage. The drainage from 0800 to 0900 is 45 mL. At which rate should the IV pump be set for the next hour?_____

56. Which assessment data would support that the client has a conductive hearing loss?
    1. The Rinne test results in air-conducted sound being louder than bone-conducted.
    2. The client is unable to hear accurately when conducting the whisper test.
    3. The Weber test results in the sound being heard better in the affected ear.
    4. The tympanogram results in the ticking watch heard better in the unaffected ear.

57. The client reports a twisting motion of the knee during a basketball game. The client is scheduled for arthroscopic surgery to repair the injury. Which information should the nurse teach the client about postoperative care?
    1. The client should begin strengthening the surgical leg.
    2. The client should take pain medication routinely.
    3. The client should remain on bed rest for two (2) weeks.
    4. The client should return to the doctor in six (6) months.

58. When preparing the client newly diagnosed with asthma for discharge, what data would indicate to the nurse that teaching about the peak flow meter has been effective?
    1. "I can continue my usual activities without medication if I am in the yellow zone."
    2. "It takes one (1) to two (2) days to establish my personal best."
    3. "When I can't talk while walking I need to take my quick-relief medicine."
    4. "When I am in the red zone, I can take my quick-relief medication and exercise."

59. Which assessment data would indicate that the client has developed a deep vein thrombosis (DVT) in the left leg?
    1. A negative Homans' sign of the left leg.
    2. Increased left leg calf circumference.
    3. Elephantiasis of the left lower leg.
    4. Brownish pigmentation of the left lower leg.

60. The 85-year-old client diagnosed with severe end-stage chronic obstructive pulmonary disease has a chest x-ray that incidentally reveals an eight (8)-cm abdominal aortic aneurysm. Which intervention should the nurse implement?
    1. Discuss possible end-of-life care issues.
    2. Prepare the client for abdominal surgery.
    3. Teach the client how to pursed-lip breathe.
    4. Talk with the family about the client's condition.

61. The unlicensed nursing assistant notifies the nurse that the client diagnosed with chronic obstructive pulmonary disease is complaining of shortness of breath and would like his oxygen level increased. Which action should the nurse implement?
    1. Notify the respiratory therapist.
    2. Ask the NA to increase the oxygen.
    3. Obtain a STAT pulse oximeter reading.
    4. Tell the NA to leave the oxygen alone.

62. Which psychosocial client problem would the nurse write for the client diagnosed with cancer of the lung and metastasis to the brain?
    1. Seizures.
    2. Grieving.
    3. Body image.
    4. Nutrition.

63. The client diagnosed with cancer of the larynx has had a partial laryngectomy. Which client problem would have the highest priority?
    1. Impaired communication.
    2. Ineffective coping.
    3. Risk for aspiration.
    4. Social isolation.

64. The client receiving a continuous heparin drip complains of sudden chest pain on inspiration and tells the nurse, "Something is really wrong with me." Which intervention should the nurse implement first?
    1. Increase the heparin drip rate.
    2. Notify the health-care provider.
    3. Assess the client's lung sounds.
    4. Apply oxygen via nasal cannula.

65. The nurse is assessing the client with a pneumothorax who has a closed chest drainage system. Which data indicates the client's condition is stable?
    1. There is fluctuation in the water seal compartment.
    2. There is blood in the drainage compartment.
    3. The trachea deviates slightly to the left.
    4. There is bubbling in the suction compartment.

66. The client is admitted to the intensive care unit diagnosed with rule out adult respiratory distress syndrome (ARDS). The client is receiving 10 L/min of oxygen via nasal cannula. Which arterial blood gas indicates the client does not have ARDS?
    1. pH 7.38, $PaO_2$ 82, $PaCO_2$ 45, $HCO_3$ 26.
    2. pH 7.35, $PaO_2$ 74, $PaCO_2$ 43, $HCO_3$ 24.
    3. pH 7.48, $PaO_2$ 90, $PaCO_2$ 34, $HCO_3$ 22.
    4. pH 7.32, $PaO_2$ 50, $PaCO_2$ 55, $HCO_3$ 28.

67. The client has gastroesophageal reflux disease. Which HCP order would the nurse question?
    1. Elevate the client's head of the bed with blocks.
    2. Administer pantoprazole (Protonix) four times a day.
    3. A regular diet with no citrus or spicy foods.
    4. Activity as tolerated and sit up in a chair for all meals.

68. The client is diagnosed with an acute exacerbation of Crohn's disease. Which assessment data would warrant immediate attention?
    1. The client's white blood cell is 10.0 ($10^3$).
    2. The client's serum amylase is 100 units/dL.
    3. The client's potassium level is 3.3 mEq/L.
    4. The client's blood glucose is 148 mg/dL.

69. Which information should the nurse discuss with the client to prevent an acute exacerbation of diverticulosis?
    1. Increase the fiber in the diet.
    2. Drink at least 1000 mL of water a day.
    3. Encourage sedentary activities.
    4. Take cathartic laxatives daily.

70. The client diagnosed with peptic ulcer disease is being discharged. Which nursing task can be delegated to the unlicensed nursing assistant?
    1. Complete the discharge instructions sheet.
    2. Remove the client's saline lock.
    3. Clean the client's room after discharge.
    4. Check the client's hemoglobin and hematocrit.

71. The client diagnosed with colon cancer tells the nurse, "All I do is sit and watch TV all day. I can barely go to the bathroom." According to the Oncology Nurse's Society's cancer fatigue scale, how would the nurse document the fatigue objectively?

**FATIGUE SCALE**
Select the number that best describes how you feel today

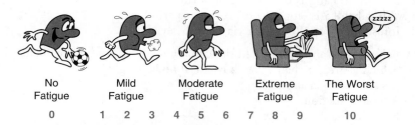

| No Fatigue | Mild Fatigue | Moderate Fatigue | Extreme Fatigue | The Worst Fatigue |
|---|---|---|---|---|
| 0 | 1  2  3 | 4  5  6 | 7  8  9 | 10 |

Reprinted with permission from the Oncology Nursing Society.

 1. Mild fatigue.
 2. Moderate fatigue.
 3. Extreme fatigue.
 4. Worst fatigue ever.

72. The home health nurse must see all of the following clients. Which client should the nurse assess first?
 1. The client who is postoperative from an open cholecystectomy who has green drainage coming from the T-tube.
 2. The client diagnosed with congestive heart failure who complains of shortness of breath while fixing meals.
 3. The client diagnosed with AIDS dementia whose family called and reported that the client is vomiting coffee grounds.
 4. The client diagnosed with end-stage liver failure who has gained three (3) pounds and is not able to wear house shoes.

73. Which data indicate the client with end-stage liver failure is improving?
 1. The client has a tympanic wave.
 2. The client is able to perform asterixis.
 3. The client is confused and lethargic.
 4. The client's abdominal girth has decreased.

74. The nurse is discussing funeral arrangements with the family of a client whose organs and tissues are being donated today. Which information should the nurse discuss with family?
 1. The family can request an open casket funeral.
 2. Your loved one must wear a long-sleeved shirt.
 3. You might want to have a private viewing only.
 4. This will not delay the timing of the funeral.

75. The public health nurse is discussing hepatitis with a client who is traveling to a Third World country in one (1) month. Which recommendation should the nurse discuss with the client?
 1. A gamma globulin injection.
 2. A hepatitis A vaccination.
 3. A PPD skin test on the left arm.
 4. A hepatitis B vaccination.

76. The client with chronic pancreatitis is admitted with an acute exacerbation of the disease. Which laboratory result would warrant immediate intervention by the nurse?
 1. The client's amylase is elevated.
 2. The client's WBC count is WNL.
 3. The client's blood glucose is elevated.
 4. The client's lipase is within normal limits.

77. The client has had an abdominal surgery and is receiving bag #5 of total parenteral nutrition (TPN) via a subclavian line infusing at 126 mL/hr. The nurse realizes that bag #6 is not on the unit and TPN number five (5) has 50 mL left to infuse. Which action should the nurse implement?
    1. Decrease the rate of bag #5 to a keep open ratWe.
    2. Prepare to hang 1000 mL bag of normal saline.
    3. When bag #5 is empty, convert to a heparin lock.
    4. Infuse $D_{10}W$ at 126 mL/hr via the subclavian line.

78. Which priority problem should the clinic nurse identify for the client who weighs 87 kg, which is greater than 15% above ideal body weight?
    1. Risk for complications.
    2. Altered nutrition.
    3. Body-image disturbance.
    4. Activity intolerance.

79. Which assessment data indicate the client with diarrhea is experiencing a complication?
    1. Moist buccal mucosa.
    2. A 3.6 mEq/L potassium level.
    3. Tented tissue turgor.
    4. Hyperactive bowel sounds.

80. The client with Type 2 diabetes mellitus asks the nurse, "What does it matter if my glucose level is high? I don't feel bad." Which statement by the nurse would be most appropriate?
    1. "The high glucose level can damage your eyes and kidneys over time."
    2. "The glucose level causes microvascular and macrovascular problems."
    3. "As long as you don't feel bad, everything will probably be all right."
    4. "A high blood glucose level will cause you to get metabolic acidosis."

81. The client with Type 1 diabetes asks the nurse, "What causes me to get dehydrated when my glucose level is elevated?" Which statement would be the nurse's best response?
    1. "The kidneys are damaged and cannot filter out the urine."
    2. "The glucose causes fluid to be pulled from the tissues."
    3. "The sweating as a result of the high glucose level causes dehydration."
    4. "You get dehydrated with a high glucose because you are so thirsty."

82. The client calls the clinic first thing in the morning and tells the nurse, "I have been vomiting and having diarrhea since last night." Which response would be appropriate for the nurse to make?
    1. Encourage the client to eat dairy products.
    2. Have the client go to the emergency room.
    3. Request the client obtain a stool specimen.
    4. Tell the client to stay on a clear liquid diet.

83. Which signs/symptoms would the nurse expect to assess in the client diagnosed with Addison's disease?
    1. Hypotension and bronze skin pigmentation.
    2. Water retention and osteoporosis.
    3. Hirsutism and abdominal striae.
    4. Truncal obesity and thin, wasted extremities.

84. The client diagnosed with neurogenic diabetes insipidus asks the nurse, "What is wrong with me? Why do I urinate so much?" Which statement by the nurse would be most appropriate?
    1. "The islet cells in your pancreas are not functioning properly."
    2. "Your pituitary gland is not secreting a necessary hormone."
    3. "Your kidneys are in failure and you are overproducing urine."
    4. "The thyroid gland is speeding up all your metabolism."

85. The client is admitted into the medical unit diagnosed with heart failure and is prescribed the thyroid hormone levothyroxine (Synthroid) orally. Which action should the nurse implement?
    1. Call the pharmacist to clarify the order.
    2. Administer the medication as ordered.
    3. Ask the client why he or she takes Synthroid.
    4. Request serum thyroid function levels.

86. Which client would be at risk for developing acute renal failure?
    1. The client diagnosed with essential hypertension.
    2. The client diagnosed with type 2 diabetes.
    3. The client who had an anaphylactic reaction.
    4. The client who had an autologous blood transfusion.

87. The client diagnosed with chronic renal failure is receiving peritoneal dialysis. Which assessment by the nurse would warrant immediate intervention?
    1. The dialysate return is cloudy.
    2. There is a greater dialysate return than input.
    3. The client complains of abdominal fullness.
    4. The client voided 50 mL during the day.

88. Which action by the unlicensed nursing assistant (NA) would require intervention by the nurse?
    1. The NA used two washcloths when washing the perineal area.
    2. The NA emptied the Foley catheter and documented the amount.
    3. The NA applied moisture barrier cream to the anal area.
    4. The NA is wiping the client's perineal area from back to front.

89. The unlicensed nursing assistant (NA) empties the indwelling urinary catheter for a client who is four (4) hours postoperative transurethral resection of the prostate and informs the nurse that the urine has blood and clots in it. Which would be the nurse's first action?
    1. Assess the client's urine output immediately.
    2. Notify the HCP that the client has gross hematuria.
    3. Explain that this is expected with this surgery.
    4. Medicate for bladder spasms to decrease bleeding.

90. The client with a history of substance abuse presents to the emergency room complaining of right flank pain and the urinalysis indicates microscopic blood. Which action should the nurse implement?
    1. Determine the last illegal drug use.
    2. Insert a #22 French Foley catheter.
    3. Give the client a back massage.
    4. Medicate the client for pain.

91. The nurse is aware that the most common sign of cancer of the bladder is which assessment data?
    1. Gross painless hematuria.
    2. Burning on urination.
    3. Terminal dribbling.
    4. Difficulty initiating the stream.

92. Which is a risk factor that predisposes the client to developing multiple sclerosis?
    1. A genetic predisposition.
    2. Living in the southern United States.
    3. Use of tobacco products.
    4. A sedentary lifestyle.

93. The elderly client from the long term care facility is admitted into the hospital diagnosed with septicemia. Which area of the body would be the most appropriate place for the nurse to assess the hydration status of the client?
    1. A
    2. B
    3. C
    4. D

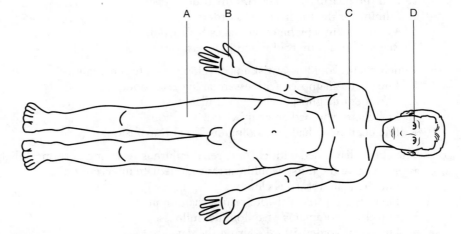

94. The student nurse accidentally punctured his finger with a contaminated needle. Which action should the student nurse take first?
    1. Notify the nursing instructor.
    2. Allow the puncture site to bleed.
    3. Report to the emergency room.
    4. Cleanse the site with Betadine.

95. Which psychosocial problem would be priority for a client diagnosed with rheumatoid arthritis?
    1. Alteration in comfort.
    2. Ineffective coping.
    3. Anxiety.
    4. Altered body image.

96. The client is admitted to the medical unit complaining of severe abdominal pain. Which intervention should the nurse implement first?
    1. Assess for complications.
    2. Medicate for pain.
    3. Turn the television on.
    4. Teach relaxation techniques.

97. The female client is admitted to the orthopedic floor with a spiral fracture of the arm and multiple contusions and abrasions covering the trunk of the body. Her husband accompanies her. During the admission interview, which action by the nurse would have priority?
    1. Notify Adult Protective Services of the client's admission.
    2. Provide privacy to discuss how the injuries occurred to the client.
    3. Refer the client to the social worker for names of women's shelters.
    4. Ask the client if she prefers the husband to stay in the room.

98. Which interventions should the nurse implement for a client who was brought to the emergency department by a friend who has an AP of 122 and a BP of 80/50? Select all that apply.
    1. Put the client in reverse Trendelenburg position.
    2. Start an intravenous line with an 18-gauge catheter.
    3. Have the client complete the admission process.
    4. Cover the client with blankets and keep warm.
    5. Request the lab draw a type and crossmatch.

99. The client is eight (8) hours postoperative small bowel resection. Which data indicate the client has had a complication from the surgery?
    1. A hard, rigid, boardlike abdomen.
    2. High-pitched tinkling bowel sounds.
    3. Absent bowel sounds.
    4. Complaints of pain at six (6) on the pain scale.

100. Which intervention will help prevent the nurse from being sued for malpractice throughout their professional practice?
    1. Keep accurate and legible documentation of client's care.
    2. A kind, caring, and compassionate bedside manner at all times.
    3. Maintain knowledge of medications for disease processes.
    4. Follow all health-care provider orders explicitly.

101. Which interventions should the nurse implement when caring for a client diagnosed with a right-sided cerebral vascular accident and stroke and who has difficulty swallowing? List the interventions in order of the nursing process.
    1. Writes the client problem of "altered tissue perfusion."
    2. Assesses the client's level of consciousness and speech.
    3. Requests dietary to send a full liquid tray with Thick-It.
    4. Instructs the UAP to elevate the head of the bed 30 degrees.
    5. Notes the amount of food consumed on the dinner tray.

1.
1. Birth control pills regulate the hormones in the body but will not cause changes in the breast tissue.
2. There is a theory that chocolate increases breast discomfort in women with fibrocystic breast changes.
3. During the menstrual cycle, pregnancy, and menopause, variations in breast tissue occur and must be distinguished from pathological disease. BSE is best performed on days five (5) to seven (7) after menses, counting the first day of menses as day one (1).
4. Sexual manipulation of the breast does not cause malignant changes in breast tissue.

2.
1. Anemia due to endometriosis occurs over time and is not an acute complication such as hemorrhaging.
2. Pain is the primary complaint of the client; the pain occurs as a result of ectopic tissue bleeding into the abdominal cavity during menses.
3. Endometriosis does not cause constipation and would not be a priority problem. The client may experience pain during a bowel movement.
4. Dyspareunia is pain during intercourse, and this client is in the hospital (and unlikely to be having sex there).

3.
1. With a remaining testicle the client will be able to maintain sexual potency, but radiation and chemotherapy may cause the client to become sterile. Therefore banking his sperm will allow him to father a child later in life.
2. Testicular cancer has a 90% cure rate with standard therapy; therefore, completing an advance directive is not priority.
3. The client will not be undergoing chemotherapy for at least six (6) weeks to allow the client to heal; therefore this is not a priority intervention.
4. This is important, but when preparing the client for surgery the priority intervention is to accomplish presurgical interventions.

4.
1. Oral sex still involves mucous membrane-to-mucous membrane contact and disease transmission is possible; herpes simplex 2 is simply herpes simplex 1 transferred to the genitalia.
2. This is a myth.
3. The more often the person engages in sexual contact and the more partners he or she has, the more likely the person will contract a STD; however, one time is enough to contract a deadly STD, such as AIDS.

4. According to developmental theories, adolescents think that they are invincible and nothing will happen to them. This attitude leads adolescents to participate in high-risk behaviors without regard to consequences.

5.
1. Kegel exercises do not have anything to do with activity endurance.
2. Kegel exercises are exercises that strengthen the perineal muscles. Multiple pregnancies weaken the pelvic muscles, resulting in bladder incontinence; a report of no stress incontinence indicates the Kegel exercises are effective.
3. Kegel exercises do not affect pregnancy.
4. Kegel exercises do not have anything to do with weight loss.

6.
1. The pelvic sonogram, which visualizes the ovary using sound waves, is a diagnostic test for an ovarian cyst, which would be suspected with the client's signs/symptoms.
2. A CBC may be ordered to rule out appendicitis, but this is not right lower abdominal pain.
3. KUB is ordered for a client with possible kidney stones.
4. A CT of the abdomen would not visualize contents in the pelvis.

7.
1. PSA is a tumor marker that may be monitored to determine the progress of the disease and treatment, but it is not monitored prior to chemotherapy.
2. Serum calcium levels may be monitored to determine metastasis to the bone, but it would not be done prior to chemotherapy.
3. The CBC is monitored to determine if the client is at risk for developing an infection or bleeding as a result of side effects of the chemotherapy medications. The chemotherapy could be held or decreased based on these results.
4. AFP is a tumor marker that may be monitored to determine the progress of the disease and treatment, but it is not monitored prior to chemotherapy.

8.
1. This client is showing signs/symptoms of hypovolemic shock and should not be assigned to an inexperienced nurse.
2. Confusion could be a sign of many complications after surgery, so this client should not be assigned to an inexperienced nurse.
3. This client is being transferred to the ICU, which indicates the client is not stable; therefore this client should not be assigned to an inexperienced nurse.

4. A myelogram is a routine diagnostic test. With minimal instruction an inexperienced nurse could care for this client.

9. 1. The nurse should encourage the client to maintain independent functioning, and delegating the NA to feed the client would be encouraging dependence.
   2. Although this is an over-the-counter medication, an NA cannot administer any medication to a client.
   3. The NA cannot assess or evaluate any of the client's diagnostic information.
   4. The NA could assist the client to ambulate to the shower room and assist with morning care.

10. 1. This would not warrant intervention because this indicates the hose are not too tight.
   2. This indicates that the hose are not too tight.
   3. There should be no wrinkles in the hose after application. Wrinkles could cause constriction in the area, resulting in clot formation or skin breakdown; therefore this would warrant immediate intervention by the charge nurse.
   4. Antiembolism hose should not be put over a wound; they would restrict the circulation to the wound and cause a decrease in wound healing.

11. 1. The nurse should suggest walking daily because bones need stress to maintain strength.
   2. Vitamin D helps the body absorb calcium.
   3. Smoking interferes with estrogen's protective effects on bones, promoting bone loss.
   4. Lack of exposure to sunlight results in decreased vitamin D, which is necessary for calcium absorption and normal bone mineralization. The client should go outside.
   5. The client is at risk for fractures; therefore a fall could result in serious complications.

12. 1. The physical therapist addresses lower-extremity strength, gait training, and transfers.
   2. The occupational therapist addresses activities of daily living and fine motor skills in the upper extremities, which would be an appropriate referral.
   3. Worker's compensation is an insurance provider for the employer and employee to cover medical expenses and loss of wages. This is not an appropriate referral by the rehabilitation nurse.
   4. The client may need this referral but after the occupational therapist has worked with the client and determined the ability to perform skills.

13. 1. The nurse would expect the client with a fractured right leg to have pain but it would not warrant immediate intervention.
   2. The nurse would assess the client's pedal or posterior tibial pulse for a client with a fractured right tibia.
   3. Any abnormal neurovascular assessment data, such as coldness, paralysis, or paresthesia, warrant immediate intervention by the nurse.
   4. Ecchymosis is bruising and would be expected in the client who has a fractured tibia.

14. 1. The client is being discharged so a self-care deficit would not be a potential complication.
   2. The client is being discharged and is ambulating; therefore impaired skin integrity should not be a problem.
   3. The client would have been taking a prophylactic anticoagulant but would not be at risk for abnormal bleeding.
   4. The client must inform all HCPs, especially the dentist, of the hip prosthesis because the client should be taking prophylactic antibiotics prior to any invasive procedure. Any bacteria that invade the body may cause an infection in the joint, and this may result in the client having the prosthesis removed.

15. 36%. Each leg is 18%, with the anterior surface (front) being 9%. Because the anterior of both legs is burned (9% each), that would be 18%. That 18% plus 18%, which is the anterior surface of the trunk, totals 36% of the total body surface burned.

16. 1. Wasting syndrome occurs in clients with protein calorie malnutrition. This syndrome leads to the pressure ulcers not healing, but it is not a complication of the pressure ulcers.
   2. Stage IV pressure ulcers frequently extend to the bone tissue, predisposing the client to developing a bone infection, osteomyelitis, which can rarely be treated effectively.
   3. Renal calculi may be a result of immobility, but they are not a complication of pressure ulcers.
   4. Cellulitis is an inflammation of the skin, which is not a complication of pressure ulcers.

17. 1. Contact dermatitis is a type of dermatitis caused by a hypersensitivity response. In this case, it is a hypersensitivity reaction to metal salts in the watch the client is wearing. Any time the nurse assesses redness or irritation in areas where jewelry (such as rings, watches, necklaces) or clothing (such as socks, shoes, or gloves) are worn, the nurse should suspect contact dermatitis.

Final Exam

2. Herpes simplex 1 virus occurs in oral or nasal mucous membranes.

3. Impetigo is a superficial infection of the skin caused by staph or strep infection and occurs on the body, face, hands, or neck.

4. Seborrheic dermatitis is a chronic inflammation of the skin that involves the scalp, eyebrows, eyelids, ear canals, nasolabial folds, axillae, and trunk.

18. 1. A bone scan would not be ordered unless a biopsy proves malignant melanoma.

2. **This is an abnormal-appearing mole on the skin, and the HCP would order a biopsy to confirm skin cancer.**

3. A CEA is a test used to mark the presence or prognosis of several cancers but not skin cancer.

4. A sonogram would not be ordered to diagnose skin cancer.

19. 1. This could be an appropriate long-term goal for the client based on the extent of injury, but it is not an appropriate short-term goal.

2. This is an appropriate long-term goal to prevent immobility complications, but it is not an appropriate short-term goal.

3. **The worse-case scenario with a closed head injury is increased intracranial pressure resulting in death. An appropriate short-term goal would be the ICP remaining within normal limits, which is 5–15 mm Hg.**

4. This is a psychosocial goal, which would not be a short-term goal, and the client may not be angry. The stem did not indicate the client is angry.

20. 1. This is negating the client's feelings and will abruptly end any conversation the client may want or need to have.

2. This is imposing the nurse's religious beliefs on the client and these are clichés, which do not address the client's feelings.

3. This is explaining why the client survived, but the client isn't really asking for any information. The client is expressing and showing emotions that should be addressed by the nurse.

4. **This is a therapeutic response that addresses the client's feelings.**

21. 1. **This statement indicates the client does not understand the discharge teaching. The client will not be able to drive until the client is seizure free for a certain period of time. The laws in each state differ.**

2. Lack of sleep is a risk factor for having seizures.

3. Noncompliance with medication is a risk factor for having a seizure.

4. If the client has a seizure in the bathtub, the client could drown.

22. 1. Using the vital sign machine to take the client's BP is an appropriate intervention.

2. **The body temperature of an unconscious client should never be taken by mouth because the client is unable to safely hold the thermometer.**

3. Verifying the blood pressure manually is an appropriate intervention if the NA questions the automatic blood pressure reading. This action should be praised.

4. Counting the respiration for 30 seconds and multiplying by two (2) is appropriate.

23. 1. This is incorrect information for radiation therapy. It is correct for chemotherapy.

2. This is a therapeutic response, which does not answer the client's question.

3. **Radiation therapy can cause permanent damage to the hair follicles and the hair may not grow back at all; the nurse should answer the client's question honestly.**

4. This is not a true statement.

24. 1. A positive Brudzinski's sign—flexion of the knees and hip when the neck is flexed—indicates the presence of meningitis. Therefore, the treatment is not effective. Sensitivity to light is a common symptom of meningitis.

2. This does not indicate whether the meningitis is resolving.

3. Kernig's sign—the leg cannot be extended when the client is lying with the thigh flexed on the abdomen—is a sign of meningitis. An elevated temperature indicates the client still has meningitis.

4. **The client does not have nuchal rigidity, which indicates the client's treatment is effective.**

25. 1. An MRI is not able to confirm the diagnosis of Parkinson's disease.

2. This is the portion of the brain where Parkinson's disease originates, but this area lies deep in the brain and cannot be biopsied.

3. This is a surgery that relieves some of the symptoms of Parkinson's disease. To be eligible for this procedure the client must have failed to achieve an adequate response with medical treatment.

4. **Many diagnostic tests are completed to rule out other diagnoses, but Parkinson's disease is diagnosed on the clinical presentation of the client and the presence of two**

of the three cardinal manifestations: tremor, muscle rigidity, and bradykinesia.

26. 1. An oral coagulant would only be ordered if the TIA was caused by atrial fibrillation, and that information is not presented in the stem.
   2. **Atherosclerosis is the most common cause of a TIA or stroke, and taking a baby aspirin every day helps prevent clot formation around plaques.**
   3. If the client had hypertension, a beta blocker may be prescribed, but this information is not in the stem.
   4. Anticonvulsant medications are not prescribed to help prevent TIAs.

27. 1. Myalgia is muscle pain, which is expected in a client diagnosed with encephalitis.
   2. **The client complaining of chest pain is priority. Remember Maslow's Hierarchy of Needs.**
   3. Refusing to eat hospital food is not a priority.
   4. The client going to the whirlpool is stable and is not a priority over chest pain.

28. 1. The client should be assessed for delirium tremens and should be assigned to a registered nurse.
   2. Palpitations indicate cardiac involvement, and because the client has a history of cocaine abuse this client should be assigned to a registered nurse.
   3. This client is at high risk for injury to self and should be assigned to a registered nurse and be on one-to-one precautions.
   4. **The client has a right to leave against medical advice (AMA), and marijuana abuse is not life threatening to him or to others. Therefore, the LPN could be assigned to this client.**

29. 1. An occasional PVC does not warrant intervention; it is normal for most clients.
   2. Less than six (6) unifocal PVCs in one (1) minute is not life threatening.
   3. **Multifocal PVCs indicate that the ventricle is irritable, and this client is at risk for a cardiac event such as ventricular fibrillation.**
   4. Atrial fibrillation is not life threatening, and the nurse would expect the client not to have a P wave when exhibiting this dysrhythmia.

30. 1. **This is a correct statement. The recommended proportions of food are 50% carbohydrates, 30% or less from fat, and 20% protein.**
   2. Only 50% of the calories should come from carbohydrates.
   3. Red meat is an excellent source of protein but should only comprise 20% of the diet, and red meat is very high in fat.
   4. Polyunsaturated fats, not the monosaturated fats, are the better fats.

31. 1. The client diagnosed with CHF will be short of breath on exertion and with activity. The significant other should report difficulty breathing that does not subside with rest or stopping the activity.
   2. **This much weight gain reflects fluid retention as a result of heart failure; a weight gain of 2–3 lbs a day or 5 lbs in one (1) week warrants notifying the HCP.**
   3. The caregiver must not administer the digoxin if the radial pulse is less than 60 bpm. The apical pulse is more difficult to assess in a client than the radial pulse.
   4. The client in end-stage CHF is dying and should not exercise daily; activity intolerance as a result of decreased cardiac output is the number-one life-limiting problem.

32. 1. Barrel chest and clubbing of the fingers are signs of chronic lung disease.
   2. Intermittent claudication and rest pain are signs of peripheral arterial disease.
   3. **Pink, frothy sputum and dyspnea on exertion are signs of congestive heart failure, which occurs when the heart can no longer compensate for the strain of an incompetent valve.**
   4. Friction rub occurs with pericarditis, and bilateral wheezing occurs with asthma.

33. 1. Once the chest incision heals the client can shower or bathe, whichever the client prefers.
   2. **Electrical devices may interfere with the functioning of the pacemaker.**
   3. **This alerts any HCP as to the presence of a pacemaker.**
   4. **The client should be taught to take the radial pulse for one (1) full minute before getting out of bed. If there is a change of more than five (5) bpm less than the preset rate, the HCP should be notified immediately because this may indicate the pacemaker is malfunctioning.**
   5. The client should notify the HCP if there is a difference of five (5) bpm less than preset rate. This may indicate pacemaker malfunction.

34. 1. Having a history of a myocardial infarction is not a risk factor for developing infective endocarditis.
   2. **Cardiac valve replacement and valve disorders are risk factors for developing infective endocarditis. This is why clients must**

receive prophylactic antibiotic treatment before dental work and invasive procedures.

3. A personal history of rheumatic fever, not a family history, increases the risk of developing infective endocarditis.

4. NSAIDs have no effect on the development of infective endocarditis.

35. 1. The client's pedal pulse does not evaluate the effectiveness of this medication.

2. This medication is not administered to help decrease blood pressure.

3. **This medication inhibits platelet aggregation and is considered effective when there is a decrease in atherosclerotic events, an example of which is a stroke.**

4. This medication will not help the pain that is associated with arterial occlusive disease.

36. 1. Sublingual nitroglycerin is the medication of choice for angina, but it is not the first intervention.

2. Applying oxygen is appropriate, but it is not the first intervention.

3. A STAT ECG should be ordered, but it is not the first intervention.

4. **Stopping the client from whatever activity is the first intervention because this decreases the oxygen demands of the heart muscle and may decrease or eliminate the chest pain.**

37. 1. This client is unstable and received medication for chest pain. The nurse cannot delegate any task on a client who is unstable.

2. The NA cannot notify the HCP because NAs are not allowed to take verbal or telephone orders.

3. **The NA can take routine vital signs. The nurse must evaluate the vital signs and take action if needed. The nurse should not delegate teaching, assessing, evaluating, or any client who is unstable.**

4. This is outside the level of an NA's expertise.

38. 1. This might be what the nurse wants to do, but the nurse should teach the client about the disease process.

2. **Elevating the legs above the heart as much as possible will help decrease edema.**

3. There are no surgical procedures to correct venous insufficiency.

4. Losing weight and walking are excellent lifestyle modifications, but there is no guarantee that the venous insufficiency will resolve.

39. 1. Cervical lymph node enlargement would indicate Hodgkin's lymphoma.

2. An asymmetrical dark-purple nevus would indicate malignant melanoma.

3. Petechiae covering the trunk and legs is one of the indicators of bone marrow problems, which could be leukemia.

4. Brownish-purple nodules on the face indicate Kaposi's sarcoma, a complication of AIDS.

40. 1. This statement does not represent the anger stage of grieving.

2. This statement does not represent the denial stage of grieving.

3. This statement does not represent the bargaining stage of grieving.

4. **This statement indicates the client is ready to die and is in the acceptance stage of the grieving process.**

41. 1. **Brown rice, dried fruit, and oatmeal are sources of nonheme iron. Nonheme iron comes from vegetable sources.**

2. Beef, chicken, and pork are sources of heme iron or animal sources of iron.

3. Broccoli, asparagus, and kidney beans are sources of folic acid.

4. Liver, cheese, and eggs are sources of vitamin $B_{12}$.

42. 1. **Heparin interferes with the clotting cascade and may prevent further clotting factor consumption resulting from uncontrolled thromboses formation.**

2. Assessment is an independent intervention; it is not collaborative and does not require an HCP's order.

3. Assessment is an independent intervention; it is not collaborative and does not require an HCP's order.

4. TPN is not a treatment for a client with DIC.

43.      **150 mL/hr.** The nurse should infuse the blood in two (2) hours because the client does not have signs/symptoms of fluid volume overload.

44. 1. This is a false statement. The client could have the sickle cell trait.

2. This should be discussed with her fiancé, but it is not the most important information.

3. **Referral to a genetic counselor is the most important information to give the client. If she and her fiancé both have the sickle cell trait, there is a 25% chance of a child having sickle cell disease with each pregnancy.**

4. Adoption may be a choice, but at this time the most important information is to refer the couple to a genetic counselor.

45. 1. **The nurse should stay at home because the nurse will expose all other personnel and clients to the illness. Flu, especially with a fever, places the nurse at risk for a secondary pneumonia.**

2. The nurse is ill, and many errors are made when the nurse is not functioning at 100%.

3. Even if the nurse doesn't have direct client care, the nurse will expose other employees to the virus.

4. OTC medications will not prevent the transmission of flu to others, nor will it prevent the nurse from developing a secondary pneumonia.

46. 1. The nurse should not administer antibiotics until the culture specimen is obtained.

2. **The sputum must be collected first to identify the infectious organism so that appropriate antibiotics can be prescribed. Administering broad-spectrum antibiotics prior to collecting sputum could alter the C&S results.**

3. This is not priority over sputum culture and getting the antibiotic started.

4. Always treat the client first.

47. 1. **Medical client problems indicate the nurse and the HCP must collaborate to care for the client; the client must have medications for heart failure.**

2. Without an HCP's order the nurse can instruct the client to pace activities and teach about rest versus activity.

3. This is a psychosocial client problem that does not require an HCP's order to effectively care for the client.

4. Anticipatory grieving is the nurse addressing issues that will occur based on the knowledge of the poor prognosis of this disease.

48. 1. **Cellulitis is the most common infectious cause of limb edema as a result of bacterial invasion of the subcutaneous tissue. This assessment would make the nurse suspect this condition.**

2. Intravenous drug use can cause cellulitis, but the description did not include track marks or needle insertion sites.

3. Raynaud's phenomenon is a form of intermittent arteriolar vasoconstriction that results in coldness, pain, and pallor of fingertips or toes. The client should keep warm to prevent vasoconstriction of extremities.

4. Buerger's disease (thromboangiitis obliterans) is a relatively uncommon occlusive disease limited to medium and small arteries and veins. The cause is unknown, but there is a strong association with tobacco use.

49. 1. This step is the first step in BSE.

2. This is step three (3) in the BSE process.

3. This is included in steps four (4) and five (5) and is described as using a systematic process of examining the breast. Using circular motions

and dividing the breast into wedges or vertical strips to palpate the entire breast is encouraged. This step was described in the stem as having been completed.

4. **The last step of BSE after palpation is to express the nipple by gently squeezing the nipple. Any discharge should be brought to the attention of an HCP. Nipple discharge can be caused by many factors such as carcinoma, papilloma, pituitary adenoma, cystic breasts, and some medications.**

50. 1. Changes in pupil size are a late sign of a neurological deficit.

2. **A change in level of consciousness is the first and most critical indicator of any neurological deficit.**

3. A decrease in motor function occurs with a neurological deficit, but it is not the most critical indicator.

4. Numbness of the extremities occurs with a neurological deficit, but it is not the most critical indicator.

51. 1. **The nurse must make a decision on the amount of blood to infuse per hour. If the client is showing any sign of heart or lung compromise, the nurse would infuse the blood at the slowest possible rate.**

2. **Blood products require the client to give specific consent to receive blood.**

3. The IV should be started with an 18-gauge if possible; the smallest possible catheter is a 20-gauge. Smaller gauge catheters break down the blood cells.

4. Blood is not compatible with $D_5W$; the nurse should hang 0.9% normal saline (NS) to keep open.

5. **The nurse should verify the HCP's order before having the client sign the consent form.**

52. 1. **Most clients with psoriasis have red, raised plaques with silvery white scales.**

2. A burning, prickling row of vesicles located along the torso is the description of herpes zoster.

3. Raised, flesh-colored papules with a rough surface area is a description of a wart.

4. An overgrowth of tissue with an excessive amount of collagen is the definition of keloids.

53. 1. **The cause of GB is unknown, but a precipitating event usually occurs one (1) to three (3) weeks prior to the onset. The precipitating event may be a respiratory or gastrointestinal viral or bacterial infection.**

2. These are not precipitating events or risk factors for developing GB.

3. Smoking is not a risk factor for developing GB.
4. GB is not more prominent in foreign countries than in the United States.

54. 1. A normal hemoglobin is 12–15 g/dL, and normal hematocrit is 36%–45%.
2. A normal SED rate is between 1 and 20 mm/hr for a female client.
3. A normal albumin level is between 3.5 and 5.0 g/dL.
4. **The client with SLE is at an increased risk for infection, and this WBC indicates an infection that requires medical intervention.**

55. 170 mL/hour. 125 + 45 = 170. The IV pump should be set at this rate.

56. 1. The Rinne test result indicates a normal hearing; in conductive hearing loss bone-conducted sound is heard as long as or longer than air-conducted sound.
2. The whisper test is used to make a general estimation of hearing, but it is not used to specifically diagnose for conductive hearing loss.
3. **The Weber test uses bone conduction to test lateralization of sound by placing a tuning fork in the middle of the skull or forehead. A normal test results in the client hearing the sound equally in both ears.**
4. The tympanogram (impedance audiometry) measures middle-ear muscle reflex to sound stimulation and compliance of the tympanic membrane by changing air pressure in a sealed ear canal. It does not specifically support the diagnosis of conductive hearing loss.

57. 1. **The client should begin exercises that will strengthen the surgical leg as soon as the surgery is completed.**
2. Pain medication should be taken as needed, not routinely.
3. The client may ambulate with the restrictions ordered by the surgeon.
4. The client will return to see the surgeon prior to six (6) months. The surgeon will need to monitor for healing and complications.

58. 1. Yellow means caution. The client should follow some, but not all, usual activities.
2. The client's personal best takes two (2) to three (3) weeks to establish.
3. **When a client can't talk while walking, there is shortness of breath. The client needs to take the quick-relief medication. If there is no relief in 15 minutes, the client should contact the health-care provider or go to the nearest hospital.**

4. When the client is in the red zone, the client should take the quick-relief medication and should not exercise or follow regular routines.

59. 1. A positive Homans' sign would indicate a DVT.
2. **The calf with deep vein thrombosis becomes edematous, so there is an increase in the size of the calf when compared to the other leg.**
3. Elephantiasis is characterized by tremendous edema usually of the external genitalia and legs and is not associated with DVT. Elephantiasis is a lymphatic problem, not a venous problem.
4. The brownish discoloration is a sign/symptom of chronic venous insufficiency.

60. 1. **The client with end-stage COPD would not be a candidate for an AAA repair, although the size of the aneurysm places the client at risk for rupture. Although many nurses do not like to address end-of-life issues, this would be an important and timely intervention.**
2. The client is not a surgical candidate because of the comorbid condition and age.
3. The client should know how to purse-lip breathe at this point in the disease process.
4. Although the client is 85 years old, the nurse should discuss all health-care issues with the client and not the family. This is a violation of HIPAA.

61. 1. The nurse can take care of this situation and does not need to notify the RT.
2. The NA cannot increase oxygen. The nurse should treat oxygen as a medication. Also, increasing the oxygen level could cause the client to stop breathing as a result of carbon dioxide narcosis.
3. The pulse oximeter reading will be low because the client has COPD.
4. **The oxygen level for a client with COPD must remain between 2 and 3 L/min because the client's stimulus for breathing is low blood oxygen levels. If the client receives increased oxygen, the stimulus for breathing will be removed and the client will stop breathing.**

62. 1. This is a physiological problem and the stem asks for a psychosocial problem.
2. **Metastasis indicates advanced disease, and the client should be allowed to express feelings of loss and grieving; the client is dying.**
3. Body image is a psychosocial problem but would not be applicable in this scenario.
4. Nutrition is a physiological problem and the stem asks for a psychosocial problem.

63. 1. The client has a partial laryngectomy and the voice quality may change, but the client can still speak.
   2. This is a psychosocial problem, but it is not priority over a potential physiological problem.
   3. **As a result of the injury to the musculature of the throat area, this client is at high risk for aspirating.**
   4. This is a psychosocial problem, but it is not priority over a potential physiological problem.

64. 1. The heparin drip may be increased because the client has now thrown a pulmonary embolus, but this needs an HCP's order.
   2. The HCP will be notified because the client has a suspected embolus, but it is not the first intervention.
   3. The client has probably thrown a pulmonary embolus, and assessing the lungs will not do anything for a client who may die. PEs are life threatening, and assessing the client is not priority in a life-threatening situation.
   4. **The client probably has a pulmonary embolus, and the priority is to provide additional oxygen so that oxygenation of tissues can be maintained.**

65. 1. **Fluctuation with respirations in the water seal compartment indicates the system is working properly and the client is stable.**
   2. Blood in the drainage compartment indicates there is a problem because the client is diagnosed with a pneumothorax and there should not be any bleeding.
   3. Any deviation of the trachea indicates a tension pneumothorax, a potentially life-threatening complication.
   4. Bubbling in the suction compartment does not indicate a stable or unstable client.

66. 1. **These are normal ABGs, which would not be expected if the client has ARDS.**
   2. This client has an oxygen level below 80–100; therefore this client may be developing early ARDS.
   3. This is respiratory alkalosis, which would not be expected in a client with ARDS.
   4. These are the expected ABGs of a client with ARDS. There is a low oxygen level despite high oxygen administration.

67. 1. The HOB is elevated to prevent reflux of stomach contents into the esophagus.
   2. Proton pump inhibitors are only administered one or twice a day; they should not be given four (4) times a day because the medication decreases gastric acidity and the stomach needs some gastric acid to digest foods. **The nurse would question this order.**
   3. The client is not prescribed any special diet; limiting spicy and citrus foods decreases acid in the stomach.
   4. Sitting upright after all meals decreases the reflux of stomach contents into the esophagus.

68. 1. This WBC level is WNL and would not warrant immediate intervention.
   2. This amylase level is within normal limits (50–180 units/dL).
   3. **This potassium level is low as a result of excessive diarrhea and puts the client at risk for cardiac dysrhythmias. Therefore these assessment data warrant immediate intervention.**
   4. The client's blood glucose level is elevated, but it would not warrant immediate intervention for a client with Crohn's disease that has hypokalemia.

69. 1. **Increasing fiber will help prevent constipation, the number-one reason for an acute exacerbation of diverticulosis, which results in diverticulitis.**
   2. The client should increase fluid intake to prevent constipation, to at least 2500 mL/day.
   3. The client should exercise daily to prevent constipation.
   4. The client should take bulk-forming laxatives, which helps prevent constipation by adding bulk to the stool. Cathartic laxatives are harsh colonic stimulants and should not be taken on a daily basis.

70. 1. The discharge instruction sheet is teaching, which cannot be delegated to an NA.
   2. **The NA can remove a saline lock from a stable client.**
   3. The NA does not clean hospital rooms; this is the housekeeping department's responsibility.
   4. The nurse cannot delegate evaluation, which is checking the client's laboratory data prior to discharge; this is out of the NA's area of expertise.

71. 1. Mild fatigue represents fatigue that the client has only occasionally.
   2. Moderate fatigue would be fatigue occurring about 40% to 60% of the time.
   3. **Extreme fatigue occurs 70% to 90% of the time, which is indicated by the client still being able to watch TV and get to the bathroom.**
   4. The worst fatigue ever occurs all the time and the client spends most of the day sleeping and is not able to stay awake to watch television.

72. 1. The T-tube is inserted into the common bile duct to drain bile until healing occurs and bile is green, so this is expected.
 2. The client with CHF would be expected to experience dyspnea on exertion.
 3. **Coffee-ground emesis indicates gastrointestinal bleeding, and this client should be seen first.**
 4. The client in end-stage liver failure is unable to assimilate protein from the diet, which leads to fluid volume retention and resulting weight gain. This is expected for this client.

73. 1. The tympanic wave indicates ascites, which is not an indicator of improving health.
 2. Asterixis is a flapping of the hands, which indicates an elevated ammonia level.
 3. Confusion and lethargy indicate increased ammonia level.
 4. **A decrease in the abdominal girth indicates an improvement in the ascitic fluid.**

74. 1. **The organs/tissues procured from the client will not be noticeable if there is an open casket funeral.**
 2. There is no reason for the client to wear long-sleeved shirts because skin is not removed from the arms.
 3. There is no reason that there has to be a private viewing as a result of the organ/tissue donation.
 4. The funeral may or may not have to be delayed depending on when the procurement team can make arrangements; the nurse should not give false information to the family.

75. 1. A gamma globulin injection is administered to provide passive immunity to clients who have been exposed to hepatitis.
 2. **Hepatitis A is contracted through the fecal/oral route of transmission; poor sanitary practices in Third World countries place the client at risk for hepatitis A.**
 3. This is a test to determine exposure to tuberculosis and does not have anything to do with hepatitis.
 4. The hepatitis B vaccination must be administered in three injections over a six (6)-month period.

76. 1. The client's amylase would be elevated in an acute exacerbation of pancreatitis.
 2. The WBC count is not elevated in this disease process.
 3. **In client's with chronic pancreatitis, the beta cells of the pancreas are affected and therefore insulin production is affected. An elevated glucose level would warrant the nurse assessing the client.**

4. Lipase is an enzyme that is excreted by the pancreas. Normal lipase levels indicate a normal functioning pancreas.

77. 1. The client could experience hypoglycemia if the rate of infusion is decreased. TPN must be tapered when discontinuing.
 2. Normal saline does not have glucose so the client would be at risk for hypoglycemia.
 3. The client must be tapered off TPN to prevent hypoglycemia; therefore the line cannot be converted to a heparin lock.
 4. **Dextrose 10% has enough glucose to prevent hypoglycemia and should be administered until bag #6 arrives to the unit.**

78. 1. This client is overweight but not morbidly obese, which would place the client at risk for complications.
 2. **Altered nutrition: more than body requirements is an appropriate client problem for a client that weighs 175 pounds.**
 3. This is a psychosocial problem, which is not priority over a physiological problem.
 4. The client may or may not be active, but altered nutrition is priority.

79. 1. A moist mouth indicates the client is not dehydrated.
 2. This is within normal limits for potassium—3.5 to 5.5 mEq/L.
 3. **Tented tissue turgor indicates dehydration, which is a complication of diarrhea.**
 4. Hyperactive bowel sounds would be expected in a client who has diarrhea.

80. 1. **The long-term complications of increased blood glucose levels to organs are the primary reasons for keeping the blood glucose level controlled.**
 2. This is the medical explanation for keeping the glucose under control, but this answer is not appropriate for laypeople.
 3. The client with Type 2 diabetes often doesn't feel bad, but the organs are still being damaged as a result of increased blood glucose levels.
 4. Metabolic acidosis occurs in clients with type 1 diabetes, not type 2. Clients with type 2 diabetes have hyperglycemic hyperosmolar nonketotic syndrome (HHNS).

81. 1. This is not the rationale as to why the client becomes dehydrated.
 2. **The glucose in the bloodstream is hyperosmolar, which causes water from the extracellular space to be pulled into the vessels, resulting in dehydration.**
 3. The client has diaphoresis in hypoglycemia, not hyperglycemia.

4. The dehydration causes the client to be thirsty; the thirst does not cause the dehydration.

82. 1. Dairy products contain milk and increase flatus and peristalsis. These products should be discouraged.
2. Symptoms lasting less than 24 hours would not warrant the client going to the emergency department; if anything, an appointment at a clinic would be appropriate.
3. A stool specimen may be needed at some point but not this early in the disease process.
4. **A clear liquid diet is recommended because it maintains hydration without stimulating the gastrointestinal tract; diarrhea/vomiting lasting longer than 24 hours, along with dehydration and weakness, would warrant the client being evaluated.**

83. 1. **These are signs/symptoms of Addison's disease, which is adrenal cortex insufficiency.**
2. These are signs/symptoms of Cushing syndrome, which is adrenal cortex hyperfunction.
3. These are signs/symptoms of Cushing syndrome, which is adrenal cortex hyperfunction.
4. These are signs/symptoms of Cushing syndrome, which is adrenal cortex hyperfunction.

84. 1. This would cause the client to have diabetes mellitus.
2. **The pituitary gland secretes vasopressin, which is the antidiuretic hormone (ADH) that causes the body to conserve water, and if the pituitary is not secreting ADH, the body will produce large volumes of dilute urine.**
3. There are two types of diabetes insipidus: neurogenic DI and nephrogenic DI. In neurogenic DI, the pituitary gland fails to produce ADH; in nephrogenic DI, the kidneys fail to respond to ADH.
4. The thyroid gland has nothing to do with DI.

85. 1. There is no reason to question or clarify this order; the nurse is responsible for clarifying the order with the HCP, not the pharmacist.
2. **Many elderly clients have comorbid conditions that require daily medications that are not the primary reason for admission into the hospital.**
3. The nurse should know why the client is taking this medication; this medication is prescribed for only one reason, hypothyroidism.
4. The serum thyroid function levels are monitored by the HCP usually yearly after maintenance doses have been established.

86. 1. The client diagnosed with essential hypertension is at risk for chronic renal failure.

2. The client diagnosed with diabetes type 2 is at risk for chronic renal failure.
3. **Anaphylaxis leads to circulatory collapse, which decreases perfusion of the kidneys and can lead to acute renal failure.**
4. This is a transfusion of the client's own blood, which should not cause a reaction.

87. 1. **A cloudy dialysate indicates an infection and must be reported immediately to prevent peritonitis.**
2. The dialysate should be greater than the intake so that fluid is being removed from the body.
3. After infusing 1000 mL of dialysate, abdominal fullness is not unexpected.
4. The client voiding any amount does not warrant immediate intervention.

88. 1. Using two washcloths to clean the client's perineal area is an appropriate action to prevent a urinary tract infection.
2. This action does not require intervention.
3. Moisture barrier cream is not considered a medication and can be applied by the NA after the perineum is cleaned.
4. **The NA should wipe the area from front to back to prevent fecal contamination of the urinary meatus, which could result in a urinary tract infection.**

89. 1. This is a normal postoperative expectation with this procedure.
2. This is gross hematuria, but it is expected with this type of surgery and the nurse should not call the surgeon.
3. **The client has a three (3)-way Foley catheter inserted in surgery. This type of catheter instills an irrigant into the bladder to flush the clots and blood from the bladder; bloody urine is expected after this surgery.**
4. The stem does not indicate the client is having bladder spasms and bladder spasms are not causing the bleeding. Clots left in the bladder and not flushed out can cause bladder spasms.

90. 1. This is not pertinent to the client's current situation.
2. The nurse should strain all the client's urine, but a large Foley catheter does not need to be inserted into this client; this isn't a bladder stone, it is a ureteral stone.
3. A back massage is a nice thing to do, but it will not help renal colic caused by ureteral calculi.
4. **The client should be medicated for pain, which is excruciating, and the client's history of substance abuse should not be an issue.**

91. 1. **This is the most common presenting symptom of bladder cancer.**

2. Burning on urination is a symptom of a urinary tract infection.
3. Terminal dribbling is a symptom of benign prostatic hypertrophy.
4. Difficulty initiating a urine stream is a symptom of benign prostatic hypertrophy or neurogenic bladder.

92. 1. **A genetic predisposition exists and is indicated by the presence of a specific cluster of human leukocyte antigens on the cell wall.**
2. There is a higher incidence of MS in people who live in the northeastern United States and Canada, but there is no known reason for this occurrence.
3. Tobacco use is a risk factor for many diseases, but not MS.
4. A sedentary lifestyle does not predispose a person to develop MS.

93. 1. The client's thigh area is not the best place to assess for skin turgor.
2. The client's hand has decreased subcutaneous tissue and has been exposed to the sun, which results in decreased tissue elasticity, so this is not the best place to assess for skin turgor.
3. **The tissue on the chest is protected from sun exposure and has adequate subcutaneous tissue to provide a more accurate assessment of hydration status.**
4. The eyeball will lose its elasticity secondary to dehydration, but most people do not like the eyes being touched.

94. 1. The nursing instructor must be notified, but it is not the first action.
2. **Allowing the site to bleed allows any pathogen to bleed out; do not apply pressure or attempt to stop the flow of blood.**
3. This would be done to document the occurrence and start early prophylaxis if necessary, but it is not the first intervention.
4. This is an appropriate intervention once the wound is allowed to bleed; this is a needle stick, so the nursing student will not bleed to death.

95. 1. Alteration in comfort is a client problem, but it not a psychosocial problem.
2. Ineffective coping is a problem that is not applicable to all clients with rheumatoid arthritis and is a very individualized problem; the test taker would need more information before selecting this as a correct answer.
3. Anxiety is a problem that is not applicable to all clients with rheumatoid arthritis and is a very individualized problem; the test taker would

need more information before selecting this as a correct answer.
4. **Altered body image is an expected psychosocial problem for all clients with rheumatoid arthritis because of the joint deformities.**

96. 1. **The nurse must rule out any complication that requires immediate intervention before masking the pain with medication. Pain indicates a problem in some instances; pain is expected after surgery, but complications should always be ruled out.**
2. The nurse should not medicate for pain until ruling out complications.
3. The television provides distraction, but it is not the first intervention. Assessment is the first intervention.
4. Teaching relaxation techniques will help the client's pain, but the first intervention must be assessment to rule out any complication.

97. 1. The APS or police should be notified of the admission unless the client refuses to have this reported, but it is not the first action.
2. **The nurse must ensure that the husband cannot hear the client discussing how she was injured. The client needs to feel safe when answering these questions because a spiral fracture indicates a twisting motion and the bruises are all in areas that can be covered with clothing. The nurse should suspect abuse with these types of injuries.**
3. The nurse should refer to the social worker if it is determined the client has been abused, but the nurse should not refer during the admission interview.
4. The nurse should make every attempt to interview the client without the possible abuser present; the client will probably be afraid to tell the nurse she wants the husband to leave the room if he is the abuser.

98. 1. The client would be placed in the Trendelenburg position, which is with the head lower than the feet.
2. **The client is in shock and may need blood transfusions; therefore, a large-bore catheter should be started to infuse fluids, plasma expanders, and possible blood.**
3. The admission process cannot be completed by the client because the condition is life threatening.
4. **The client will be cold as a result of vasoconstriction of the periphery resulting from a low pulse and blood pressure.**
5. **The client will more than likely need blood**

transfusions that require a type and cross-match.

99. 1. A hard, rigid, boardlike abdomen is the hallmark sign of peritonitis, which is a life-threatening complication of abdominal surgery.
    2. This occurs when the client has a nasogastric tube that is connected to suction and has minimal peristalsis and would not be a complication of the surgery.
    3. The client has had general anesthesia for this surgery, and absent bowel sounds at eight (8) hours postoperative would not indicate a complication.
    4. The client with this type of surgery would be expected to have pain at a six (6) or higher on a one (1) to ten (10) scale and would not be considered a complication.

100. 1. Documentation can help the nurse defend his or her actions if a lawsuit occurs, but it will not help prevent a lawsuit.
    2. Research indicates that nurses that form a trusting nurse–client relationship are less likely to be sued; if the nurse were to make an error, the client and family are often more forgiving.
    3. Knowledge of medications will prevent medication errors but will not keep the nurse from being sued. Nurses are human and can make mistakes with medications even if they are knowledgeable.
    4. The nurse is a client advocate and is legally, morally, and ethically required to question the HCP's orders when caring for assigned clients.

101.    In order of the nursing process: 2, 1, 3, 4, 5.
    2. This is the assessment step, the first step of the nursing process.
    1. Diagnosis is the second step in the nursing process. In this case, it is "altered tissue perfusion."
    3. Planning is the third step of the nursing process.
    4. Implementation is the fourth step in the nursing process.
    5. Evaluation is the last step of the nursing process.

# Glossary of English Words Commonly Encountered on Nursing Examinations

**Abnormality**—defect, irregularity, anomaly, oddity

**Absence**—nonappearance, lack, nonattendance

**Abundant**—plentiful, rich, profuse

**Accelerate**—go faster, speed up, increase, hasten

**Accumulate**—build up, collect, gather

**Accurate**—precise, correct, exact

**Achievement**—accomplishment, success, reaching, attainment

**Acknowledge**—admit, recognize, accept, reply

**Activate**—start, turn on, stimulate

**Adequate**—sufficient, ample, plenty, enough

**Angle**—slant, approach, direction, point of view

**Application**—use, treatment, request, claim

**Approximately**—about, around, in the region of, more or less, roughly speaking

**Arrange**—position, place, organize, display

**Associated**—linked, related

**Attention**—notice, concentration, awareness, thought

**Authority**—power, right, influence, clout, expert

**Avoid**—keep away from, evade, let alone

**Balanced**—stable, neutral, steady, fair, impartial

**Barrier**—barricade, blockage, obstruction, obstacle

**Best**—most excellent, most important, greatest

**Capable**—able, competent, accomplished

**Capacity**—ability, capability, aptitude, role, power, size

**Central**—middle, mid, innermost, vital

**Challenge**—confront, dare, dispute, test, defy, face up to

**Characteristic**—trait, feature, attribute, quality, typical

**Circular**—round, spherical, globular

**Collect**—gather, assemble, amass, accumulate, bring together

**Commitment**—promise, vow, dedication, obligation, pledge, assurance

**Commonly**—usually, normally, frequently, generally, universally

**Compare**—contrast, evaluate, match up to, weigh or judge against

**Compartment**—section, part, cubicle, booth, stall

**Complex**—difficult, multifaceted, compound, multipart, intricate

**Complexity**—difficulty, intricacy, complication

**Component**—part, element, factor, section, constituent

**Comprehensive**—complete, inclusive, broad, thorough

**Conceal**—hide, cover up, obscure, mask, suppress, secrete

**Conceptualize**—to form an idea

**Concern**—worry, anxiety, fear, alarm, distress, unease, trepidation

**Concisely**—briefly, in a few words, succinctly

**Conclude**—make a judgment based on reason, finish

**Confidence**—self-assurance, certainty, poise, self-reliance

**Congruent**—matching, fitting, going together well

**Consequence**—result, effect, outcome, end result

**Constituents**—elements, components, parts that make up a whole

**Contain**—hold, enclose, surround, include, control, limit

**Continual**—repeated, constant, persistent, recurrent, frequent

**Continuous**—constant, incessant, nonstop, unremitting, permanent

**Contribute**—be a factor, add, give

**Convene**—assemble, call together, summon, organize, arrange

**Convenience**—expediency, handiness, ease

**Coordinate**—organize, direct, manage, bring together

**Create**—make, invent, establish, generate, produce, fashion, build, construct

**Creative**—imaginative, original, inspired, inventive, resourceful, productive, innovative

**Critical**—serious, grave, significant, dangerous, life threatening

**Cue**—signal, reminder, prompt, sign, indication

**Curiosity**—inquisitiveness, interest, nosiness, snooping

**Damage**—injure, harm, hurt, break, wound

**Deduct**—subtract, take away, remove, withhold

**Deficient**—lacking, wanting, underprovided, scarce, faulty

**Defining**—important, crucial, major, essential, significant, central

**Defuse**—resolve, calm, soothe, neutralize, rescue, mollify

**Delay**—hold up, wait, hinder, postpone, slow down, hesitate, linger

**Demand**—insist, claim, require, command, stipulate, ask

**Describe**—explain, tell, express, illustrate, depict, portray

**Design**—plan, invent, intend, aim, propose, devise

**Desirable**—wanted, pleasing, enviable, popular, sought after, attractive, advantageous

**Detail**—feature, aspect, element, factor, facet

**Deteriorate**—worsen, decline, weaken

**Determine**—decide, conclude, resolve, agree on

**Dexterity**—skillfulness, handiness, agility, deftness

**Dignity**—self-respect, self-esteem, decorum, formality, poise

**Dimension**—aspect, measurement

**Diminish**—reduce, lessen, weaken, detract, moderate

**Discharge**—release, dismiss, set free

**Discontinue**—stop, cease, halt, suspend, terminate, withdraw

**Disorder**—complaint, problem, confusion, chaos

**Display**—show, exhibit, demonstrate, present, put on view

**Dispose**—to get rid of, arrange, order, set out

**Dissatisfaction**—displeasure, discontent, unhappiness, disappointment

**Distinguish**—to separate and classify, recognize

**Distract**—divert, sidetrack, entertain

**Distress**—suffering, trouble, anguish, misery, agony, concern, sorrow

**Distribute**—deliver, spread out, hand out, issue, dispense

**Disturbed**—troubled, unstable, concerned, worried, distressed, anxious, uneasy

**Diversional**—serving to distract

**Don**—put on, dress oneself in

**Dramatic**—spectacular

**Drape**—cover, wrap, dress, swathe

**Dysfunction**—abnormal, impaired

**Edge**—perimeter, boundary, periphery, brink, border, rim

**Effective**—successful, useful, helpful, valuable

**Efficient**—not wasteful, effective, competent, resourceful, capable

**Elasticity**—stretch, spring, suppleness, flexibility

**Eliminate**—get rid of, eradicate, abolish, remove, purge

**Embarrass**—make uncomfortable, make self-conscious, humiliate, mortify

**Emerge**—appear, come, materialize, become known

**Emphasize**—call attention to, accentuate, stress, highlight

**Ensure**—make certain, guarantee

**Environment**—setting, surroundings, location, atmosphere, milieu, situation

**Episode**—event, incident, occurrence, experience

**Essential**—necessary, fundamental, vital, important, crucial, critical, indispensable

**Etiology**—assigned cause, origin

**Exaggerate**—overstate, inflate

**Excel**—to stand out, shine, surpass, outclass

**Excessive**—extreme, too much, unwarranted

**Exhibit**—show signs of, reveal, display

**Expand**—get bigger, enlarge, spread out, increase, swell, inflate

**Expect**—wait for, anticipate, imagine

**Expectation**—hope, anticipation, belief, prospect, probability

**Experience**—knowledge, skill, occurrence, know-how

**Expose**—lay open, leave unprotected, allow to be seen, reveal, disclose, exhibit

**External**—outside, exterior, outer

**Facilitate**—make easy, make possible, help, assist

**Factor**—part, feature, reason, cause, think, issue

**Focus**—center, focal point, hub

**Fragment**—piece, portion, section, part, splinter, chip

**Function**—purpose, role, job, task

**Furnish**—supply, provide, give, deliver, equip

**Further**—additional, more, extra, added, supplementary

**Generalize**—to take a broad view, simplify, to make inferences from particulars

**Generate**—make, produce, create

**Gentle**—mild, calm, tender

**Girth**—circumference, bulk, weight

**Highest**—uppermost, maximum, peak, main

**Hinder**—hold back, delay, hamper, obstruct, impede

**Humane**—caring, kind, gentle, compassionate, benevolent, civilized

**Ignore**—pay no attention to, disregard, overlook, discount

**Imbalance**—unevenness, inequality, disparity

**Immediate**—insistent, urgent, direct

**Impair**—damage, harm, weaken

**Implantation**—to put in

**Impotent**—powerless, weak, incapable, ineffective, unable

**Inadvertent**—unintentional, chance, unplanned, accidental

**Include**—comprise, take in, contain

**Indicate**—point out, sign of, designate, specify, show

**Ineffective**—unproductive, unsuccessful, useless, vain, futile

**Inevitable**—predictable, to be expected, unavoidable, foreseeable

**Influence**—power, pressure, sway, manipulate, affect, effect

**Initiate**—start, begin, open, commence, instigate

**Insert**—put in, add, supplement, introduce

**Inspect**—look over, check, examine

**Inspire**—motivate, energize, encourage, enthuse

**Institutionalize**—to place in a facility for treatment

**Integrate**—put together, mix, add, combine, assimilate

**Integrity**—honesty

**Interfere**—get in the way, hinder, obstruct, impede, hamper

**Interpret**—explain the meaning of, to make understandable

**Intervention**—action, activity

**Intolerance**—bigotry, prejudice, narrowmindedness

Involuntary—instinctive, reflex, unintentional, automatic, uncontrolled

Irreversible—permanent, irrevocable, irreparable, unalterable

Irritability—sensitivity to stimuli, fretful, quick excitability

Justify—explain in accordance with reason

Likely—probably, possible, expected

Logical—using reason

Longevity—long life

Lowest—inferior in rank

Maintain—continue, uphold, preserve, sustain, retain

Majority—the greater part of

Mention—talk about, refer to, state, cite, declare, point out

Minimal—least, smallest, nominal, negligible, token

Minimize—reduce, diminish, lessen, curtail, decrease to smallest possible

Mobilize—activate, organize, assemble, gather together, rally

Modify—change, adapt, adjust, revise, alter

Moist—slightly wet, damp

Multiple—many, numerous, several, various

Natural—normal, ordinary, unaffected

Negative—no, harmful, downbeat, pessimistic

Negotiate—bargain, talk, discuss, consult, cooperate, settle

Notice—become aware of, see, observe, discern, detect

Notify—inform, tell, alert, advise, warn, report

Nurture—care for, raise, rear, foster

Obsess—preoccupy, consume

Occupy—live in, inhabit, reside in, engage in

Occurrence—event, incident, happening

Odorous—scented, stinking, aromatic

Offensive—unpleasant, distasteful, nasty, disgusting

Opportunity—chance, prospect, break

Organize—put in order, arrange, sort out, categorize, classify

Origin—source, starting point, cause, beginning, derivation

Pace—speed

Parameter—limit, factor, limitation, issue

Participant—member, contributor, partaker, applicant

Perspective—viewpoint, view, perception

Position—place, location, point, spot, situation

Practice—do, carry out, perform, apply, follow

Precipitate—to cause to happen, to bring on, hasten, abrupt, sudden

Predetermine—fix or set beforehand

Predictable—expected, knowable

Preference—favorite, liking, first choice

Prepare—get ready, plan, make, train, arrange, organize

Prescribe—set down, stipulate, order, recommend, impose

Previous—earlier, prior, before, preceding

Primarily—first, above all, mainly, mostly, largely, principally, predominantly

Primary—first, main, basic, chief, most important, key, prime, major, crucial

Priority—main concern, giving first attention to, order of importance

Production—making, creation, construction, assembly

Profuse—a lot of, plentiful, copious, abundant, generous, prolific, bountiful

Prolong—extend, delay, put off, lengthen, draw out

Promote—encourage, support, endorse, sponsor

Proportion—ratio, amount, quantity, part of, percentage, section of

Provide—give, offer, supply, make available

Rationalize—explain, reason

Realistic—practical, sensible, reasonable

Receive—get, accept, take delivery of, obtain

Recognize—acknowledge, appreciate, identify, aware of

Recovery—healing, mending, improvement, recuperation, renewal

Reduce—decrease, lessen, ease, moderate, diminish

Reestablish—reinstate, restore, return, bring back

Regard—consider, look upon, relate to, respect

Regular—usual, normal, ordinary, standard, expected, conventional

Relative—comparative, family member

Relevance—importance of

Reluctant—unwilling, hesitant, disinclined, indisposed, averse

Remove—take away, get rid of, eliminate, eradicate

Reposition—move, relocate, change position

Require—need, want, necessitate

Resist—oppose, defend against, keep from, refuse to go along with, defy

Resolution—decree, solution, decision, ruling, promise

Resolve—make up your mind, solve, determine, decide

Response—reply, answer, reaction, retort

Restore—reinstate, reestablish, bring back, return to, refurbish

Restrict—limit, confine, curb, control, contain, hold back, hamper

Retract—take back, draw in, withdraw, apologize

Reveal—make known, disclose, divulge, expose, tell, make public

Review—appraisal, reconsider, evaluation, assessment, examination, analysis

Ritual—custom, ceremony, formal procedure

Rotate—turn, go around, spin, swivel

Routine—usual, habit, custom, practice

Satisfaction—approval, fulfillment, pleasure, happiness

Satisfy—please, convince, fulfill, make happy, gratify

**Secure**—safe, protected, fixed firmly, sheltered, confident, obtain

**Sequential**—chronological, in order of occurrence

**Significant**—important, major, considerable, noteworthy, momentous

**Slight**—small, slim, minor, unimportant, insignificant, insult, snub

**Source**—basis, foundation, starting place, cause

**Specific**—exact, particular, detail, explicit, definite

**Stable**—steady, even, constant

**Statistics**—figures, data, information

**Subtract**—take away, deduct

**Success**—achievement, victory, accomplishment

**Surround**—enclose, encircle, contain

**Suspect**—think, believe, suppose, guess, deduce, infer, distrust, doubtful

**Sustain**—maintain, carry on, prolong, continue, nourish, suffer

**Synonymous**—same as, identical, equal, tantamount

**Thorough**—careful, detailed, methodical, systematic, meticulous, comprehensive, exhaustive

**Tilt**—tip, slant, slope, lean, angle, incline

**Translucent**—see-through, transparent, clear

**Unique**—one and only, sole, exclusive, distinctive

**Universal**—general, widespread, common, worldwide

**Unoccupied**—vacant, not busy, empty

**Unrelated**—unconnected, unlinked, distinct, dissimilar, irrelevant

**Unresolved**—unsettled, uncertain, unsolved, unclear, in doubt

**Various**—numerous, variety, range of, mixture of, assortment of

**Verbalize**—express, voice, speak, articulate

**Verify**—confirm, make sure, prove, attest to, validate, substantiate, corroborate, authenticate

**Vigorous**—forceful, strong, brisk, energetic

**Volume**—quantity, amount, size

**Withdraw**—remove, pull out, take out, extract

# Index